Oxidants, Antioxidants, and Impact of the Oxidative Status in Male Reproduction

Oxidants, Antioxidants, and Impact of the Oxidative Status in Male Reproduction

Edited by

Ralf Henkel

Luna Samanta

Ashok Agarwal

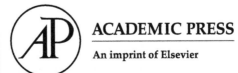

ACADEMIC PRESS

An imprint of Elsevier

Academic Press is an imprint of Elsevier
125 London Wall, London EC2Y 5AS, United Kingdom
525 B Street, Suite 1650, San Diego, CA 92101, United States
50 Hampshire Street, 5th Floor, Cambridge, MA 02139, United States
The Boulevard, Langford Lane, Kidlington, Oxford OX5 1GB, United Kingdom

Notices

Knowledge and best practice in this field are constantly changing. As new research and experience broaden our understanding, changes in research methods, professional practices, or medical treatment may become necessary.

Practitioners and researchers must always rely on their own experience and knowledge in evaluating and using any information, methods, compounds, or experiments described herein. In using such information or methods they should be mindful of their own safety and the safety of others, including parties for whom they have a professional responsibility.

To the fullest extent of the law, neither the Publisher nor the authors, contributors, or editors, assume any liability for any injury and/or damage to persons or property as a matter of products liability, negligence or otherwise, or from any use or operation of any methods, products, instructions, or ideas contained in the material herein.

Library of Congress Cataloging-in-Publication Data
A catalog record for this book is available from the Library of Congress

British Library Cataloguing-in-Publication Data
A catalogue record for this book is available from the British Library

ISBN: 978-0-12-812501-4

For information on all Academic Press publications visit our website at
https://www.elsevier.com/books-and-journals

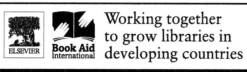

Working together
to grow libraries in
developing countries

www.elsevier.com • www.bookaid.org

Publisher: Stacy Masucci
Acquisition Editor: Tari K. Broderick
Editorial Project Manager: Sam W. Young
Production Project Manager: Mohanapriyan Rajendran
Designer: Christian J. Bilbow

Typeset by TNQ Technologies

Contents

Part I
Basic Aspects

1.1 Life Under Aerobic Conditions

Kristian Leisegang

1.2 The Oxidant Paradox

Nicholas N. Tadros and Sarah C. Vij

1.3 From Past to Present: An Historical Overview of the Concept of Spermatozoa, Reactive Oxygen Species, and Male-Factor Infertility

*Mark A. Baker, Jacob Netherton and
R. John Aitken*

Part II
Clinical Aspects

2.1 Epidemiology of Oxidative Stress in Male Fertility

Michael Owyong and Ranjith Ramasamy

2.2 Role of Oxidative Stress in the Etiology of Male Infertility and the Potential Therapeutic Value of Antioxidants

R. John Aitken, Geoffrey N. De Iuliis and Joel R. Drevet

2.3 Male Genital Tract Infections and Leukocytospermia

Shu-Jian Chen and Gerhard Haidl

2.4 Varicocele

Nicholas N. Tadros and Edmund Sabanegh, Jr.

2.5 Malnutrition and Obesity

Kristian Leisegang

2.6 Role of Reactive Oxygen Species in Diabetes-Induced Male Reproductive Dysfunction

Luís Rato, Pedro F. Oliveira, Mário Sousa, Branca M. Silva and Marco G. Alves

2.7 Thyroid Dysfunction and Testicular Redox Status: An Intriguing Association

Dipak Kumar Sahoo, Srikanta Jena and Gagan B.N. Chainy

2.8 Aging

Sezgin Gunes and Gülgez Neslihan Hekim Taskurt

Part IV
Current Approaches: The OMICS

Contributors

Ashok Agarwal, American Center for Reproductive Medicine, Cleveland Clinic, Cleveland, OH, United States

R. John Aitken, The University of Newcastle (UoN), University drive, Callaghan, NSW, Australia

Marco G. Alves, Institute of Biomedical Sciences Abel Salazar, University of Porto, Porto, Portugal

Mark A. Baker, The University of Newcastle (UoN), University drive, Callaghan, NSW, Australia

Albert D. Bui, American Center for Reproductive Medicine, Cleveland Clinic, Cleveland, OH, United States

Meaghanne Caraballo, American Center for Reproductive Medicine, Cleveland Clinic, Cleveland, OH, United States

Gagan B.N. Chainy, Utkal University, Bhubaneswar, Odisha, India

Shu-Jian Chen, Rheinische Friedrich-Wilhelms University, Bonn, Germany

Julie W. Cheng, Loma Linda University Medical Center, Loma Linda, CA, United States

Chak-Lam Cho, Union Hospital, Hong Kong, China

Geoffrey N. De Iuliis, The University of Newcastle (UoN), University drive, Callaghan, NSW, Australia

Joel R. Drevet, Université Clermont Auvergne (UCA), Clermont-Ferrand, France

Damayanthi Durairajanayagam, Universiti Teknologi MARA, Sungai Buloh, Selangor, Malaysia

Nicolás Garrido, IVI Foundation, Valencia, Spain

Sezgin Gunes, Ondokuz Mayis University, Samsun, Turkey

Sajal Gupta, American Center for Reproductive Medicine, Cleveland Clinic, Cleveland, OH, United States

Gerhard Haidl, Rheinische Friedrich-Wilhelms University, Bonn, Germany

Ralf R. Henkel, University of the Western Cape, Bellville, South Africa

James M. Hotaling, University of Utah, Salt Lake City, UT, United States

Soumya Ranjan Jena, Ravenshaw University, Cuttack, Odisha, India

Srikanta Jena, Ravenshaw University, Cuttack, Odisha, India

Edmund Y. Ko, Loma Linda University Medical Center, Loma Linda, CA, United States

Kristian Leisegang, School of Natural Medicine, University of the Western Cape, Bellville, South Africa

Asli M. Mahmutoglu, Ondokuz Mayis University, Samsun, Turkey

Jasmine Nayak, Ravenshaw University, Cuttack, Odisha, India

Jacob Netherton, The University of Newcastle (UoN), University drive, Callaghan, NSW, Australia

Pedro F. Oliveira, Institute of Biomedical Sciences Abel Salazar, University of Porto, Porto, Portugal

Michael Owyong, University of Miami Miller School of Medicine, Miami, FL, United States

Manesh Kumar Panner Selvam, American Center for Reproductive Medicine, Cleveland Clinic, Cleveland, OH, United States

Biren V. Patel, University of Utah, Salt Lake City, UT, United States

Ranjith Ramasamy, University of Miami Miller School of Medicine, Miami, FL, United States

Luís Rato, (CICS-UBI) Health Sciences Research Centre, University of Beira Interior, Covilhã, Portugal

Rocío Rivera, Instituto Universitario IVI Valencia, València, Spain

Edmund Sabanegh, Jr., Cleveland Clinic Foundation, Cleveland, OH, United States

Dipak Kumar Sahoo, Iowa State University, Ames, IA, United States

Luna Samanta, Ravenshaw University, Cuttack, Odisha, India

Rakesh Sharma, American Center for Reproductive Medicine, Cleveland Clinic, Cleveland, OH, United States

Suresh C. Sikka, Tulane University, New Orleans, LA, United States

Branca M. Silva, University of Beira Interior, Covilhã, Portugal

Michael C. Solomon, Jr., University of the Western Cape, Bellville, South Africa

Mário Sousa, Institute of Biomedical Sciences Abel Salazar, University of Porto, Porto, Portugal

Nicholas N. Tadros, Southern Illinois University, Springfield, IL, United States

Gülgez Neslihan Hekim Taşkurt, Ondokuz Mayis University, Samsun, Turkey

Jaideep S. Toor, Tulane University, New Orleans, LA, United States

Kelton Tremellen, Flinders University, Bedford Park, SA, Australia

Eva Tvrda, Slovak University of Agriculture in Nitra, Nitra, Slovak Republic

Sarah C. Vij, Cleveland Clinic Foundation, Cleveland, OH, United States

Foreword

It is estimated that a male factor is identified in up to half of infertile couples. The etiology of male factor infertility is multifactorial yet studies have found that oxidative stress (OS) is a common mediator in the pathophysiology of this disease. It has been shown that 25% of unselected infertile men possess high levels of semen reactive oxygen species (ROS), whereas fertile men do not have high levels of ROS in semen. A controlled production of these ROS is required for normal sperm physiology (e.g., sperm hyperactivation, capacitation, and acrosome reaction) and for natural fertilization but the excessive production of ROS by immature germ cells and leukocytes causes sperm dysfunction (lipid peroxidation, loss of motility, and sperm DNA damage). Seminal OS is believed to be caused by an imbalance between ROS production and ROS scavenging by seminal antioxidants. However, whether it is an excess ROS production or a deficiency in antioxidant capacity that is the primary cause of semen OS remains a subject of controversy.

Spermatozoa are particularly susceptible to oxidative injury due to the abundance of plasma membrane polyunsaturated fatty acids. These unsaturated fatty acids provide fluidity that is necessary for membrane fusion events (e.g., the acrosome reaction and sperm—egg interaction) and for sperm motility. However, the unsaturated nature of these molecules predisposes them to free radical attack and lipid peroxidation of the sperm plasma membrane. Once this process has been initiated, accumulation of lipid peroxides occurs on the sperm surface (this results in loss of sperm motility) and oxidative damage to DNA can ensue. Natural protection from semen OS is afforded by sperm antioxidants and, to a greater extent, by seminal plasma, a fluid rich in both enzymatic and nonenzymatic antioxidants.

In this textbook, *Oxidants, Antioxidants, and Impact of the Oxidative Status in Male Reproduction*, co-editors Henkel, Samanta, and Agarwal have gathered an impressive group of experts (biologists and clinicians) to share their knowledge on the topic of OS. The drive to study OS in the male reproductive tract can be traced back to the research of Claude Gagnon and John Aitken, both pioneers in this field. The book is divided into three sections that cover this important area of reproductive biology: basic aspects, clinical aspects, and current approaches to OS. In the first section of the textbook, the biology of aerobic systems and the oxidant paradox is discussed. This is followed by several chapters that describe the etiology, physiology, and pathophysiology of OS in the male reproductive system, an active area of research.

A better understanding of the pathophysiology of male infertility and, in particular, the role of OS in male reproduction may help us more accurately define the causes of this condition. An ongoing area of research in the field of clinical andrology is the question of how specific health conditions (e.g., diabetes) contribute to male infertility. In the second section of the textbook, experts in the field discuss the epidemiology of OS and the clinical factors associated with OS in male reproduction. The techniques used to determine OS are also presented in this section. A detailed presentation on the role of in vivo and in vitro antioxidants is also explored. Antioxidant therapy remains a widely debated topic in male infertility. To date, studies suggest that antioxidants may be of benefit to infertile men although additional studies are needed to define the ideal antioxidant regimen and confirm the true advantage of this form of therapy. In the last section of the textbook, novel approaches to study ROS-mediated sperm function are presented. The interplay between OS in male reproductive health and genomics, epigenetics, and metabolomics are discussed. This ongoing area of research will help define the influence of OS on the metabolic profile of semen and sperm, the assembly and organization of the sperm chromatin, and the genomic integrity of sperm.

In order to better diagnose and treat male factor infertility we must further our understanding of the pathophysiology of this condition and, in particular, the role of OS in male reproductive health. The editors and authors of this book have done a superb job in assembling the most complete resource to date on the subject of oxidative stress in male reproduction and its clinical relevance. This textbook will undoubtedly be an important reference work that will guide biologists and clinicians on how to interpret and further investigate OS in male reproductive health.

Armand Zini, MD, FRCSC
Professor of Surgery, Department of Surgery, McGill University
Associate Professor of Obstetrics and Gynecology University of Montreal
Montreal, Canada
(Email: ziniarmand@yahoo.com)

Preface

Male infertility is a global health concern because it affects not only the physical well-being of individual patients, but also the psychological health of couples who want to have children. It also has significant negative societal implications. In certain societies, for a man to not be able to father children means that he will suffer from ridicule, low self-esteem, and marginalization. On the other hand, in many male-dominated societies, women carry the burden of reproduction, including the blame if a marriage is barren. Generally, male infertility is the sole cause of a couple's infertility in 30% of cases, and in more than 50% of the cases if a female factor is also taken into consideration. Despite this large prevalence, male infertility, as a major public health concern, is not properly addressed, and the problem is not only underestimated by the patients themselves, but also by many health-care professionals. Even to this day, too many clinicians limit their evaluation of male infertility to the standard semen analysis, which has clearly been shown to be insufficient in predicting the fertilizing capacity of male germ cells. Consequently, many clinicians too often offer expensive assisted reproduction techniques instead of properly examining and treating problems of male infertility. Up to 40%–50% of male infertility cases in general and up to 80% in men with idiopathic infertility are due to an imbalance between oxidants and antioxidants in their male reproductive system in favor of the oxidants, thus causing oxidative stress. Although in recent years, scientists and clinicians have discovered that oxidative stress is a major cause and contributing factor in many cases of male infertility, the knowledge and understanding of its pathology and possible treatment options are lagging behind. This has the potential for unsatisfactory diagnoses and treatment of male infertility.

The book is organized in three main sections: basic aspects, clinical aspects, and current approaches. Renowned experts from 12 countries wrote 24 state-of-the-art chapters selected for this book. Thus our book provides detailed information on the role of reactive oxygen species in sperm physiology and pathology with essential, up-to-date, basic, and clinical information on these highly reactive compounds and oxidative stress. While the first part of the book provides basic, up-to-date background on the topic, including the chemical nature of reactive oxygen species, antioxidants, the antioxidant paradox, oxidative stress, and reductive stress, the second part deals with the clinical aspects, providing insightful information in the pathophysiological role of reactive oxygen species in various diseases such as aging, malnutrition, diabetes, and thyroid dysfunction. Furthermore, the most common diagnostic tests to determine oxidative stress are described in a simple and practical manner.

In light of the fact that many patients routinely take various dietary antioxidants in an uncontrolled manner as these are very much extolled for their beneficial effects, we included chapters on treatment options of oxidative stress in vitro and in vivo as well as on so-called reductive stress, which is due to an overdosage of antioxidants and is as dangerous as oxidative stress. While the latter is a new concept in andrology and an additional way of thinking and explaining certain aspects of male infertility, we also included practical diagnostic aspects and rounded these topics off with very recent developments using the omics platform. We feel that this book provides current and comprehensive information that addresses the physiology and pathology of oxidative stress as a cause of male infertility. This combination of basic and clinical information makes our book well suited for fertility practitioners, andrologists, urologists, medical doctors, reproductive professionals, and research students.

We are grateful to our contributors, who are distinguished leaders in the field with extensive experience from around the world.

This book would not have been possible without the excellent support of Elsevier. We are thankful to Tari Broderick, Senior Acquisition Editor, for her constant support, and Samuel Young, Editorial Project Manager, for managing this project. The editors are grateful to their families for their love and support.

We genuinely hope that this volume will support and enrich your practice in clinical andrology.

Ralf Henkel, BEd, PhD, Habil
Bellville, South Africa

Luna Samanta, PhD
Cuttack, India

Ashok Agarwal, PhD, HCLD (ABB), EMB (ACE)
Cleveland, OH, USA

Introduction

R. John Aitken

University of Newcastle, Callaghan, NSW, Australia

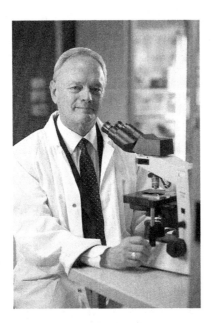

Oxidants, Antioxidants, and Impact of the Oxidative Status in Male Reproduction provides readers with a definitive up-to-date account of our current understanding of the role played by oxidative stress in the etiology of male infertility. Within the pages of this book, Ralf Henkel, Luna Samanta, and Ashok Agarwal have orchestrated a thoughtful collection of authoritative reviews that demonstrate just how important the redox status of the ejaculate is in defining the quality of the human ejaculate. While the individual chapters reveal a fair level of consensus in terms of the overall clinical importance of reactive oxygen species (ROS) generation in the germ line, this accord is balanced by some enduring uncertainties over the source, nature, and detection of reactive oxygen metabolites as well as the significance of antioxidant supplementation in countering the oxidative stress they induce. Some differences of opinion in such a rapidly developing field are as inevitable as they are insightful. In order to understand the challenges being faced by this field the reader is initially presented with clear, well-articulated accounts of the fundamental chemistry of oxidative stress and then led through some of the hot spots of debate in the application of this knowledge to one of nature's most intractable problems—what factors are responsible for the very high levels of male infertility seen in our species?

It has been quite a journey. The initial steps on this long and winding road were taken by Tosic and Walton who, as long ago as 1946, published a paper in *Nature*, highlighting the sensitivity of bovine spermatozoa to hydrogen peroxide toxicity [1]. This was then succeeded by a much more extensive paper [2] in which they showed that bovine spermatozoa possess an aromatic L-amino acid oxidase (LAAO) system that in the presence of oxygen will affect the processes of deamination and dehydrogenation to generate H_2O_2 and ammonia [2]. Similar LAAO activity has been described in ram and stallion spermatozoa [3] where it may also play a role in creating oxidative stress, particularly in the presence of egg-yolk extenders containing high concentrations of aromatic amino acids (particularly phenylalanine). While a similar system is present in human spermatozoa it does not appear to play a significant role in the spontaneous generation of excess ROS by these cells [4]. Indeed, there is still great uncertainty in the field as to the sources of ROS that might contribute to disruption of human sperm function.

The answer to this question is unlikely to be simple. Several chapters in this volume allude to the significance of leukocyte contamination in defining the redox status human semen samples. There can be no doubt that in unfractionated ejaculates, leukocytes comprise the most significant source of ROS; however, the potential of these molecules to cause damage is countered by the antioxidant properties of seminal plasma. Indeed seminal plasma has probably evolved to perform just this role. At the moment of ejaculation spermatozoa will suddenly be exposed to an increase in oxygen tension and the ROS generated by leukocytes originating from the urethra, seminal vesicles, or prostate. Normally this oxidative attack is short-lived and the spermatozoa are protected by the powerful antioxidant properties of seminal plasma during the hiatus between ejaculation and colonization of the female reproductive tract. However, the seminal antioxidant pool may become exhausted if levels of leukocytic infiltration are high, leaving the spermatozoa vulnerable to a leukocyte-mediated oxidative attack. The degree of stress experienced by the spermatozoa under these circumstances will ultimately depend on the number of infiltrating leukocytes (particularly neutrophils and macrophages), their state of activation, and the details of how, when, and where they became activated. Measuring the balance of ROS generation within the ejaculate and the level of residual antioxidant protection offered by seminal plasma is an excellent approach to capturing this redox balance [5]. In making such measurements, we might reflect on whether the transient sojourn of spermatozoa in seminal plasma depleted of its antioxidant reserve is actually sufficient to compromise sperm function directly. Is it also possible that, in vivo, the presence of leukocytes in the ejaculate provides an indirect indication of long-term proinflammatory conditions prevailing in the male reproductive tract (or even systemically) that are actually responsible for the loss of sperm function seen in oxidative stress patients? There are many conditions where the level of oxidative stress in the ejaculate is reflective of a more generalized stress as in patients suffering from obesity, exposure to cigarette smoke, high alcohol intake, exposure to organic pesticides and herbicides, radiation, and other conditions. Moreover, several of the chapters in this volume highlight a growing range of clinical conditions including diabetes, chronic kidney disease, β-thalassemia, thyroid dysfunction, and hyperhomocysteinemia, which appear to be associated with a systemic oxidative stress of such intensity that fertility is compromised. In this context, oxidatively damaged spermatozoa may be the "canaries in the coal mine," reflecting underlying conditions that influence an individual's entire health trajectory, including the ultimate risk of malignancy [6].

Once the spermatozoa have been separated from seminal plasma and purified, attention switches (or should switch) to gametes. Too many studies in this field have been compromised by a failure to account for the impact of contaminating leucocytes on the generation of ROS in washed sperm suspensions. Most commonly used sperm isolation techniques (including swim-up and discontinuous gradient density gradient centrifugation) do not succeed in removing all the leukocytes. The leukocyte-derived redox signals generated under such circumstances tend to overwhelm the limited ROS-generating capacity of spermatozoa, leading to potential errors in the literature in defining the source of ROS in spermatozoa. This has, for example, potentially impacted our view of the significance of NADPH oxidases in spermatozoa. At present, most evidence points to the sperm mitochondria as a major source of ROS [7] possibly supplemented with the activity of cytoplasmic enzymes such as the lipoxygenase, ALOX15 [8].

Another challenge that has plagued the field is the development of detection methods to determine the ROS-generating capacity of the ejaculate. Techniques such as chemiluminescence or nitroblue tetrazolium reduction are certainly sensitive but they do not report on a defined chemical entity and cannot readily discriminate the relative contributions from spermatozoa and leukocytes. Flow cytometry has the power to focus exclusively on the sperm population but specificity is again a problem. Most commonly used flow cytometry probes, such as dihydroethidium or dihydrodichlorofluorescein, are highly redox sensitive, but do not report on specific ROS. While we await the development of more specific probes we might focus on measuring the consequences of oxidative stress by assessing the products of lipid peroxidation. This could be achieved by flow cytometry mediated measurements of lipid oxidation products such as 4-hydroxynonenal, 4-hydroxyhexanal, acrolein, or malondiadhyde. A systematic analysis of the lipid peroxidation breakdown products generated as a consequence of an oxidative attack on human spermatozoa would be valuable in selecting an appropriate marker (see Chapter 1).

The role of oxidative stress in damaging sperm DNA and thereby influencing the mutational load subsequently carried by any offspring is another area of investigation highlighted in this book that has important implications for assisted reproductive technologies. It is particularly relevant to the increasing use of intracytoplasmic sperm injection (ICSI) as the default insemination technique, since the inadvertent fertilization of oocytes with oxidatively damaged spermatozoa is inevitable with this approach. The consequences of such action, in terms of the normality and health trajectory of the offspring, will be an important focus for future studies in this area. A recent study demonstrating an increase in autism spectrum disorder in offspring conceived by ICSI [9] may be a harbinger for bad news yet to come.

Ultimately ROS are a two-edged sword as far as the cell biology of human spermatozoa is concerned. On the positive side, they are important modulators of sperm capacitation, but when the antioxidant factors that protect these vulnerable cells are overwhelmed, they are mediators of cell senescence and death. For these and other aspects of oxidative stress in the male germ line this book provides expert comprehensive coverage and should be read by anybody interested in this rapidly emerging field.

REFERENCES

[1] Tosic J, Walton A. Formation of hydrogen peroxide by spermatozoa and its inhibitory effect on respiration. Nature 1946;158:485.

[2] Tosic J, Walton A. Metabolism of spermatozoa. The formation and elimination of hydrogen peroxide by spermatozoa and effects on motility and survival. Biochem J 1950;47:199−212.

[3] Aitken JB, Naumovski N, Curry B, Grupen CG, Gibb Z, Aitken RJ. Characterization of an L-amino acid oxidase in equine spermatozoa. Biol Reprod 2015;92:125.

[4] Houston B, Curry B, Aitken RJ. Human spermatozoa possess an IL4I1 l-amino acid oxidase with a potential role in sperm function. Reproduction 2015;149:587−96.

[5] Sharma RK, Pasqualotto FF, Nelson DR,Thomas Jr AJ, Agarwal A. The reactive oxygen species-total antioxidant capacity score is a new measure of oxidative stress to predict male infertility. Hum Reprod 1999;14:2801−7.

[6] Hanson BM, Eisenberg ML, Hotaling JM. Male infertility: a biomarker of individual and familial cancer risk. Fertil Steril 2018;109:6−19.

[7] Koppers AJ, De Iuliis GN, Finnie JM, McLaughlin EA, Aitken RJ. Significance of mitochondrial reactive oxygen species in the generation of oxidative stress in spermatozoa. J Clin Endocrinol Metab 2008;93:3199−207.

[8] Bromfield EG, Mihalas BP, Dun MD, Aitken RJ, McLaughlin EA, Walters JL, Nixon B. Inhibition of arachidonate 15-lipoxygenase prevents 4-hydroxynonenal-induced protein damage in male germ cells. Biol Reprod 2017;96:598−609.

[9] Kissin DM, Zhang Y, Boulet SL, Fountain C, Bearman P, Schieve L, Yeargin-Allsopp M, Jamieson DJ. Association of assisted reproductive technology (ART) treatment and parental infertility diagnosis with autism in ART-conceived children. Hum Reprod 2015;2015(30):454−65.

Part I

Basic Aspects

Chapter 1.1

Life Under Aerobic Conditions

Kristian Leisegang

School of Natural Medicine, University of the Western Cape, Bellville, South Africa

INTRODUCTION

Biology on earth has had a significant impact on planetary evolution. This is prominently evident through planetary redox evolution due to changing atmospheric and oceanic gaseous environments [1]. In the modern era, climate change is based on the evolutionary recent rapid rise of CO_2 in the atmosphere, significantly driven by *Homo sapiens'* influence through industrialization and unrestricted utilization of fossil fuel (carbonaceous) resources [2]. However, in the ancient organic rich environment of the late Archean (4–2.5 Ga: *giga anuum* = 1 billion years ago) and Proterozoic (2.5–0.5 Ga) periods, significant climate change occurred in which the atmosphere was being polluted by rising oxygen (O_2) concentrations [2]. Although a rapid rise of O_2 is evident in the records, it remains a challenge for geobiologists to fully understand the role of biological life in the oxygenation of the planet. This is due to scarce access to the well-preserved rocks from these times as well as a poor biological record of early biota [1]. However, it is evident that biological life significantly contributed to the changing environment, in which aerobic respiration evolved as a prominent event for the development of multicellular organisms due to the ability to produce energy more efficiently [1,2].

THE GREAT OXYGENATION EVENT

The early biosphere of earth, around 3.8 Ga in which life arose, is generally accepted to have been a low O_2 environment [2] dominated by carbon dioxide (CO_2) and nitrogen (N_2). This chemical composition would have created an environment with mild reducing conditions, providing the main energy source for exclusively unicellular organisms consisting mainly of hyperthermophiles [1,3]. These organisms utilized chemical sources of energy through metabolic CO_2 assimilation mechanisms, and from this photosynthesis appears to have arisen early in the evolution of life. O_2 is a toxic molecular by-product of this anaerobic respiration [3]. Following this, geographical evidence suggests a significant global rise in atmospheric O_2 approximately 2.3 Ga, known as the Great Oxygenation Event (GOE) [4]. In addition to biological life, environmental and climatic events such as glaciations and intense continental weathering that resulted in oxidation of the ocean surface water also contributed to the rise in O_2 levels [5].

However, as early as 3 Ga, there was an atmospheric change in which oxygenic photosynthesis (oxygenic phototrophy) evolved through ancient cyanobacteria as a significant microbial biochemical innovation, providing the most significant source of modern atmospheric O_2 concentrations [6]. Following the GOE, a final rise in atmospheric O_2 was observed approximately 0.5 Ga [1].

It is clear, therefore, that the biological production of O_2 dramatically modified the environment into the Proterozoic period, resulting in more oxidizing conditions compared to that of the Archean period [1,7]. Importantly, the associated change in the environmental redox state modified the bioavailability of metals, including iron, copper and molybdenum [8]. The bioavailability of O_2 provided early biota with an oxidant environment, which arguably necessitated the evolution of aerobic respiration [8].

BIOLOGICAL LIFE AND ENVIRONMENTAL EVOLUTION

The emergence of O_2 in the evolution of Earth required at least one biological pathway to have been active and present, as abiotic generation of O_2 (e.g., photodissociation of water vapor with hydrogen escaping to space) would have been too ineffective [9]. With abiotic production of O_2 from water via UV light considered as a minor contributor, it is proposed that biological photosynthesis in cyanobacteria and photosynthetic eukaryotes greatly contributed to modern atmospheric O_2 levels [10].

In addition to oxygenic photosynthesis, biological sources of O_2 generation include reactive oxygen species (ROS) detoxification, chlorate generation, and nitrogen-driven anaerobic methane oxidation [9]. O_2 production from detoxification of ROS is generally regarded to have evolved after oxygenic photosynthesis, and initial mechanisms of defense to ROS were physical barriers as opposed to enzymatic antioxidant systems [11]. Although there is some debate, aerobic respiration would have likely evolved after that of oxygen photosynthesis [1]. However, prior to this evolution, O_2 may have been produced by chemosynthetic sources, such as possible nitrite anaerobic methane oxidation by oxygenic bacteria, primordial chlorate metabolism by microbial chlorate dismutation, catalase-like enzymes converting radioactivity produced peroxides, or via nitric oxide dismutation on volcanic nitric oxide in the presence of abundant oceanic iron to release environmental oxygen [12]. Increased subaerial volcanic activity further provided oxidized gases such as CO_2 and SO_2, whereas submarine volcanoes provided more reducing gases such as H_2, CO, CH_4, and H_2S [1]. Although surface oceanic water may have become oxygen-rich earlier, the deep oceans remained anoxic until atmospheric O_2 reached near present-day levels around 0.5 Ga [1]. This period ended the dominance of prokaryotes on earth and allowed complex and multicellular life to evolve [1].

With the evolution of oxygenic phototrophs, molecular O_2 became the major electron acceptor on Earth [12]. Other electron acceptors exist; for example nitrate, which has an oxidative potential that is similar to that of O_2 through the process of denitrification [12]. Both aerobic respiration and denitrification reactions share some common machinery and enzyme mediators, resulting in the production of potentially damaging highly reactive molecules [12].

Although there is more research required for geochemists to refine the understanding of earth's redox evolution in atmospheric and oceanic gasses [1,6], particularly the timing of oxygenation and the GOE currently dated at 2.3 Ga [1,4,6], the increasing generation of O_2 in the atmosphere during this period was in fact a major atmospheric pollutant that affected biological life on earth [13]. Increasing atmospheric O_2 led to the development of aerobic niches for advanced eukaryote organisms to develop into more complex multicellular life observed in the present-day biosphere [3].

AEROBIC RESPIRATION AND THE MITOCHONDRIA

Fundamental to cellular activity, respiration critically involves a molecular series of redox reactions. This consists of the transfer of electrons through membrane-associated cofactors and protein complexes, from an electron donor to an electron acceptor [10]. Aerobic respiration appears to have evolved after O_2 increased in the atmosphere following climate transformation via anaerobic life forms [10]. The evolution of aerobic respiration was therefore driven by the increasing environmental source of O_2 [12].

All known eukaryotes either have mitochondria or evolved from ancestors with mitochondria. With the energy demands of multicellular life being very high, aerobic respiration was a critical step in the development of biological evolution [10]. Aerobic respiration is in fact the most effective exergonic biological process known. Furthermore, this process plays central roles in molecular cycles of carbon, nitrogen, and sulfur in addition to oxygen [14]. In mitochondrial-driven aerobic respiration, the electron transfer is to the dioxygen molecule, driven via the oxygen reductase members of the heme-copper oxidoreductase family, which conserves some of the free energy released from O_2 reduction [15]. The energy released in this biological process leads to the generation of an electrochemical gradient, known as the mitochondrial membrane potential (MMP), required for adenosine triphosphate (ATP) production [10].

Mitochondria are cytoplasmic organelles found in all eukaryote cells, and through cellular aerobic respiration (oxidative phosphorylation) provide the principle molecular energy supply in ATP. This happens primarily via the metabolism of simple sugars and long chain fatty acids [16]. In addition to energy production and recycling of adenosine diphosphate (ADP) into ATP, steroid hormones (pregnenolone) and lipids are synthesized. Ancient and distinct mitochondrial DNA (mtDNA) is replicated and hundreds of biochemical processes essential for human life occur [17]. Furthermore, mitochondria have significant roles in molecular signaling, cellular differentiation, cellular growth and division, immune signaling, and apoptosis [17].

Energy producing metabolic pathways originated very early during the evolution of life, and proteins associated with aerobic respiration chains have been found in early bacteria and Archaea, and may have arisen from a common ancestor [18]. Mitochondria themselves are considered to be of bacterial origin, arising from α-proteobacteria [19]. It has been argued that mitochondria, as well as chloroplasts, evolved from free-living bacteria within the eukaryotic cell as a symbiotic relationship (endosymbiont hypothesis) [20]. However, a significant amount of the mitochondrial proteome appears to have evolved outside α-proteobacteria, and has followed diverse evolutionary pathways through different eukaryote lineages creating a genomic and functional mosaic [19]. Hence, a debate remains whether mitochondria evolved after eukaryote cells arose or originated at the same time as the cells containing these organelles [19], with two fundamentally different themes: (1) the *archezoan scenario*, where primitive mitochondria were hosted in a hypothetical primitive eukaryote termed archezoan; and (2) the *symbiogenesis scenario*, where a single endosymbiotic event occurred, leading to the development of the mitochondria [19].

Including the double membrane, mitochondrial structure is divided into four compartments: the outer membrane, intermembrane space, inner membrane (folded into cristae), and matrix. The inner membrane is folded into cristae, where ATP synthase and protein complexes that regulate cellular respiration occur [17]. Rather than a static producer of energy, the mitochondria are dynamic, and the mitochondrial membrane is continuously remodeled in response to cellular signaling [17]. However, it is important to note that mitochondria across different species show significant variations in morphological appearance, coding capacity, and modes of expression [19]. In mammals, mtDNA has been sequenced from numerous species. In addition to ATP synthase, mtDNA encodes approximately 13 protein subunits of the mitochondrial electron transport chain as well as rRNA and tRNA units for the mitochondrial translation system [19]. Only the most ancestral mtDNAs encode for almost all of this gene set, for example *Reclinomonas americana* [21], with other organisms using as little as only three protein genes (e.g., mtDNA of *Plasmodium falciparum*).

The mitochondrial biomachinery and related redox activity is operated by five mitochondrial protein complexes [22]. These consist of nicotinamide adenine dinucleotide (NADH) dehydrogenase (complex I), the quinine pool, bc_1 complex (complex III), and cytochrome *c* as the back bone for aerobic respiratory chain, with complex IV as a terminal oxidase [12]. Furthermore, based on the membrane associated bioelectrical gradient, the MMP is an important and reliable marker for mitochondrial function. A range of -136 to -140 mV is considered optimal for ATP production in all living organisms [23]. However, a detailed understanding of MMP generation has still not been completely elicited. Under normal cellular conditions, this potential appears to be exclusively generated by electron flow through electron transport chain complexes I–IV, terminating as a direct electrical current that terminates in subunit II of complex IV that gradually charges the MMP [23].

REDOX BIOLOGY AND THE PARADOXICAL NATURE OF AEROBIC LIFE

Following the GOE and the environment becoming O_2-rich, the molecule has become critical for aerobic life on Earth, specifically through ATP-generation via oxidative phosphorylation [24]. However, it is apparent that this molecule is paradoxical in nature, as excessive free radical generation is detrimental to biological life. During aerobic respiration, O_2 is metabolized into various molecules termed ROS [24,25]. Although ROS is considered an umbrella term for highly reactive O_2 derivatives associated with both cellular regulatory roles and pathophysiological mechanism of disease, it is important to consider that not all ROS are free radicals [26,27]. The term ROS specifically defines molecules that have one or more unpaired electrons in the outer molecular orbits, making them unstable. Examples include superoxide ($\cdot O_2^-$) and peroxide molecules [28]. Hydrogen peroxide (H_2O_2), however, is not an unstable radical although it is termed a ROS [28]. In this context, we also must consider that O_2 itself is a diradical, a characteristic that explains its chemical reactivity.

Endogenous ROS are generated via a series of redox reactions via the transfer of electrons through the mitochondrial protein complexes. As a result, there is a measureable leakage of electrons, specifically from protein complexes I and III, generating $\cdot O_2^-$ at a rate of approximately 0.2%–2.0% of the O_2 consumed. Superoxide dismutase (SOD)1 and SOD2 then further metabolize $\cdot O_2^-$ in the mitochondria, producing H_2O_2 (a major cellular regulator of redox sensing and signaling) [22]. H_2O_2 may undergo reduction to produce a hydroxyl radical ($\cdot OH^-$). ROS can also be generated via enzyme activity or via metal catalyzed from $\cdot O_2^-$ [26,29]. The highly reactive and detrimental peroxynitrite is produced via nitric oxide activity on $\cdot O_2^-$ [30].

ROS are known to regulate various cellular functions, such as apoptosis, ion transport systems, immune regulation and inflammatory responses, cellular responses to growth factor signaling, and regulation of genetic expression [28]. These small reactive molecules can further react with and damage cellular macromolecules, particularly proteins and lipids [28]. Molecular redox (phosphorylation/dephosphorylation) switches are the adaption mechanisms for physiological concentrations of ROS, which then function as mechanisms of cellular signaling [31]. Oxidative stress (OS) is therefore defined as a state of excess ROS production and/or the reduction in savaging antioxidants, which results in pathophysiological changes similar to the general adaption syndrome of cellular stressors [22,31].

ENDOGENOUS ANTIOXIDANTS AND OXIDATIVE STRESS

As excessive ROS production is toxic to cellular molecules and structures, a balance between ROS generation and metabolism by endogenous and exogenous antioxidants is crucial. Internal and external disturbances to this balance can lead to OS within cells and broader biological systems [27]. Over time, OS induces cellular damage that may accumulate, which is increasingly associated with complex pathophysiology known to mediate chronic disease. This includes a prominent role in ageing and age-related chronic diseases, including but not limited to obesity, metabolic syndrome, and associated type-2 diabetes mellitus, cardiovascular diseases, various malignancies, and neurodegenerative diseases including Alzheimer's disease [28]. OS has also been implicated as major cause or contributing factor of male infertility [32,33].

Due to the potentially detrimental effects of OS, cells have evolved defense mechanisms through the scavenging and neutralizing properties of endogenous antioxidants that reduced ROS with various cofactors. These regulating enzymes include catalase, glutathione peroxidase, and the SOD family [13]. Members of the SOD family include SOD1 (copper and zinc), SOD2 (Manganese), and the extracellular SOD3. Additional examples of well-studied endogenous antioxidant families include peroxiredoxins, glutaredoxins, and thioredoxins [13,34].

Contrary to the concept of OS, reductive stress (RS) involves a cellular shift of the redox status into the reduced state, which is also detrimental for cells as they are not able to induce regulatory redox switches [35]. RS is considered as dangerous for cells as OS [36], associated with cardiac damage, neurological diseases [37], and dysregulations of embryogenesis [38]. RS is also increasingly associated with male infertility [39,40].

MITOCHONDRIAL DYSFUNCTION

Through the production of ATP via aerobic respiration, mitochondria are a significant source for the generation of excessive ROS, which further results in mitochondrial damage and dysfunction [41]. Underlying this dysfunction are the minor variations in MMP, which results in a dramatic reduction in ATP synthesis and a further increase in ROS production, thus reflecting the concept of mitochondrial dysfunction [23].

Mitochondrial dysfunction is receiving increasing attention and is associated with a wide range of human pathology, particularly involving non-communicable chronic and degenerative diseases. This includes obesity, metabolic syndrome, type-2 diabetes mellitus, cardiovascular disease, numerous cancers, and neurodegeneration [42,43]. Furthermore, mitochondrial dysfunction and associated OS is considered to be a major underlying mechanism of the ageing process, including negative impact on spermatogenesis and steroidogenesis in males [41,43]. However, there is evidence to suggest that ROS are not always deleterious, and may even promote longevity pathways, and therefore play a complex role in health and disease [41].

CONCLUSION

The evolution of aerobic respiration was necessitated by the toxic evolution of the planet due to oxygen generated as a by-product of prokaryote-based anaerobic respiration. This allowed for the evolution of aerobic respiration and a significant increase in energy generation for cellular activities, and multicellular eukaryote life evolved. In this process, mitochondria have emerged as a significant organelle associated with numerous cellular activities beyond energy production. Due to leakage of electrons in aerobic respiration, physiologically critical yet potentially toxic molecules termed ROS arise. It is important for a cellular redox steady state to be maintained for appropriate cellular functioning, with numerous endogenous antioxidants having evolved for this regulation. Oxidative and reductive stress arise out of an imbalance between ROS and total antioxidant capacity (TAC), and the understanding of this relationship in the molecular pathology across a wide range of diseases is of critical importance. Additionally, dysfunctional mitochondria and changes in MMP are associated with cellular or tissue ROS:TAC mismatch, and is emerging as an important mediator in numerous disease processes.

GLOSSARY

Aerobic respiration Process of developing cellular energy involving oxygen.
Anaerobic respiration Cellular respiration in the absence of oxygen.
Antioxidant Any molecule that inhibits oxidation and scavenges free radicals and reactive oxygen species.
Archaea Microorganisms that are similar in morphology to bacteria with different molecular organization that constitute an ancient group between bacteria and eukaryotes.

Archean period Denoting the eon that constitutes the early to middle Precambrian period in which there was no life on Earth.

Cyanobacteria A division of prokaryote microorganisms related to bacteria that are capable of photosynthesis, representing the earliest known form of life on Earth.

Exergonic A chemical or metabolic process accompanied by the release of energy.

Eukaryote Cells that have genetic material in the form of DNA, including all living organisms except eubacteria and archaea.

Free radical An uncharged highly reactive and short-lived molecule having an unpaired valence electron.

Geobiology The study of interactions that occur between the living organisms and their biological products (biosphere) and the geosphere.

Great Oxygenation Event The appearance of dioxygen in the Earth's atmosphere induced predominantly by biological activities of living organisms.

Oxidative stress An imbalance between increased free radicals and/or reduced antioxidant scavengers that contributes to cellular cytotoxicity.

Oxygenic phototrophy Metabolic respiration process using photons for energy generation (photosynthesis) that releases oxygen as a by-product, found in some plants, algae, and cyanobacteria.

Prokaryote Microscopic single-cell organism with no distinct nucleus or other specialized organelles, including bacteria and cyanobacteria.

Proterozoic period The eon that constitutes the later part of the Precambrian, between the Archean eon and the Cambrian period, in which the earliest forms of life evolved.

Proteobacteria The largest and most diverse group (phylum) of bacteria that are gram-negative that show metabolic diversity including chemoautotrophic, chemoorganotrophic, and phototrophic. This phylum includes a variety of pathogens such as Escherichia, Salmonella, Vibrio, Helicobacter, and others.

Reactive oxygen species (ROS) Chemically reactive molecules containing oxygen that are formed as a normal by-product of aerobic respiration.

Redox (reduction-oxidation) The chemical processes of oxidation (process of losing or donating one or more electrons) and reduction (process of gaining or accepting one or more electrons) considered together as complementary processes.

Redox reaction One atom or molecule receives electrons from another atom or compound.

Reductive stress An imbalance between reduced free radicals and/or increased antioxidant scavengers that contributes to cellular cytotoxicity.

LIST OF ACRONYMS AND ABBREVIATIONS

ADP adenosine diphosphate
AMP adenosine monophosphate
ATP adenosine triphosphate
CO_2 carbon dioxide molecule
Ga Giga-anuum (one billion years ago)
H_2O_2 hydrogen peroxidase
N_2 nitrogen molecule
MMP mitochondrial membrane potential
mtDNA mitochondrial DNA
mV millivolts
NADH nicotinamide adenine dinucleotide
NO nitrous oxide
O_2 oxygen molecule
O_2^- superoxide radical
OH hydroxyl radical
OS oxidative stress
ROS reactive oxygen species
SO_2 sulphide
SOD superoxide dismutase

REFERENCES

[1] Hamilton TL, Bryant DA, Macalady JL. The role of biology in planetary evolution: cyanobacterial primary production in low-oxygen Proterozoic oceans. Environ Microbiol 2016;18(2):325–40.

[2] Crowe SA, Døssing LN, Beukes NJ, Bau M, Kruger SJ, Frei R, Canfield DE. Atmospheric oxygenation three billion years ago. Nature 2013;501(7468):535–8.

[3] Des Marais DJ. Earth's early biosphere. Gravit Space Biol Bull 1998;11(2):23–30.

[4] Luo G, Ono S, Beukes NJ, Wang DT, Xie S, Summons RE. Rapid oxygenation of Earth's atmosphere 2.33 billion years ago. Sci Adv 2016;2(5):e1600134.

[5] Holland HD. The oxygenation of the atmosphere and oceans. Phil Trans Biol Sci 2006;361(1470):903–15.

[6] Lyons TW, Reinhard CT, Planavsky NJ. The rise of oxygen in Earth's early ocean and atmosphere. Nature 2014;506(7488):307–15.

[7] Kump LR. The rise of atmospheric oxygen. Nature 2008;451(7176):277—8.

[8] Anbar AD. Oceans. Elements and evolution. Science 2008;322(5907):1481—3.

[9] Ettwig KF, Butler MK, Le Paslier DL, Pelletier E, Mangenot S, Kuypers MMM, et al. Nitrite-driven anaerobic methane oxidation by oxygenic bacteria. Nature 2010;464:543—8.

[10] Brochier-Armanet C, Talla E, Gribaldo S. The multiple evolutionary histories of dioxygen reductases: implications for the origin and evolution of aerobic respiration. Mol Biol Evol 2009;26(2):285—97.

[11] Bilinski T. Oxygen toxicity and microbial evolution. Biosystems 1991;24:305—12.

[12] Chen J, Strous M. Denitrification and aerobic respiration, hybrid electron transport chains and co-evolution. Biochim Biophys Acta 2013;1827(2):136—44.

[13] Cabiscol E, Tamarit J, Ros J. Oxidative stress in bacteria and protein damage by reactive oxygen species. Int Microbiol 2000;3(1):3—8.

[14] Falkowski PG, Fenchel T, Delong E. The microbial engines that drive Earth's biogeochemical cycles. Science 2008;320:1034—9.

[15] Han H, Hemp J, Pace LA, Ouyang H, Ganesan K, Roh JH, Daldal F, Blanke SR, Gennis RB. Adaptation of aerobic respiration to low O_2 environments. Proc Natl Acad Sci USA 2011;108(34):14109—14.

[16] Henze K, Martin W. Evolutionary biology: essence of mitochondria. Nature 2003;426:127—8.

[17] McBride HM, Neuspiel M, Wasiak S. Mitochondria: more than just a powerhouse. Curr Biol 2006;16(14):R551—60.

[18] Castresana J, Saraste M. Evolution of energetic metabolism: the respiration-early hypothesis. Trends Biochem Sci 1995;20(11):443—8.

[19] Gray MW. Mitochondrial evolution. Cold Spring Harb Perspect Biol 2012;4(9):a011403.

[20] Margulis L. Origin of eukaryotic cells. New Haven, CT: Yale University Press; 1970.

[21] Gray MW, Lang BF, Burger G. Mitochondria of protists. Annu Rev Genet 2004;38:477—524.

[22] Sies H. Hydrogen peroxide as a central redox signalling molecule in physiological oxidative stress: oxidative eustress. Redox Biol 2017;11:613—9.

[23] Bagkos G, Koufopoulos K, Piperi C. ATP synthesis revisited: new avenues for the management of mitochondrial diseases. Curr Pharm Des 2014;20(28):4570—9.

[24] Greabu M, Battino M, Mohora M, Olinescu R, Totan A, Didilescu A. Oxygen, a paradoxical element? Rom J Intern Med 2008;46(2):125—35.

[25] Hayyan M, Hashim MA, Alnashef IM. Superoxide ion: generation and chemical implications. Chem Rev 2016;116(5):3029—85.

[26] Tremellen K. Oxidative stress and male infertility — a clinical perspective. Hum Reprod Update 2008;14(3):243—58.

[27] Lushchak VI. Free radicals, reactive oxygen species, oxidative stresses and their classifications. Ukr Biochem J 2015;87(6):11—8.

[28] Morrell CN. Reactive oxygen species. Circ Res 2008;103:571—2.

[29] Turrens JF. Mitochondrial formation of reactive oxygen species. J. Physiol 2003;552:335—44.

[30] Lee D-Y, Wauquier F, Eid AA, Roman LJ, Ghosh-Choudhury G, Khazim K, Block K, Gorin Y. Nox4 NADPH oxidase mediates peroxynitrite-dependent uncoupling of endothelial nitric-oxide synthase and fibronectin expression in response to angiotensin II: role of mitochondrial reactiveoxygen species. J Biol Chem 2013;288(40):28668—86.

[31] Sies H. Oxidative stress: a concept in redox biology and medicine. Redox Biol 2015;4:180—3.

[32] Aitken RJ, Smith TB, Jobling MS, Baker MA, De Iuliis GN. Oxidative stress and male reproductive health. Asian J Androl 2014;16:31—8.

[33] Agarwal A, Virk G, Ong C, du Plessis SS. Effect of oxidative stress on male reproduction. World J Mens Health 2014;32:1—17.

[34] Li X, Fang P, Mai J, Choi ET, Wang H, Yang X. Targeting mitochondrial reactive oxygen species as novel therapy for inflammatory diseases and cancers. J Hematol Oncol 2013;6:19.

[35] Wendel A. Measurement of in vivo lipid peroxidation and toxicological significance. Free Radic Biol Med 1987;3:355—8.

[36] Castagné V, Lefèvre K, Natero R, Clarke PG, Bedker DA. An optimal redox status for the survival of axotomized ganglion cells in the developing retina. Neuroscience 1999;93:313—20.

[37] Brewer A, Banerjee Mustafi S, Murray TV, Namakkal Soorappan R, Benjamin I. Reductive stress linked to small HSPs, G6PD and NRF2 pathways in heart disease. Antioxid Redox Signal 2013;18:1114—27.

[38] Ufer C, Wang CC, Borchert A, Heydeck D, Kuhn H. Redox control in mammalian embryo development. Antioxid Redox Signal 2010;13:833—75.

[39] Henkel R. Leukocytes and oxidative stress: dilemma for sperm function and male fertility. Asian J Androl 2011;13:43—52.

[40] Chen SJ, Allam JP, Duan YG, Haidl G. Influence of reactive oxygen species on human sperm functions and fertilizing capacity including therapeutical approaches. Arch Gynecol Obstet 2013;288:191—9.

[41] Wang Y, Hekimi S. Mitochondrial dysfunction and longevity in animals: untangling the knot. Science 2015;350(6265):1204—7.

[42] Bagkos G, Koufopoulos K, Piperi C. A new model for mitochondrial membrane potential production and storage. Med Hypotheses 2014b;83(2):175—81.

[43] Leisegang K, Henkel R, Agarwal A. Redox regulation of fertility in aging male and the role of antioxidants: a savior or stressor. Curr Pharm Des 2017;23(30):4438—50.

Chapter 1.2

The Oxidant Paradox

Nicholas N. Tadros[1] and Sarah C. Vij[2]
[1]Southern Illinois University, Springfield, IL, United States; [2]Cleveland Clinic Foundation, Cleveland, OH, United States

INTRODUCTION

Oxygen is essential for all life as we know it, yet oxygen is also inherently dangerous to all aerobic organisms as well. This has come to be known as the Oxygen Paradox [1]. The deleterious effects of oxygen stem from the fact that each oxygen atom has one unpaired electron in its outer valence shell, and molecular oxygen (O_2) has two unpaired electrons, making even O_2 a free radical. Reactive oxygen species (ROS), the group of molecules that are responsible for the damage caused by oxidative stress (OS), all stem from the inherent radical nature of O_2.

O_2 undergoes enzymatic reduction in the relatively efficient electron transport chain within the mitochondria. Some oxygen escapes this process and can participate in unique oxidative/reductive chemistry via the nonenzymatic reduction pathways: The addition of one electron to oxygen results in the creation of the superoxide anion radical ($\cdot O_2^-$), an ROS. The addition of two electrons (and two protons) to oxygen creates hydrogen peroxide (H_2O_2), another ROS despite the fact that all its outer valence electrons are paired. A third electron addition will create the highly reactive hydroxyl radical ($\cdot OH$) and a hydroxide ion (OH^-). Finally, addition of the fourth electron creates a water molecule.

Phagocytic cells (neutrophils and macrophages) also produce ROS intentionally as part of their defense mechanisms. This is important in fertility in the setting of leukocytospermia [2]. To maintain adequate oxidative homeostasis, cells have developed a variety of antioxidant molecules that can be produced or obtained from the diet as well as antioxidant enzymatic mechanisms to counteract ROS [3]. While the antioxidant defense mechanisms are relatively effective, our cells have also evolved enzymes and mechanisms to repair oxidative damage to proteins, lipids, and DNA [4].

In this chapter, we will explore the role of antioxidants in infertility and other disease states and discuss the antioxidant paradox. This paradox refers to the observation that administering antioxidants does not always improve OS-related disease states. We will also discuss the risks of antioxidant overload.

REACTIVE OXYGEN SPECIES AND FERTILITY

ROS are an important part of male fertility, and not just for their detrimental effects. Small amounts of ROS are essential for normal sperm physiology. Specifically, the superoxide anion, hydrogen peroxide and nitric oxide (NO), induce sperm hyperactivation, capacitation, and the acrosome reaction in vitro [5]. Human sperm capacitation and acrosome reactions are associated with extracellular production of superoxide anions. The lipid membrane oxidation that results from these low concentrations of ROS promote binding to the *zona pellucida*. The fine balance between ROS production and destruction as well as the right timing and location of the production seem to be very important for proper fertilizing capacity.

Capacitation

Sperm capacitation is the penultimate step in sperm maturation, which occurs after ejaculation and usually within the female reproductive tract in vivo, but can also occur in vitro in certain environments. ROS has been shown to promote capacitation in hamster, mouse, rat, bull, horse, and human sperm [6,7]. De Lamirande and Gagnon showed that the addition of xanthine, xanthine oxidase, and xanthine catalase (to generate a superoxide anion) increased the number of sperm undergoing capacitation and hyperactivation by threefold (15.4% vs 5.4%). The addition of the antioxidant superoxide dismutase prevented this increase [6].

Sperm Maturation

The majority of testicular sperm do not exhibit progressive motility or the ability to capacitate until their passage through the epididymis. In addition to gaining motility, the maturation of sperm also includes completion of nuclear condensation and changes in the expression of molecules on the sperm membrane [8]. ROS play an important role in these events by generating lipid peroxides, which act as a substrate for phospholipid hydroperoxide glutathione peroxidase, which facilitates nuclear condensation [9]. ROS may also initiate motility by enhancing protein phosphorylation [10].

In addition to these effects, ROS also play a role in chemotaxis, binding to zona pellucida, acrosome reaction, and subsequent sperm−oocyte fusion. But despite ROS serving an important role in sperm physiology, excess ROS production in semen has been associated with loss of sperm motility, decreased capacity for sperm−oocyte fusion, and loss of fertility [11].

In 1943, MacLeod was the first to observe that sperm suffered when exposed to ROS. He found that this oxygen overload would cause the profound depression of sperm motility as well as the development of ROS [12]. But it was not until many decades later that the important effects of OS on our health was realized [13]. In the intervening years, OS has been implicated in a myriad of pathologic processes including neurodegenerative diseases, cardiovascular disease, inflammation, cancer, and aging [14].

OXIDATIVE STRESS

Any system that tips its balance away from oxidative-reductive homeostasis in favor of oxidation is said to be under OS. This stress is caused by the effects of free radicals and other ROS at the molecular level. As mentioned previously, the most common and reactive oxygen derived free radical is the hydroxyl radical, created as part of the immune response by macrophages and other immune cells to kill pathogens as well as a by-product of cellular metabolism. These radicals are incredibly short-lived (10^{-9} s) but remain highly reactive and can damage all types of macromolecules including carbohydrates, DNA, lipids, and amino acids [15]. Unlike many other ROS, the hydroxyl radical cannot be eliminated by an enzymatic reaction. Antioxidants can scavenge hydroxyl radicals before they cause damage to cell structures and these mechanisms will be discussed later. The hydroxyl radical as well as the other major ROS are produced through oxidative phosphorylation of adenosine triphosphate via the electron transport chain within mitochondria. During this process, electrons are passed through a series of proteins via oxidation-reduction reactions, the last destination for an electron being an oxygen molecule. In normal conditions, the oxygen is completely reduced to produce water, but in a small percentage, the electrons passing through the chain will directly bond to oxygen (specifically in Complex III) to produce a superoxide radical [16].

NO, another known ROS, is synthesized from L-arginine by nitric oxide synthase (NOS). The inducible form of NOS (iNOS) is responsible for the majority of NO overproduction. NO readily diffuses into the cells and reacts with superoxide anions to produce oxidative metabolites such as peroxynitrite and peroxynitrous acid [17]. Peroxynitrite (sometimes called peroxonitrite), an unstable structural isomer of nitrate is not in itself a free radical, but a powerful oxidant. Its oxidizing properties can damage a wide array of molecules.

In summary, OS likely causes damage in one of four ways [18]:

- damage to DNA or RNA
- oxidation of polyunsaturated fatty acids in lipids (lipid peroxidation)
- oxidation of amino acids
- oxidative deactivation of specific enzymes by oxidation of cofactors

This damage can cause or contribute to a wide array of pathology and disease states. Male infertility is but a small potential consequence of increased OS in the human body. The free radical theory of aging postulates that organisms age because cells accumulate increased free radical damage over time [19]. This theory, first proposed by Dr. Harman [20], was one of the first to recognize that free radicals were not too unstable to be biologically active. Since 1956, the free-radical theory has expanded to include not only aging, but also age-related diseases.

Cancer

It was shown as early as 1984 that exposure of mouse fibroblasts to ROS can lead to malignant transformation [21]. Other mouse studies have shown that knockout mice missing copper- and zinc-containing superoxide dismutase (a scavenger of ROS) have increased rates of liver cancer [22]. Mice with only 50% normal manganese-containing superoxide dismutase showed increased risk of developing lymphomas, adenocarcinomas, and pituitary adenomas [23]. Other studies have found an increased rate of intestinal cancers [24], sarcomas, and adenomas [25] in mouse knockout models for various enzymes that help to break down ROS. The actual mechanism for how ROS causes cancer is complex and likely involves a combination of direct DNA damage, cell proliferation, and decreased apoptosis [26].

Neurodegenerative Disease

OS is particularly important in the brain and neuronal tissues as the metabolism of neurotransmitters produce ROS. These ROS attack postmitotic glial cells and neurons, which are particularly sensitive to free radicals [27]. OS has a suspected role in many neurodegenerative diseases including amyotrophic lateral sclerosis, Parkinson's disease, Alzheimer's disease, Huntington's disease, and multiple sclerosis [28]. In Alzheimer's disease, amyloid plaques are formed by chelation with copper and iron ions. This causes alteration in the oxidation state of both metals, producing hydrogen peroxide and free radicals [29]. While Parkinson's disease, unlike Alzheimer's disease, is characterized by motor dysfunction and decreased dopamine in the substantia nigra of the midbrain, these patients still exhibit many classic findings of OS, including lipid peroxidation, nucleic acid and protein oxidation, and changes in antioxidant concentrations [30]. In fact, studies have found that the deposition of inclusion (Lewy) bodies is stabilized by increased oxidation [31]. Excessive ROS generation by macrophages has been implicated as a mediator of demyelination and axonal damage in multiple sclerosis and other autoimmune encephalomyelitis [32].

Reperfusion Injury in Cardiovascular Disease

Following ischemia and reperfusion, ROS formation is greatly increased and the normal antioxidant mechanisms are overwhelmed. This can eventually lead to further cellular injury after the ischemia has resolved. This was first described in 1973 when they demonstrated that reoxygenation of hypoxic rat hearts resulted in significant damage rather than improvement [33]. This is of particular interest in humans as acute revascularization with thrombolytics or interventional procedures has emerged as the standard treatment for patients with acute myocardial infarction [34]. After revascularization of coronary arteries, ROS cause lipid peroxidation that results in cell membrane breakdown and resultant swelling. Increased ROS also result in the chemotaxis of neutrophils that in turn can lead to further microvascular plugging of capillaries. In addition, these white cells produce more ROS, causing the cycle to repeat [35]. These pathways contribute to potential reperfusion injuries. Furthermore, research has shown that if you prevent oxidative damage during reperfusion by inhibiting ROS production or increasing antioxidant content, you can have improved recovery of myocardial contractile function and reduced infarct size [36,37].

DIABETES

Increasing evidence in both basic science and clinical studies indicates that OS plays a major role in the pathogenesis of diabetes mellitus. Free radicals are formed by glucose oxidation and the nonenzymatic glycation and oxidative degradation of proteins. This leads to high concentrations of free radicals and the development of insulin resistance and its complications (coronary artery disease, nephropathy, and stroke) in type 2 diabetes. There is even evidence that OS is present in patients with type 1 diabetes [38]. Patients with diabetes have been found to have alterations in glutathione peroxidase, glutathione reductase, superoxide dismutase, and catalase activity, as well as a decrease in antioxidant vitamin concentrations [39]. Research has also shown that the apolipoprotein component of low-density lipoprotein can form insoluble aggregates due to hydroxyl radical-induced cross-linkage between apo-B monomers that may be responsible for some diabetic complications [40].

Definition of Antioxidant

If OS contributes to many human diseases and to the human aging process, then antioxidants should be of therapeutic benefit for many of these diseases [41]. Despite widespread use of various antioxidants, true clinical benefits have not been shown across many disease categories. It is likely that the mechanism of antioxidants is not fully understood and there may be paradoxical effects depending on dosing. Halliwell and Gutteridge defined antioxidant as "any substance that, when present at low concentrations compared with those of an oxidizable substrate, significantly delays or prevents oxidation of that substrate" [42]. Many different compounds fall into this category. The human body's antioxidant defenses are both enzymatic and nonenzymatic. Nonenzymatic defenses include vitamins C and E, coenzyme Q10, glutathione, and B-carotene, which have intrinsic antioxidant properties. Vitamin E (alpha-tocopherol) quenches lipid peroxidation and captures free hydroxyl radicals and superoxide. Glutathione reconstructs thiol groups of proteins that are eliminated by OS, contributing to its antioxidant activity [43].

Enzymatic defenses include superoxide dismutases, catalases, peroxidases, and many others discussed earlier and in other chapters. Superoxide dismutases are a class of enzymes that catalyze the dismutation reactions of the superoxide anion. Catalases aid in the conversion of hydrogen peroxide to oxygen and water. Glutathione peroxidase catalyzes the reduction of hydrogen peroxide and organic peroxides. These directly scavenge free radicals [44]. Compounds with free sulfhydryls are antioxidants but are not used clinically. The free sulfhydryl can absorb free electrons and thus react with ROS. Also, compounds with highly conjugated double bonds can bond with electrons and neutralize ROS. Examples of clinically utilized highly conjugated systems include retinoids and carotenoids [45].

Antioxidant Paradox

Despite the fact that ROS and free radicals are involved in several human diseases, administering antioxidants to human subjects has failed to show benefits across many human disease states. This phenomenon has been termed the antioxidant paradox. The idea that OS is uniformly bad and that antioxidants minimize OS is pervasive among the public, but this way of thinking is largely oversimplified at best and dangerous at worst. ROS may be beneficial at low concentrations and harmful at higher concentrations [46]. Innumerable clinical studies have been performed on several antioxidants in several disease states without overwhelming findings. This is likely due to the fact that the mechanism of antioxidants is dose-dependent and host-dependent.

Several large-scale studies have demonstrated lack of efficacy of antioxidants. The Alpha-Tocopherol, Beta-Carotene (ATBC) Lung Cancer Prevention Study is a well-known randomized, double-blind, placebo-controlled chemoprevention trial that examined whether increased intake of alpha-tocopherol and/or beta-carotene contributed to prevention of lung cancer among male smokers in Finland. This study enrolled over 29,000 men and ultimately showed that the intake of alpha-tocopherol and beta-carotene did not reduce the incidence of lung cancer. In fact, men taking beta-carotene had a high risk of developing lung cancer and a higher rate of ischemic heart disease. The authors concluded that the intake of these antioxidants may be harmful but further study is needed. They also found a reduced incidence of prostate cancer in men on alpha-tocopherol but reported that this may have been due to chance [47].

The Nutritional Prevention of Cancer trial is a clinical trial studying the effect of selenium supplementation on nonmelanoma skin cancer with second endpoints of lung, prostate, and colorectal cancer incidence. This study was a randomized, double-blind, placebo-controlled trial in 1312 participants from low-selenium areas of the United States. All subjects had a history of nonmelanoma skin cancer within the year before randomization. This study did not find a reduced incidence of nonmelanoma skin cancer; however, prostate cancer incidence was reduced in a statistically significant manner in patients with low baseline selenium levels. Prostate cancer incidence was not a primary endpoint in this study and therefore study participants were not systematically screened or diagnosed. Additionally, the introduction of prostate-specific antigen as a screening test occurred during the study period (1983–1991), which likely complicated diagnosis of prostate cancer in the study [48].

The findings of the ATBC Cancer Prevention Study prompted the design of the SELECT trial, which studied the effects of vitamin E and/or selenium supplementation on the risk of prostate cancer. This trial is a phase 3 randomized, placebo-controlled trial of selenium 200 μg, vitamin E 400 International Units (IU), or both for prostate cancer prevention with minimum follow-up of 7 years with goal follow-up of 12 years. The primary endpoint was prostate cancer incidence. The study was terminated 7 years early due to the finding that the supplements had no impact of incidence of prostate cancer whether given alone or in combination. A nonstatistically significant increased incidence of prostate cancer was observed in the vitamin E alone group. A total of 35,533 men were randomized in this study, which is a major strength; however, varied doses of the supplements were not studied [49].

The Physicians Health Study II examined the effect of a daily multivitamin in a randomized, double-blinded, placebo-controlled trial on the incidence of cancer. Over 14,000 male physicians were enrolled in this study and total cancer incidence was the primary outcome. This study found a modest but statistically significant reduction in total cancer incidence in men taking multivitamins but no statistically significant reduction in site-specific cancers [50]. Vitamin E supplementation did not reduce the incidence of prostate cancer when compared to placebo in this study population [51]. A metaanalysis by Miller et al. examined the relationship between vitamin E supplementation and total mortality based on 19 randomized controlled trials. Notably, this analysis revealed that high-dosage vitamin E supplementation increased all-cause mortality. Many of the high-dose vitamin E trials involved small numbers of patients with chronic diseases; however, this finding should raise some concern and highlight the need for further study [52]. Bjelakovic et al. performed a metaanalysis for randomized trials comparing the effect of beta-carotene, vitamin A, vitamin C, vitamin E, and selenium either alone or in combination with placebo on all-cause mortality. Their data suggest that beta-carotene, vitamin A, and vitamin E may increase mortality in a statistically significant manner [53]. Additionally, Vivekananthan et al. examined eight randomized trials of beta-carotene treatment and found a small but significant increase in all-cause mortality with beta-carotene (7.4% vs 7.0%) [54]. The trials included in this study used commonly found preparations of beta-carotene, which is concerning.

Oxidative damage to sperm DNA has been implicated in the etiology of male infertility in many cases. Spermatozoa are particularly sensitive to negative effects of ROS as a result of high concentration of unsaturated fatty acids in their cell membranes that can be oxidized. Their cytoplasm has limited concentration of enzymes able to neutralize the resultant ROS. ROS can cause sperm DNA damage, accelerate apoptosis, and alter motility. Semen contains superoxide dismutase, glutathione, and thioredoxin, all of which are naturally occurring antioxidants [55]. Evidence suggests that activity of superoxide dismutase and glutathione peroxidase are reduced in infertile men [56]. Additionally, total antioxidant capacity has been shown to be lower in both the blood and seminal plasma of infertile males as compared to fertile males [57]. Administering antioxidants to male infertility patients is therefore rational to improve sperm quality. Unfortunately, high-quality evidence showing that administering antioxidants improves live birth rates is lacking. Like other studies referenced in this chapter, even sperm may not be immune to the potential negative effects of antioxidant use. Menezo et al. treated 58 men with idiopathic infertility with vitamins C and E (400 mg each), β-carotene (18 mg), zinc (500 μmol), and selenium (1 μmol) for 90 days. After treatment, their DNA fragmentation improved by a mean of 19.1% ($P < 0.0004$), suggesting some role for the treatment of OS in these patients. However, it also led to an unexpected finding: an increase in sperm decondensation by 22.8% ($P < 0.0009$). The authors postulate that this may be caused by the opening of interchain disulphide bridges in protamines, which can be caused by antioxidants such as vitamin C, which can interfere with paternal gene activity during preimplantation development. This observation might explain the discrepancy observed concerning the role of these antioxidant treatments in improving male fertility [58].

Selenium is an essential component of redox enzymes and has been shown to play a role in sperm motility [59]. Increased ROS decreases fertility potential by decreasing the viability of sperm [60]. It has been proposed that selenium reduces ROS by increasing glutathione-peroxidase activity [61]. Glutathione peroxidase aids in the destruction of hydrogen peroxide and organic hydroperoxides [62]. N-acetyl-cysteine is known to be a strong oxygen-free radical scavenger and has been shown to decrease ROS in human semen [63]. Safarinejad and Safarinejad studied the effects of oral selenium daily and/or N-acetyl-cysteine oral daily on hormonal profiles and semen quality measured by sperm concentration, sperm motility, and percent normal morphology in a population of infertile men with idiopathic oligoasthenoteratospermia. They found that taking both selenium and N-acetyl-cysteine daily resulted in decreased follicle-stimulating hormone and increased serum testosterone and inhibin. Additionally, sperm concentration, sperm motility, and percent normal morphology all improved in the men on both supplements. The improvements in semen quality were modest in this study though, and pregnancy rates were not evaluated.

Numerous clinical studies have been performed to elucidate the positive effects of various antioxidants on semen parameters and fertility potential. Ross et al. analyzed 17 such trials including a total of 1665 men. Despite significant variation across the trials in terms of study population, endpoints, antioxidant studied, and dose selected, antioxidant therapy did lead to improvement in sperm quality in 14 out of 17 trials [64]. A Cochrane review performed by Showell et al. examined 48 randomized controlled trials studying single and combined antioxidants with placebo in subfertile men. They reported an increased rate of live birth rates and clinical pregnancy rates, but the evidence was considered low quality [65]. Many of these trials enrolled small numbers of men, and great inconsistency exists across trials. Adverse events were rarely reported. Robust clinical trials are still needed in this arena in order to fully support the use of antioxidant therapy in infertile male patients. Further studies will help identify the type and dose of antioxidants needed to minimize harm and maximize benefits to fertility.

Theories

Many large-scale randomized clinical trials have failed to support the experimental and observational evidence of a health benefit of antioxidant use. There are many theories as to why antioxidants seem to have little effect on OS-related diseases and occasionally even cause harm. The association of OS with different disease states may not be causative in many cases. In fact, some of the very disease processes that are most closely associated with OS (such as atherosclerosis and inflammation) also use ROS as part of the natural inflammation process: As discussed, ROS can cause tissue damage, but also act as a normal modulator of inflammation at certain levels to help treat the inflammation faster [26].

Many antioxidants only operate in their antioxidant role at a given dose. If the appropriate dose was not selected in clinical trials, there will not be an improvement in the OS in a tissue- or cell-specific manner. There may be a dose-dependent effect, with positive and negative effects seen at opposite ends of the dosing spectrum. Some compounds that can induce an antioxidant effect (polyphenols and ascorbate) at one dose for example, can also exert prooxidant effects at different doses due to the presence of transition metals that can catalyze oxidative reactions [66]. ROS inhibition may be insufficient to stop the complex cascade of signaling pathways and processes that cause infertility. This phenomenon is seen in cancer studies where antioxidants alone will not cause the tumor to die or regress by itself, but require sequential introduction of therapeutic agents for maximal effect [45]. The endogenous antioxidant defenses in the human body are complex, interdependent, and carefully regulated. Increasing the intake of antioxidants may be an oversimplification of treatment for what is a very complex and highly regulated system in the human body. For example, many flavonoids have considerable antioxidant activity in vitro. Despite this, there are no real studies that show that polyphenols can exert any antioxidant effects in vivo [67].

Finally, there is a lack of a standardized method for quantification of redox status as well as baseline nutritional status that may have caused the inconclusive findings of many clinical trials, though this does not necessarily mean that antioxidants are ineffective in those disease states. If the patients are well nourished with optimal levels of antioxidants at baseline, then giving more antioxidants will likely not show any effect. A better method is needed to evaluate the whole patient's overall OS levels to better understand the effects of treatment with antioxidants. Some advances in the male infertility specialty include the use of oxidation-reduction potential, which measures the relationship between oxidants and reductants (antioxidants) to provide a more comprehensive measure of OS [68].

Conclusions

The theory that antioxidants may have a positive impact on several human diseases derives from the fact that OS is harmful and plays a part in many disease processes. Although this makes theoretical sense, proving a direct cause and effect is very difficult in human subjects. Existing trials examining several antioxidants at varied doses across several disease states are thus far ambiguous in terms of the succinct conclusions that can be drawn for their use. It is notable that several trials have shown negative effects of antioxidants that challenge the assumption that this is a low-risk, potentially high-reward treatment paradigm across several disease states including infertility. The doses used in studies vary and it is difficult to control for the fact that each individual host may be harboring varying levels of OS, reductive potential, and adequate nutrition at any given time. Ideally, the ability to directly measure OS in real time in human tissue will enable the study of direct biological effects of antioxidant administration and possibly the development of more effective antioxidant treatments.

REFERENCES

[1] Davies KJ. Oxidative stress: the paradox of aerobic life. Biochem Soc Symp 1995;61:1−31.
[2] Villegas J, Schulz M, Soto L, Iglesias T, Miska W, Sánchez R. Influence of reactive oxygen species produced by activated leukocytes at the level of apoptosis in mature human spermatozoa. Fertil Steril 2005;83(3):808−10.
[3] Irshad M, Chaudhuri PS. Oxidant-antioxidant system: role and significance in human body. Indian J Exp Biol 2002;40(11):1233−9.
[4] Mates JM, Perez-Gomez C, Nunez de Castro I. Antioxidant enzymes and human diseases. Clin Biochem 1999;32(8):595−603.
[5] de Lamirande E, Jiang H, Zini A, Kodama H, Gagnon C. Reactive oxygen species and sperm physiology. Rev Reprod 1997;2(1):48−54.
[6] de Lamirande E, Gagnon C. Human sperm hyperactivation and capacitation as parts of an oxidative process. Free Radic Biol Med 1993;14(2):157−66.
[7] Ford WC. Regulation of sperm function by reactive oxygen species. Hum Reprod Update 2004;10(5):387−99.
[8] Cooper TG. Role of the epididymis in mediating changes in the male gamete during maturation. Adv Exp Med Biol 1995;377:87−101.
[9] Aitken RJ, Vernet P. Maturation of redox regulatory mechanisms in the epididymis. J Reprod Fertil Suppl 1998;53:109−18.
[10] Aitken RJ. Possible redox regulation of sperm motility activation. J Androl 2000;21(4):491−6.
[11] Griveau JF, Le Lannou D. Reactive oxygen species and human spermatozoa: physiology and pathology. Int J Androl 1997;20(2):61−9.
[12] MacLeod J. The role of oxygen in the metabolism and motility of human spermatozoa. Am J Physiol 1943;138(3):512−8.
[13] Davies KJA. The Oxygen Paradox, oxidative stress, and ageing. Arch Biochem Biophys 2016;595:28−32.
[14] Mariani E, Polidori MC, Cherubini A, Mecocci P. Oxidative stress in brain aging, neurodegenerative and vascular diseases: an overview. J Chromatogr B 2005;827(1):65−75.

[15] Sies H. Strategies of antioxidant defense. Eur J Biochem 1993;215(2):213−9.

[16] Li X, Fang P, Mai J, Choi ET, Wang H, Yang XF. Targeting mitochondrial reactive oxygen species as novel therapy for inflammatory diseases and cancers. J Hematol Oncol 2013;6:19.

[17] Jourd'heuil D, Jourd'heuil FL, Kutchukian PS, Musah RA, Wink DA, Grisham MB. Reaction of superoxide and nitric oxide with peroxynitrite. Implications for peroxynitrite-mediated oxidation reactions in vivo. J Biol Chem 2001;276(31):28799−805.

[18] Brooker RJ. Genetics: analysis & principles. 4th ed. New York: McGraw-Hill; 2012. xviii, 761, 85 pp.

[19] Hekimi S, Lapointe J, Wen Y. Taking a "good" look at free radicals in the aging process. Trends Cell Biol 2011;21(10):569−76.

[20] Harman D. Aging: a theory based on free radical and radiation chemistry. J Gerontol 1956;11(3):298−300.

[21] Zimmerman R, Cerutti P. Active oxygen acts as a promoter of transformation in mouse embryo C3H/10T1/2/C18 fibroblasts. Proc Natl Acad Sci Unit States Am 1984;81(7):2085−7.

[22] Elchuri S, Oberley TD, Qi W, Eisenstein RS, Jackson Roberts L, Van Remmen H, et al. CuZnSOD deficiency leads to persistent and widespread oxidative damage and hepatocarcinogenesis later in life. Oncogene 2005;24(3):367−80.

[23] Van Remmen H, Ikeno Y, Hamilton M, Pahlavani M, Wolf N, Thorpe SR, et al. Life-long reduction in MnSOD activity results in increased DNA damage and higher incidence of cancer but does not accelerate aging. Physiol Genom 2003;16(1):29−37.

[24] Chu F-F, Esworthy RS, Chu PG, Longmate JA, Huycke MM, Wilczynski S, et al. Bacteria-induced intestinal cancer in mice with disrupted Gpx1 and Gpx2 genes. Cancer Res 2004;64(3):962−8.

[25] Neumann CA, Krause DS, Carman CV, Das S, Dubey DP, Abraham JL, et al. Essential role for the peroxiredoxin Prdx1 in erythrocyte antioxidant defence and tumour suppression. Nature 2003;424(6948):561−5.

[26] Halliwell B. Oxidative stress and cancer: have we moved forward? Biochem J 2007;401(1):1−11.

[27] Uttara B, Singh AV, Zamboni P, Mahajan RT. Oxidative stress and neurodegenerative diseases: a review of upstream and downstream antioxidant therapeutic options. Curr Neuropharmacol 2009;7(1):65−74.

[28] Patel VP, Chu CT. Nuclear transport, oxidative stress, and neurodegeneration. Int J Clin Exp Pathol 2011;4(3):215−29.

[29] Opazo C, Huang X, Cherny RA, Moir RD, Roher AE, White AR, et al. Metalloenzyme-like activity of Alzheimer's disease beta-amyloid. Cu-dependent catalytic conversion of dopamine, cholesterol, and biological reducing agents to neurotoxic H(2)O(2). J Biol Chem 2002;277(43):40302−8.

[30] Jenner P, Olanow CW. Oxidative stress and the pathogenesis of Parkinson's disease. Neurology 1996;47(6 Suppl. 3):S161−70.

[31] Klein JA, Ackerman SL. Oxidative stress, cell cycle, and neurodegeneration. J Clin Invest 2003;111(6):785−93.

[32] Gilgun-Sherki Y, Melamed E, Offen D. The role of oxidative stress in the pathogenesis of multiple sclerosis: the need for effective antioxidant therapy. J Neurol 2004;251(3):261−8.

[33] Hearse DJ, Humphrey SM, Chain EB. Abrupt reoxygenation of the anoxic potassium-arrested perfused rat heart: a study of myocardial enzyme release. J Mol Cell Cardiol 1973;5(4):395−407.

[34] Hansen PR. Myocardial reperfusion injury: experimental evidence and clinical relevance. Eur Heart J 1995;16(6):734−40.

[35] Rosen H, Klebanoff SJ. Hydroxyl radical generation by polymorphonuclear leukocytes measured by electron spin resonance spectroscopy. J Clin Invest 1979;64(6):1725−9.

[36] Ambrosio G, Weisfeldt ML, Jacobus WE, Flaherty JT. Evidence for a reversible oxygen radical-mediated component of reperfusion injury: reduction by recombinant human superoxide dismutase administered at the time of reflow. Circulation 1987;75(1):282−91.

[37] Hano O, Thompson-Gorman SL, Zweier JL, Lakatta EG. Coenzyme Q10 enhances cardiac functional and metabolic recovery and reduces Ca^{2+} overload during postischemic reperfusion. Am J Physiol 1994;266(6 Pt 2):H2174−81.

[38] Marra G, Cotroneo P, Pitocco D, Manto A, Di Leo MA, Ruotolo V, et al. Early increase of oxidative stress and reduced antioxidant defenses in patients with uncomplicated type 1 diabetes: a case for gender difference. Diabetes Care 2002;25(2):370−5.

[39] Maritim AC, Sanders RA, Watkins 3rd JB. Diabetes, oxidative stress, and antioxidants: a review. J Biochem Mol Toxicol 2003;17(1):24−38.

[40] Pham-Huy LA, He H, Pham-Huy C. Free radicals, antioxidants in disease and health. Int J Biomed Sci 2008;4(2):89−96.

[41] Halliwell B, Whiteman M. Measuring reactive species and oxidative damage in vivo and in cell culture : how should you do it and what do the results mean ? Br J Pharmacol 2004;142(2):231−55.

[42] Halliwell B, Gutteridge J. Free radicals in biology and medicine. 1999.

[43] Walczak-Jedrzejowska R, Wolski JK, Slowikowska-Hilczer J. The role of oxidative stress and antioxidants in male fertility. Cent Eur J Urol 2013;66(1):60−7.

[44] Scandalios JG. Oxidative stress: molecular perception and transduction of signals triggering antioxidant gene defenses. Braz J Med Biol Res 2005;38(7):995−1014.

[45] Bonner MY, Arbiser JL. The antioxidant paradox: what are antioxidants and how should they be used in a therapeutic context for cancer. Future Med Chem 2014;6(12):1413−22.

[46] Greabu M, Battino M, Mohora M, Olinescu R, Totan A, Didilescu A. Oxygen, a paradoxical element. Rom J Intern Med 2008;46(2):125−35.

[47] Heinonen OP, Huttunen JK, Albanes D. The effect of vitamin E and beta carotene on the incidence of lung cancer and other cancers in male smokers. N Engl J Med 1994;330:1029−35.

[48] Duffield-Lillico AJ, Dalkin BL, Reid ME, Turnbull BW, Slate EH, Jacobs ET, et al. Selenium supplementation, baseline plasma selenium status and incidence of prostate cancer: an analysis of the complete treatment period of the Nutritional Prevention of Cancer Trial. BJU Int 2003;91(7):608−12.

[49] Lippman SM, Klein EA, Goodman PJ, Lucia MS, Thompson IM, Ford LG, et al. Effect of selenium and vitamin E on risk of prostate cancer and other cancers: the Selenium and Vitamin E Cancer Prevention Trial (SELECT). J Am Med Assoc 2009;301(1):39−51.

[50] Gaziano JM, Sesso HD, Christen WG, Bubes V, Smith JP, MacFadyen J, et al. Multivitamins in the prevention of cancer in men: the Physicians' Health Study II randomized controlled trial. J Am Med Assoc 2012;308(18):1871–80.

[51] Gaziano JM, Glynn RJ, Christen WG, Kurth T, Belanger C, Macfadyen J, et al. Vitamins E and C in the prevention of prostate and total cancer in men: the Physicians' Health Study II, a randomized controlled trial. J Am Med Assoc 2010;301:52–62.

[52] Miller ERI, Pastor-barriuso R, Dalal D, Riemersma RA. Review meta-analysis : high-dosage vitamin E supplementation may increase all cause mortality. Ann Intern Med 2005;142(1):37–46.

[53] Bjelakovic G, Nikolova D, Gluud LL, Simonetti RG, Gluud C. Mortality in randomized trials of antioxidant supplements for primary and secondary prevention: systematic review and meta-analysis. J Am Med Assoc 2007;297(8):842–57.

[54] Vivekananthan DP, Penn MS, Sapp SK, Hsu A, Topol EJ. Use of antioxidant vitamins for the prevention of cardiovascular disease: meta-analysis of randomised trials. Lancet 2003;361(9374):2017.

[55] Jung JH, Seo JT. Empirical medical therapy in idiopathic male infertility: promise or panacea? Clin Exp Reprod Med 2014;41(3):108–14.

[56] Dorostghoal M, Kazeminejad SR, Shahbazian N, Pourmehdi M, Jabbari A. Oxidative stress status and sperm DNA fragmentation in fertile and infertile men. Andrologia 2017;49.

[57] Benedetti S, Tagliamonte MC, Catalani S, Primiterra M, Canestrari F, De Stefani S, et al. Differences in blood and semen oxidative status in fertile and infertile men, and their relationship with sperm quality. Reprod Biomed Online 2012;25(3):300–6.

[58] Ménézo YJ, Hazout A, Panteix G, Robert F, Rollet J, Cohen-Bacrie P, et al. Antioxidants to reduce sperm DNA fragmentation: an unexpected adverse effect. Reprod Biomed Online 2007;14.

[59] Ursini F, Heim S, Kiess M, Maiorino M, Roveri A, Wissing J, et al. Dual function of the selenoprotein PHGPx during sperm maturation. Science 1999;285(5432):1393–6.

[60] Safarinejad MR, Safarinejad S. Efficacy of selenium and/or N-acetyl-cysteine for improving semen parameters in infertile men: a double-blind, placebo controlled, randomized study. J Urol 2009;181(2):741–51.

[61] Irvine DS. Glutathione as a treatment for male infertility. Rev Reprod 1996;1(1):6–12.

[62] Rotruck JT, Pope AL, Ganther HE, Swanson AB, Hafeman DG, Hoekstra WG. Selenium: biochemical role as a component of glutathione peroxidase. Science 1973;179(4073):588–90.

[63] Oeda T, Henkel R, Ohmori H, Schill WB. Scavenging effect of N-acetyl-L-cysteine against reactive oxygen species in human semen: a possible therapeutic modality for male factor infertility? Andrologia 1997;29(3):125–31.

[64] Ross C, Morriss A, Khairy M, Khalaf Y, Braude P, Coomarasamy A, et al. A systematic review of the effect of oral antioxidants on male infertility. Reprod Biomed Online 2010;20(6):711–23.

[65] Showell MG, Mackenzie-Proctor R, Brown J, Yazdani A, Stankiewicz MT, Hart RJ. Antioxidants for male subfertility. Cochrane Database Syst Rev 2014;12:CD007411.

[66] Halliwell B, Zhao K, Whiteman M. The gastrointestinal tract: a major site of antioxidant action? Free Radic Res 2000;33(6):819–30.

[67] Niki E. Assessment of antioxidant capacity in vitro and in vivo. Free Radic Biol Med 2010;49(4):503–15.

[68] Agarwal A, Roychoudhury S, Sharma R, Gupta S, Majzoub A, Sabanegh E. Diagnostic application of oxidation-reduction potential assay for measurement of oxidative stress: clinical utility in male factor infertility. Reprod Biomed Online 2017;34(1):48–57.

Chapter 1.3

From Past to Present: An Historical Overview of the Concept of Spermatozoa, Reactive Oxygen Species, and Male-Factor Infertility

Mark A. Baker, Jacob Netherton and R. John Aitken
The University of Newcastle (UoN), University drive, Callaghan, NSW, Australia

In this chapter we outline the history of reactive oxygen species (ROS) and spermatozoa, starting with some of the foundation experiments conducted by John MacLeod in 1943. Historically, we have seen that if ROS come into contact with spermatozoa in high enough concentrations, they trigger peroxidative damage that culminates in aldehyde by-products that are detrimental to cell function. This can be demonstrated in a number of ways, but for the most part, this has been achieved by external addition of ROS or exposure to ROS-generating in vitro systems. We also discuss the many challenges that await this field, including the various pitfalls associated with measuring ROS that make it difficult to ascertain if these metabolites are causally involved in the etiology of male-factor infertility or whether they are just playing a passive role. Today, with improved methods of measuring ROS, together with a better knowledge of the pathways associated with peroxidative damage, the involvement of oxidative stress on sperm function should become clearer.

DEFINITION OF REACTIVE OXYGEN SPECIES

A free radical by definition is any chemical species that contains an unpaired electron in its outer orbit [1]. The unpaired electron makes free radicals highly reactive with lipids, proteins, carbohydrates, and nucleic acids. In biology, the free radicals of interest are ROS, which, by definition, are oxygen-centered free radicals. This includes superoxide anion and hydroxyl radical. A third component of ROS is hydrogen peroxide, which is technically not a free radical as it does not contain an unpaired electron. However, hydrogen peroxide does break down into hydroxyl free radicals when it interacts with transition metals including iron and copper.

THE FOUNDATION OF THE THEORY OF REACTIVE OXYGEN SPECIES IN HUMAN SPERM EJACULATES

The earliest citation for ROS in spermatozoa appears to have come from the laboratory of John MacLeod [2]. In 1943, MacLeod states that his work was inspired by the observation that the metabolism of human spermatozoa was exclusively dependent on glycolysis and that oxygen consumption was "being of such small magnitude that it could not properly be interpreted as true respiration" (cited from MacLeod [2]). In other words, spermatozoa appeared to have very little to no detectable mitochondrial activity. MacLeod used methylene blue, a redox sensor that turns blue in an oxidizing environment, and determined that in the presence of either glucose or succinate, sperm were able to reduce the dye. The

Oxidants, Antioxidants, and Impact of the Oxidative Status in Male Reproduction. https://doi.org/10.1016/B978-0-12-812501-4.00003-1

idea of using these sugar sources is that they ultimately drive metabolism by feeding into different parts of the mitochondrial electron transport chain.

This was the first piece of evidence that sperm cells did have active mitochondria, or, as better phrased by MacLeod, that within the samples he was measuring there was evidence for an "active cytochrome" system. Why did he say this? Today, we understand that addition of either glucose or succinate to most cells will also increase the output of nicotinamide adenine dinucleotide (NADH). The main contributor in the reduction of redox dyes like methylene blue are cytochrome enzymes, such as cytochrome $b5$ reductase (CYB5R), which use NADH as the electron donor. As an example, methylene blue is often used to measure methemoglobinemia, a disease that appears in subjects lacking CYB5R [3]. When added to normal red blood cells, it turns the characteristic blue color. However, in a patient lacking CYB5R, their red blood cells are unable to reduce methylene blue [3], demonstrating that this is the main source of dye reduction. We can only presume that at that time, MacLeod also (reasonably) assumed that other cytochrome systems within the mitochondria could also be responsible. Therefore, MacLeod furthered his work by looking at the impact that high oxygen levels had on sperm cells. For this purpose, he raised the oxygen levels from 5% to 95%. Under these conditions, it was very clear that sperm lost motility [2]. However, when these conditions were repeated in the presence of catalase, an enzyme that converts hydrogen peroxide into water and oxygen, cells were able to retain their motility [2].

The notion here is that when forced to use oxidative phosphorylation, a toxic by-product is created in the form of hydrogen peroxide. So, how did catalase prevent the inhibition of sperm motility? We can assume that MacLeod reasoned that either the sperm mitochondria made hydrogen peroxide directly, or (as we understand today) that two molecules of superoxide anion reacted with each other (dismutation) to form hydrogen peroxide, which breaks down into oxygen radicals that are consequently detrimental to sperm. Thus the fundamental concept that ROS can have a detrimental impact on spermatozoa was laid [4–7].

A key issue that MacLeod faced, and one that persists to this present day, is the source of the ROS detected in his experiments. MacLeod reasoned that spermatozoa were the major source of ROS and indeed many others have also stated this [4,6,8,9]. However, in a repeat of the experiment, Whittington and Ford decided to investigate the contribution of leukocyte contamination with the MacLeod experiment [10]. The majority of men have leukocytes present in their semen, something MacLeod may not have known at that time. Whittington and Ford also used Percoll gradients to isolate sperm populations free of both precursor germ cells, and more importantly, leukocytes [10]. Leukocytes contain an NADPH (NAD phosphate)-oxidase (NOX) that generates superoxide anion through oxidation of NADPH on the cytosolic side and reduction of oxygen across the membrane [11]. One of the main roles of this enzyme is to destroy bacteria [11]. However, the enzyme is so active that spermatozoa can be immobilized by as little as 6×10^5 stimulated leukocytes [12]. When leukocyte-free populations of spermatozoa were incubated in MacLeods' initial conditions (95% oxygen), they were less affected by the high oxygen tensions and remained motile for over 6 h. However, a significant loss of curvilinear velocity was still observed (54.7 vs. 64.1 µM/s) in leukocyte free samples albeit these samples were stimulated with Phorbol Myristate Acetate or n-Formylmethionine-leucyl-phenylalanine [10]. Thus in the original experiment by MacLeod it appears that leukocytes were the main contributor.

Spermatozoa and Their Susceptibility Toward Reactive Oxygen Species

What the work of John MacLeod did achieve was to inspire a generation of andrologists to look at the susceptibility of spermatozoa toward ROS. Arguably, Thaddeus Mann was one of the first to realize the potential clinical significance of this association, in a landmark paper with Roy Jones and Dick Sherins published in 1979 [13]. Jones et al. took suspensions of pure fatty acids (arachidonic, linoleic, and linolenic acids) and exposed them to ultraviolet light [13]. These suspensions were then added to sperm in the presence of ascorbate and ferrous sulphate. Under these conditions, it was very clear that sperm lost motility. But why? The use of UV light catalyses the oxidation of pure unsaturated fatty acids and the extent of this oxidation can be measured either as peroxide or aldehyde formation [14].

Unsaturated aldehydes (such as acrolein, malondialdehyde (MDA), or 4-hydroxy-2-nonenal (4-HNE)) react with lysine, cysteine, and histidine through a Michael-type addition [15]. Thus, Jones et al. were inducing the production of aldehydes that would then form a covalent bond with the nearest (relevant) amino acid. Given enough aldehyde, it was inevitable that a protein involved in sperm motility (such as AKAP4 [16], dynein or enzymes involved in either the glycolytic or oxidative phosphorylation pathways [17,18]) will form an adduct with such lipid aldehydes. The consequence of this would be a loss of protein function, leading to sperm immobilization [19]. Indeed, Jones et al. could show that MDA—one of the by-products of lipid peroxidation—was produced within these samples [14]. Interestingly, these authors were also able to show that higher levels of MDA were measured in patients presenting with necrozoospermia [14]. Thus, one interpretation of these data is that pathological necrozoospermic samples produce higher levels of MDA compared to normozoospermic samples. Interestingly enough, this appears to have sparked a major interest in the field of ROS and defective spermatozoa and for the first time offered a mechanism into why spermatozoa might be infertile.

Following from this work, others have clearly shown that either ROS or aldehydes are detrimental to sperm function. The common theme with the majority of these approaches, something that can be easily overlooked, is that in most cases there is either (1) an external source of ROS/aldehyde added to the cells or (2) spermatozoa are forced to generate ROS by inhibiting the mitochondria. Much of the earlier work involved the use of ascorbate plus ferrous ion [13,20,21], which initiates a cascade of reactions that produces superoxide anion radical, hydrogen peroxide, and hydroxyl radicals. In the presence of such, sperm of many species lose motility [13,20]. Other examples include the external addition of xanthine-xanthine oxidase [22—27], hydrogen peroxide [28], glucose plus glucose oxidase a [29], nitric oxide radical [24,30], and 4-HNE [18,19], all of which have been reported to exert detrimental effects on spermatozoa.

The pathway by which this occurs is the same pathway Jones investigated earlier, where an unsaturated fatty acid becomes oxidized upon interaction with an oxygen radical, leading to aldehyde formation. In high enough doses, the aldehyde will inhibit sperm motility [19]. Yet, while it is clear that external addition of these compounds are detrimental to sperm, what remains a challenge to the field is the in vivo significance, or spontaneous lipid peroxidation. In the case of the horse, an increase in the level for 4-HNE from 52.6% to 85.8% occurs over a 24 h period. Of particular interest is that over this same time period, a loss in total progressive motility from 43.9% to 15.0% is seen [31]. Strikingly in the horse, both glutathione transferase and aldehyde dehydrogenase appear to play a role in detoxifying any aldehyde build up [31]. However, in both rabbit and mouse, studies have shown that this process is slow and takes place at a rate equivalent to the lifetime of the sperm cell [32]. The same has been shown to be true for human spermatozoa, even though the lifetime of a human sperm inside the female reproductive tract can be several days [18,19].

Interestingly, by putting human sperm cells in a high Na^+ medium, motility within different ejaculates can be lost from 1 to 11 h [33]. The loss in motility was highly correlated to the level of superoxide dismutase (SOD) activity (r = 0.92) [33]. This strongly suggests that peroxidation involving superoxide anion plays not just a significant role, but perhaps the *major* role when it comes to loss of sperm motility over time. However, this is in complete contrast with another report, which shows that the level of SOD activity is negatively correlated with human sperm motility [34]. By isolating sperm on Percoll fractions, lower density sperm contained more SOD and had less motility than their higher density counterparts [34]. Furthermore, by looking at the total percentage motility after 24 h, it was noted that a negative correlation existed between SOD activity and motility (r = 0.303) [34]. Although there were differences in the way SOD activity was measured—one uses acetylated ferricytochrome [33], the other uses lucigenin [34]—this cannot really account for the contrasting data.

Sperm and Their High Amount of Polyunsaturated Fatty Acids

It is quite clear, historically speaking, that no matter what source of exogenous ROS are applied to sperm cells, they will eventually lose motility. Questions that deserve consideration in this context ask why is this the case and why are spermatozoa vulnerable in this regard? One argument put forward is that "mammalian spermatozoa membranes are very sensitive to free radical induced damage" (cited from [35]) due to their high levels of polyunsaturated fatty acids (PUFAs). So what exactly are the levels of PUFAs within spermatozoa and how do they compare to other cell types?

In the whole ejaculate, the overall PUFA content in spermatozoa is between 36% and 39%, while in Percoll purified sperm, this level increases to 48%—52% [36]. In comparison, cancer cells grown in culture typically contain 20%—30% PUFAs [37] and as such, if sperm are compared to somatic cells, they do contain higher percentages of PUFAs. These levels of PUFAs, however, are not unique to sperm cells, since similar percentages are also seen in other cells, such as melanocytes [36]. Furthermore, a comparison of Percoll-purified sperm to red blood cells shows that spermatozoa contain a lower percentage of almost all PUFAs [36,38], with the exception of n-3 docosahexaenoic acid, which accounts for around 35% of total sperm fatty acid composition [36,38]. Such a high level of this one PUFA, to date, is unique to the sperm cell. When looking at the more abundant PUFAs in spermatozoa, the second and third most prevalent ones vulnerable to oxidation are linoleic acid (18:3; present around ~7.8%—10.5% of total fatty acid content) and arachidonic acid (20:4, present around 4.7%—10.5% of total fatty acid content), both of which can generate 4-HNE (6-carbon aldehyde), whereas the latter can also form 4-hydroxy, 6-dodecadienal 4-hydroxyhexenal. As outline earlier, the formation of 4-HNE in spermatozoa has been looked at in stallion [39,40] and human [18,19] spermatozoa and in the case of humans takes around 3 days to appear [18,19] and is associated with a concomitant loss in motility. Both datasets suggest that loss of sperm motility in vitro (in both horse and human) may be a result of 4-HNE accumulation [18,19].

A second aldehyde that has been studied in humans is MDA (3-carbon aldehyde), which is derived from the lipid peroxidation of the omega-3 and omega-6 fatty acids and is often tested due to its facile reaction with thiobarbituric acid (TBA). However, before proceeding it should be noted that reliability of this test has been questioned by many, with one article stating that the "MDA assay is not able to provide valid analytical data for biological samples due to its high reactivity and possibility of various cross-reactions with co-existing biochemicals" [41].

The fatty-acid MDA breakdown products relevant to sperm include eicosatetraenoic acid (present at 10.5% of PUFAs) and docosahexaenoic acid (22:6). Certainly, MDA levels have been found to be higher within infertile sperm [42–45], however in all cases the TBA assay has been used and hence further work is necessary to confirm these findings. Finally, the major PUFA present in sperm, certainly the one that makes the cell quite unusual, is docosahexaenoic acid (DHA, C22:6). This fatty acid is so important that in male mice depleted of the delta-6 desaturase (such mice are unable to synthesize arachidonic acid, DHA, and n6-docosapentaenoic acid) animals are infertile but when fed on a diet of DHA all fertility is restored [46]. The oxidized product of DHA is 4-hydroxyhexanal (4-HHE). However, the level of either induced or spontaneous production of 4-HHE, surprisingly, has never been examined in human sperm cells, yet it may be a sensitive marker of oxidative stress.

Leukocytes and Their Contribution Toward Reactive Oxygen Species and Male-Factor Infertility

Throughout the history of ROS, there has always been concern over the contribution of contaminating leukocytes and whether they are a contributing source of ROS that affects sperm function. Approximately 10%–20% of infertile men produce an excess amount of white blood cells (WBCs) within their ejaculate [47]. According to the WHO standard, the term "excess" is defined as greater than 1×10^6 per ml [48]. As such, many have argued that the presence of leukocytes or WBCs is a confounding factor for male infertility [49–52]. The rationale is logical and suggests that WBCs are able to produce superoxide anion, hydroxyl radical, and hydrogen peroxide, all of which would be detrimental to spermatozoa. Yet how confident are we that WBC within the sperm ejaculate contribute to poor sperm quality? While some have reported a damaging role for WBCs by correlating sperm dysfunction with the amount of WBCs present in an ejaculate [53,54], others have shown this correlation does not exist [55,56]. In an intriguing study that looked at WBCs from fertile men who had fathered a child in the last year it was shown that concentrations ranging from 0.5 to 16.6×10^6 per ml were normal [57]. Many of these were well above the WHO excess criteria of 1×10^6 per ml.

Data on leukocyte numbers in semen are always hard to interpret because we have no idea when the leukocytes entered the seminal compartment, whether they were activated, when they were activated, and how they were activated. In all probability, the first time that spermatozoa see large numbers of leukocytes is at the moment of ejaculation because significant numbers of leukocytes are rarely seen in the lumina of the seminiferous or epididymal tubules. At the moment of ejaculation, spermatozoa will be protected by the antioxidants present in seminal plasma [58]. Of course, as soon as the seminal plasma is removed, the leukocytes are able to attack the spermatozoa with impunity; it is for this reason that strong associations exist between the presence of leukocytes in washed sperm preparations and fertilization rates in an in vitro fertilization setting [59].

WHAT KIND OF OXIDASE ARE WE DEALING WITH?

One of the most interesting questions relating to the relationships between spermatozoa, ROS, and male-factor infertility concerns the exact nature of the enzyme systems responsible for generating the free radicals. One major review at the time summed up the situation saying, "Spermatozoa may generate ROS in two ways: (1) the nicotinamide adenine dinucleotide phosphate (NADPH) oxidase system at the level of the sperm plasma membrane and (2) the NADH-dependent oxido-reductase (diaphorase) at the level of mitochondria" (cited from [60], which has over 500 citations).

The NADPH-oxidase concept idea was based upon two main experimental results. First, the addition of the ionophore A23187 to oligozoospermic samples produced a luminol-dependent chemiluminescent signal [61]. These data were explained by the presence of a Ca^{2+}-dependent NADPH-oxidase [61–63]. Second, the external addition of NADH or NADPH to suspensions of human spermatozoa resulted in the generation of superoxide anion [63], which could be measured by lucigenin or nitro blue tetrazolium (NBT) [64,65]. Furthermore, the NADPH-dependent lucigenin signal was effectively inhibited by the addition of copper, zinc, diphenyleneiodonium (DPI), and SOD1, a specific scavenger of $O_2^{\cdot}$ [66,67]. However, the external addition of NADPH to human spermatozoa did not stimulate a chemiluminescent signal using another superoxide-dependent probe, namely 2-methyl-6-(p-methoxyphenyl)-3,7-dihydroimidazo [1,2-a] pyrazine-3-one (MCLA) [63]. Moreover, no $O_2^{\cdot}$ production was found using electron spin measurements upon addition of NADPH [68]. If $O_2^{\cdot}$ was being produced by spermatozoa upon addition of NADH or NADPH then it must be detected by *all* probes capable of detecting superoxide anion. This paradox was resolved when the enzymes responsible for the NADPH-dependent lucigenin response were identified as cytochrome-p450 reductase [69] and cytochrome b5-reductase [70]. In the case of the former, NADPH was the preferred cofactor, whereas cytochrome b5-reductase had a higher affinity toward NADH. These enzymes are capable of a direct, one-electron reduction of either lucigenin or NBT, which explained why these probes evoked a signal in these systems but failed to give a true superoxide anion response in the case of MCLA and electron spin resonance. Furthermore, both CP450R and CB5R can be inhibited with DPI since they are flavoproteins.

Finally, what of the observation that SOD inhibits NADPH-dependent lucigenin chemiluminescence or tetrazolium salt formation? The generation of lucigenin-dependent chemiluminescence in the absence of ROS generation can be explained by a biochemical process initiated by the one electron reduction of lucigenin (L^{2+}) to generate a lucigenin radical ($LH^{+}\cdot$). $LH^{+}\cdot$ is unstable and reverts to L^{2+} with the concomitant release of an electron to oxygen, thereby generating $O_2^{-\cdot}$. $LH^{+}\cdot$ then combines with $O_2^{-\cdot}$ to generate the oxygenated dioxetane that subsequently decomposes with the emission of light [69]. If SOD1 is added to this reaction, it inhibits the generation of light.

The same principle holds true for NBT and is explained elsewhere [70]. Despite the fact that NADPH-dependent reduction of either lucigenin or tetrazolium salts is artefactual [68], many have used this approach to report the presence of ROS and correlate with human semen quality [71], DNA damage of infertile men [72], the presence of ROS in equine sperm [26], as involvement of ROS for human capacitation [73], hyperactivation [27], DNA integrity, and apoptosis [74] among others. Yet probably for all these reports, they were simply looking at the presence of cytochrome B5/P450-reductases.

What About Other Sources of Reactive Oxygen Species in Sperm?

Given the correlations with ROS and poor sperm function, more work needs to be done to determine if other enzymes that can use oxygen as a final sink are potentially playing a role. Indeed cyclooxygenases and lipoxygenases [75] are capable of producing ROS and are present in spermatozoa. However, a formal role in the process of either sperm maturation (capacitation) and/or male-factor infertility is yet to be documented.

The Potential for NOX5-Involvement in a NADPH-ROS Generating System

In 2002, Musset and colleagues demonstrated that spermatozoa contain an NADPH-oxidase (NOX5) system [76]. Their evidence was extraction of mRNA from a testicular homogenate followed by measurement of sperm using a luminol/horseradish peroxidase (HRP)-based chemiluminescent assay [76]. Such a system showed the same characteristics of what others had already reported [61], in that a calcium ionophore stimulated an ROS signal, which could be inhibited by SOD and DPI. Unfortunately, like many of their predecessors, this same group also failed to purify the sperm cells and simply used washed ejaculates. As such, the contribution of leukocytes to their assay cannot be ruled out [10,68]. However, this same group also produced an immunoblot against NOX5 in which two cross-reacting bands were shown, including a 65 kDa and an 80 kDa protein, neither of which matches to the predicted size of NOX5 itself (55 kDa) [76]. To explain this, the authors speculate that an alternate-splicing isoform was found by the antibody, yet to date, no further ratification of this idea has come forward [76]. Immunofluorescence using the NOX5 antibody demonstrated cross-reactivity in the flagellum, neck, and acrosome regions. Yet, doubt remains over the abundant presence of NOX5 in spermatozoa, since it fails to appear in the many proteomic lists available on human spermatozoa [77–79]. If NOX5 is present as an alternatively spliced isoform, this situation should be clarified and its contribution to ROS generation by spermatozoa determined.

The Involvement of Mitochondria in Reactive Oxygen Species and Spermatozoa

Although sperm contain only very few mitochondria [80], there has been much effort to link mitochondrial ROS production to sperm dysfunction. Mitochondria produce superoxide radicals in two positons. In complex I, superoxide anion is produced on the matrix side by the oxidation of reduced flavin or flavin semiquinone [81]. A second site within the cytochrome $bc1$ complex of mitochondria has also been shown to produce superoxide anion, albeit this would be produced within the intermembrane space [82]. Although in his original publication, MacLeod makes note that by using traditional biochemistry he could not detect mitochondrial function in spermatozoa, this does not mean they are not active. The fact that the addition of the complex 1 inhibitors antimycin A or rotenone stimulates ROS production in sperm cells [82] strongly suggests that despite the small number of mitochondria, they can still produce enough free radicals to cause sperm dysfunction.

There is evidence to suggest that in the horse, the generation of ROS from the mitochondria results in a positive correlation between oxidative stress and sperm function [75]. However, in other species such as the human, where metabolism is more focused on glycolysis, the role of the mitochondria in ROS generation by the spermatozoa is less obvious.

OTHER MEASUREMENTS OF REACTIVE OXYGEN SPECIES: THE CHALLENGE IN MOVING THE FIELD FORWARD AND WHY WE CANNOT CONTINUE TO DO AS WE HAVE DONE

Clearly, as we navigate through the history of sperm and ROS there are many areas of controversy that no doubt will be examined and rectified. However, before this occurs, it is worth mentioning common probes for the measurements of ROS and presenting the challenges to the field that need to be overcome. The use of NADPH in conjunction with either lucigenin or tetrazolium salts has already been discussed, with the main concern here being that cytochrome reductases have the ability to directly reduce both of these probes, giving incorrect interpretations on the presence of ROS. An ideal probe would be one that is highly reactive, specific, and without other reactivity. Unfortunately, currently, no such probe exists and as such, potentially false conclusions are being drawn. As this area is discussed extensively elsewhere in great detail (see [83]), we will limit this discussion to two other probes that are used extensively in field of spermatozoa and ROS; these include luminol/HRP and dihydroethidium (DHE; and a derivative that is packaged as MitoSOX red).

Luminol/Horseradish Peroxidase

Due to the increased sensitivity it offers, researchers have chosen to use luminol with the catalyst HRP [84]. Several warnings have appeared in the literature on the use of this probe for measurement of oxygen radicals. For example, "Luminol is known to elicit chemiluminescence under almost an unlimited variety of conditions" [85], or "luminol-dependent chemiluminescence used in biological systems is prone to many interferences, which are difficult to control" [85], and finally, "luminol … can neither serve to study the formation kinetics nor be used as a valid continues assay of ROS" [85].

The main area of concern is that luminol cannot react directly with superoxide anion, but must first be converted into a radical. This is achieved through addition of HRP. While this luminol radical is capable of reacting with superoxide anion, it will also react with many compounds capable of donating an electron. This principle is demonstrated around the world on a daily basis when luminol-dependent immunoblotting is performed. Herein, the antibody (attached to HRP) oxidizes luminol (often referred to as solution one), and in the presence of any reduced substances (often a phenol-based substrate) will emit light. Thus there are many compounds that the luminol-radical may interact with in a cellular environment. Therefore, trying to ascertain the contribution of superoxide anion from the other reacting compounds cannot be achieved.

Using the luminol/HRP-based system, many publications have arisen suggesting that pathological spermatozoa generate higher amounts of ROS than controls (for examples see [86,87]). Perhaps one of the most pertinent observations in this field is the idea that ROS, or really luminol-enhanced chemiluminescence, is highly correlated with poor sperm morphology, including amorphous heads, damaged acrosomes, and retained cytoplasmic droplets [88]. Another interpretation of this data is that luminol/HRP reacts with sperm containing luminol−reactive metabolites that are, as yet, unspecified.

Dihydroethidium

DHE, hydroethidium, or hexyl triphenylphosphonium cation (MitoSOX Red) have all been branded as selective ROS reactive reagents or, in the case of the latter, mitochondrial ROS probes. Investigations into the chemistry of DHE have shown that if superoxide anion is present, then 2-hydroxyethidium can be produced [89]. However, DHE suffers from a similar drawback as the luminol/HRP assay, since nonspecific oxidation leads to the formation of ethidium. Both ethidium and 2-hydroxyethidium emit red fluorescence, exciting at 510 nm. Of concern, many publications that use this compound have simply added DHE to cells and then measured red fluorescence. However, in doing so, they record both ethidium and 2-hydroxyethidium products. Despite this, many authors assume that all the fluorescence is contributed by the superoxide−mediated product 2-hydroxyethidium (i.e., ROS) and ignore any potential contribution created by the oxidation of DHE via alternative pathways [90−92]. The beauty of DHE as a probe is that there is a way to work around it. Using High Performance Liquid chromatography and a reversed phase column, the ethidium and 2-hydroxyethidium peaks can be separated and resolved [93]. In this manner, the contribution of superoxide anion to the overall signal can be deciphered. However, to our knowledge this analysis has been performed only in menadione-treated spermatozoa [93]; it has never been used to compare spontaneous levels of ROS generation in normal and pathological sperm cells.

DNA Oxidation and Its Measurement of Reactive Oxygen Species

The earlier difficulties encountered in achieving the direct measurement of ROS from spermatozoa should serve as a warning to future researchers. Encouragingly, indirect measurements of oxidative stress do appear to show that abnormal sperm cells may have had significant ROS exposure. For example, higher levels of 8-oxo-7,8-dihydro-2′-deoxyguanosine (a DNA adduct formed in the presence of ROS) have been shown within infertile men in comparison to their fertile counterparts [94]. Of particular note, higher levels of DNA damage were found in sperm compared with leukocytes collected from the blood of the same patients [94]. This suggests that either sperm are more sensitive to DNA damage or the testis may harbor an environment with more oxidative stress. However, if this is the case, such oxidative stress is occurring well before the production of a sperm cell and unfortunately can be used only as an endpoint of spermatogenesis.

CONCLUSION

In concluding this chapter, we paraphrase Georg Wilhelm Friedrich Hegel, who said the only thing "we learn from history, (is) that we do not learn from history." To some degree this applies to our consideration of ROS and spermatozoa. In looking forward in this field, there are a few lessons that we need take into account. First, leukocytes must be removed. Their presence will always cast doubt as to the true interpretation of the data as clearly evidenced from the work of John MacLeod. Second, the choice of probe: Many publications cite ROS and its involvement in sperm biology and correlate the putative generation of these metabolites in connection with human semen quality [71], DNA damage of infertile men [72], equine sperm behavior [26], human capacitation [73], hyperactivation [27], and apoptosis [74], among others. Yet, all of these reports involve a potential misinterpretation of the probes employed for ROS detection. If possible, actual measurements of DNA adducts or the correct use of probes such as DHE should be applied. Finally, the in vivo relevance of ROS needs further clarity. More studies using refined methodologies to look at the level of spontaneous ROS generation or lipid peroxidation in fertile and infertile males are required. In addition to this, while measurements of aldehydes such as 4-HNE or MDA have been performed, perhaps the most important aldehyde product of all, 4-HHE, still needs to be evaluated. It is our hope that history does not repeat itself, but more definitive experiments need to be performed around the concept of ROS and male-factor infertility.

REFERENCES

[1] Aprioku JS. Pharmacology of free radicals and the impact of reactive oxygen species on the testis. J Reprod Infertil 2013;14(4):158.

[2] MacLeod J. The role of oxygen in the metabolism and motility of human spermatozoa. Am J Physiol 1943;138:512–8.

[3] Saraswat M, et al. Human spermatozoa quantitative proteomic signature classifies normo- and asthenozoospermia. Mol Cell Proteomics 2017;16(1):57–72.

[4] Tremellen K. Oxidative stress and male infertility—a clinical perspective. Hum Reprod Update 2008;14(3):243–58.

[5] Aitken RJ. Free radicals, lipid peroxidation and sperm function. Reprod Fertil Dev 1995;7(4):659–68.

[6] Aitken J, Fisher H. Reactive oxygen species generation and human spermatozoa: the balance of benefit and risk. Bioessays 1994;16(4):259–67.

[7] Ko EY, Sabanegh ES, Agarwal A. Male infertility testing: reactive oxygen species and antioxidant capacity. Fertil Steril 2014;102(6):1518–27.

[8] Aitken RJ, et al. Relative impact of oxidative stress on the functional competence and genomic integrity of human spermatozoa. Biol Reprod 1998;59(5):1037–46.

[9] Bánfi B, et al. A Ca2+-activated NADPH oxidase in testis, spleen, and lymph nodes. J Biol Chem 2001;276(40):37594–601.

[10] Whittington K, Ford W. The effect of incubation periods under 95% oxygen on the stimulated acrosome reaction and motility of human spermatozoa. Mol Hum Reprod 1998;4(11):1053–7.

[11] Baehner RL, Nathan DG. Leukocyte oxidase: defective activity in chronic granulomatous disease. Science 1967;155(3764):835–6.

[12] Kovalski NN, de Lamirande E, Gagnon C. Reactive oxygen species generated by human neutrophils inhibit sperm motility: protective effect of seminal plasma and scavengers. Fertil Steril 1992;58(4):809–16.

[13] Jones R, Mann T, Sherins R. Adverse effects of peroxidized lipid on human spermatozoa. Proc R Soc Lond B Biol Sci 1978;201(1145):413–7.

[14] Kenaston CB, Wilbur KM, Ottolenghi A, Bernheim F. Comparison of methods for determining fatty acid oxidation produced by ultraviolet irradiation. J Am Oil Chem Soc 1955;32(1):33–5.

[15] Esterbauer H, Schaur RJ, Zollner H. Chemistry and biochemistry of 4-hydroxynonenal, malonaldehyde and related aldehydes. Free Radic Biol Med 1991;11(1):81–128.

[16] Brown PR, Miki K, Harper DB, Eddy EM. A-kinase anchoring protein 4 binding proteins in the fibrous sheath of the sperm flagellum. Biol Reprod 2003;68(6):2241–8.

[17] Welch JE, et al. Human glyceraldehyde 3-phosphate dehydrogenase-2 gene is expressed specifically in spermatogenic cells. J Androl 2000;21(2):328–38.

[18] Aitken RJ, et al. Electrophilic aldehydes generated by sperm metabolism activate mitochondrial reactive oxygen species generation and apoptosis by targeting succinate dehydrogenase. J Biol Chem 2012;287(39):33048–60.

[19] Baker MA, et al. Defining the mechanism by which the reactive oxygen species by-product, 4-hydroxynonenal, affects human sperm cell function. Biol Reprod 2015;92(4):108—12.

[20] Jones R, Mann T. Lipid peroxidation in spermatozoa. Proc R Soc Lond B Biol Sci 1973;184(1074):103—7.

[21] Aitken RJ, Clarkson JS, Fishel S. Generation of reactive oxygen species, lipid peroxidation, and human sperm function. Biol Reprod 1989;41(1):183—97.

[22] De Lamirande E, Gagnon C. Reactive oxygen species and human spermatozoa: I. Effects on the motility of intact spermatozoa and on sperm axonemes. J Androl 1992;13:368—78.

[23] Aitken R, Buckingham D, Harkiss D. Use of a xanthine oxidase free radical generating system to investigate the cytotoxic effects of reactive oxygen species on human spermatozoa. J Reprod Fertil 1993;97(2):441—50.

[24] Mitropoulos D, et al. Nitric oxide synthase and xanthine oxidase activities in the spermatic vein of patients with varicocele: a potential role for nitric oxide and peroxynitrite in sperm dysfunction. J Urol 1996;156(6):1952—8.

[25] Nissen H, Kreysel H. Superoxide dismutase in human semen. Klin Wochenschr 1983;61(1):63—5.

[26] Baumber J, Ball BA, Gravance CG, Medina V, Davies-Morel MC. The effect of reactive oxygen species on equine sperm motility, viability, acrosomal integrity, mitochondrial membrane potential, and membrane lipid peroxidation. J Androl 2000;21(6):895—902.

[27] de Lamirande E, Cagnon C. Human sperm hyperactivation and capacitation as parts of an oxidative process. Free Radic Biol Med 1993;14(2):157—66.

[28] Duru NK, Morshedi M, Oehninger S. Effects of hydrogen peroxide on DNA and plasma membrane integrity of human spermatozoa. Fertil Steril 2000;74(6):1200—7.

[29] Bize I, Santander G, Cabello P, Driscoll D, Sharpe C. Hydrogen peroxide is involved in hamster sperm capacitation in vitro. Biol Reprod 1991;44(3):398—403.

[30] Zini A, Lamirande E, Gagnon C. Low levels of nitric oxide promote human sperm capacitation in vitro. J Androl 1995;16(5):424—31.

[31] Gibb Z, Lambourne SR, Curry BJ, Hall SE, Aitken RJ. Aldehyde dehydrogenase plays a pivotal role in the maintenance of stallion sperm motility. Biol Reprod 2016;94(6):133.

[32] Alvarez JG, Storey BT. Spontaneous lipid peroxidation in rabbit epididymal spermatozoa: its effect on sperm motility. Biol Reprod 1982;27(5):1102—8.

[33] Alvarez JG, Touchstone JC, Blasco L, Storey BT. Spontaneous lipid peroxidation and production of hydrogen peroxide and superoxide in human spermatozoa Superoxide dismutase as major enzyme protectant against oxygen toxicity. J Androl 1987;8(5):338—48.

[34] Aitken RJ, Buckingham DW, Carreras A, Irvine DS. Superoxide dismutase in human sperm suspensions: relationship with cellular composition, oxidative stress, and sperm function. Free Radic Biol Med 1996;21(4):495—504.

[35] Maneesh M, Jayalekshmi H. Role of reactive oxygen species and antioxidants on pathophysiology of male reproduction. Indian J Clin Biochem 2006;21(2):80—9.

[36] Lenzi A, Picardo M, Gandini L, Dondero F. Lipids of the sperm plasma membrane: from polyunsaturated fatty acids considered as markers of sperm function to possible scavenger therapy. Hum Reprod Update 1996;2(3):246—56.

[37] Spector A, Mathur S, Kaduce T. Lipid nutrition and metabolism of cultured mammalian cells. Prog Lipid Res 1980;19(3—4):155—86.

[38] Sanocka D, Kurpisz M. Reactive oxygen species and sperm cells. Reprod Biol Endocrinol 2004;2(1):12.

[39] MartinMuñoz P, et al. Depletion of intracellular thiols and increased production of 4-hydroxynonenal that occur during cryopreservation of stallion spermatozoa lead to caspase activation, loss of motility, and cell death. Biol Reprod 2015;93(6):143.

[40] Aitken RJ, et al. Sperm motility is lost in vitro as a consequence of mitochondrial free radical production and the generation of electrophilic aldehydes but can be significantly rescued by the presence of nucleophilic thiols. Biol Reprod 2012;87(5).

[41] Khoubnasabjafari M, Ansarin K, Jouyban A. Reliability of malondialdehyde as a biomarker of oxidative stress in psychological disorders. Bioimpacts 2015;5(3):123.

[42] Suleiman SA, Ali ME, Zaki Z, El-Malik E, Nasr M. Lipid peroxidation and human sperm motility: protective role of vitamin E. J Androl 1996;17(5):530—7.

[43] Keskes-Ammar L, et al. Sperm oxidative stress and the effect of an oral vitamin E and selenium supplement on semen quality in infertile men. Arch Androl 2003;49(2):83—94.

[44] Rao B, Soufir J, Martin M, David G. Lipid peroxidation in human spermatozoa as related to midpiece abnormalities and motility. Mol Reprod Dev 1989;24(2):127—34.

[45] Tavilani H, Doosti M, Saeidi H. Malondialdehyde levels in sperm and seminal plasma of asthenozoospermic and its relationship with semen parameters. Clin Chim Acta 2005;356(1):199—203.

[46] Roqueta-Rivera M, et al. Docosahexaenoic acid supplementation fully restores fertility and spermatogenesis in male delta-6 desaturase-null mice. J Lipid Res 2010;51(2):360—7.

[47] Patil PS, Humbarwadi RS, Patil AD, Gune AR. Immature germ cells in semen—correlation with total sperm count and sperm motility. J Cytol 2013;30(3):185.

[48] WHO. WHO laboratory manual for the examination of human semen and sperm-cervical mucus interaction. United Kingdom: Cambridge University Press; 2010.

[49] Saleh RA, Held AA. Oxidative stress and male infertility: from research bench to clinical practice. J Androl 2002;23(6):737—52.

[50] Makker K, Agarwal A, Sharma R. Oxidative stress & male infertility. Indian J Med Res 2009;129(4):357—67.

[51] Wolff H, et al. Leukocytospermia is associated with poor semen quality. Fertil Steril 1990;53(3):528—36.

[52] Kaleli S, Öçer F, Irez T, Budak E, Aksu MF. Does leukocytospermia associate with poor semen parameters and sperm functions in male infertility?: the role of different seminal leukocyte concentrations. Eur J Obstet Gynecol Reprod Biol 2000;89(2):185−91.

[53] Auroux M, Collin C, Couvillers M. Do nonspermatozoal cells mainly stem from spermiogenesis? Study of 106 fertile and 102 subfertile men. Arch Androl 1985;14(1):73−80.

[54] Wolff H, Anderson DJ. Immunohistologic characterization and quantitation of leukocyte subpopulations in human semen. Fertil Steril 1988;49(3):497−504.

[55] El-Demiry M, et al. Leucocytes in the ejaculate from fertile and infertile men. BJU Int 1986;58(6):715−20.

[56] Kung A, Ho P, Wang C. Seminal leucocyte subpopulations and sperm function in fertile and infertile Chinese men. Int J Androl 1993;16(3):189−94.

[57] Harrison P, Barratt C, Robinson A, Kessopoulou E, Cooke I. Detection of white blood cell populations in the ejaculates of fertile men. J Reprod Immunol 1991;19(1):95−8.

[58] Aitken RJ, Baker MA. Oxidative stress, spermatozoa and leukocytic infiltration: relationships forged by the opposing forces of microbial invasion and the search for perfection. J Reprod Immunol 2013;100(1):11−9.

[59] Krausz C, Mills C, Rogers S, Tan S, Aitken RJ. Stimulation of oxidant generation by human sperm suspensions using phorbol esters and formyl peptides: relationships with motility and fertilization in vitro. Fertil Steril 1994;62(3):599−605.

[60] Agarwal A, Saleh RA, Bedaiwy MA. Role of reactive oxygen species in the pathophysiology of human reproduction. Fertil Steril 2003;79(4):829−43.

[61] Aitken RJ, Clarkson JS, Hargreave TB, Irvine DS, Wu FC. Analysis of the relationship between defective sperm function and the generation of reactive oxygen species in cases of oligozoospermia. J Androl 1989;10(3):214−20.

[62] de Lamirande E, Jiang H, Zini A, Kodama H, Gagnon C. Reactive oxygen species and sperm physiology. Rev Reprod 1997;2(1):48−54.

[63] Lamirande E, Harakat A, Gagnon C. Human sperm capacitation induced by biological fluids and progesterone, but not by NADH or NADPH, is associated with the production of superoxide anion. J Androl 1998;19(2):215−25.

[64] Aitken RJ, et al. Reactive oxygen species generation by human spermatozoa is induced by exogenous NADPH and inhibited by the flavoprotein inhibitors diphenylene iodonium and quinacrine. Mol Reprod Dev 1997;47(4):468−82.

[65] Aitken RJ, Ryan AL, Baker MA, McLaughlin EA. Redox activity associated with the maturation and capacitation of mammalian spermatozoa. Free Radic Biol Med 2004;36(8):994−1010.

[66] Aitken RJ, Vernet P. Maturation of redox regulatory mechanisms in the epididymis. J Reprod Fertil Suppl 1998;53:109−18.

[67] Vernet P, Fulton N, Wallace C, Aitken RJ. Analysis of reactive oxygen species generating systems in rat epididymal spermatozoa. Biol Reprod 2001;65(4):1102−13.

[68] Richer SC, Ford WC. A critical investigation of NADPH oxidase activity in human spermatozoa. Mol Hum Reprod 2001;7(3):237−44.

[69] Baker MA, Krutskikh A, Curry BJ, McLaughlin EA, Aitken RJ. Identification of cytochrome P450-Reductase as the enzyme responsible for NADPH-dependent lucigenin and tetrazolium salt reduction in rat epididymal sperm preparations. Biol Reprod 2004;71(1):307−18.

[70] Baker MA, Krutskikh A, Curry BJ, Hetherington L, Aitken RJ. Identification of cytochrome-b5 reductase as the enzyme responsible for NADH-dependent lucigenin chemiluminescence in human spermatozoa. Biol Reprod 2005;73(2):334−42.

[71] Said TM, et al. Human sperm superoxide anion generation and correlation with semen quality in patients with male infertility. Fertil Steril 2004;82(4):871−7.

[72] Said TM, Agarwal A, Sharma RK, Thomas AJ, Sikka SC. Impact of sperm morphology on DNA damage caused by oxidative stress induced by β-nicotinamide adenine dinucleotide phosphate. Fertil Steril 2005;83(1):95−103.

[73] Donà G, et al. Evaluation of correct endogenous reactive oxygen species content for human sperm capacitation and involvement of the NADPH oxidase system. Hum Reprod 2011;26(12):3264−73.

[74] Tunc O, Thompson J, Tremellen K. Development of the NBT assay as a marker of sperm oxidative stress. Int J Androl 2010;33(1):13−21.

[75] Bromfield EG, et al. Inhibition of arachidonate 15-lipoxygenase prevents 4-hydroxynonenal-induced protein damage in male germ cells. Biol Reprod 2017;96(3):598−609.

[76] Musset B, et al. NOX5 in human spermatozoa expression, function, and regulation. J Biol Chem 2012;287(12):9376−88.

[77] Wang G, et al. In-depth proteomic analysis of the human sperm reveals complex protein compositions. J Proteom 2013;79:114−22.

[78] Baker MA, et al. Head and flagella Sub-compartmental proteomic analysis of human spermatozoa. Proteomics 2013;13(1):61−74.

[79] Baker MA, et al. Identification of gene products present in Triton X-100 soluble and insoluble fractions of human spermatozoa lysates using LC-MS/MS analysis. Proteomics Clin Appl 2007;1(5):524−32.

[80] Ankel-Simons F, Cummins JM. Misconceptions about mitochondria and mammalian fertilization: implications for theories on human evolution. Proc Natl Acad Sci Unit States Am 1996;93(24):13859−63.

[81] Kussmaul L, Hirst J. The mechanism of superoxide production by NADH: ubiquinone oxidoreductase (complex I) from bovine heart mitochondria. Proc Natl Acad Sci Unit States Am 2006;103(20):7607−12.

[82] Dröse S, Brandt U. The mechanism of mitochondrial superoxide production by the cytochrome bc1 complex. J Biol Chem 2008;283(31):21649−54.

[83] Wardman P. Fluorescent and luminescent probes for measurement of oxidative and nitrosative species in cells and tissues: progress, pitfalls, and prospects. Free Radic Biol Med 2007;43(7):995−1022.

[84] Merényi G, Lind J, Eriksen TE. Luminol chemiluminescence: chemistry, excitation, emitter. Luminescence 1990;5(1):53−6.

[85] Vilim V, Wilhelm J. What do we measure by a luminol-dependent chemiluminescence of phagocytes? Free Radic Biol Med 1989;6(6):623−9.

[86] Durak I, Kacmaz M, Cimen MB, Avci A, Biri H. Re: reactive oxygen species production by the spermatozoa of patients with idiopathic infertility: relationship to seminal plasma antioxidants. J Urol 1999;161(5):1583−4.

[87] Gil-Guzman E, et al. Differential production of reactive oxygen species by subsets of human spermatozoa at different stages of maturation. Hum Reprod 2001;16(9):1922−30.

[88] Aziz N, et al. Novel association between sperm reactive oxygen species production, sperm morphological defects, and the sperm deformity index. Fertil Steril 2004;81(2):349−54.

[89] Zhao H, et al. Superoxide reacts with hydroethidine but forms a fluorescent product that is distinctly different from ethidium: potential implications in intracellular fluorescence detection of superoxide. Free Radic Biol Med 2003;34(11):1359−68.

[90] Espinoza J, Schulz M, Sánchez R, Villegas J. Integrity of mitochondrial membrane potential reflects human sperm quality. Andrologia 2009;41(1):51−4.

[91] Burnaugh L, Sabeur K, Ball B. Generation of superoxide anion by equine spermatozoa as detected by dihydroethidium. Theriogenology 2007;67(3):580−9.

[92] Aitken RJ, Hanson AR, Kuczera L. Electrophoretic sperm isolation: optimization of electrophoresis conditions and impact on oxidative stress. Hum Reprod 2011;26(8):1955−64.

[93] De Iuliis GN, Wingate JK, Koppers AJ, McLaughlin EA, Aitken RJ. Definitive evidence for the nonmitochondrial production of superoxide anion by human spermatozoa. J Clin Endocrinol Metab 2006;91(5):1968−75.

[94] Guz J, et al. Comparison of oxidative stress/DNA damage in semen and blood of fertile and infertile men. PLoS One 2013;8(7):e68490.

Chapter 1.4

Basic Aspects of Oxidative Stress in Male Reproductive Health

Michael C. Solomon, Jr. [1], Chak-Lam Cho [2] and Ralf R. Henkel [1]

[1] University of the Western Cape, Bellville, South Africa; [2] Union Hospital, Hong Kong, China

INTRODUCTION

Male factors play a significant role in approximately 15% of infertile couples of reproductive age and are of paramount importance in human reproduction [1]. Oxidative stress (OS) represents a common mediator in the pathogenesis of male infertility related to a number of medical conditions and diseases including varicocele, obesity and male genital tract infections/inflammations.

Oxygen is essential in sustaining and maintaining life, and spermatozoa, like all other aerobic cells, are constantly subjected to the oxygen paradox [2]. On one hand oxygen is essential for cells to live, but on the other hand, too much exposure to oxygen-derived oxidants results in cellular stress and cell death through OS. OS occurs as a result of an imbalance between reactive oxygen species (ROS) and antioxidants in the body [3]: either an increase in ROS or decrease in antioxidants, or both. Oxygen-derived oxidants including hydroxyl ion ($\cdot OH^-$), superoxide ($\cdot O_2^-$), hydrogen peroxide (H_2O_2), peroxyl radical ($\cdot ROO^-$), and hypochlorite ion (ClO^-) are the most common ROS [4]. Elevated levels of ROS are known to negatively impact sperm maturation and function [5].

Indeed, ROS may exert different roles in various systems at different levels. Previous studies have provided evidence that low or physiological levels of ROS are vital in the activation of intracellular pathways responsible for spermatozoa maturation, capacitation, hyperactivation, acrosome reaction, and chemotactic processes as well as fusion with the female gamete [6−10]. On the other hand, ROS have been implicated in the origin and progression of diseases such as cancer and neurodegenerative , or deleterious effects in embryo development [11−14].

PATHOLOGICAL EFFECTS OF OXIDATIVE STRESS ON SPERMATOZOA AND THEIR FUNCTIONAL CAPACITY

Lipid Peroxidation

Considered the most susceptible macromolecules, lipids are present in the plasma membrane in the form of polyunsaturated fatty acids (PUFAs), which are fatty acids containing more than two carbon-carbon double bonds [15]. ROS attack PUFAs in the cell membrane, contributing toward a cascade of chemical reactions known as lipid peroxidation (LPO) (Fig. 1). The cascade of reactions of LPO occurs in three stages: initiation, propagation, and termination, in sequence.

Most membrane PUFAs consist of unconjugated double bonds separated by methylene groups. Furthermore, the presence of a double bond adjacent to a methylene group weakens the methylene C−H bonds, enhancing the susceptibility of oxidative assault and abstraction of a hydrogen atom. Subsequent to this abstraction, a radical is produced, which is stabilized by the reconfiguration of double bonds, resulting in the formation of a lipid radical, which in turn can be oxidized by oxygen leading to a lipid peroxyl radical. Therefore, lipids are particularly susceptible to peroxidation as a result of the large number of methylene-interrupted bonds present [16]. The process is then propagated as a radical chain reaction

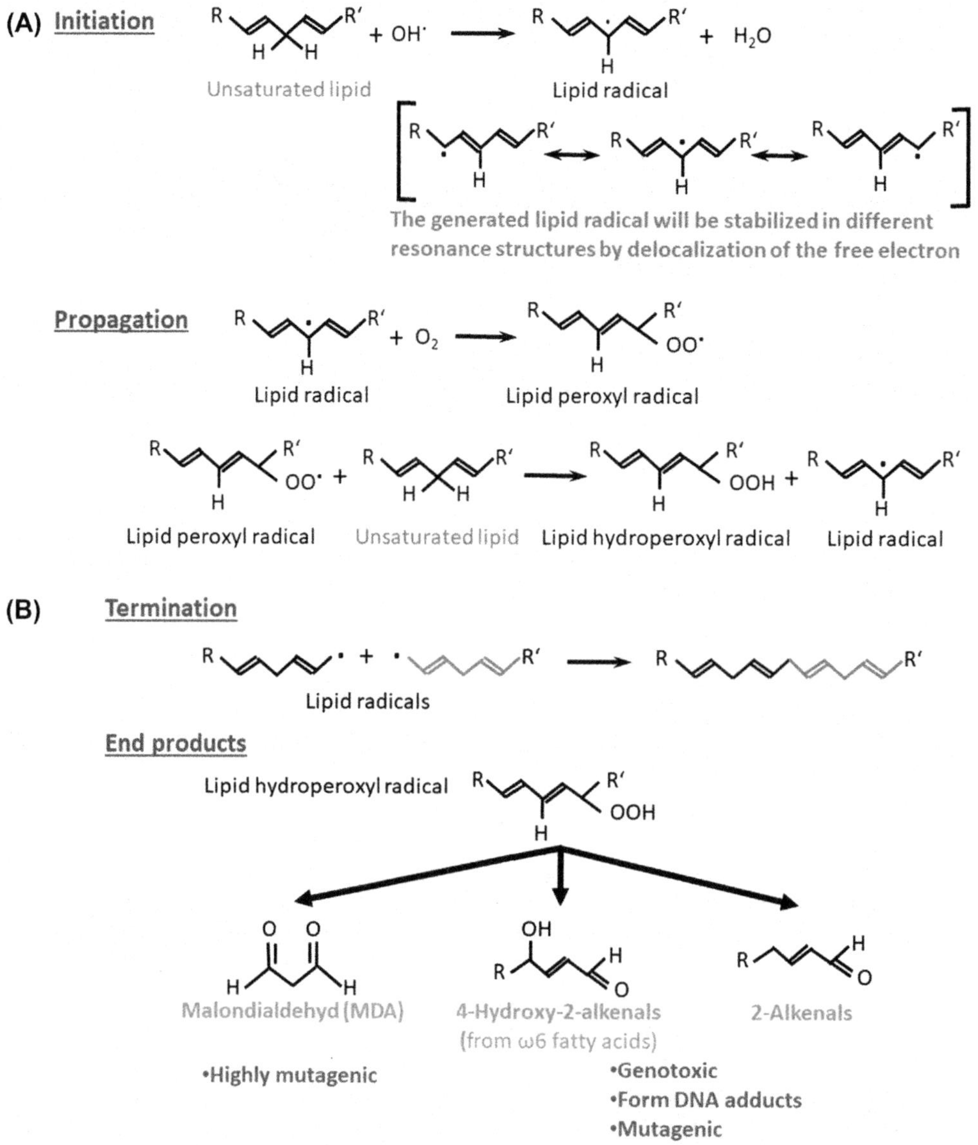

FIGURE 1 Mechanism and phases of lipid peroxidation. This process is a radical chain reaction that can be separated into three phases: initiation, propagation, and termination (A). At the end of this detrimental process highly mutagenic and genotoxic compounds are formed (B).

through the reaction of the lipid peroxyl radical with neighboring unsaturated lipids, a process whereby the free unpaired electron is further transferred to other lipid molecules until two radicals react with one another, thereby terminating this chain reaction.

In this instance, spermatozoa are not only prone to oxidative damage given the large quantities of PUFAs (predominantly 22:6) in their plasma membrane [17], but also as a result of the low concentration of scavenging enzymes and other antioxidants contained within their cytoplasm [8,18−20]. Spermatozoa also exhibit no capacity for membrane repair and possess a significant ability to generate ROS, chiefly superoxide anion and hydrogen peroxide [18,21,22]. Additionally, intracellular enzymes become compromised due to oxidative damage, thus providing limited protection to the plasma membrane that surrounds the acrosome and tail [23]. Hence, spermatozoa are dependent on the limited intrinsic antioxidant defenses provided by seminal plasma to counteract LPO [23,24].

Malondialdehyde (MDA) is a highly mutagenic end product of LPO [25], and has been used in biochemical assays to monitor the degree of oxidative damage in spermatozoa [19,26]. This assay provides insight into male infertility as a result of oxidative damage and is thought to indicate the correlation between the impairment of sperm function, sperm motility, and the capacity for sperm-oocyte fusion [27]. Nevertheless, the validity and reliability of this test has been questioned as MDA is highly reactive and has the ability to react with other biomolecules [28,29]. The unstable nature of MDA attributes to the poor reproducibility of the assays due to variations in the production rate in biological fluids, sample storage, derivatization rate, and analytical methods.

Apoptosis

Necrosis (damage caused by external injury) and apoptosis (programmed cell death induced by internal or external stimuli) are the two major mechanisms of cell death. The latter consists of intricate and sophisticated energy-dependent cascade mechanisms that occur via the extrinsic or intrinsic pathways. Apoptosis is a naturally occurring and programmed cell death process, which has an essential role in the normal development and homeostasis of all multicellular organisms by eliminating damaged, infected, or neoplastic cells. However, it may result in adverse biological consequences when the delicate balance of apoptotic cell death is not maintained [30]. When stimulated, the intrinsic or mitochondrial pathway leads to the release of cytochrome c from the mitochondria and the activation of the death signal [31].

The Bcl-2 family of proteins are the most important regulators of the intrinsic pathway, and include anti-apoptotic markers that block the release of cytochrome c, and pro-apoptotic (Bax, Bak, Bad, Bcl-Xs, Bid, Bik, Bim, Hrk) markers promote apoptosis. Subsequent to the activation of the death signal, these pro-apoptotic proteins undergo post-translational modification, resulting in their activation and translocation to the mitochondria, leading to apoptosis [31]. The outer mitochondrial membrane becomes permeable due to apoptotic stimuli, and releases cytochrome c into the cytosol. Cytochrome c then interacts with apoptotic protease activating factor 1 (Apaf-1), resulting in the activation of caspase 9 proenzymes. Active caspase 9 then continues to activate caspase 3, and the domino effect is the activation of the rest of the caspase cascade that drives apoptosis [32].

Within the context of male reproduction, apoptosis plays a key role in the elimination of abnormal spermatozoa, as germ cells constantly proliferate and differentiate to become mature spermatozoa during spermatogenesis [33]. In order to achieve alignment with the supporting capability of Sertoli cells during spermatogenesis, proliferation of germ cells is optimized via selective apoptosis. This is important in order to maintain a precise germ cell population while complying with the nursing capacity of Sertoli cells [33,34]. Selective apoptosis further ensures that no defective germ cells are allowed to differentiate into spermatozoa [35].

Generally, cell surface proteins such as Fas (APO-1, CD95) may induce apoptosis in sperm by ROS-independent pathways [36]. Fas is a type-1 transmembrane protein in the tumor necrosis factor—nerve growth receptor family that mediates apoptosis [37]. If Fas binds to Fas-ligand (FasL), which is expressed in Sertoli cells [36], Fas-expressing cells are induced to undergo apoptosis [38] in a process in regulating and limiting the number of spermatozoa that can be supported by the Sertoli cells. However, in case Sertoli cells express insufficient levels of FasL as found in patients with abnormal sperm parameters, Fas-positive sperm can appear in the ejaculate [39], a process called "abortive apoptosis" (Fig. 2).

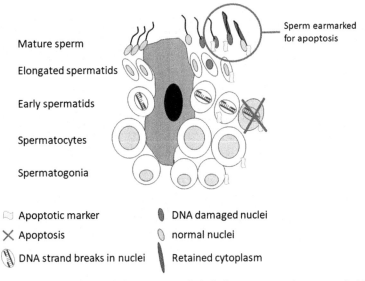

FIGURE 2 Mechanism of abortive apoptosis. Under normal circumstances cells including spermatogonia are earmarked for apoptosis if these cells failed to repair DNA strand breaks. In case this process of the elimination of defective cells is not functioning properly or the earmarked cells cannot properly be identified, this will lead to their escape from the mechanism. As a result, such sperm cells with damaged DNA will appear in the ejaculate.

Studies in various species, including human spermatozoa, have also shown that apoptosis inducing factor is released in response to mitochondrial exposure to ROS, which directly interacts with the DNA, resulting in DNA fragmentation [40,41].

Sperm Motility

Elevated levels of ROS have been correlated with a reduction in sperm motility [42−44]. Yet, the indiscernible link between ROS and declining motility remains controversial as numerous mechanisms of action have been previously proposed [45]. One such hypothesis is that H_2O_2 diffuses across the membranes into cells and is then inhibiting the activity of glucose-6-phosphate dehydrogenase (G6PD) via the hexose monophosphate shunt that regulates the availability of NADPH. Spermatozoa, in turn, use this as a source of electrons to fuel the generation of ROS by NADPH oxidase [46]. Since motility is closely linked with the membrane lipid content, however, it may also be that extrinsic ROS damage the sperm plasma membrane and thereby negatively affect motility [47]. Another theory suggests that a decrease in axonemal protein phosphorylation and sperm immobilization, both of which are associated with a reduction in membrane fluidity that is essential for sperm-oocyte fusion [48], may further impair fertility outcome in assisted reproductive techniques (ARTs) including in vitro fertilization (IVF) and intracytoplasmic sperm injection (ICSI).

Sperm DNA Damage

A major consequence associated with elevated ROS levels is sperm DNA damage, which is closely linked to male infertility and poor embryo development [49−51]. An array of endogenous and exogenous factors that may induce DNA damage to the male germ cell line include apoptosis, improper DNA packaging during spermatogenesis, sperm maturation, and OS [52−56]. Studies have shown that the rate of DNA fragmentation is higher in men with poor semen quality [57,58]. Since physiological barriers for sperm entry into the oocyte are bypassed in ARTs, particularly ICSI, the impact of DNA-damaged spermatozoa may be higher when these techniques are employed. Furthermore, the resultant sperm DNA damage has been linked to lower fertilization rates subsequent to IVF, lower embryo quality and pregnancy rates, and higher rates of miscarriage, malformations, and childhood cancers [59].

OS compromises the integrity of sperm DNA by inducing a higher frequency of single- and double-stranded DNA breaks [60,61]. ROS may further elicit point mutations and polymorphism, resulting in decreased sperm quality [62,63]. Moreover, most of these factors affect the integrity of sperm chromatin through the induction of OS. Mechanisms such as denaturation and base-pair oxidation may also be implicated as a result of this cellular stress, allowing the generation of oxidized DNA base adducts such as 8-hydroxy-2′-deoxyguanosine (8-OHdG), which is prevalent particularly in areas of the genome that are not heavily protaminated [64,65]. 8-OHdG assay is available and is considered one of the biomarkers of oxidative DNA damage [66].

DIFFERENCE IN OXIDATIVE STRESS BETWEEN FERTILE AND INFERTILE MEN

Male factor infertility is solely and partially implicated in 20%−50% of cases of infertility [67]. There is a significant proportion (10%−30%) of infertile men who have normal semen analysis and are classified as unexplained male infertility (UMI) [68]. It is well known that conventional semen parameters (sperm concentration, motility, and morphology) does not guarantee normal functions of sperm, and studies have further identified a significant overlap in the semen parameters between fertile and infertile men [69,70]. Numerous factors have been associated with UMI, which include the presence of antisperm antibodies [71], sperm DNA damage [64], elevated levels of ROS [72,73], and sperm dysfunction [74,75].

Elevated levels of ROS are believed to be a major contributing factor. Increased seminal ROS levels can induce pathophysiological changes in spermatozoa [76,77] and have been implicated as a cause of infertility in up to 20%−40% of infertile men [46,78].

Iwasaki and Gagnon (1992) observed elevated ROS levels in up to 40% of semen samples from infertile men, whereas no ROS were detected in control and azoospermic patients. ROS were significantly and negatively correlated with the ejaculate volume, motility, and linearity for both unprocessed semen and washed sperm after density gradient centrifugation. Simple washing of spermatozoa resulted in ROS production up to 20−50 times higher than in the native semen sample [26]. The results observed by these authors can either be due to increased ROS production or reduced seminal antioxidant capacity. In fact, it was repeatedly shown that seminal total antioxidant capacity (TAC) in infertile men is lower compared to fertile men [69,79] and has significant predictive power as diagnostic parameter [80]. In asthenozoospermic men, the presence of ROS activity in infertile men is coupled with lower levels of chain-braking antioxidants [69,81]. Later studies, using different and novel methods such as the MiOXSYS System for the evaluation of the oxidation-reduction potential (ORP) [82], obtained similar results in identifying higher OS levels in infertile patients [83].

ROLE OF OXIDATIVE STRESS ASSAYS IN UNEXPLAINED MALE INFERTILITY

In an estimate of 15% of the cases of male infertility, with reports ranging from 6% to 50% [84,85], normal results of routine semen analysis cannot explain the cause of the infertility. These infertile men are referred to as suffering from UMI [84]. ROS and OS are possible factors that cause or significantly contribute to UMI [84]. OS can be the result of either elevated production of ROS by leukocytes or the spermatozoa [45,47,86,87] or a depleted antioxidant capacity, which normally scavenges excessive amounts of ROS [69,88]. Excessive ROS production, antioxidant capacity, and OS have repeatedly been shown to have diagnostic value for UMI [84,85,88].

OS was determined by measuring ROS via a chemiluminescence assay, which directly measures, depending on the methodology, both intra- and extracellular ROS, and records the intensity of light produced from the chemiluminescent probe (luminol, lucigenin, etc.) with ROS in relative light units [84]. Alternatively, either the breakdown products of LPO, MDA [89,90], or the TAC as measure of ROS-counteracting activity in seminal plasma have obtained some clinical relevance [83,91]. For MDA assay, however, its reliability and reproducibility have been questioned [82,83]. After all, these methods are complex, time-consuming, and need larger amounts of the respective samples.

A novel method detecting OS has been developed recently. OS is measured in terms of ORP by using the galvanostat-based MiOXSYS analyzer, which expresses the sum of all oxidants and reductants available in the seminal fluid. This methodology has been shown to be a reliable, reproducible, and cost-effective way in determining seminal OS [92] within 5 min in a clinical setup. The correlation between high ORP and poor semen parameters has been reported [93].

SELECTION OF NON-DNA DAMAGED SPERM

Selection of healthy spermatozoa capable of fertilizing oocytes plays a vital role in the success of ART. The aim of sperm selection is to minimize the risk of fertilizing the ovum by abnormal spermatozoon. Thus, the ideal procedure should optimally eliminate nonviable and poor quality spermatozoa, leukocytes, bacteria, and other sources of contamination as these cells are potent producers or initiators of excessive ROS that damage functional spermatozoa [94]. Therefore, the elimination thereof is of paramount importance since otherwise sperm functions to fertilize oocytes would be severely compromised [77,95−97]. The selection process essentially depends on the type of ART that is to be employed. According to Henkel (2012), the criteria for good sperm selection are as follows: elimination of seminal plasma, decapitation factors and debris, ROS-producing sperm, leukocytes, bacteria, enrichment of functional sperm, cost-effectiveness, and ease and speed at which assays are performed [98]. For IVF and intrauterine insemination, mainly swim-up and density gradient centrifugation are used as these methods are able to process larger volumes of ejaculates. More advanced and sophisticated techniques include annexin V magnetic activated cell separation, based on the externalization of phosphatidylserine [99], hyaluronic acid (HA$^-$) mediated sperm selection based on the presence of HA receptors [100], electrophoretic isolation [101,102], and the zeta method based on sperm electric charge [92].

On the other hand, for ICSI, single sperm selection methods such as the standard microscopical selection, intra-cytoplasmic morphologically selected sperm injection (IMSI), or picked spermatozoa for ICSI are used as they are thought to obtain better-quality sperm, which achieve higher pregnancy rates by selection of DNA-intact sperm [103−105]. The principle of the techniques is based on the fact that nuclear vacuoles are thought to contain a higher percentage of damaged DNA [106,107]. On the other hand, a more recent study indicates that there is no such relationship [108,109]. Yet, it appears that patients with a high percentage of sperm DNA damage who had special interventions such as IMSI had better clinical outcomes as compared to patients where such procedures were not performed [110].

Several studies have been conducted with controversy as to whether density gradient centrifugation or the swim-up method should be recommended in obtaining normal functioning sperm [72,92,111−113]. In fact, the use of apoptotic or DNA-damaged sperm during ARTs contributes toward suboptimal fertilization results [56,114,115]. According to Bungum et al. (2007), ICSI should be performed if the DNA fragmentation index exceeds 30% [116]. While embryonic development will not continue with a damaged male genome theoretically, it is not fully understood why the high proportion of DNA-damaged sperm in a semen sample can successfully bypass the physiological barrier and achieve fertilization. The only reason why the success rate of ICSI in these cases could be higher is due to the selection of morphologically most normally appearing sperm in the microscope at normal magnification [117].

Since a strong relationship between DNA methylation levels and normal sperm morphology has been revealed, it appears that epigenetic conditions play a significant role in the successful onset of pregnancy [108,118]. Thus, for ICSI to be successful, it is imperative not only to select the most motile spermatozoa, but the most competent ones too. Functional competence of individual sperm cannot be assessed using normal light microscopy. Therefore, specific sperm functional tests including testing for DNA fragmentation should be performed [119,120].

REVERSAL OF OXIDATIVE STRESS

To remedy elevated levels of ROS, antioxidant supplementation is often recommended based on its capability in stabilizing and deactivating free radicals. This is achieved via the enzymatic and nonenzymatic antioxidant systems [2], and lastly via metal-binding proteins [121]. While superoxide dismutase, catalase, and glutathione peroxidase form the enzymatic system, vitamin C, vitamin E, urate, pyruvate, glutathione, lycopene, β-carotene, taurine, and hypotaurine constitute the nonenzymatic system. In seminal plasma, antioxidants such as vitamins C and E, folate, zinc, selenium, carnitine, and carotenoids are readily available scavengers that can counteract the elevated levels of ROS under normal circumstances.

Studies have enumerated the widespread effect of antioxidant supplementation in andrology. Antioxidant supplementation at the recommended daily dosage, prescribed by clinicians, has been shown to improve semen parameters (concentration, motility, morphology) [122], reduce seminal OS [123], reduce sperm DNA fragmentation [124], improve clinical pregnancy rate [91], improve live birth rate [125], and provide protection for sperm in vitro against the deleterious effects of incubation time and freeze-thawing [126]. However, the use of antioxidant in management of male infertility is still highly debated as both positive and negative results have been reported [91,124,127–130]. The reason for this discrepancy could lie in the ignorance of the normal ranges of redox levels in the body in general, and the seminal plasma specifically. The delicate balance between oxidants and antioxidants that are necessary for triggering the essential physiological sperm functions and the normal scavenging of ROS is largely unknown. This could lead to an excessive amount of antioxidants, which may lead to infertility due to reductive stress that can be as dangerous as OS [131].

CONCLUSION

ROS have both physiological and pathophysiological roles in sperm functionality. If the ROS levels exceed the scavenging capacity of the antioxidants available in the male genital tract and seminal fluid, OS is generated, which is detrimental to sperm function. The pathological mechanisms of OS are mediated by an excessive amount of ROS, whereby sperm functionality is compromised at several levels, namely the plasma membrane through oxidation of the membrane lipids or direct oxidation of mitochondrial and nuclear DNA. The role of ROS assays may be particularly useful in UMI in which conventional semen analysis fails to identify any abnormality. As a remedy to correct OS, antioxidants may possibly restore and maintain the redox balance in order to achieve successful pregnancy outcome and restore fertility of the infertile males. However, the risk of overdose should not be overlooked before better understanding of the redox state is revealed by further research.

REFERENCES

[1] Jarow JP, Sharlip ID, Belker AM, Lipshultz LI, Sigman M, Thomas AJ, Schlegel PN, Howards SS, Nehra A, Damewood MD, Overstreet JW. Best practice policies for male infertility. J Urol 2002;167(5):2138–44.

[2] Sies H. Strategies of antioxidant defense. FEBS J 1993;215(2):213–9.

[3] Agarwal A, Makker K, Sharma R. Clinical relevance of oxidative stress in male factor infertility: an update. Am J Reprod Immunol 2008;59(1):2–11.

[4] Agarwal A, Said TM. Oxidative stress, DNA damage and apoptosis in male infertility: a clinical approach. Br J Urol Int 2005;95(4):503–7.

[5] Makker K, Agarwal A, Sharma R. Oxidative stress & male infertility. Indian J Med Res 2009:357–67.

[6] Aitken RJ. A free radical theory of male infertility. Reprod Fertil Dev 1994;6(1):19–23.

[7] de Lamirande E, Jiang H, Zini A, Kodama H, Gagnon C. Reactive oxygen species and sperm physiology. Rev Reprod 1997;2(1):48–54.

[8] de Lamirande E, Gagnon C. Impact of reactive oxygen species on spermatozoa: a balancing act between beneficial and detrimental effects. Hum Reprod 1995;10(Suppl. 1):15–21.

[9] Aitken RJ, Irvine DS, Wu FC. Prospective analysis of sperm-oocyte fusion and reactive oxygen species generation as criteria for the diagnosis of infertility. Am J Obstet Gynecol 1991;164(2):542–51.

[10] Sánchez R, Sepúlveda C, Risopatrón J, Villegas J, Giojalas LC. Human sperm chemotaxis depends on critical levels of reactive oxygen species. Fertil Steril 2010;93(1):150–3.

[11] Aitken RJ, Baker MA, Sawyer D. Oxidative stress in the male germ line and its role in the aetiology of male infertility and genetic disease. Reprod Biomed Online 2003;7:65–70.

[12] Aitken RJ, Smith TB, Jobling MS, Baker MA, De Iuliis GN. Oxidative stress and male reproductive health. Asian J Androl 2014;16:31–8.

[13] Baker MA, Aitken RJ. Reactive oxygen species in spermatozoa: methods for monitoring and significance for the origins of genetic disease and infertility. Reprod Biol Endocrinol 2005;3:67.

[14] Klaunig JE, Kamendulis LM, Hocevar BA. Oxidative stress and oxidative damage in carcinogenesis. Toxicol Pathol 2010;38:96–109.

[15] Halliwell B. Tell me about free radicals, doctor: a review. J R Soc Med 1989;82(12):747.

[16] Blake DR, Allen RE, Lunec J. Free radicals in biological systems—a review orientated to inflammatory processes. Br Med Bull 1987;43(2):371–85.

[17] Alvarez JG, Storey BT. Differential incorporation of fatty acids into and peroxidative loss of fatty acids from phospholipids of human spermatozoa. Mol Reprod Dev 1995;42(3):334–46.

[18] Jones R, Mann T, Sherins R. Peroxidative breakdown of phospholipids in human spermatozoa, spermicidal properties of fatty acid peroxides, and protective action of seminal plasma. Fertil Steril 1979;31(5):531–7.

[19] Aitken J, Fisher H. Reactive oxygen species generation and human spermatozoa: the balance of benefit and risk. Bioessays 1994;16(4):259–67.

[20] Sharma RK, Agarwal A. Role of reactive oxygen species in male infertility. Urology 1996;48(6):835–50.

[21] Aitken RJ, Clarkson JS. Cellular basis of defective sperm function and its association with the genesis of reactive oxygen species by human spermatozoa. J Reprod Fertil 1987;81(2):459–69.

[22] Alvarez JG, Touchstone JC, Blasco L, Storey BT. Spontaneous lipid peroxidation and production of hydrogen peroxide and superoxide in human spermatozoa superoxide dismutase as major enzyme protectant against oxygen toxicity. J Androl 1987;8(5):338–48.

[23] Iwasaki A, Gagnon C. Formation of reactive oxygen species in spermatozoa of infertile patients. Fertil Steril 1992;57(2):409–16.

[24] Zini A, Lamirande E, Gagnon C. Reactive oxygen species in semen of infertile patients: levels of superoxide dismutase-and catalase-like activities in seminal plasma and spermatozoa. Int J Androl 1993;16(3):183–8.

[25] Luczaj W, Skrzydlewska E. DNA damage caused by lipid peroxidation products. Cell Mol Biol Lett 2003;8:391–413.

[26] John Aitken R, Clarkson JS, Fishel S. Generation of reactive oxygen species, lipid peroxidation, and human sperm function. Biol Reprod 1989;41(1):183–97.

[27] Aitken RJ, Harkiss D, Buckingham DW. Analysis of lipid peroxidation mechanisms in human spermatozoa. Mol Reprod Dev 1993;35(3):302–15.

[28] Khoubnasabjafari M, Ansarin K, Jouyban A. Reliability of malondialdehyde as a biomarker of oxidative stress in psychological disorders. Bioimpacts 2015;5:123–7.

[29] Azizi S, Shahrisa A, Khoubnasabjafari M, Ansarin K, Khoubnasabjafari M, Soleymani J, Jouyban A. A possible reason for the low reproducibility of malondialdehyde determinations in biological samples. Bioanalysis 2016;8:2179–81.

[30] Nagata S. Fas-mediated apoptosis. Adv Exp Biol 1996:119–24.

[31] Scorrano L, Korsmeyer SJ. Mechanisms of cytochrome c release by proapoptotic BCL-2 family members. Biochem Biophys Res Commun 2003;304(3):437–44.

[32] Reed JC. Cytochrome c: can't live with it—can't live without it. Cell 1997;91(5):559–62.

[33] Mclachlan RI, Wreford NG, Meachem SJ, De Kretser DM, Robertson DM. Effects of testosterone on spermatogenic cell populations in the adult rat. Biol Reprod 1994;51(5):945–55.

[34] Hikim AS, Swerdloff RS. Hormonal and genetic control of germ cell apoptosis in the testis. Rev Reprod 1999;4(1):38–47.

[35] Shukla KK, Mahdi AA, Rajender S. Apoptosis, spermatogenesis and male infertility. Front Biosci 2012;4:746–54.

[36] Lee J, Richburg JH, Younkin SC, Boekelheide K. The Fas system is a key regulator of germ cell apoptosis in the testis. Endocrinology 1997;138(5):2081–8.

[37] Krammer PH, Behrmann I, Daniel P, Dhein J, Debatin KM. Regulation of apoptosis in the immune system. Curr Opin Immunol 1994;6(2):279–89.

[38] Suda T, Takahashi T, Golstein P, Nagata S. Molecular cloning and expression of the Fas ligand, a novel member of the tumor necrosis factor family. Cell 1993;75:1169–78.

[39] Sakkas D, Mariethoz E, St John JC. Abnormal sperm parameters in humans are indicative of an abortive apoptotic mechanism linked to the Fas-mediated pathway. Exp Cell Res 1999;251:350–5.

[40] Paasch U, Sharma RK, Gupta AK, Grunewald S, Mascha EJ, Thomas Jr AJ, Glander HJ, Agarwal A. Cryopreservation and thawing is associated with varying extent of activation of apoptotic machinery in subsets of ejaculated human spermatozoa. Biol Reprod 2004;71(6):1828–37.

[41] Candé C, Cecconi F, Dessen P, Kroemer G. Apoptosis-inducing factor (AIF): key to the conserved caspase-independent pathways of cell death? J Cell Sci 2002;115(24):4727–34.

[42] Lenzi A, Lombardo F, Gandini L, Alfano P, Dondero F. Computer assisted sperm motility analysis at the moment of induced pregnancy during gonadotropin treatment for hypogonadotropic hypogonadism. J Endocrinol Invest 1993;16(9):683–6.

[43] Agarwal AS, Ikemoto IS, Loughlin KR. Relationship of sperm parameters with levels of reactive oxygen species in semen specimens. J Urol 1994;152(1):107–10.

[44] Armstrong JS, Rajasekaran M, Chamulitrat W, Gatti P, Hellstrom WJ, Sikka SC. Characterization of reactive oxygen species induced effects on human spermatozoa movement and energy metabolism. Free Radic Biol Med 1999;26(7):869–80.

[45] Henkel R. Leukocytes and oxidative stress: dilemma for sperm function and male fertility. Asian J Androl 2011;13:43–52.

[46] Aitken RJ, Fisher HM, Fulton N, Gomez E, Knox W, Lewis B, Irvine S. Reactive oxygen species generation by human spermatozoa is induced by exogenous NADPH and inhibited by the flavoprotein inhibitors diphenylene iodonium and quinacrine. Mol Reprod Dev 1997;47(4):468–82.

[47] Henkel R, Kierspel E, Stalf T, Mehnert C, Menkveld R, Tinneberg HR, Schill WB, Kruger TF. Effect of reactive oxygen species produced by spermatozoa and leukocytes on sperm functions in non-leukocytospermic patients. Fertil Steril 2005;83:635–42.

[48] de Lamirande E, Gagnon CL. Reactive oxygen species and human spermatozoa: I. Effects on the motility of intact spermatozoa and on sperm axonemes. J Androl 1992;13:368.

[49] Saleh A, Agarwal A, Nelson DR, Nada EA, El-Tonsy MH, Alvarez JG, Thomas AJ, Sharma RK. Increased sperm nuclear DNA damage in normozoospermic infertile men: a prospective study. Fertil Steril 2002;78:313−8.

[50] Zini A, Meriano J, Kader K, Jarvi K, Laskin CA, Cadesky K. Potential adverse effect of sperm DNA damage on embryo quality after ICSI. Hum Reprod 2005;20:3476−80.

[51] Simon L, Murphy K, Shamsi MB, Liu L, Emery B, Aston KI, Hotaling J, Carrell DT. Paternal influence of sperm DNA integrity on early embryonic development. Hum Reprod 2014;29:2402−12.

[52] Aitken RJ, Curry BJ. Redox regulation of human sperm function: from the physiological control of sperm capacitation to the etiology of infertility and DNA damage in the germ line. Antioxidants Redox Signal 2011;14(3):367−81.

[53] McPherson SM, Longo FJ. Localization of DNase I-hypersensitive regions during rat spermatogenesis: stage-dependent patterns and unique sensitivity of elongating spermatids. Mol Reprod Dev 1992;31(4):268−79.

[54] Gomez E, Buckingham DW, Brindle J, Lanzafame F, Irvine DS, Aitken RJ. Development of an image analysis system to monitor the retention of residual cytoplasm by human spermatozoa: correlation with biochemical markers of the cytoplasmic space, oxidative stress, and sperm function. J Androl 1996;17(3):276−87.

[55] Sakkas D, Mariethoz E, Manicardi G, Bizzaro D, Bianchi PG, Bianchi U. Origin of DNA damage in ejaculated human spermatozoa. Rev Reprod 1999;4(1):31−7.

[56] Henkel R, Hajimohammad M, Stalf T, Hoogendijk C, Mehnert C, Menkveld R, Gips H, Schill WB, Kruger TF. Influence of deoxyribonucleic acid damage on fertilization and pregnancy. Fertil Steril 2004;81(4):965−72.

[57] Saleh RA, Agarwal A, Nada EA, El-Tonsy MH, Sharma RK, Meyer A, Nelson DR, Thomas AJ. Negative effects of increased sperm DNA damage in relation to seminal oxidative stress in men with idiopathic and male factor infertility. Fertil Steril 2003;79:1597−605.

[58] Erenpreiss J, Elzanaty S, Giwercman A. Sperm DNA damage in men from infertile couples. Asian J Androl 2008;10(5):786−90.

[59] Lewis SE. Sperm DNA fragmentation and base oxidation. In: Genetic damage in human spermatozoa. New York: Springer; 2014. p. 103−16.

[60] Hughes CM, Lewis SE, McKelvey-Martin VJ, Thompson W. A comparison of baseline and induced DNA damage in human spermatozoa from fertile and infertile men, using a modified comet assay. Mol Hum Reprod: Basic Science of Reproductive Medicine 1996;2(8):613−9.

[61] Twigg JP, Irvine DS, Aitken RJ. Oxidative damage to DNA in human spermatozoa does not preclude pronucleus formation at intracytoplasmic sperm injection. Hum Reprod (Oxf) 1998;13(7):1864−71.

[62] Sharma RK, Said T, Agarwal A. Sperm DNA damage and its clinical relevance in assessing reproductive outcome. Asian J Androl 2004;6(2):139−48.

[63] Spiropoulos J, Turnbull DM, Chinnery PF. Can mitochondrial DNA mutations cause sperm dysfunction? Mol Hum Reprod: Basic Science of Reproductive Medicine 2002;8(8):719−21.

[64] De Iuliis GN, Thomson LK, Mitchell LA, Finnie JM, Koppers AJ, Hedges A, Nixon B, Aitken RJ. DNA damage in human spermatozoa is highly correlated with the efficiency of chromatin remodeling and the formation of 8-hydroxy-2'-deoxyguanosine, a marker of oxidative stress. Biol Reprod 2009;81(3):517−24.

[65] Noblanc A, Damon-Soubeyrand C, Karrich B, Henry-Berger J, Cadet R, Saez F, Guiton R, Janny L, Pons-Rejraji H, Alvarez JG, Drevet JR. DNA oxidative damage in mammalian spermatozoa: where and why is the male nucleus affected? Free Radic Biol Med 2013;65:719−23.

[66] Helbock HJ, Beckman KB, Shigenaga MK, Walter PB, Woodall AA, Yeo HC, Ames BN. DNA oxidation matters: the HPLC−electrochemical detection assay of 8-oxo-deoxyguanosine and 8-oxo-guanine. Proc Natl Acad Sci Unit States Am 1998;95(1):288−93.

[67] Jarow JP. Diagnostic approach to the infertile male patient. Endocrinol Metab Clin N Am 2007;36(2):297−311.

[68] Hamada A, Esteves SC, Agarwal A. Unexplained male infertility: potential causes and management. Hum Androl 2011;1(1):2−16.

[69] Lewis SEM, Boyle PM, McKinney KA, Young IS, Thompson W. Total antioxidant capacity of seminal plasma is different in fertile and infertile men. Fertil Steril 1995;64:868−70.

[70] Van der Steeg JW, Steures P, Eijkemans MJ, Habbema JDF, Hompes PG, Kremer JA, van der Leeuw-Harmsen L, Bossuyt PM, Repping S, Silber SJ, Mol BW, van der Veen F, Collaborative Effort for Clinical Evaluation in Reproductive Medicine Study Group. Role of semen analysis in subfertile couples. Fertil Steril 2011;95:1013−9.

[71] Haidl G. Characterization of fertility related antisperm antibodies- a step towards casual treatment of immunological infertility and immune-contraception. Asian J Androl 2010;12:793−4.

[72] Sakkas D, Manicardi GC, Tomlinson M, Mandrioli M, Bizzaro D, Bianchi PG, Bianchi U. The use of two density gradient centrifugation techniques and the swim-up method to separate spermatozoa with chromatin and nuclear DNA anomalies. Hum Reprod 2000;15(5):1112−6.

[73] Henkel R. The impact of oxidants on sperm function. Andrologia 2005;37:205−506.

[74] Ahmad G, Agarwal A. Pathological effects of elevated reactive oxygen species on sperm function. In: Ahmad SI, editor. Reactive oxygen species in biology and human Health. Boca Raton, Ann Arbor, London, Tokyo: CRC Press; 2016. p. 409−20.

[75] Bisht S, Faiq M, Tolahunase M, Dada R. Oxidative stress and male infertility. Nat Rev Urol 2017;14:470−85.

[76] Aitken RJ, Gordon E, Harkiss D, Twigg JP, Milne P, Jennings Z, Irvine DS. Relative impact of oxidative stress on the functional competence and genomic integrity of human spermatozoa. Biol Reprod 1998;59(5):1037−46.

[77] Aitken RJ. The Amoroso Lecture. The human spermatozoon−a cell in crisis? J Reprod Fertil 1999;115(1):1−7.

[78] Gil-Guzman E, Ollero M, Lopez MC, Sharma RK, Alvarez JG, Thomas Jr AJ, Agarwal A. Differential production of reactive oxygen species by subsets of human spermatozoa at different stages of maturation. Hum Reprod 2001;16(9):1922−30.

[79] Smith R, Vantman D, Ponce J, Escobar J, Lissi E. Total antioxidant capacity of human seminal plasma. Hum Reprod 1996;11:1655—60.

[80] Mahfouz R, Sharma R, Sharma D, Sabanegh E, Agarwal A. Diagnostic value of the total antioxidant capacity (TAC) in human seminal plasma. Fertil Steril 2009;91:805—11.

[81] Baker HG, Brindle J, Irvine DS, Aitken RJ. Protective effect of antioxidants on the impairment of sperm motility by activated polymorphonuclear leukocytes. Fertil Steril 1996;65(2):411—9.

[82] Agarwal A, Sharma R, Roychoudhury S, Du Plessis S, Sabanegh E. MiOXSYS: a novel method of measuring oxidation reduction potential in semen and seminal plasma. Fertil Steril 2016;106:566—73.

[83] Agarwal A, Arafa M, Chandrakumar R, Majzoub A, AlSaid S, Elbardisi H. A multicenter study to evaluate oxidative stress by oxidation-reduction potential, a reliable and reproducible method. Andrology 2017;5(5):939—45. https://doi.org/10.1111/andr.12395 [Epub 2017 Jul 20].

[84] Hamada A, Esteves SC, Nizza M, Agarwal A. Unexplained male infertility: diagnosis and management. Int Braz J Urol 2012;38:576—94.

[85] Mayorga-Torres BJM, Camargo M, Cadavid AP, du Plessis SS, Cardona Maya WD. Are oxidative stress markers associated with unexplained male infertility? Andrologia 2017;49(5). https://doi.org/10.1111/and.12659 [Epub 2016 Aug 10].

[86] Pasqualotto FF, Sharma RK, Kobayashi H, Nelson DR, Thomas Jr AJ, Agarwal A. Oxidative stress in normospermic men undergoing infertility evaluation. J Androl 2001;22:316—22.

[87] Colavitti R, Pani G, Bedogni B, Anzevino R, Borrello S, Waltenberger J, Galeotti T. Reactive oxygen species as downstream mediators of angiogenic signaling by vascular endothelial growth factor receptor-2/KDR. J Biol Chem 2002;277:3101—8.

[88] Roychoudhury S, Sharma R, Sikka S, Agarwal A. Diagnostic application of total antioxidant capacity in seminal plasma to assess oxidative stress in male factor infertility. J Assist Reprod Genet 2016;33:627—35.

[89] Gomez E, Irvine DS, Aitken RJ. Evaluation of a spectrophotometric assay for the measurement of malondialdehyde and 4-hydroxyalkenals in human spermatozoa: relationships with semen quality and sperm function. Int J Androl 1998;21:81—94.

[90] Agarwal R, Chase SD. Rapid, fluorimetric-liquid chromatographic determination of malondialdehyde in biological samples. J Chromatogr B 2002;775:121—6.

[91] Tremellen K, Miari G, Froiland D, Thompson J. A randomised control trial examining the effect of an antioxidant (Menevit) on pregnancy outcome during IVF-ICSI treatment. Aust N Z J Obstet Gynaecol 2007;47(3):216—21.

[92] Chan PJ, Jacobson JD, Corselli JU, Patton WC. A simple zeta method for sperm selection based on membrane charge. Fertil Steril 2006;85(2):481—6.

[93] Agarwal A, Henkel R, Sharma R, Tadros NN, Sabanegh E. Determination of seminal oxidation-reduction potential (ORP) as an easy and cost-effective clinical marker of male infertility. Andrologia 2018;50(3). https://doi.org/10.1111/and.12914. Epub 2017 Oct 23.

[94] Kheirollahi-Kouhestani M, Razavi S, Tavalaee M, Deemeh MR, Mardani M, Moshtaghian J, Nasr-Esfahani MH. Selection of sperm based on combined density gradient and Zeta method may improve ICSI outcome. Hum Reprod 2009;24(10):2409—16.

[95] Twigg J, Fulton N, Gomez E, Irvine DS, Aitken RJ. Analysis of the impact of intracellular reactive oxygen species generation on the structural and functional integrity of human spermatozoa: lipid peroxidation, DNA fragmentation and effectiveness of antioxidants. Hum Reprod (Oxf) 1998;13(6):1429—36.

[96] Kodama H, Yamaguchi R, Fukuda J, Kasai H, Tanaka T. Increased oxidative deoxyribonucleic acid damage in the spermatozoa of infertile male patients. Fertil Steril 1997;68(3):519—24.

[97] Duru NK, Morshedi M, Oehninger S. Effects of hydrogen peroxide on DNA and plasma membrane integrity of human spermatozoa. Fertil Steril 2000;74(6):1200—7.

[98] Henkel R. Sperm separation: state-of-the-art-physiological aspects and application of advanced sperm separation methods. Asian J Androl 2012;14(2):260.

[99] Said TM, Agarwal A, Grunewald S, Rasch M, Glander HJ, Paasch U. Evaluation of sperm recovery following annexin V magnetic-activated cell sorting separation. Reprod Biomed Online 2006;13(3):336—9.

[100] Nasr-Esfahani MH, Razavi SH, Vahdati AA, Fathi F, Tavalaee M. Evaluation of sperm selection procedure based on hyaluronic acid binding ability on ICSI outcome. J Assist Reprod Genet 2008;25(5):197—203.

[101] Ainsworth C, Nixon B, Aitken RJ. Development of a novel electrophoretic system for the isolation of human spermatozoa. Hum Reprod 2005;20(8):2261—70.

[102] Fleming SD, Ilad RS, Griffin AG, Wu Y, Ong KJ, Smith HC, Aitken RJ. Prospective controlled trial of an electrophoretic method of sperm preparation for assisted reproduction: comparison with density gradient centrifugation. Hum Reprod 2008;23(12):2646—51.

[103] Parmegiani L, Cognigni GE, Bernardi S, Troilo E, Ciampaglia W, Filicori M. "Physiologic ICSI": hyaluronic acid (HA) favors selection of spermatozoa without DNA fragmentation and with normal nucleus, resulting in improvement of embryo quality. Fertil Steril 2010;93:598—604.

[104] Hammoud I, Boitrelle F, Ferfouri F, Vialard F, Bergere M, Wainer B, Bailly M, Albert M, Selva J. Selection of normal spermatozoa with a vacuole-free head (x6300) improves selection of spermatozoa with intact DNA in patients with high sperm DNA fragmentation rates. Andrologia 2013;45:163—70.

[105] Maettner R, Sterzik K, Isachenko V, Strehler E, Rahimi G, Alabart JL, Sanchez R, Mallmann P, Isachenko E. Quality of human spermatozoa: relationship between high-magnification sperm morphology and DNA integrity. Andrologia 2014;46:547—55.

[106] Franco Jr JG, Mauri AL, Petersen CG, Massaro FC, Silva LF, Felipe V, Cavagna M, Pontes A, Baruffi RL, Oliveira JB, Vagnini LD. Large nuclear vacuoles are indicative of abnormal chromatin packaging in human spermatozoa. Int J Androl 2012;35:46—51.

[107] Boitrelle F, Guthauser B, Alter L, Bailly M, Wainer R, Vialard F, Albert M, Selva J. The nature of human sperm head vacuoles: a systematic literature review. Basic Clin Androl 2013;23:3.

[108] McDowell S, Kroon B, Ford E, Hook Y, Glujovsky D, Yazdani A. Advanced sperm selection techniques for assisted reproduction. Cochrane Database Syst Rev 2014;28:CD010461.

[109] Fortunato A, Boni R, Leo R, Nacchia G, Liguori F, Casale S, Bonassisa P, Tosti E. Vacuoles in sperm head are not associated with head morphology, DNA damage and reproductive success. Reprod Biomed Online 2016;32:154−61.

[110] Bradley CK, McArthur SJ, Gee AJ, Weiss KA, Schmidt U, Toogood L. Intervention improves assisted conception intracytoplasmic sperm injection outcomes for patients with high levels of sperm DNA fragmentation: a retrospective analysis. Andrology 2016;4:903−10.

[111] Spano M, Cordelli E, Leter G, Lombardo F, Lenzi A, Gandini L. Nuclear chromatin variations in human spermatozoa undergoing swim-up and cryopreservation evaluated by the flow cytometric sperm chromatin structure assay. Mol Hum Reprod 1999;5(1):29−37.

[112] Zini A, Finelli A, Phang D, Jarvi K. Influence of semen processing technique on human sperm DNA integrity. Urology 2000;56(6):1081−4.

[113] Younglai EV, Holt D, Brown P, Jurisicova A, Casper RF. Sperm swim-up techniques and DNA fragmentation. Hum Reprod 2001;16(9):1950−3.

[114] Lopes S, Sun JG, Jurisicova A, Meriano J, Casper RF. Sperm deoxyribonucleic acid fragmentation is increased in poor-quality semen samples and correlates with failed fertilization in intracytoplasmic sperm injection. Fertil Steril 1998;69:528−32.

[115] Bungum M, Spano M, Humaidan P, Eleuteri P, Rescia M, Giwercman A. Sperm chromatin structure assay parameters measured after density gradient centrifugation are not predictive for the outcome of ART. Hum Reprod 2008;23(1):4−10.

[116] Bungum M, Humaidan P, Axmon A, Spano M, Bungum L, Erenpreiss J, Giwercman A. Sperm DNA integrity assessment in prediction of assisted reproduction technology outcome. Hum Reprod 2007;22:174−9.

[117] Daris B, Goropevsek A, Hojnik N, Vlaisavljevic V. Sperm morphological abnormalities as indicators of DNA fragmentation and fertilization in ICSI. Arch Gynecol Obstet 2010;281:363−7.

[118] Cassuto NG, Montjean D, Siffroi JP, Bouret D, Marzouk F, Copin H, Benkhalifa M. Different levels of DNA methylation detected in human sperms after morphological selection using high magnification microscopy. BioMed Res Int 2016:6372171. https://doi.org/10.1155/2016/6372171 [Epub 2016 Apr 11].

[119] Opuwari CS, Henkel RR. An update on oxidative damage to spermatozoa and oocytes. BioMed Res Int 2016:9540142. https://doi.org/10.1155/2016/9540142. Epub 2016 Jan 28.

[120] Cho CL, Agarwal A, Majzoub A, Esteves SC. Clinical utility of sperm DNA fragmentation testing: concise practice recommendations. Transl Androl Urol 2017;6(Suppl. 4):S366−73.

[121] Agarwal A, Nallella KP, Allamaneni SS, Said TM. Role of antioxidants in treatment of male infertility: an overview of the literature. Reprod Biomed Online 2004;8(6):616−27.

[122] Gharagozloo P, Aitken RJ. The role of sperm oxidative stress in male infertility and the significance of oral antioxidant therapy. Hum Reprod 2011;26(7):1628−40.

[123] Zini A, Al-Hathal N. Antioxidant therapy in male infertility: fact or fiction? Asian J Androl 2011;13(3):374.

[124] Greco E, Iacobelli M, Rienzi L, Ubaldi F, Ferrero S, Tesarik J. Reduction of the incidence of sperm DNA fragmentation by oral antioxidant treatment. J Androl 2005;26(3):349−53.

[125] Showell MG, Mackenzie-Proctor R, Brown J, Yazdani A, Stankiewicz MT, Hart RJ. Antioxidants for male subfertility. The Cochrane Library; 2014.

[126] Sierens J, Hartley JA, Campbell MJ, Leathem AJ, Woodside JV. In vitro isoflavone supplementation reduces hydrogen peroxide-induced DNA damage in sperm. Teratog Carcinog Mutagen 2002;22(3):227−34.

[127] Ten J, Vendrell FJ, Cano A, Tarín JJ. Dietary antioxidant supplementation did not affect declining sperm function with age in the mouse but did increase head abnormalities and reduced sperm production. Reprod Nutr Dev 1997;37:481−92.

[128] Donnelly ET, McClure N, Lewis SEM. Antioxidant supplementation in vitro does not improve human sperm motility. Fertil Steril 1999;72:484−95.

[129] Lanzafame FM, La Vignera S, Vicari E, Calogero AE. Oxidative stress and medical antioxidant treatment in male infertility. Reprod Biomed Online 2009;19:638−59.

[130] Busetto GM, Agarwal A, Virmani A, Antonini G, Ragonesi G, Del Guidice F, Micic S, Gentile V, De Berardinis E. Effect of metabolic and antioxidant supplementation on sperm parameters in oligo-astheno-teratozoospermia, with and without varicocele: a double-blind placebo-controlled study. Andrologia 2018;50(3). https://doi.org/10.1111/and.12927.

[131] Castagne V, Lefevre K, Natero R, Clarke PG, Bedker DA. An optimal redox status for the survival of axotomized ganglion cells in the developing retina. Neuroscience 1999;93:313−20.

Chapter 1.5

Leukocytes as a Cause of Oxidative Stress

Ralf R. Henkel and Michael C. Solomon, Jr.
University of the Western Cape, Bellville, South Africa

ORIGIN AND FUNCTION OF SEMINAL LEUKOCYTES

In 1943, MacLeod observed that spermatozoa rapidly lose their motility when incubated with oxygen [1]. Given the high content of polyunsaturated fatty acids (PUFAs), chiefly docosahexaenoic acid (DHA), sperm plasma membranes are prone to oxidation and thus damage of cellular integrity and function [2−4]. This impairment of sperm function either due to exposure to oxidants or reduced availability of protective antioxidative mechanisms in the reproductive organs or the semen is of pathophysiological importance in male factor fertility.

The main sources of these reactive oxygen species (ROS) include immature spermatozoa exhibiting an excess amount of residual cytoplasm and particularly seminal leukocytes [5], which normally appear in semen, even in that of healthy fertile men without a genital tract infection [6]. Considering their essential role in the body in immune surveillance and phagocytosis of pathogens including defective sperm [7], leukocytes produce large amounts of ROS, accounting for 1000 times higher production of ROS than that of spermatozoa [8,9] at capacitation [10]. However, in approximately 20%−30% of infertile men, the number of seminal leukocytes is elevated, resulting in a significantly higher ROS production as a concurrent result of genital tract infection, inflammatory , and cellular defense mechanisms [11]. The distribution profile of the different types of leukocytes depends on the individual and the type of infection. While polymorphonuclear (PMN) granulocytes are the most prevalent type of white blood cell in semen (50%−60%), macrophages and T-lymphocytes occur with 20%−30% and 2%−5%, respectively, much less. Whereas granulocytes originate predominantly from the prostate and seminal vesicles, other types of white blood cells derive predominantly from the epididymis and rete testis [6].

Comparing the seminal leukocyte concentration in fertile and infertile men shows generally lower white blood cell counts in fertile men. However, the extremely wide and overlapping ranges of leukocyte counts in fertile (mean: 0.17×10^6/mL; range: 0.009×10^6/mL to 20.52×10^6/mL) and infertile men (mean: 1.035×10^6/mL; range: 0.043×10^6/mL to 104.58×10^6/mL) [6] make it difficult to use the seminal white blood cell count as diagnostic parameter for male infertility. It also points to the importance of functionality and status of activation of leukocytes, which dictates the amount of active oxidants that are released. According to the World Health Organization in its latest Laboratory Manual for the Examination and Processing of Human Semen [12], a clinical cut-off value of 1×10^6/mL is recommended. On the one hand, a number of studies [13−16] have questioned this value as being too high. On the other hand, some authors suggested that the even higher leukocyte counts would have no effect on male fertility potential [17] or would have beneficial effects in supporting the induction of sperm acrosome reaction [18]. Barraud-Lange and coworkers [19] associated leukocyte levels less than 1×10^6 leukocytes/mL with increased fertilization rates and pregnancy outcomes. Yet recent literature, though not consenting to a certain cut-off value, rather indicates that elevated leukocyte counts have detrimental effects [20−22].

The question whether or not elevated numbers of leukocytes have detrimental effects on male fertility remains unanswered by clinical studies and the clinical significance of leukocytospermia on fertility is unclear. Clinical association between male genital tract infections/inflammations and oligozoospermia, asthenozoospermia, or even azoospermia [23,24] suggest deleterious effects of leukocytospermia on sperm function and integrity [25−27]. However, the negative implication of leukocytes on fertilization and pregnancy was not observed in the setting of assisted reproduction clinics [19,28,29]. Indeed, the effect and outcome of leukocytospermia may vary among patients. It has been reported that activated leukocytes in bacterial infections elicit more detrimental effects on fertility-compromised patients [30]. Activated leukocytes infiltrate the infected organs and release high amounts of ROS, resulting in infertility by membrane lipid peroxidation (LPO) via oxidative stress (OS) [31−33]. Thus, further studies are needed to clarify the effects of leukocytes on the male fertility potential.

SECRETIONS OF LEUKOCYTES

Immature spermatozoa and leukocytes (consisting of neutrophils and macrophages) in the male genital tract are known to generate ROS. The introduction of bacterial microorganisms elicits the host's defenses at the site of tissue entry (testis, epididymis, prostate gland, and seminal vesicles) via specific or nonspecific immunity [34]. In seminal plasma, spermatozoa are in contact with leukocytes for a relatively short period of time, namely from the point of ejaculation until the entry of the male germ cells into the cervix.

PMN granulocytes and macrophages destroy foreign material and cells by secreting oxidants including hydrogen peroxide and superoxide and phagocytosing the pathogens. PMNs further potentiate phagocytosis [35] in infections/inflammations, and together with macrophages are powerful producers of ROS [6,36,37]. In addition, these leukocytes secrete cytokines, a group of small proteins important for cell signaling. Generally, cytokines are broadly categorized in proinflammatory and antiinflammatory cytokines and further divided into chemokines, interferons, lymphokines, tumor necrosis factors, and interleukins (ILs), the latter of which are molecules that mediate communication between leukocytes and other cells involved in immune reactions (e.g., macrophages).

Macrophages located at tissue entry sites will release proteases, neutrophil chemotactic factors, and ROS signaling endothelial cells lining the blood vessels to present certain chemicals on the inner walls of the blood vessels upon activation. In turn, each WBC produces large amounts of ROS to combat infections from invading pathogens by stimulating the activity of G6PDH, generating high amounts of nicotinamide adenine dinucleotide phosphate (NADPH). NADPH oxidase further removes an electron from NADPH to convert oxygen into superoxide anion [38].

Cytokines occupy an important role in immunological and inflammatory mechanisms in response to host infections [39]. Agents such as ILs act by modulating leukocytes to produce an inflammatory response, and by downregulating inflammatory cells [40]. Excessive ROS generated due to infiltrating pathogens will activate cytokines CXCL, CXCL8, IL-6, and IL-8 [21,41]. The production of IL-8 from macrophages [42] exerts a negative effect on the fertilizing potential of spermatozoa [43]. The resulting infections also induce tissue damage, which stimulates the generation of IL-1 in the surrounding environment [44]. In turn, PMN neutrophils and macrophages secrete IL-6, which interacts with B-lymphocytes that become antibody-producing cells [45], which may further interfere with sperm function [46]. IL-2 is produced by T-cells in response to mitogen alloantigen antigen, potentiating the inflammatory response via the proliferation of T-cells. Moreover, numerous studies have shown a correlation between decreased sperm function and elevated levels of IL-6, IL-8, and tumor necrosis factor in seminal plasma, all of which contribute to sperm cell membrane LPO [47,48]. Therefore, an imbalance exists between antioxidants and seminal ROS levels, leading to OS-induced infertility [49]. High concentrations of seminal leukocytes reduce sperm/concentration and motility, and induce abnormal sperm morphology [25,50].

NATURE AND FEATURES OF REACTIVE OXYGEN SPECIES

Free atmospheric and dissolved oxygen appears as a molecule (O_2), not as a single atom, but it has two unpaired electrons with parallel spins in its outer molecular orbits, which renders it as paramagnetic biradical. Nevertheless, because of its unusual electronic structure, molecular oxygen is kinetically relatively inert. However, if O_2 reacts in oxidation reactions with other atoms or molecules, this process can only involve one electron at a time (Fig. 1). Thus, three types of reactions can take place leading to superoxide radical ($^{\bullet}O_2^-$) and related species, peroxyl radicals (ROO$^{\bullet}$), and singlet oxygen ($^1O_2$).

Chemically, ROS are highly reactive oxygen derivatives, which can be either radical or nonradical in nature. Chemical radicals are molecules such as superoxide ($^{\bullet}O_2^-$) or the hydroxyl radical ($\bullet$OH) that have one or more unpaired electrons in their outer orbit, which causes the molecule to be electronically unstable. As a result, such molecules are chemically unstable and highly reactive with extremely short half-life times ranging from milliseconds (10^{-3} s) to as low as nanoseconds (10^{-9} s) [51], depending on the specific oxygen derivative. Therefore, these molecules will react immediately after their generation at the site of generation. On the other hand, nonradical ROS such as hydrogen peroxide (H_2O_2) are highly reactive compounds, but are not radicals, meaning that these molecules have paired electrons with antiparallel spin

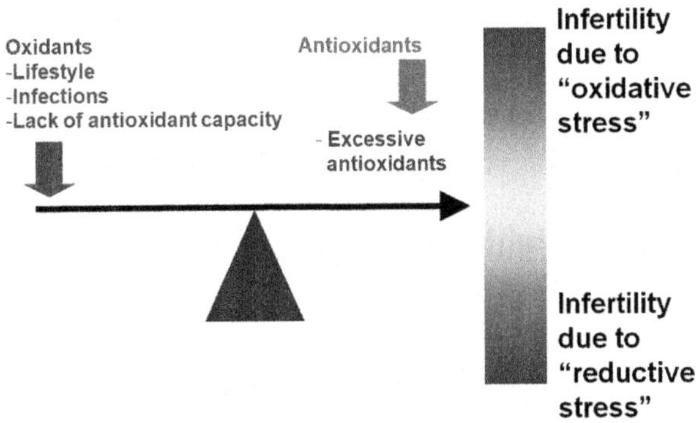

FIGURE 1 In a healthy body, oxidants and reductants (antioxidants) are in a finely balanced equilibrium, which ensures all cellular functions can be executed optimally. In case of oxidative stress, the amount of oxidants overwhelms the available antioxidants. Contrary, if antioxidants are available in surplus, the redox status of cells is forced into reductive stress. Both oxidative stress and reductive stress can cause male infertility, either due to overstimulation of sperm functions resulting in premature cellular actions, or in the inhibition thereof as a small physiological amount of ROS is necessary to induce capacitation and acrosome reaction, for example.

in their outer orbit [52]. The problem that arises with longer-living ROS (few of the ROS even show half-life times in the second range; RO•: 7 s) and those that are electronically uncharged such as hydrogen peroxide is that they are rather persistent, and can freely penetrate plasma membranes and travel longer distances and then exert their actions at other target sites. Consequently, H_2O_2, which is released by activated leukocytes, is not only able to damage the sperm plasma membrane, but also structures including the DNA inside the sperm cells [10,53,54]. Contrarily, charged molecules such as superoxide cannot penetrate the plasma membrane.

In light of the extreme high chemical reactivity of ROS, these compounds are generally thought to have detrimental effects on biological systems, hence are a cause of aging, dysfunction, disease, and infertility. On the other hand, various studies revealed that ROS are also essential triggers of important physiological cellular functions including hyperactivation, capacitation, and acrosome reaction [55–57].

In addition to oxygen derivatives, nitrogen (N_2) free radical derivatives also play biologically important roles. These compounds are referred to as reactive nitrogen species.

OXIDATIVE STRESS

From a chemical point of view, a reduced redox state is essential for normal cellular function. Although the exact redox balance varies depending on the respective physiological state of a cell, any cell produces its own ROS in the electron transfer chain in the mitochondria by leakage of up to 5% of the consumed oxygen, which is converted into free radicals [58,59], resulting in OS. In addition to intrinsic ROS production in sperm, extrinsic ROS production (e.g., by leukocytes, drugs, smoking, diabetes, or cancer) further poses challenges in maintaining a physiological redox balance [60,61]. Under normal circumstances, nonenzymatic scavengers (e.g., vitamins C and E, glutathione, L-carnitine ubiquinol) and enzymes (e.g., catalase or glutathione-peroxidase) play a major role in counterbalancing the OS. Studies also showed that albumin and carotenes may also relieve OS [62]. Consequently, oxidation and reduction results in a very finely balanced equilibrium, which enables cells to function properly and spermatozoa to fertilize oocytes [63]. In case this finely balanced cellular system is experiencing either an overexposure to oxidants or an undersupply of ;antioxidants, this will result in a condition referred to as OS, a concept in redox biology, which was coined by Sies [64].

Cells are able to neutralize OS through different principles—prevention, interception, and repair [65]—whereby prevention refers to the nonrelease of ROS through relevant enzymes and chelation of metal ions to control the process of LPO. ROS can also be neutralized by enzymatic or nonenzymatic elimination of the free radicals, thereby preventing these highly reactive compounds from chemically interacting with other molecules. The last resort, however, for any cell to counteract the damaging effects of ROS is their ability to repair damage to all relevant biomolecules including DNA. As a result, cells are constantly exposed to the interplay of oxidation and reduction and the swing in both directions, either leading to OS or to reductive stress (Fig. 1), which is as dangerous as OS [66], will have serious consequences for cellular function, individual wellbeing and health, and will include infertility and cancer. Both of the latter can be caused by DNA damage and the failure of cells to induce apoptotic pathways, which would normally eliminate cancerous cells.

EFFECT OF OXIDATIVE STRESS ON SPERM FUNCTIONS AND MALE FERTILITY

The most obvious effects of OS are either the direct oxidation and thereby damage of plasma membrane lipids or damage of DNA. In addition, in view of small amounts of ROS triggering essential physiological events such as capacitation, these functions can be overstimulated, leading to overreaction or premature triggering.

Oxidative Damage to Membrane Lipids

Considering that the plasma membrane of sperm contains an extraordinarily high amount of PUFAs [4,67,68] and a lack of cytoplasm with a relevant content of protective antioxidative enzymes, OS is particularly detrimental to sperm. In view of this dilemma that sperm are facing, antioxidative protection is normally provided by the seminal plasma, which contains high activities of superoxide dismutase (SOD) and catalase. The activity of these enzymes was found to be positively correlated with sperm progressive motility [69]. Significantly lower SOD levels were observed in seminal plasma of infertile patients [70] with the seminal total antioxidant capacity being recognized as a diagnostic parameter for male infertility [71].

PUFAs are lipids that have many conjugated carbon-carbon double-bonds in the molecules, which delocalize electrons over a wider area of the molecule and are therefore very prone to oxidation. When ROS attack these PUFAs they are initiating LPO, whereby the PUFAs are oxidatively degraded via lipid peroxyl and lipid hydroperoxyl radicals and eventually form genotoxic (4-hydroxy-2-alkenales such as 4-hydroxy-nonenal, resulting from $\omega6$ fatty acids like DHA, and 2-alkenales) and mutagenic (malondialdehyde) end products [72,73]. These by-products, in turn, pose a significant additional threat to the male germ cells as they damage the DNA through formation of DNA adducts (mainly pyrimido [1,2-*a*]purin-10(*3H*)-one), thereby indirectly damaging the DNA [74]. The direct damage of LPO to the membrane lipids leads to a decrease in membrane fluidity of both plasma and organelle membranes. Since sperm functions rely on membrane function, membrane ion gradients and receptor-mediated signal transduction are compromised [75,76]. Ultimately, these processes result in a loss of the sperm cell's functional ability, including fertilizing capacity [77,78]. In this connection, it appears that the site of the ROS generation seems to play a role as ROS deriving from leukocytes (i.e., outside of sperm) rather affect the plasma membrane and its functions, while sperm-derived ROS seem to affect the sperm nuclear DNA integrity [16]. In addition, sperm-derived ROS might also directly attack the mitochondrial membrane potential and mitochondrial DNA integrity [79–81].

Oxidative Damage to DNA

Apart from directly damaging the membrane lipids with the relevant indirect consequences for the DNA and genome, OS also causes significant direct damage to both nuclear (nDNA) [31,82–84] and mitochondrial (mtDNA) DNA [85,86], particularly the strong negative association between nuclear DNA fragmentation and male infertility indicators such as normal sperm morphology and motility [87,88]. Its relation to poor success rates with assisted reproduction has also been reported repeatedly, in original studies as well as in metaanalyses [89–92]. Yet by comparing different techniques to determine sperm nDNA damage (sperm chromatin structure assay, SCSA; sperm chromatin dispersion test, SCD; terminal deoxynucleotidyl transferase-mediated deoxyuridine triphosphate nick end labeling, TUNEL; single cell gel electrophoresis assay, Comet) as well as different methods of assisted reproduction (in vitro fertilization, IVF; intracytoplasmic sperm injection, ICSI; mixed cycles), it appears that determination of sperm DNA fragmentation has better prognostic value if it is measured with the TUNEL assay; prediction with the SCSA seemed to be ineffective or only poor [92,93]. On the other hand, it also appears that the connection between sperm nDNA damage caused by OS is without doubt for intrauterine insemination and IVF [31,94]. For ICSI, however, the relationship of DNA damage with fertilization and pregnancy is controversial [95,96]; reasons for this are still unknown.

Cells not only contain nuclear DNA, but also DNA (mtDNA) in the mitochondria, which is about 100 times more susceptible to assaults causing damage and mutations than nDNA [97] because mtDNA is not protected by histones and protamines. In addition, mtDNA replicates faster without appropriate proofreading and has only very basic DNA repair mechanisms [98], which renders this DNA especially vulnerable to OS. In this context, St. John et al. [99] indicated a potential risk of abnormal mtDNA transmission for patients undergoing assisted reproductive technique. More recently, Kao et al. [100], Shamsi et al. [101], and Venkatesh et al. [80] reported that ROS, mutations of mtDNA, and mtDNA depletion would be a major etiological factor for male infertility. Furthermore, Spiropoulos et al. [102] showed that high levels of mtDNA mutations strongly correlate with poor sperm motility. While in oligoasthenozoospermic patients mitochondrial DNA defects seems to be defective and unavailable for amplification, mitochondria were functional in motile sperm [85]. Treulen and coworkers [103] basically confirmed the idea that a breakdown in the mitochondrial membrane potential increases sperm ROS production, resulting in OS with decreased motility. By the same token, OS due to leukocytospermia would damage mitochondrial function by decreasing the mitochondrial membrane potential, which in turn would lead to a vicious cycle with even more intracellular ROS production [104].

A report by Bonanno et al. [105] indicated that asthenozoospermic patients not only show elevated ROS levels, but also a significantly increased number of mtDNA copies and decreased mtDNA integrity and mitochondrial membrane potential. The latter parameters were also closely associated with elevated ROS levels. Yet, nDNA fragmentation was increased in only 20% of the patients. From the available data it remains unclear whether or not this patient group with increased nuclear DNA damage represents an endpoint due to an extended or increased exposure of these spermatozoa to elevated levels of OS.

The debate on the role of mtDNA goes on with opposing results reported from other studies. Lim et al. [106] indicated that the oxidative damage to mtDNA would not be extensive and not higher than that in nuclear DNA. Yet in an analysis from a complete mtDNA sequencing of asthenozoospermic males, Pereira et al. [107] showed no evidence for a role of mtDNA in sperm motility, indicating that the hypothesis of the role of mitochondrial involvement in germ cell selection [108,109] would have to be treated very cautiously. Bandelt [110] highlighted that a misanalysis would have given a false association of mtDNA mutations with male infertility.

CONCLUSION

In light of the abundant evidence available indicating that OS is a major contributing factor to male infertility, numerous studies on its origins and molecular mechanisms of action are on the way. Leukocytes, as major ROS-producing cells in the ejaculate and a possible cause of infertility in a number of infertile men, have been widely studied. Nonetheless, the exact role of leukocytes is still a matter of dispute. The clinical cut-off value of leukocytospermia is not standardized. Yet it appears that the status of activation of leukocytes may be more important than their quantity in determining the potential damaging effect on spermatozoa. Likewise, more research is necessary, investigating not only the mechanisms by which the damage occurs but also how the damage can be avoided and treated. Different types of treatment of leukocytospermia and infections are discussed in Chapters 2.3.1 and 2.5.

REFERENCES

[1] MacLeod J. The role of oxygen in the metabolism and motility of human spermatozoa. Am J Physiol—Legacy Content 1943;138:512—8.

[2] Jones R, Mann T, Sherins R. Peroxidative breakdown of phospholipids in human spermatozoa, spermicidal properties of fatty acid peroxides, and protective action of seminal plasma. Fertil Steril 1979;31:531—7.

[3] Storey BT. Biochemistry of the induction and prevention of lipoperoxidative damage in human spermatozoa. Mol Hum Reprod 1997;3:203—13.

[4] Zalata AA, Christophe AB, Depuydt CE, Schoonjans F, Comhaire FH. The fatty acid composition of phospholipids of spermatozoa from infertile patients. Mol Hum Reprod 1998;4:111—8.

[5] Henkel RR. Leukocytes and oxidative stress: dilemma for sperm function and male fertility. Asian J Androl 2011;13:43—52.

[6] Wolff H. The biologic significance of white blood cells in semen. Fertil Steril 1995;63:1143—57.

[7] Plant TMEK, Neill JD. Knobil and Neill's physiology of reproduction. Amsterdam: Academic Press; 2015.

[8] Ford WC, Whittington K, Williams AC. Reactive oxygen species in human sperm suspensions: production by leukocytes and the generation of NADPH to protect sperm against their effects. Int J Androl 1997;20:44—9.

[9] Plante M, de Lamirande E, Gagnon C. Reactive oxygen species released by activated neutrophils, but not by deficient spermatozoa, are sufficient to affect normal sperm motility. Fertil Steril 1994;62:387—93.

[10] de Lamirande E, Gagnon C. Capacitation-associated production of superoxide anion by human spermatozoa. Free Radic Biol Med 1995;18:487—95.

[11] Henkel R, Maass G, Jung A, Haidl G, Schill W-B, Schuppe HC. Age-related changes in seminal polymorphonuclear elastase in men with asymptomatic inflammation of the genital tract. Asian J Androl 2007;9:299—304.

[12] WHO. WHO laboratory manual for the examination and processing of human semen. 5th ed. Switzerland: WHO Press; 2010.

[13] Aitken RJ, Paterson M, Fisher H, Buckingham DW, van Duin M. Redox regulation of tyrosine phosphorylation in human spermatozoa and its role in the control of human sperm function. J Cell Sci 1995;108:2017—25.

[14] Sharma RK, Pasqualotto AE, Nelson DR, Thomas Jr AJ, Agarwal A. Relationship between seminal white blood cell counts and oxidative stress in men treated at an infertility clinic. J Androl 2001;22:575—83.

[15] Punab M, Loivukene K, Kermes K, Mändar R. The limit of leucocytospermia from the microbiological viewpoint. Andrologia 2003;35:271—8.

[16] Henkel R, Kierspel E, Stalf T, Mehnert C, Menkveld R, Tinneberg HR, Schill WB, Kruger TF. Effect of reactive oxygen species produced by spermatozoa and leukocytes on sperm functions in non-leukocytospermic patients. Fertil Steril 2005;83:635—42.

[17] Yanushpolsky EH, Politch JA, Hill JA, Anderson DJ. Is leukocytospermia clinically relevant? Fertil Steril 1996;66:822—5.

[18] Kaleli S, Öcer F, Irez T, Budak E, Aksu MF. Does leukocytospermia associate with poor semen parameters and sperm functions in male infertility? The role of different seminal leukocyte concentrations. Eur J Obstet Gynecol Reprod Biol 2000;89:185–91.

[19] Barraud-Lange V, Pont JC, Ziyyat A, Pocate K, Sifer C, Cedrin-Durnerin I, Fechtali B, Ducot B, Wolf JP. Seminal leukocytes are Good Samaritans for spermatozoa. Fertil Steril 2011;96:1315–9.

[20] Lackner JE, Märk I, Sator K, Huber J, Sator M. Effect of leukocytospermia on fertilization and pregnancy rates of artificial reproductive technologies. Fertil Steril 2008;90:869–71.

[21] Sandoval JS, Raburn D, Muasher S. Leukocytospermia: overview of diagnosis, implications, and management of a controversial finding. Middle East Fertil Soc J 2013;18:129–34.

[22] Fraczek M, Hryhorowicz M, Gill K, Zarzycka M, Gaczarzewicz D, Jedrzejczak P, Bilinska B, Piasecka M, Kurpisz M. The effect of bacteriospermia and leukocytospermia on conventional and nonconventional semen parameters in healthy young normozoospermic males. J Reprod Immunol 2016;118:18–27.

[23] Weidner W, Colpi GM, Hargreave TB, Papp GK, Pomerol JM. EAU working group on male infertility. EAU guidelines on male infertility. Eur Urol 2002;42:313–22.

[24] Schuppe HC, Meinhardt A, Allam JP, Bergmann M, Weidner W, Haidl G. Chronic orchitis: a neglected cause of male infertility? Andrologia 2008;40:84–91.

[25] Aziz N, Saleh RA, Sharma RK, Lewis-Jones I, Esfandiari N, Thomas AJ, Agarwal A. Novel association between sperm reactive oxygen species production, sperm morphological defects, and the sperm deformity index. Fertil Steril 2004;81:349–54.

[26] Lackner JE, Herwig R, Schmidbauer J, Schatzl G, Kratzik C, Marberger M. Correlation of leukocytospermia with clinical infection and the positive effect of antiinflammatory treatment on semen quality. Fertil Steril 2006;86:601–5.

[27] Tomlinson MJ, White A, Barratt CLR, Bolton AE, Cooke ID. The removal of morphologically abnormal sperm forms by phagocytes: a positive role for seminal leukocytes? Hum Reprod 1992;7:517–22.

[28] Cavagna M, Oliveira JB, Petersen CG, Mauri AL, Silva LF, Massaro FC, Baruffi RL, Franco Jr JG. The influence of leukocytospermia on the outcomes of assisted reproductive technology. Reprod Biol Endocrinol 2012;10:44.

[29] Ricci G, Granzotto M, Luppi S, Giolo E, Martinelli M, Zito G, Borelli M. Effect of seminal leukocytes on in vitro fertilization and intracytoplasmic sperm injection outcomes. Fertil Steril 2015;104:87–93.

[30] Moretti E, Capitani S, Figura N, Pammolli A, Federico MG, Giannerini V, Collodel G. The presence of bacteria species in semen and sperm quality. J Assist Reprod Genet 2009;26:47–56.

[31] Henkel R, Hajimohammad M, Stalf T, Hoogendijk C, Mehnert C, Menkveld R, Gips H, Schill W-B, Kruger TF. Influence of deoxyribonucleic acid damage on fertilization and pregnancy. Fertil Steril 2004;81:965–72.

[32] Aitken RJ, Clarkson JS, Hargreave TB, Irvine DS, Wu FC. Analysis of the relationship between defective sperm function and the generation of reactive oxygen species in cases of oligozoospermia. J Androl 1989;10:214–20.

[33] Martínez P, Proverbio F, Camejo MI. Sperm lipid peroxidation and pro-inflammatory cytokines. Asian J Androl 2007;9:102–7.

[34] Ochsendorf FR. Infections in the male genital tract and reactive oxygen species. Hum Reprod Update 1999;5:399–420.

[35] Fantone JC, Ward PA. Role of oxygen-derived free radicals and metabolites in leukocyte-dependent inflammatory reactions. Am J Pathol 1982;107:395–418.

[36] Wolff H, Anderson DJ. Immunohistologic characterization and quantitation of leukocyte subpopulations in human semen. Fertil Steril 1988;49:497–504.

[37] Fedder J, Askjaer SA, Hjort T. Nonspermatozoal cells in semen: relationship to other semen parameters and fertility status of the couple. Arch Androl 1993;31:95–103.

[38] Agarwal A, Rana M, Qiu E, AlBunni H, Bui AD, Henkel R. Role of oxidative stress, infection and inflammation in male infertility. Andrologia 2018 [submitted for publication].

[39] Solomon M, Henkel R. Semen culture and the assessment of genitourinary tract infections. Ind J Urol 2017;33:188–93.

[40] Comhaire FH, Mahmoud AMA, Depuydt CE, Zalata AA, Christophe AB. Mechanisms and effects of male genital tract infection on sperm quality and fertilizing potential: the andrologist's viewpoint. Hum Reprod Update 1999;5:393–8.

[41] Comhaire F, Bosmans E, Ombelet W, Punjabi U, Schoonjans F. Cytokines in semen of normal men and of patients with andrological diseases. Am J Reprod Immunol 1994;31:99–103.

[42] Yoshimura T, Matsushima K, Oppenheim JJ, Leonard EJ. Neutrophil chemotactic factor produced by lipopolysaccharide (LPS)-stimulated human blood mononuclear leukocytes: partial characterization and separation from interleukin 1 (IL1). J Immunol 1987;139:788–93.

[43] Yamauchi-Takihara K, Ihara Y, Ogata A, Yoshizaki K, Azuma J, Kishimoto T. Hypoxic stress induces cardiac myocyte–derived interleukin-6. Circulation 1995;91:1520–4.

[44] Arend WP, Dayer J. Naturally occurring inhibitors of cytokines. In: Davies ME, Dingle JT, editors. Immunopharmacology of joints and connective tissue. London: Academic Press; 1994. p. 129.

[45] Hirano T, Akira S, Taga T, Kishimoto T. Biological and clinical aspects of interleukin 6. Immunol Today 1990;11:443–9.

[46] Depuydt C, Zalata A, Christophe A, Mahmoud A, Comhaire F. Mechanisms of sperm deficiency in male accessory gland infection. Andrologia 1998;30(S1):29–33.

[47] Nandipati KC, Pasqualotto FF, Thomas AJ, Agarwal A. Relationship of interleukin-6 with semen characteristics and oxidative stress in vasectomy reversal patients. Andrologia 2005;37:131–4.

[48] Lavranos G, Balla M, Tzortzopoulou A, Syriou V, Angelopoulou R. Investigating ROS sources in male infertility: a common end for numerous pathways. Reprod Toxicol 2012;34:298−307.

[49] Agarwal A, Saleh RA, Bedaiwy MA. Role of reactive oxygen species in the pathophysiology of human reproduction. Fertil Steril 2003;79:829−43.

[50] Saleh RA, Agarwal A, Kandirali E, Sharma RK, Thomas AJ, Nada EA, Evenson DP, Alvarez JG. Leukocytospermia is associated with increased reactive oxygen species production by human spermatozoa. Fertil Steril 2002;78:1215−24.

[51] Halliwell B, Gutteridge JMC. Free radicals in biology and medicine. 2nd ed. Oxford: Clarendon Press; 1989.

[52] Cadenas E. Biochemistry of oxygen toxicity. Annu Rev Biochem 1989;58:79−110.

[53] Tosic J, Walton A. Metabolism of spermatozoa: the formation and elimination of hydrogen peroxide by spermatozoa and effects on motility and survival. Biochem J 1950;47:199−202.

[54] Griveau JF, Dumont E, Renard P, Callegari JP, le Lannou D. Reactive oxygen species, lipid peroxidation and enzymatic defence systems in human spermatozoa. J Reprod Fertil 1995;103:17−26.

[55] de Lamirande E, Gagnon C. A positive role for the superoxide anion in triggering hyperactivation and capacitation of human spermatozoa. Int J Androl 1993;16:21−5.

[56] de Lamirande E, Jiang H, Zini A, Kodama H, Gagnon C. Reactive oxygen species and sperm physiology. Rev Reprod 1997;2:48−54.

[57] O'Flaherty CM, Beorlegui NB, Beconi MT. Reactive oxygen species requirements for bovine sperm capacitation and acrosome reaction. Theriogenology 1999;52:289−301.

[58] Boveris A, Chance B. The mitochondrial generation of hydrogen peroxide. General properties and effect of hyperbaric oxygen. Biochem J 1973;134:707−16.

[59] Chance B, Sies H, Boveris A. Hydroperoxide metabolism in mammalian organs. Physiol Rev 1979;59:527−605.

[60] Agarwal A, Prabakaran SA, Sikka SC. Clinical relevance of oxidative stress in patients with male factor infertility: evidence-based analysis. AUA Update Ser 2007;26(Lesson 1):1−12.

[61] Sharma R, Biedenharn KR, Fedor JM, Agarwal A. Lifestyle factors and reproductive health: taking control of your fertility. Reprod Biol Endocrinol 2013;11:66.

[62] Zini A, Al-Hathal N. Antioxidant therapy in male infertility: fact or fiction? Asian J Androl 2011;13:374−81.

[63] Garrido N, Meseguer M, Simon C, Pellicer A, Remohi J. Pro-oxidative and anti-oxidative imbalance in human semen and its relation with male fertility. Asian J Androl 2004;6:59−65.

[64] Sies H. Oxidative stress: introductory remarks. In: Sies H, editor. Oxidative stress. London: Academic Press; 1985. p. 1−8.

[65] Sies H. Strategies of antioxidant defense. Eur J Biochem 1993;215:213−9.

[66] Castagne V, Lefevre K, Natero R, Clarke PG, Bedker DA. An optimal redox status for the survival of axotomized ganglion cells in the developing retina. Neuroscience 1999;93:313−20.

[67] Parks JE, Lynch DV. Lipid composition and thermotropic phase behavior of boar, bull, stallion, and rooster sperm membranes. Cryobiology 1992;29:255−66.

[68] Sanocka D, Kurpisz M. Reactive oxygen species and sperm cells. Reprod Biol Endocrinol 2004;2:12.

[69] Macanovic B, Vucetic M, Jankovic A, Stancic A, Buzadzic B, Garalejic E, Korac A, Korac B, Otasevic V. Correlation between sperm parameters and protein expression of antioxidative defense enzymes in seminal plasma: a pilot study. Dis Markers 2015:436236. https://doi.org/10.1155/2015/436236 [Epub 2015 Jan 27].

[70] Murawski M, Saczko J, Marcinkowska A, Chwiłkowska A, Gryboś M, Banaś T. Evaluation of superoxide dismutase activity and its impact on semen quality parameters of infertile men. Folia Histochem Cytobiol 2007;45(Suppl. 1):S123−6.

[71] Roychoudhury S, Sharma R, Sikka S, Agarwal A. Diagnostic application of total antioxidant capacity in seminal plasma to assess oxidative stress in male factor infertility. J Assist Reprod Genet 2016;33:627−35.

[72] Esterbauer H. Cytotoxicity and genotoxicity of lipid-oxidation products. Am J Clin Nutr 1993;57(5 Suppl.):779S−85S.

[73] Luczaj W, Skrzydlewska E. DNA damage caused by lipid peroxidation products. Cell Mol Biol Lett 2003;8:391−413.

[74] Marnett LJ. Lipid peroxidation-DNA damage by malondialdehyde. Mutat Res 1999;424:83−95.

[75] Sikka SC, Rajasekaran M, Hellstrom WJ. Role of oxidative stress and antioxidants in male infertility. J Androl 1995;16:464−8.

[76] Sikka SC. Relative impact of oxidative stress on male reproductive function. Curr Med Chem 2001;8:851−62.

[77] Carpino A, Siciliano L, Petroni MF, De Stefano C, Aquila S, Ando S, Petroni MF. Low seminal zinc bound to high molecular weight proteins in asthenozoospermic patients: evidence of increased sperm zinc content in oligoasthenozoospermic patients. Hum Reprod 1998;13:111−4.

[78] Veaute C, Andreoli MF, Racca A, Bailat A, Scalerandi MV, Bernal C, Malan Borel I. Effects of isomeric fatty acids on reproductive parameters in mice. Am J Reprod Immunol 2007;58:487−96.

[79] Wang X, Sharma RK, Gupta A, George V, Thomas AJ, Falcone T, Agarwal A. Alterations in mitochondria membrane potential and oxidative stress in infertile men: a prospective observational study. Fertil Steril 2003;80(Suppl. 2):844−50.

[80] Venkatesh S, Deecaraman M, Kumar R, Shamsi MB, Dada R. Role of reactive oxygen species in the pathogenesis of mitochondrial DNA (mtDNA) mutations in male infertility. Indian J Med Res 2009;129:127−37.

[81] Sousa AP, Amaral A, Baptista M, Tavares R, Caballero Campo P, Caballero Peregrín P, Freitas A, Paiva A, Almeida-Santos T, Ramalho-Santos J. Not all sperm are equal: functional mitochondria characterize a subpopulation of human sperm with better fertilization potential. PLoS One 2011;6:e18112.

[82] De Jonge C. The clinical value of sperm nuclear DNA assessment. Hum Fertil 2002;5:51−3.

[83] Seli E, Gardner DK, Schoolcraft WB, Moffatt O, Sakkas D. Extent of nuclear DNA damage in ejaculated spermatozoa impacts on blastocyst development after in vitro fertilization. Fertil Steril 2004;82:378—83.

[84] Shamsi MB, Kumar R, Dada R. Evaluation of nuclear DNA damage in human spermatozoa in men opting for assisted reproduction. Indian J Med Res 2008;127:115—23.

[85] Carra E, Sangiorgi D, Gattuccio F, Rinaldi AM. Male infertility and mitochondrial DNA. Biochem Biophys Res Commun 2004;322:333—9.

[86] Wai T, Ao A, Zhang X, Cyr D, Dufort D, Shoubridge EA. The role of mitochondrial DNA copy number in mammalian fertility. Biol Reprod 2010;83:52—62.

[87] Zribi N, Chakroun NF, Elleuch H, Abdallah FB, Ben Hamida AS, Gargouri J, Fakhfakh F, Keskes LA. Sperm DNA fragmentation and oxidation are independent of malondialdheyde. Reprod Biol Endocrinol 2011;9:47.

[88] Sa R, Cunha M, Rocha E, Barros A, Sousa M. Sperm DNA fragmentation is related to sperm morphological staining patterns. Reprod Biomed Online 2015;31:506—15.

[89] Zini A, Boman JM, Belzile E, Ciampi A. Sperm DNA damage is associated with an increased risk of pregnancy loss after IVF and ICSI: systematic review and meta-analysis. Hum Reprod 2008;23:2663—8.

[90] Osman A, Alsomait H, Seshadri S, El-Toukhy T, Khalaf Y. The effect of sperm DNA fragmentation on live birth rate after IVF or ICSI: a systematic review and meta-analysis. Reprod Biomed Online 2015;30:120—7.

[91] Simon L, Zini A, Dyachenko A, Ciampi A, Carrell DT. A systematic review and meta-analysis to determine the effect of sperm DNA damage on in vitro fertilization and intracytoplasmic sperm injection outcome. Asian J Androl 2017;19:80—90.

[92] Cissen M, Wely MV, Scholten I, Mansell S, Bruin JP, Mol BW, Braat D, Repping S, Hamer G. Measuring sperm DNA fragmentation and clinical outcomes of medically assisted reproduction: a systematic review and meta-analysis. PLoS One 2016;11:e0165125.

[93] Li Z, Wang L, Cai J, Huang H. Correlation of sperm DNA damage with IVF and ICSI outcomes: a systematic review and meta-analysis. J Assist Reprod Genet 2006;23:367—76.

[94] Duran EH, Morshedi M, Taylor S, Oehninger S. Sperm DNA quality predicts intrauterine insemination outcome: a prospective cohort study. Hum Reprod 2002;17:3122—8.

[95] Speyer BE, Pizzey AR, Ranieri M, Joshi R, Delhanty JD, Serhal P. Fall in implantation rates following ICSI with sperm with high DNA fragmentation. Hum Reprod 2010;7:1609—18.

[96] Anifandis G, Bounartzi T, Messini CI, Dafopoulos K, Markandona R, Sotiriou S, Tzavella A, Messinis IE. Sperm DNA fragmentation measured by Halosperm does not impact on embryo quality and ongoing pregnancy rates in IVF/ICSI treatments. Andrologia 2015;47:295—302.

[97] Pesole G, Gissi C, De Chirico A, Saccone C. Nucleotide substitution rate of mammalian mitochondrial genomes. J Mol Evol 1999;48:427—34.

[98] Croteau DL, Stierum RH, Bohr VA. Mitochondrial DNA repair pathways. Mutat Res 1999;434:137—48.

[99] St John JC, Lloyd R, El Shourbagy S. The potential risks of abnormal transmission of mtDNA through assisted reproductive technologies. Reprod Biomed Online 2004;8:34—44.

[100] Kao SH, Chao HT, Liu HW, Liao TL, Wei YH. Sperm mitochondrial DNA depletion in men with asthenospermia. Fertil Steril 2004;82:66—73.

[101] Shamsi MB, Kumar R, Bhatt A, Bamezai RN, Kumar R, Gupta NP, Das TK, Dada R. Mitochondrial DNA mutations in etiopathogenesis of male infertility. Indian J Urol 2008;24:150—4.

[102] Spiropoulos J, Turnbull DM, Chinnery PF. Can mitochondrial DNA mutations cause sperm dysfunction? Mol Hum Reprod 2002;8:719—21.

[103] Treulen F, Uribe P, Boguen R, Villegas JV. Mitochondrial outer membrane permeabilization increases reactive oxygen species production and decreases mean sperm velocity but is not associated with DNA fragmentation in human sperm. Mol Hum Reprod 2015;30:767—76.

[104] Henkel R. ROS and DNA integrity—implications of male accessory gland infections. In: Björndahl L, Giwercman A, Tournaye H, Weidner W, editors. Clinical andrology. Informa Healthcare (incorporating Parthenon Publishing, Marcel Dekker, and Taylor & Francis Medical (London)); 2010. p. 324—8.

[105] Bonanno O, Romeo G, Asero P, Pezzino FM, Castiglione R, Burrello N, Sidoti G, Frajese GV, Vicari E, D'Agata R. Sperm of patients with severe asthenozoospermia show biochemical, molecular and genomic alterations. Reproduction 2016;152:695—704.

[106] Lim KS, Jeyaseelan K, Whiteman M, Jenner A, Halliwell B. Oxidative damage in mitochondrial DNA is not extensive. Ann N Y Acad Sci 2005;1042:210—20.

[107] Pereira L, Goncalves J, Franco-Duarte R, Silva J, Rocha T, Arnold C, Richards M, Macaulay V. No evidence for an mtDNA role in sperm motility: data from complete sequencing of asthenozoospermic males. Mol Biol Evol 2007;24:868—74.

[108] Moore FL, Reijo-Pera RA. Male sperm motility dictated by mother's mtDNA. Am J Hum Genet 2000;67:543—8.

[109] Giannelli F. Mitochondria and the quality of human gametes. Am J Hum Genet 2001;68:1535—7.

[110] Bandelt HJ. Misanalysis gave false association of mtDNA mutations with infertility. Int J Androl 2008;31:450—3.

Chapter 1.6

Human Spermatozoa and Interactions With Oxidative Stress

Jaideep S. Toor and Suresh C. Sikka
Tulane University, New Orleans, LA, United States

INTRODUCTION

Physiological levels of reactive oxygen species (ROS) play a crucial role in spermatogenesis, as well as in the sperm physiological processes like capacitation, hyperactivation, and ova penetration. However, the overproduction of ROS leads to oxidative stress (OS), which damages the sperm membrane, DNA, and mitochondria, leading to decreased sperm motility, and also reduces the chances of fusion between sperm and oocyte. The contribution of ROS to male infertility is estimated to be between 30% and 80% [1].

OS reflects the imbalance of ROS (free radicals), which modulates various biological processes by activating several signal-transduction pathways. These free radicals, which include highly reactive molecules with unpaired electrons, serve as second messengers/signaling molecules. Free radicals can alter the DNA methylation pattern, which regulates the expression of various genes via DNA methyltransferase and transcription factors regulating signal transduction cascades. High ROS levels can influence cellular activities via calcium signaling pathways (calcium influx and store mobilization), protein phosphorylation, and various protein-kinase signaling pathways, which include the mitogen-activated protein kinase pathways and tumorigenic signaling pathway (phosphoinositide 3-kinase (PI3K)) [2]. Another important function of ROS is the induction of tumor necrosis factor and interleukins, followed by the increased expression of transcription factor NF-κB (nuclear factor kappa-light-chain-enhancer of activated B cells), which inhibits apoptosis and promotes cell survival, possibly linking OS with male infertility [2−4]. Many such signals are redox-sensitive, which requires maintaining an optimal balance between ROS levels and cellular function. This chapter briefly relates to such interaction between ROS and sperm function.

WHAT ARE REACTIVE OXYGEN SPECIES?

ROS refer to a pool of reactive oxygen molecules, which include free radicals and derivatives capable of inducing oxidative changes within the cell. These oxidizing agents are generated by endogenous (e.g., mitochondrial electron transport chain (ETC), lipoxygenases, peroxisomes, nicotinamide adenine dinucleotide phosphate (NADPH) oxidase (NOX), and cytochrome P450) as well as exogenous factors (e.g., ionizing radiation, ultraviolet light, drugs, xenobiotics, inflammatory cytokines, and many environmental toxins) (Table 1) [5−7].

The superoxide anion ($O_2^{\bullet-}$) radical is the most important widespread ROS formed by enzymatic processes, auto-oxidation reactions, and a nonenzymatic electron transfer reaction, in which an electron is transferred to molecular oxygen. The generation of superoxide radical from oxygen (O_2) is mediated by; (1) NOX complex, (2) xanthine oxidase, and/or (3) peroxidases. Once formed, it is involved in several reactions that, in turn, generate hydroxyl radical (OH•), hydrogen peroxide (H_2O_2), peroxynitrite ($ONOO^-$), and hypochlorous acid (HOCl). H_2O_2 (a nonradical) is produced by multiple oxidase enzymes, (e.g., amino acid oxidase and xanthine oxidase). The hydroxyl radical (OH•) is the most reactive among all the free radical species in vivo and is generated by reaction of $O_2^{\bullet-}$ with H_2O_2, with Fe^{2+} or Cu^+ as a reaction catalyst (Fenton reaction) [8−14] (Fig. 1). Superoxide anions interact with nitric oxide (NO•), resulting in the formation of

TABLE 1 Source of Reactive Oxygen Species

Endogenous	Exogenous
Mitochondria (by-products of electron transport)	Chemotherapeutics
Inflammation (neutrophils, macrophages)	Dietary factors
Peroxisomal fatty acid metabolism (peroxisomes, lipoxygenases)	Inflammatory cytokines (macrophages, neutrophils)
Cytochrome P450 reactions	Ionizing radiation (X−, γ−, UV)
Oxidases (Oxidase-catalyzed reactions)	Cigarette smoke
Arginine metabolism	Industrial solvent
NADPH oxidase (NOX)	Pesticides

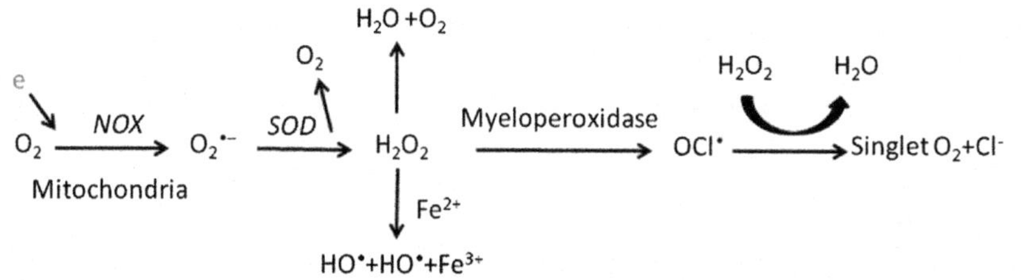

FIGURE 1 Diagrammatic representation of generation of ROS. *NOX*, NADPH oxidase; *ROS*, reactive oxygen species; *SOD*, superoxide dismutase.

TABLE 2 Two Common Forms of Free Radicals: (1) Reactive Oxygen Species (ROS) That Are Considered to Be Oxidizing Agents Generated as a Result of Metabolism of Oxygen and (2) Reactive Nitrogen Species (RNS) That Are Considered to Be a Subclass of ROS

Reactive Oxygen Species		Reactive Nitrogen Species	
Free radical	Structural formula	Free radical	Structural formula
Superoxide anion	$O_2^{\bullet-}$	Nitric oxide	$NO^\bullet$
Hydrogen peroxide	H_2O_2	Nitrous oxide	N_2O
Hydroxyl radical	OH^-	Peroxynitrite	$ONOO^-$
Peroxyl radical	ROO^-	Nitroxyl anion	$HNO^\bullet$
Alkoxyl radical	RO^-	Nitrogen dioxide	NO_2

peroxynitrite ($ONOO^-$). The reactive nitrogen species (nitrogen radicals) are a subclass of ROS (Table 6.2). The nitrogen species derived from $NO^\bullet$ and peroxynitrite anion ($ONOO^-$) are important for reproduction and fertilization. NO is an oxygen-free radical that is generated from the oxidation of the amino acids L-arginine to L-citrulline by NAPDH-dependent NO synthases (NOS) [15].

The most abundant major type of ROS are superoxide anion, hydrogen peroxide, and hydroxyl radicals, each of which has distinct biological targets based on its chemical properties (chemical reactivity, half-life, and lipid solubility). ROS have two different actions.

● First, with their unstable and highly reactive chemical nature, ROS react and can cause damage to proteins, lipids, carbohydrates, and DNA [16,17], affecting different cellular processes (apoptosis, necrosis, autophagy, and senescence) related to aging, various disease, and cell death (Fig. 2) [18].
● Second, ROS act as a stimulating agent for biological processes within the cell. At normal physiological levels, ROS directly interacts with critical signaling molecules involved in cellular homeostatic functions such as proliferation and survival via heat-shock transcription factor 1, NF-κB, p53, tyrosine phosphatases, Nrf-2, PI3K, and MAP kinase pathways [9,19].

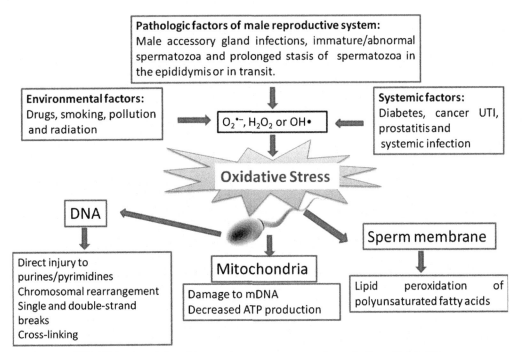

FIGURE 2 Association of increased reactive oxygen species production with infertility.

PHYSIOLOGICAL ROLES OF REACTIVE OXYGEN SPECIES IN SEMINAL PLASMA

ROS exhibit a dual role on sperm function, which can lead to both beneficial and detrimental effects, depending on the nature, strength, and duration of its exposure. Its levels must be tightly regulated by continuous inactivation while allowing normal cell function. Excessive generation of ROS in semen may cause damage to spermatozoa due to the fact that the sperm plasma membrane contains high contents of ROS attack sensitive polyunsaturated fatty acid, which gives the sperm cell the needed fluidity for membrane fusion during fertilization. This results in decreased sperm motility (due to loss of adenosine triphosphate (ATP) production leading to axonemal damage), decreased sperm viability, and midpiece sperm morphological defects [20].

The male germ cells start producing small amount of ROS from the earliest stages of the development [21]. In this phase, ROS plays an important role in sperm chromatin condensation and controlling germ cell number by regulating apoptosis or proliferation of spermatogonia [22]. In mature spermatozoa, low levels of ROS have been shown to be essential for fertilization, capacitation/acrosome reaction (AR), mitochondrial stability, and progressive sperm motion [10,23]. ROS also help transmit signals by increasing the influx of calcium ions and inducing chain reactions leading to increased production of ATP [24].

REACTIVE OXYGEN SPECIES GENERATION IN SPERMATOZOA

In 1943, John Macleod was the first to demonstrate the ability of human sperm to produce ROS [25]. Forty-five years later, by using the chemiluminescent probe luminol, Aitken and Clarkson (1987) confirmed such ROS production by human sperm [26]. Since then, multiple studies have shown that ROS play an important sperm physiological role [27,28]. It can induce spermatozoa capacitation and AR via cAMP-induced tyrosine phosphorylation of nuclear factor NF-κB p105 subunit and ezrin proteins [2,29]. The ability of H_2O_2 to suppress tyrosine-phosphatase activity results in ROS-induced tyrosine phosphorylation and an increase in cAMP levels. This is comparable to the effects of bicarbonate, which activates soluble adenylyl cyclase in sperm [29]. Hydrogen peroxide enhances adenylyl cyclase activity to produce cAMP and protein kinase A-dependent tyrosine phosphorylation. Oxidative phosphorylation in the inner mitochondrial membrane releases energy used to produce ATP. ROS are generated mainly as a by-product of mitochondrial respiration, resulting in a decrease in sperm motility and fusion with the vitelline membrane of the oocyte. This redox biology referring to low/steady production of ROS initiates capacitation. However, if ROS levels go higher or the spermatozoa are exposed to exogenous or endogenous ROS generated by morphological abnormal spermatozoa, precursor germ cells, and leukocytes (e.g., in leukocytospermia), then a state of OS can be readily induced.

Spermatozoa, characterized by high polyunsaturated fatty acid content, which is required to provide the plasma membrane with the fluidity essential for fertilization, are particularly vulnerable to such stress and their limited store of antioxidant enzymes such as superoxide dismutase or glutathione peroxidase [22]. These characteristics make spermatozoa functionally incompetent when exposed to ROS generated by xanthine oxidase at levels having a negligible effect on somatic cells and, importantly, this effect can be reversed by the addition of catalase [30,31]. Similar studies have demonstrated the damaging effect of ROS not only in functional aspects but also the genomic integrity of human spermatozoa [32,33]. This is also related to the human paternal diseases where endogenous ROS produced by spermatozoa have a direct effect on the spermatozoa functional competence and its nuclear DNA [34].

MECHANISM OF REACTIVE OXYGEN SPECIES PRODUCTION BY SPERMATOZOA

In spermatozoa, there are multiple sources of ROS that mainly include intracellular oxidases/peroxidases like NOX enzyme complex present in the sperm plasma membrane and leakage of electrons from the ETC within the mitochondria [35,36]. Production of superoxide, the major ROS of human spermatozoa, involves an enzyme NADH oxido-reductase (diaphorase) located within the midpiece of spermatozoa together with the mitochondrial respiratory chain [37]. Immature or infertile spermatozoa with impaired morphology (excessive cytoplasmic residue) have greater ROS production than normal spermatozoa [38,39]. Also, maturing spermatozoa during spermatogenesis and when passing through the epididymis produce different levels of ROS [40,41].

NADPH OXIDASES GENERATED REACTIVE OXYGEN SPECIES BY SPERMATOZOA: ROLE IN CAPACITATION

The involvement of ROS in physiological and pathological processes in spermatozoa is well defined, but the identification of ROS-producing enzyme systems remains a matter of speculation. NADPH-dependent generation of ROS is related to the NOX family [42,43]. NOX1 was the first candidate for $O_2^{\bullet-}$ generation in human spermatozoa; however, the characteristics of $O_2^{\bullet-}$ production (measured by chemiluminescence using the $O_2^{\bullet-}$-specific probe MCLA) between the sperm oxidase and NOX1 from neutrophils are completely different [44]. Few important differences that had questioned the presence of NOX1 were as follows:

1. Spermatozoa produced three times less superoxide during capacitation in comparison to activated neutrophils. The superoxide production takes place over a period of hours in spermatozoa instead of the $O_2^{\bullet-}$ burst seen in 30–40 min in leukocytes.
2. Zinc (Zn^{2+}) or semenogelin (Sg) have a greater inhibitory effect on $O_2^{\bullet-}$ production in spermatozoa than that produced in neutrophils.
3. Kinases such as PKC, PTK, and ERK, which activate NOX1, have no influence on production of $O_2^{\bullet-}$ by human spermatozoa [45–47].

Studies using immunocytochemistry and immunoblotting confirmed the absence of NOX1, NOX2, and NOX4 in human spermatozoa. NOX5 is expressed in the testis and may also generate ROS in spermatozoa [48–50]. NOX5 is activated by calcium and is associated with sperm motility [8,51]. However, because of its localization—mostly in the flagellum and midpiece—as well as its regulation by PKC, it is unlikely that this isoform is the source of $O_2^{\bullet-}$ required for sperm capacitation.

Regardless of the identity of the sperm oxidase, NADPH is essential to generate either $O_2^{\bullet-}$ or NO• (Fig. 3) [52]. The isoform C4 of lactate dehydrogenase is specific to testis and spermatozoa, and is seen in several species [53,54].

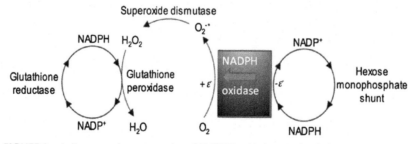

FIGURE 3 A diagrammatic representation of NADPH oxidation reaction in human spermatozoa.

It generates NADH upon oxidation of lactate into pyruvate and is found in the cytosol, mitochondria, and the plasma membrane of many species. This isoform of the enzyme represents more than 80% of lactate dehydrogenase activity in spermatozoa [54]. The addition of NADPH has been associated with the production of $O_2^{\bullet-}$ in human spermatozoa [55,56]. The in vivo supply of NADPH could be accomplished by two different enzymes: isocitrate dehydrogenase (ICDH) and glucose 6-phosphate dehydrogenase (G6PDH). Both enzymes are present in the cytosol of spermatozoa, as confirmed by various proteomic studies [46,57–59]. Whether the ICDH is involved in human sperm capacitation remains unknown.

NITRIC OXIDE SYNTHASE GENERATED REACTIVE NITROGEN SPECIES BY SPERMATOZOA DURING CAPACITATION

Nitric oxide (NO•), is produced from L-arginine via NOS. The reaction takes place in the presence of oxygen and other cofactors (e.g., NADPH, flavin mononucleotide (FMN), flavin adenine dinucleotide, calmodulin, and calcium), resulting in the production of NO and L-citrulline [60,61]. Human spermatozoa express three NOS isoforms (neuronal, endothelial, and inducible NOS), located in the head and/or flagellum of the sperm [45,62,63]. Physiological levels of NO• are important for various sperm functions such as capacitation, acrosomal reaction, zona pellucida binding, and also in maintaining sperm motility, morphology, and viability [44,61,64].

Specific inhibitors of NOS such as N^G-monomethyl-L-arginine (L-NMMA) or N^G-nitro-L-arginine methyl ester (L-NAME) prevent sperm capacitation, suggesting the role of NO in this process [44,65,66]. Human spermatozoa incubated with diethyl amine (DA)-NONOate (a NO• donor) and superoxide dismutase (SOD), a scavenger of $O_2^{\bullet-}$, or with the xanthine–xanthine oxidase (X–XO) system, a well-known $O_2^{\bullet-}$ generator, and either L-NAME or L-NMMA, were unable to undergo capacitation. Moreover, the addition of DA-NONOate triggered the production of $O_2^{\bullet-}$ while the production of NO• was stimulated by the X–XO system. These series of experiments demonstrate that the production of $O_2^{\bullet-}$ depends on NO•, and vice versa [46].

REACTIVE OXYGEN SPECIES AND IMMATURE SPERMATOZOA

Subsets of human spermatozoa at different stages of development and maturation can produce ROS. Morphologically abnormal spermatozoa are very active in ROS production [67,68]. Sperm with residual cytoplasm or cytoplasmic droplet are considered the most important in ROS production [67,68]. During normal spermiogenesis, the majority of cytoplasm is extruded from the maturing spermatozoa. The remaining cytoplasmic droplet in the midpiece contains enzymes required for energy production such as glucose-6-phosphate dehydrogenase and creatinine kinase and helps in the reduction of $NADP^+$ to NADPH leading to production of ROS by NOX [69]. It is thought that excess residual cytoplasm remaining from defective spermiogenesis increases the amount of G6PDH, leading to increased ROS production. For this reason, immature spermatozoa, or incorrectly matured spermatozoa are a major source of ROS production in OS and may cause DNA damage in mature spermatozoa during transit in the epididymis [39,67,68] (Fig. 4).

APOPTOSIS AND THE ROLE OF REACTIVE OXYGEN SPECIES GENERATION

Apoptosis in spermatozoa represents a default process and is largely intrinsically induced. Since not every spermatozoon in the ejaculate is capable of fertilizing, many undergo an apoptotic death. The compartmentalized physical structure of the human spermatozoa makes this pathway distinct from the conventional intrinsic apoptotic cascade. This involves the ability of cytotoxic aldehydes like 4-hydroxynonenal to activate mitochondrial ROS production. Due to this apoptotic cascade, a rapid loss of mitochondrial membrane potential ensues affecting caspase activation, exteriorization of phosphatidylserine, lipid peroxidation, and sperm motility [70,71].

ANTIOXIDANT EXPRESSION IN SPERMATOZOA

OS is caused due to high production of ROS and low antioxidant activity in a biological system, creating a redox imbalance. ROS produced by spermatozoa as a by-product of electron transfer chain in mitochondria is mainly composed of O_{2-} and H_2O_2 molecules [72]. These are neutralized by antioxidants, mainly SOD, glutathione peroxidase, and catalase located within the mitochondria and in the secretions of the reproductive tract [73,74].

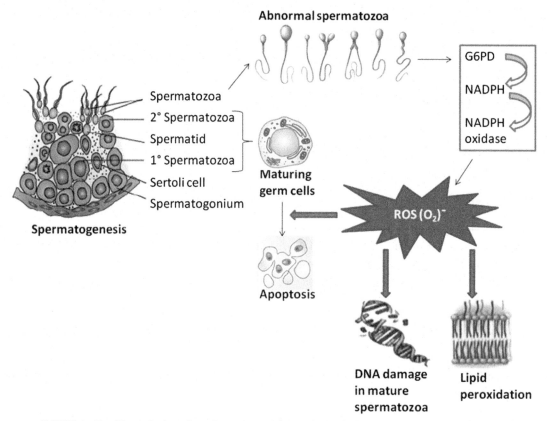

FIGURE 4 Possible mechanism of reactive oxygen species production by immature or abnormal spermatozoa.

Superoxide anion is a moderately reactive ROS with a short half-life. $O_2^{\bullet-}$ can be converted into a strong oxidant ROS, H_2O_2, either spontaneously or by an enzymatic reaction catalyzed by SOD (see below). SOD scavenges both extracellular and intracellular superoxide, thus affecting lipid peroxidation, hyperactivation, and capacitation.

$$2(O_2^{\bullet-}) + 2H^+ \xrightarrow{\text{SOD}} H_2O_2 + O_2$$
$$H_2O_2 \xrightarrow{\text{Catalase}} H_2O + \tfrac{1}{2}\,O_2$$

Hydrogen peroxide is a more stable ROS and has been shown to be highly toxic for human spermatozoa. The first candidate is catalase, which can detoxify intracellular and extracellular H_2O_2 and convert it to water and O_2. Also catalase activates NO-induced sperm capacitation that involves H_2O_2. Thus, both antioxidants (SOD and catalase) help remove excessive ROS to protect sperm from oxidative damage.

Another enzyme capable of removing H_2O_2 is the glutathione peroxidase/reductase system, which prevents lipid peroxidation of the sperm plasma membrane by scavenging lipid peroxides. Glutathione peroxidase (Se-GSH-Px) with the help of glutathione (GSH) serving as the electron donor removes these peroxyl radicals. Reduced GSH regenerates glutathione reductase (GSH-red) from GSSG (glutathione disulfide) as a part of progressive chain reaction shown in the following equation:

$$2GSH + H_2O_2 \xrightarrow{\text{Se-GSH-Px}} GSSH + 2H_2O$$

$$GSSH + NADPH + H^+ \xrightarrow{\text{GSH-Red}} 2GSH + NADP^+$$

Thus a steady supply of NADPH in the presence of Se-GSH-Px scavenges H_2O_2, which is responsible for the initiation of lipid peroxidation, thereby preventing sperm damage.

CONCLUSION

In light of the present knowledge, it is clear that controlled production of low ROS is important for normal sperm physiological processes (e.g., sperm capacitation, hyperactivation, ARs) to ensure normal fertilization. If fertilization does not occur, as is usually the case for an individual spermatozoon where ROS activates the intrinsic apoptosis cascade, it results in arrest of sperm movement with increased phosphatidylserine expression. These activities promote phagocytosis of spermatozoa by female neutrophils and macrophages. The increased susceptibility of spermatozoa to increased OS in the presence of low cellular antioxidant capacity becomes more evident over time. Aging sperm exhibit lower activity of Se-GSH-Px and SOD. This ROS-antioxidant equilibrium plays a pivotal role in physiological and pathological events of spermatozoa preventing damage. A properly maintained balance ensures normal physiological functions and success of fertilization.

REFERENCES

[1] Agarwal A, Sharma RK, Nallella KP, Thomas Jr AJ, Alvarez JG, Sikka SC. Reactive oxygen species as an independent marker of male factor infertility. Fertil Steril October 2006;86(4):878−85.

[2] Bisht S, Faiq M, Tolahunase M, Dada R. Oxidative stress and male infertility. Nat Rev Urol August 2017;14(8):470−85.

[3] Cindrova-Davies T, Yung HW, Johns J, Spasic-Boskovic O, Korolchuk S, Jauniaux E, et al. Oxidative stress, gene expression, and protein changes induced in the human placenta during labor. Am J Pathol October 2007;171(4):1168−79.

[4] Mukherjee TK, Mukhopadhyay S, Hoidal JR. The role of reactive oxygen species in TNFalpha-dependent expression of the receptor for advanced glycation end products in human umbilical vein endothelial cells. Biochim Biophys Acta June 30, 2005;1744(2):213−23.

[5] Huang H, Manton KG. The role of oxidative damage in mitochondria during aging: a review. Front Biosci May 1, 2004;9:1100−17.

[6] Migliore L, Coppede F. Environmental-induced oxidative stress in neurodegenerative disorders and aging. Mutat Res March 31, 2009;674(1−2):73−84.

[7] Finkel T, Holbrook NJ. Oxidants, oxidative stress and the biology of ageing. Nature November 9, 2000;408(6809):239−47.

[8] Armstrong JS, Bivalacqua TJ, Chamulitrat W, Sikka S, Hellstrom WJ. A comparison of the NADPH oxidase in human sperm and white blood cells. Int J Androl August 2002;25(4):223−9.

[9] Droge W. Free radicals in the physiological control of cell function. Physiol Rev January 2002;82(1):47−95.

[10] Genestra M. Oxyl radicals, redox-sensitive signalling cascades and antioxidants. Cell Signal September 2007;19(9):1807−19.

[11] Kumar S, Pandey AK. Chemistry and biological activities of flavonoids: an overview. Sci World J 2013;2013:162750.

[12] Pacher P, Beckman JS, Liaudet L. Nitric oxide and peroxynitrite in health and disease. Physiol Rev January 2007;87(1):315−424.

[13] Pizzino G, Irrera N, Cucinotta M, Pallio G, Mannino F, Arcoraci V, et al. Oxidative stress: harms and benefits for human health. Oxid Med Cell Longev 2017;2017:8416763.

[14] Valko M, Izakovic M, Mazur M, Rhodes CJ, Telser J. Role of oxygen radicals in DNA damage and cancer incidence. Mol Cell Biochem November 2004;266(1−2):37−56.

[15] Agarwal A, Makker K, Sharma R. Clinical relevance of oxidative stress in male factor infertility: an update. Am J Reprod Immunol January 2008;59(1):2−11.

[16] Glasauer A, Chandel NS. ROS. Curr Biol February 4, 2013;23(3):R100−2.

[17] Hayyan M, Hashim MA, AlNashef IM. Superoxide ion: generation and chemical implications. Chem Rev March 9, 2016;116(5):3029−85.

[18] Valko M, Leibfritz D, Moncol J, Cronin MT, Mazur M, Telser J. Free radicals and antioxidants in normal physiological functions and human disease. Int J Biochem Cell Biol 2007;39(1):44−84.

[19] Lander HM. An essential role for free radicals and derived species in signal transduction. FASEB J February 1997;11(2):118−24.

[20] Cocuzza M, Sikka SC, Athayde KS, Agarwal A. Clinical relevance of oxidative stress and sperm chromatin damage in male infertility: an evidence based analysis. Int Braz J Urol September−October 2007;33(5):603−21.

[21] Fisher HM, Aitken RJ. Comparative analysis of the ability of precursor germ cells and epididymal spermatozoa to generate reactive oxygen metabolites. J Exp Zool April 1, 1997;277(5):390−400.

[22] Aitken RJ. The Amoroso Lecture. The human spermatozoon—a cell in crisis? J Reprod Fertil January 1999;115(1):1−7.

[23] Agarwal A, Nallella KP, Allamaneni SS, Said TM. Role of antioxidants in treatment of male infertility: an overview of the literature. Reprod Biomed Online June 2004;8(6):616−27.

[24] Tvrda E, Knazicka Z, Bardos L, Massanyi P, Lukac N. Impact of oxidative stress on male fertility—a review. Acta Vet Hung December 2011;59(4):465−84.

[25] Macleod J. The role of oxygen in the metabolism and motility of human spermatozoa. Am J Physiol 1943;138:512−8.

[26] Aitken RJ, Clarkson JS. Cellular basis of defective sperm function and its association with the genesis of reactive oxygen species by human spermatozoa. J Reprod Fertil November 1987;81(2):459−69.

[27] Aitken RJ, Whiting S, De Iuliis GN, McClymont S, Mitchell LA, Baker MA. Electrophilic aldehydes generated by sperm metabolism activate mitochondrial reactive oxygen species generation and apoptosis by targeting succinate dehydrogenase. J Biol Chem September 21, 2012;287(39):33048−60.

[28] Homa ST, Vessey W, Perez-Miranda A, Riyait T, Agarwal A. Reactive Oxygen Species (ROS) in human semen: determination of a reference range. J Assist Reprod Genet May 2015;32(5):757–64.

[29] Aitken RJ, Harkiss D, Knox W, Paterson M, Irvine DS. A novel signal transduction cascade in capacitating human spermatozoa characterised by a redox-regulated, cAMP-mediated induction of tyrosine phosphorylation. J Cell Sci March 1998;111(Pt 5):645–56.

[30] Aitken RJ, Buckingham D, Harkiss D. Use of a xanthine oxidase free radical generating system to investigate the cytotoxic effects of reactive oxygen species on human spermatozoa. J Reprod Fertil March 1993;97(2):441–50.

[31] Griveau JF, Dumont E, Renard P, Callegari JP, Le Lannou D. Reactive oxygen species, lipid peroxidation and enzymatic defence systems in human spermatozoa. J Reprod Fertil January 1995;103(1):17–26.

[32] Lopes S, Jurisicova A, Sun JG, Casper RF. Reactive oxygen species: potential cause for DNA fragmentation in human spermatozoa. Hum Reprod April 1998;13(4):896–900.

[33] Aitken RJ, Gordon E, Harkiss D, Twigg JP, Milne P, Jennings Z, et al. Relative impact of oxidative stress on the functional competence and genomic integrity of human spermatozoa. Biol Reprod November 1998;59(5):1037–46.

[34] Baker MA, Aitken RJ. Reactive oxygen species in spermatozoa: methods for monitoring and significance for the origins of genetic disease and infertility. Reprod Biol Endocrinol November 29, 2005;3:67.

[35] Chance B, Sies H, Boveris A. Hydroperoxide metabolism in mammalian organs. Physiol Rev July 1979;59(3):527–605.

[36] Ford WC. Regulation of sperm function by reactive oxygen species. Hum Reprod Update September–October 2004;10(5):387–99.

[37] Fraczek M, Kurpisz M. [The redox system in human semen and peroxidative damage of spermatozoa]. Postepy Hig Med Dosw 2005;59:523–34.

[38] Aziz N, Saleh RA, Sharma RK, Lewis-Jones I, Esfandiari N, Thomas Jr AJ, et al. Novel association between sperm reactive oxygen species production, sperm morphological defects, and the sperm deformity index. Fertil Steril February 2004;81(2):349–54.

[39] Gomez E, Buckingham DW, Brindle J, Lanzafame F, Irvine DS, Aitken RJ. Development of an image analysis system to monitor the retention of residual cytoplasm by human spermatozoa: correlation with biochemical markers of the cytoplasmic space, oxidative stress, and sperm function. J Androl May–June 1996;17(3):276–87.

[40] Walczak-Jedrzejowska R, Wolski JK, Slowikowska-Hilczer J. The role of oxidative stress and antioxidants in male fertility. Cent European J Urol 2013;66(1):60–7.

[41] Henkel R, Schill WB. Sperm separation in patients with urogenital infections. Andrologia 1998;30(Suppl. 1):91–7.

[42] Lambeth JD. Nox/Duox family of nicotinamide adenine dinucleotide (phosphate) oxidases. Curr Opin Hematol January 2002;9(1):11–7.

[43] Sabeur K, Ball BA. Characterization of NADPH oxidase 5 in equine testis and spermatozoa. Reproduction August 2007;134(2):263–70.

[44] de Lamirande E, Gagnon C. Capacitation-associated production of superoxide anion by human spermatozoa. Free Radic Biol Med March 1995;18(3):487–95.

[45] de Lamirande E, Lamothe G, Villemure M. Control of superoxide and nitric oxide formation during human sperm capacitation. Free Radic Biol Med May 15, 2009;46(10):1420–7.

[46] O'Flaherty C. Redox regulation of mammalian sperm capacitation. Asian J Androl July–August 2015;17(4):583–90.

[47] Rahamim Ben-Navi L, Almog T, Yao Z, Seger R, Naor Z. A-Kinase Anchoring Protein 4 (AKAP4) is an ERK1/2 substrate and a switch molecule between cAMP/PKA and PKC/ERK1/2 in human spermatozoa. Sci Rep November 30, 2016;6:37922.

[48] Baker MA, Krutskikh A, Aitken RJ. Biochemical entities involved in reactive oxygen species generation by human spermatozoa. Protoplasma May 2003;221(1–2):145–51.

[49] Banfi B, Molnar G, Maturana A, Steger K, Hegedus B, Demaurex N, et al. A Ca(2+)-activated NADPH oxidase in testis, spleen, and lymph nodes. J Biol Chem October 5, 2001;276(40):37594–601.

[50] Cheng G, Cao Z, Xu X, van Meir EG, Lambeth JD. Homologs of gp91phox: cloning and tissue expression of Nox3, Nox4, and Nox5. Gene May 16, 2001;269(1–2):131–40.

[51] Musset B, Clark RA, DeCoursey TE, Petheo GL, Geiszt M, Chen Y, et al. NOX5 in human spermatozoa: expression, function, and regulation. J Biol Chem March 16, 2012;287(12):9376–88.

[52] Griendling KK, Sorescu D, Ushio-Fukai M. NAD(P)H oxidase: role in cardiovascular biology and disease. Circ Res March 17, 2000;86(5):494–501.

[53] Blanco A, Zinkham WH. Lactate dehydrogenases in human testes. Science February 15, 1963;139(3555):601–2.

[54] Zinkham WH, Blanco A, Clowry Jr LJ. An unusual isozyme of lactate dehydrogenase in mature testes: localization, ontogeny, and kinetic properties. Ann N Y Acad Sci December 1964;28(121):571–88.

[55] Aitken RJ, Paterson M, Fisher H, Buckingham DW, van Duin M. Redox regulation of tyrosine phosphorylation in human spermatozoa and its role in the control of human sperm function. J Cell Sci May 1995;108(Pt 5):2017–25.

[56] de Lamirande E, Harakat A, Gagnon C. Human sperm capacitation induced by biological fluids and progesterone, but not by NADH or NADPH, is associated with the production of superoxide anion. J Androl March–April 1998;19(2):215–25.

[57] Sarkar S, Nelson AJ, Jones OW. Glucose-6-phosphate dehydrogenase (G6PD) activity of human sperm. J Med Genet August 1977;14(4):250–5.

[58] Amaral A, Castillo J, Ramalho-Santos J, Oliva R. The combined human sperm proteome: cellular pathways and implications for basic and clinical science. Hum Reprod Update January–February 2014;20(1):40–62.

[59] Wang G, Guo Y, Zhou T, Shi X, Yu J, Yang Y, et al. In-depth proteomic analysis of the human sperm reveals complex protein compositions. J Proteomics February 21, 2013;79:114–22.

[60] Archer S. Measurement of nitric oxide in biological models. FASEB J February 1, 1993;7(2):349–60.

[61] Sikka SC. Relative impact of oxidative stress on male reproductive function. Curr Med Chem June 2001;8(7):851–62.

[62] de Lamirande E, Lamothe G. Reactive oxygen-induced reactive oxygen formation during human sperm capacitation. Free Radic Biol Med February 15, 2009;46(4):502−10.

[63] Herrero MB, de Lamirande E, Gagnon C. Nitric oxide is a signaling molecule in spermatozoa. Curr Pharm Des 2003;9(5):419−25.

[64] Kothari S, Thompson A, Agarwal A, du Plessis SS. Free radicals: their beneficial and detrimental effects on sperm function. Indian J Exp Biol May 2010;48(5):425−35.

[65] Herrero MB, de Lamirande E, Gagnon C. Nitric oxide regulates human sperm capacitation and protein-tyrosine phosphorylation in vitro. Biol Reprod September 1999;61(3):575−81.

[66] Herrero MB, Perez Martinez S, Viggiano JM, Polak JM, de Gimeno MF. Localization by indirect immunofluorescence of nitric oxide synthase in mouse and human spermatozoa. Reprod Fertil Dev 1996;8(5):931−4.

[67] Gil-Guzman E, Ollero M, Lopez MC, Sharma RK, Alvarez JG, Thomas Jr AJ, et al. Differential production of reactive oxygen species by subsets of human spermatozoa at different stages of maturation. Hum Reprod September 2001;16(9):1922−30.

[68] Ollero M, Gil-Guzman E, Lopez MC, Sharma RK, Agarwal A, Larson K, et al. Characterization of subsets of human spermatozoa at different stages of maturation: implications in the diagnosis and treatment of male infertility. Hum Reprod September 2001;16(9):1912−21.

[69] Dona G, Fiore C, Andrisani A, Ambrosini G, Brunati A, Ragazzi E, et al. Evaluation of correct endogenous reactive oxygen species content for human sperm capacitation and involvement of the NADPH oxidase system. Hum Reprod December 2011;26(12):3264−73.

[70] Aitken RJ, Findlay JK, Hutt KJ, Kerr JB. Apoptosis in the germ line. Reproduction February 2011;141(2):139−50.

[71] Koppers AJ, Mitchell LA, Wang P, Lin M, Aitken RJ. Phosphoinositide 3-kinase signalling pathway involvement in a truncated apoptotic cascade associated with motility loss and oxidative DNA damage in human spermatozoa. Biochem J June 15, 2011;436(3):687−98.

[72] Koppers AJ, De Iuliis GN, Finnie JM, McLaughlin EA, Aitken RJ. Significance of mitochondrial reactive oxygen species in the generation of oxidative stress in spermatozoa. J Clin Endocrinol Metab August 2008;93(8):3199−207.

[73] Starkov AA. The role of mitochondria in reactive oxygen species metabolism and signaling. Ann N Y Acad Sci December 2008;1147:37−52.

[74] Vernet P, Aitken RJ, Drevet JR. Antioxidant strategies in the epididymis. Mol Cell Endocrinol March 15, 2004;216(1−2):31−9.

Chapter 1.7

Causes of Reductive Stress in Male Reproduction

Julie W. Cheng and Edmund Y. Ko
Loma Linda University Medical Center, Loma Linda, CA, United States

INTRODUCTION

Chemical reactions within the human body need to remain in equilibrium between oxidative and reductive states. Physiologic balance is important as extremes of either oxidation or reduction can cause tissue injury. Oxidative stress arises when there is a pathologic abundance of oxidative equivalents and there is a subsequent increase in the production of reactive oxygen species (ROS). Oxidative stress has been studied extensively in male infertility as it can impair the structural and functional integrity of spermatozoa [1–3]. Antioxidants have been regarded as a form of defense against oxidative stress by acting as reducing agents that react with ROS [4]. Considering antioxidants as a defense mechanism or buffering system, however, would suggest a misconceived notion that antioxidants can only offer protection and that no harm can come from treatment.

Shifting away from an optimal environment toward the nonoxidative state is not without its risks. Reductive stress can result from an imbalance to the other extreme in which there is a pathologic abundance of reducing equivalents. The purpose of this chapter is to describe the antioxidant paradox, review the clinical implications of reductive stress, and identify reducing agents in male reproduction. As this chapter will focus on the potential causes of reductive stress in male reproduction, studies reviewing the efficacy of reducing agents as a form of treatment in male infertility will be discussed in a separate chapter.

REACTIVE OXYGEN SPECIES AND THE MALE REPRODUCTIVE SYSTEM

ROS are highly reactive molecules that can cause oxidative stress due to an unpaired electron in their outer valence shells. Despite this, ROS are important components of physiologic reactions as local oxidation is necessary in basic cellular functions. While ROS serve as signal transducers that help regulate embryologic development [5], they also contribute to the induction of apoptosis [6]. With regard to cellular functions such as protein synthesis, a more oxidizing environment within the endoplasmic reticulum is needed to allow for disulfide bond formation and proper folding in secretory proteins [7]. In fact, antioxidant supplementation with ascorbic acid can reduce the formation of disulfide bridges and impair protein folding [8].

Oxidative stress may also provide a protective function that allows for cellular adaptation [9–11]. ROS generated after an initial insult may play an essential role in protecting against ensuing episodes of injury. This has been demonstrated in an animal study in which conscious pigs were subjected to cycles of brief coronary occlusion followed by reperfusion. The initial cycle of ischemia-reperfusion resulted in a period of cardiac stunning followed by recovery. When this cycle was repeated with the same stimuli, there was an adapted response in which there were fewer changes suggestive of cardiac stunning in the control group. In contrast, this cardioprotective response was blunted in pigs that received antioxidant infusions with superoxide dismutase (SOD), catalase, and mercaptopropionyl glycine [10]. This suggests that oxidative stress, while initially damaging, may help generate a protective response against subsequent injury, and antioxidants can limit this response [10].

A human study found that ROS might contribute to the beneficial effects of exercise. Subjects underwent a 4-week period of physical exercise to monitor changes in parameters of insulin sensitivity with and without antioxidant supplementation. Daily antioxidant supplementation with 1000 mg of ascorbic acid and 400 IU of tocopherol limited the improvement in insulin sensitivity that was measured in control subjects that did not receive supplementation [11]. As supplementation negated the transient oxidative stress generated in physical exercise, this may have also limited the induction of transcription factors in regulating insulin sensitivity [11].

Spermatozoa were the first mammalian cells reported to generate ROS [12]. Human spermatozoa produce varying levels of ROS through the different stages of spermatogenesis [13]. The greatest amount of ROS production has been demonstrated in immature spermatozoa compared to lower production in mature spermatozoa and immature germ cells[13].

Superoxide anion ($\cdot O_2^-$), hydroxyl ion ($\cdot OH^-$), and hydrogen peroxide (H_2O_2) are ROS that have been identified in male infertility and are produced by seminal leukocytes and sperm cells [12,14]. With regard to oxidative stress, these molecules may interfere with spermatozoa structure and function. As there is a high proportion of polyunsaturated fatty acids in the plasma membrane of spermatozoa [15], these reproductive cells are particularly vulnerable to oxidative damage through lipid peroxidation [1,2]. Oxidative stress can also cause DNA fragmentation, which has been shown to decrease with antioxidant supplementation using combinations of ascorbic acid and tocopherol [16] or selenium and zinc [17].

ROS nevertheless contribute to physiologic reactions within the setting of male reproduction. Following ejaculation into the female tract, spermatozoa interact with uterine factors to increase calcium permeability during capacitation [18]. Increased intracellular calcium levels then increase sperm motility through hyperactivation. Low levels of $\cdot O_2^-$ are needed during capacitation and higher levels of this ROS contribute to hyperactivation [19]. As spermatozoa reach the oocyte, $\cdot O_2^-$ and H_2O_2 contribute to the acrosome reaction [20] that is necessary for a spermatozoon to fuse with the oocyte during fertilization. More details regarding the role of ROS in male reproduction will be discussed in a separate chapter.

THE ANTIOXIDANT PARADOX

The concept of the antioxidant paradox was first discussed by Halliwell in 2000 [21]. Contrary to expectations that antioxidant therapy would treat or prevent damage from oxidative stress, antioxidants may actually have detrimental effects on cellular injury and disease. Halliwell [21] discussed the conflicting outcomes regarding the impact of high-dose tocopherol supplementation in the Cambridge Heart Antioxidant Study (CHAOS) [22] and the GISSI-Prevenzione trial [23]. The CHAOS trial was a double-blind, randomized, placebo-controlled study in which high-dose tocopherol supplementation in patients with ischemic heart disease reduced the rate of a nonfatal myocardial infarction [22]. Whereas antioxidant supplementation was beneficial in the CHAOS trial, there was no benefit in daily tocopherol supplementation in preventing nonfatal myocardial infarction, stroke, or death in the GISSI-Prevenzione trial [23]. Halliwell [21] uses these conflicting results to consider the lack of benefit and even the potential harm that can result from antioxidant treatment. It was suggested that this can occur through a loss of necessary oxidative mechanisms, promotion of tissue injury in the reductive state, or a paradoxical increase in ROS production [21].

REDUCING AGENTS IN MALE REPRODUCTION

While reductive and oxidative reactions occur naturally in male reproduction, studies regarding reductive stress and male fertility are limited. Studies have yet to show that reductive stress arises from physiologic levels of enzymatic or nonenzymatic reducing agents. Pathologic abundance of reducing agents, however, may be a sequela of unregulated antioxidant supplementation. The focus of this section is to discuss the role of antioxidants as reducing agents in male reproduction that can potentially lead to reductive stress.

Antioxidants can be classified as either enzymatic or nonenzymatic reducing agents [3,4]. They can also be classified as physiologic agents that are endogenously produced or dietary agents that are consumed. Dietary antioxidants can be natural antioxidants isolated from food or synthetic agents that are chemically produced. Reducing agents identified in male reproduction are categorized in Table 1. Significant enzymatic reducing agents that have been identified in male reproduction include SOD, catalase, and glutathione peroxidase (GPX).

- **SOD** scavenges superoxide anion $\cdot O_2^-$ and catalyzes its conversion to hydrogen peroxide H_2O_2. This reducing agent exists in three isoenzymes: manganese SOD in the mitochondria, copper-zinc SOD in the cytoplasm, and extracellular SOD within extracellular fluids. SOD within the seminal plasma has been shown to protect against phospholipid

TABLE 1 Reducing Agents in Male Reproduction

Enzymatic	Non-enzymatic
	Glutathione
	N-acetylcysteine
	Ascorbic acid (vitamin C)
	Tocopherol (vitamin E)
	Folic acid
Superoxide dismutase	Selenium
Catalase	Zinc
Glutathione peroxidase	Carotenoids
	Lycopene
	Uric acid
	Thiols
	Carnitine
	Hypotaurine
	Taurine

Reducing agents (or antioxidants) can be classified as either enzymatic or nonenzymatic agents.

peroxidation on the membrane of human spermatozoa [24], decrease DNA damage in a dose-dependent manner [25], and decrease markers for oxidative stress [26].

- **Catalase** converts hydrogen peroxide H_2O_2 to water and molecular oxygen. This enzyme is also considered to contribute to male fertility and protect against oxidative damage. Infertile men with asthenozoospermia exhibited lower levels of catalase activity in their semen compared to normospermic men [27].
- **GPX** uses glutathione as an electron donor to catalyze hydrogen peroxide H_2O_2 and superoxide anion $\cdot O_2^-$. Multiple isoforms of this enzyme can be found within the cytoplasm, plasma membranes, or extracellular fluids. While the GPX3 isoform is mainly expressed in kidney, its expression has also been identified in the epididymis and testis [28,29]. This enzyme has also been found to protect against phospholipid peroxidation on the membrane of human spermatozoa [24].

Major nonenzymatic reducing agents that naturally occur in the male reproductive tract include glutathione, ascorbic acid, tocopherol, selenium, and lycopene.

- **Glutathione** is an abundant nonenzymatic reducing agent that acts as a free radical scavenger and coenzyme for enzymatic reducing agents, particularly GPX.
- **Ascorbic acid** (also known as vitamin C) is a water-soluble vitamin that has been found to neutralize ROS as a means of protection against oxidative damage [30].
- **Tocopherol** (also known as vitamin E) is a fat-soluble vitamin that reduces lipid peroxidation at the plasma membrane of spermatozoa [31].
- **Selenium** is an essential trace element that acts as a cofactor to specific isoforms of GPX [32].
- **Lycopene** is the predominant carotenoid within the testis. The small amount that is stored in the testis may serve a protective role against ischemia-reperfusion tissue injury from oxidative stress [33,34].

Reducing Agents in the Testicle and Epididymis

The distribution of reducing agents in the testicles and epididymis are shown in Fig. 1. The seminiferous tubules that are coiled within the testicles serve as the site for spermatogenesis. The germinal epithelium lines the lumen of these tubules and is comprised of Sertoli and spermatogonium germ cells. Sertoli cells encompass developing sperm cells to provide structural and functional support as these cells develop. As Sertoli cells undergo various oxidative reactions during spermatogenesis, such as phagocytosis of excess cytoplasm, there have been high levels of reducing agents reported in

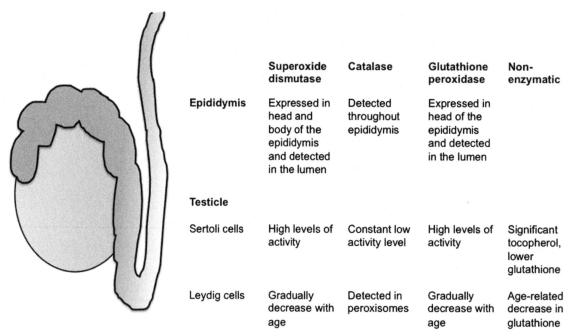

	Superoxide dismutase	Catalase	Glutathione peroxidase	Non-enzymatic
Epididymis	Expressed in head and body of the epididymis and detected in the lumen	Detected throughout epididymis	Expressed in head of the epididymis and detected in the lumen	
Testicle				
Sertoli cells	High levels of activity	Constant low activity level	High levels of activity	Significant tocopherol, lower glutathione
Leydig cells	Gradually decrease with age	Detected in peroxisomes	Gradually decrease with age	Age-related decrease in glutathione

FIGURE 1 **Reducing agents in the testicle and epididymis.** Prior to merging with seminal plasma, spermatozoa are surrounded by and exposed to reducing agents within the testicle and epididymis.

these cells [35,36]. Whereas high levels of SOD and GPX have been demonstrated [35,36], there is a constant low level of catalase activity [37]. There are also significantly higher levels of tocopherol that were found to be fourfold higher in Sertoli cells than in round spermatids [35]. Compared to other testicular components, however, Sertoli cells exhibit lower levels of glutathione [36].

The activity of individual enzymatic reducing agents in the testis can change through the development of the male reproductive system [37]. The developmental profiles of SOD, catalase, and GPX have been measured in the rat testis and liver. SOD activity in the rat testis is high early in life but declines to one-third of that level before plateauing [37]. There is a constant low level of catalase activity within the testis that is 2%−7% of that in the liver [37]. Compared to other reducing agents, GPX activity is lower in the rat testis early in life but increases with age [37].

Leydig cells, fibroblasts, and macrophages compose the peritubular and interstitial cells of the testicle. Although these cells do not directly contribute to spermatogenesis, they nevertheless contribute to the overall function and microenvironment of the testicle. While there is a high level of both selenium-dependent and total GPX activity in interstitial cells, peritubular and interstitial cells have a relatively lower level of SOD activity [36]. Catalase can be found within the peroxisomes of Leydig cells [38]. These cells also demonstrate intermediate-to-lower levels of glutathione compared to other cells within the testicle [36]. Leydig cells specifically exhibit a gradual decrease in mRNA levels, protein levels, and enzyme activities of SOD and GPX with increasing age [39]. There has also been an age-related decrease in glutathione levels measured in Leydig cells [39].

As the next component of the male reproductive tract, the epididymis serves as the site of sperm maturation and storage. Evaluation of mRNA expression of enzymatic reducing agents has shown the presence of SOD, catalase, and GPX throughout the head, body, and tail of the epididymis [40]. Region-specific mRNA expression demonstrates that GPX is produced in the epididymal head whereas SOD is expressed in both the head and body of the epididymis [40,41]. SOD enzyme activity within the lumen of the epididymis suggests that this reducing agent is secreted [41]. Animal studies have demonstrated that the epididymis also expresses and secretes significant levels of GPX from the epididymal head [25,28,29,40,42], and this reducing agent is then detected in the lumen of the body and tail [42]. Furthermore, it remains bound to spermatozoa retrieved from uterine secretions in female rats after mating, whereas virgin female rats have no GPX in their uterine secretions [42]. This suggests that GPX secreted by the epididymis continues to act as a reducing agent in both the male and female through the mating and fertilization process.

Reducing Agents in Sperm Cells

The profile of reducing agents within sperm cells changes through the stages of spermatogenesis and can be seen in Fig. 2. Spermatogonia are the germ cells from which spermatogenesis is initiated. These diploid germ cells are anchored within the basal compartment of the germinal epithelium by Sertoli cell tight junctions. Germ cells produce a relatively lower amount of ROS compared to other stages of developing sperm cells [13]. Although there is a lower level of GPX activity in these cells, there are nevertheless high levels of SOD activity [35,36].

Spermatogonia initiate spermatogenesis by undergoing mitosis. One daughter cell stays in the basal compartment to maintain the germ line and the other is released to proceed through spermatogenesis as a primary spermatocyte. Primary spermatocytes undergo meiosis to form secondary spermatocytes that then undergo meiosis to form spermatids. Spermatocytes and spermatids have been found to have a different system of reducing agents with higher SOD and glutathione compared to somatic cells within the testis [36]. Despite high glutathione levels, GPX activity is relatively lower in spermatocytes [36]. No catalase activity has been detected in developing spermatocytes and spermatids [36].

Spermatids then progress through spermiogenesis to develop into immature spermatozoa. It is at this stage that developing sperm begin to transform from a basic round cell to a specialized motile reproductive cell. There is migration of intracellular structures and the tail is formed. Mitochondria migrate to the midpiece of the tail. Cytoplasm is shed to compact the head of the spermatozoon. These cells subsequently have a limited supply of cytoplasmic reducing agents and depend on extracellular reducing agents during maturation and fertilization. Immature spermatozoa exhibit very high SOD and lower GPX activity compared to Sertoli and peritubular cells [36].

Following spermatogenesis, immature spermatozoa are shed into the lumen of the seminiferous tubules, proceed to the epididymis, and enter the male reproductive tract. Significant SOD and catalase activity has been detected in motile spermatozoa [27,43]. In fact, SOD activity within human spermatozoa correlates with motility [26]. Glutathione levels, while higher in spermatocytes and spermatids, decrease to lower levels in spermatozoa with a correspondingly low level of GPX activity [36]. GPX has nevertheless been identified in the head and midpiece of spermatozoa [42,44]. Upon

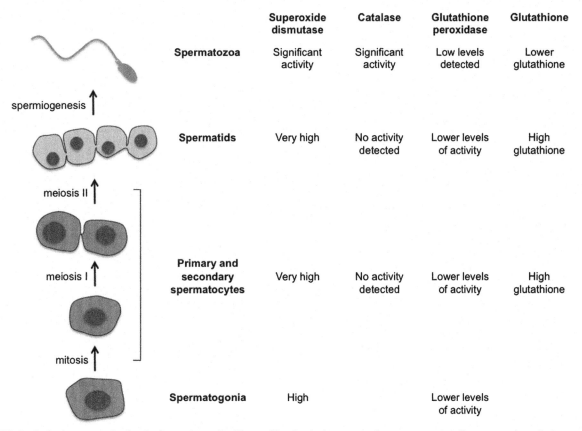

	Superoxide dismutase	Catalase	Glutathione peroxidase	Glutathione
Spermatozoa	Significant activity	Significant activity	Low levels detected	Lower glutathione
Spermatids	Very high	No activity detected	Lower levels of activity	High glutathione
Primary and secondary spermatocytes	Very high	No activity detected	Lower levels of activity	High glutathione
Spermatogonia	High		Lower levels of activity	

FIGURE 2 **Reducing agents in developing sperm cells.** The profile of reducing agents changes as sperm cells progress through the stages of spermatogenesis.

release from the epididymis, spermatozoa pass through the vas deferens before merging with seminal plasma at the ejaculatory duct.

Reducing Agents in Seminal Plasma

Seminal plasma is a combination of secretions from the seminal vesicles, prostate, and bulbourethral glands. Not only does seminal plasma need to provide optimal pH and viscosity for sperm viability and motility, it must also provide a medium of fructose and various ions for spermatozoa to function. Accessory glands of the male reproductive system individually contribute to the composition of seminal plasma. The seminal vesicles produce the majority of seminal plasma and most notably, provide fructose as an energy source for ATP production [45]. The prostate and bulbourethral glands secrete the remainder of seminal plasma in the form of ions and mucus that aid in sperm motility and lubricate the penile urethra [45,46]. A combination of seminal plasma and spermatozoa is then expelled through the prostatic and penile urethra during ejaculation.

As spermatozoa are compact cells that have limited antioxidant capacity, seminal plasma provides the majority of physiologic antioxidant protection against oxidative injury. Spermatozoa incubated in a medium without seminal plasma demonstrate a significant decrease in motility after just 2 h with an increase in markers for oxidative stress [26]. Furthermore, there is a significantly lower profile of enzymatic reducing agents in the seminal plasma of men with idiopathic infertility compared to that of fertile men [47].

In addition to fructose and ions, enzymatic reducing agents are also secreted by the accessory glands into the seminal plasma. While reducing agents have been demonstrated in epididymal secretions, there is no difference in the activity levels of each enzyme in the ejaculate of fertile men compared to that of men that had undergone a vasectomy [48]. This suggests that, regardless of epididymal secretions, there is a significant contribution of reducing agents from seminal plasma.

Although the contribution of each specific enzyme from each accessory sex gland has yet to be fully elucidated, analysis of seminal plasma demonstrates enzymatic activity of SOD, catalase, and GPX [25,27,43,48]. Although GPX activity has been detected in the seminal plasma [25], little-to-no glutathione has been detected [48]. This may suggest that GPX, while present, may have limited activity in the seminal plasma. Significant levels of SOD and catalase are nevertheless present in the seminal plasma [25,27,43].

Nonenzymatic reducing agents identified in the seminal plasma include ascorbic acid, tocopherol, uric acid, thiols, carotenoids, folate, selenium, zinc, carnitine, hypotaurine, and taurine. Ascorbic acid in seminal plasma may protect against endogenous oxidative DNA damage in sperm [30]. Significantly lower levels of this reducing agent correspond with greater ROS activity [49]. There are significant levels of ascorbic acid in the seminal plasma, as there is twice as much compared to uric acid and three times as much compared to thiols in semen samples from fertile men [49]. While lycopene has been localized in the prostate [34], it may not be secreted as analysis of seminal plasma did not detect its presence [49].

REDUCTIVE STRESS AND THE MALE REPRODUCTIVE SYSTEM

Reductive stress occurs when there is an excess of reducing equivalents that offset the balance of physiologic reactions. This phenomenon can occur with an irregularly higher ratio of reducing agents relative to oxidizing agents, such as NADH-to-NAD$^+$ or reduced glutathione-to-oxidized glutathione. Reducing agents may cause additional harm through loss of oxidative mechanisms, further promoting tissue injury, or a paradoxical increase in ROS production as suggested by Halliwell when describing the antioxidant paradox [21].

Within the cellular environment, reductive stress from glutathione may trigger mitochondrial oxidation and cytotoxicity [50]. In an in vitro animal study, a reductive environment with excess glutathione levels and increased reductive potential was generated through pharmacologic *N*-acetylcysteine administration or genetic overexpression of the catalytic subunit of glutamate cysteine ligase (GCL) or the GCL modifier subunit. Although there was a decrease in ROS levels, there was also an increase in mitochondrial oxidation as well as a dose-dependent decrease in cell viability in embryonic rat cardiomyocytes [50].

Reductive stress can also result in a paradoxical increase in ROS despite the ROS scavenging system associated with antioxidants [51,52]. Recombinant antioxidant nicotinamide adenine dinucleotide phosphate reductases have been shown to generate ROS by leaking electrons from reduced flavoproteins to O_2 when the availability of natural electron acceptors is limited [51]. Mitochondria and cardiomyocytes isolated from guinea pig hearts were subjected to an oxidative or reductive environment and an imbalance in ROS developed at either extreme [52]. At greater oxidative potentials, there was an expected depletion of ROS scavengers that then allowed for ROS overflow. Greater reduction potentials, in contrast, allowed for and favored the production of ROS. This resulted in an overproduction of ROS that gradually exceeded antioxidant scavenger capacity [52].

The emerging clinical impact of reductive stress has been demonstrated by animal studies of the cardiovascular system [53,54]. Heat-shock protein 27 was used as a cardiac-specific antioxidant expressed at varying levels in transgenic mice. A reductive state was demonstrated by an increased ratio of reduced glutathione-to-oxidized glutathione and decreased ROS levels. This reduced state recapitulated the development of cardiomyopathy as these mice demonstrated decreased cardiac function and an overall lower survival rate [53]. Furthermore, inhibition of the reducing enzyme GPX actually attenuated the development of cardiac dysfunction [53]. In a similar study, overexpression of glucose-6-phosphate dehydrogenase, glutathione reductase, and GPX subjected mouse hearts to reductive stress and also recapitulated cardiomyopathy [54].

The potential impact of reductive stress has also been demonstrated in studies of the nervous system [55−57]. High concentrations of antioxidants have not conferred protection to the nervous system and may even be detrimental to neurons [55]. In an animal study, endothelial cells from mouse brains were incubated and exposed to various concentrations of antioxidants sourced from fermented rooibos tea. These cells demonstrated dose-dependent decreases in cellular proliferation [56]. Furthermore, there was also decreased permeability across the blood−brain barrier associated with antioxidant exposure [56]. Fisher and Mentor attributed these changes to reductive stress from excess antioxidant exposure [57]. They suggested that reductive stress could limit the ability of the brain microenvironment to repair capillaries and respond to injury through suppression of cellular proliferation, membrane transport, and mitochondrial function [57].

Within the setting of the male reproductive system, antioxidant supplementation may impact physiologic reactions through the loss of oxidative mechanisms. As previously discussed, cellular functions, such as protein folding and disulfide bridge formation, can be altered with ascorbic acid supplementation [8]. Furthermore, the addition of SOD to in vitro media has been shown to prevent capacitation through inhibition of local oxidation in spermatozoa [19], and the addition of excess SOD and catalase can prevent the acrosome reaction [20].

Ascorbic acid has been used in the treatment of male infertility. Seminal concentrations of ascorbic acid respond to dietary depletion or repletion of this reducing agent [58]. However, dietary ascorbic acid depletion in the semen may not necessarily impact spermatic function in healthy fertile men [58]. Furthermore, high-dose supplementation with 1000 mg of daily ascorbic acid and 800 mg of daily tocopherol does not improve semen parameters or sperm survival in patients with asthenozoospermia or reduced sperm concentration [59].

Ascorbic acid may actually act as a prooxidant that can promote cellular damage [60−62]. Studies have demonstrated that 500 mg of daily ascorbic acid supplementation for 6 weeks in healthy volunteers resulted in a significant increase in DNA damage in lymphocytes [60]. Another study demonstrated that cosupplementation of ascorbic acid with iron also promoted a transient rise in oxidative DNA damage [61].

The role of ascorbic acid as an antioxidant or a prooxidant may be influenced by its dosing. Male subjects supplemented with various doses of ascorbic acid ranging from 50 to 4000 μmol underwent semen analysis for sperm motility, sperm viability, and lipid peroxidation. Dosing below 1000 μmol resulted in a dose-dependent improvement in motility and viability as well as a decrease in lipid peroxidation [63]. High doses of ascorbic acid above the 1000 μmol threshold, however, paradoxically increased ROS levels, decreased sperm motility and viability, and increased lipid peroxidation [63].

In addition to dosing levels, the protective versus damaging effect of ascorbic acid may also depend on the timing of its administration within the setting of oxidative damage. In a study evaluating the role of antioxidant supplementation in oxidative stress, ascorbic acid was protective if administered before the initiation of cellular injury [62]. However, if ascorbic acid was administered after damaged cells had already released free transition metal ions, it generated a more reductive state that worsened the extent of injury [62].

Other reducing agents used for antioxidant supplementation may also act through the antioxidant paradox and cause additional harm. Although selenium and zinc supplementation has been shown to reduce DNA fragmentation, there was also DNA decondensation in spermatozoa that can be attributed to the high reducing potential of these two trace elements [17]. Similar outcomes were observed in patients supplemented with modified SOD [17]. These studies demonstrate that antioxidant supplementation is not without its risks. In an attempt to treat oxidative stress in male infertility, antioxidants can result in an imbalance to the other extreme and can lead to paradoxical injury through reductive stress.

CONCLUSION

While oxidative stress is commonly recognized with the modern-day lifestyle, antioxidant supplementation is not without its risks. As there is a lack of dosing guidelines or regulations for antioxidant treatment, there is potential for oversupplementation. The overuse of reducing agents has the potential to cause reductive stress that can, as part of the antioxidant paradox, result in a loss of needed oxidative mechanisms, perpetuated cellular injury in a reduced environment, and a paradoxical increase in ROS. As our understanding of oxidative and reductive reactions affecting male fertility continues to develop, more studies are needed to elucidate the phenomenon of reductive stress and its effect on male reproduction.

LIST OF ACRONYMS AND ABBREVIATIONS

GPX Glutathione peroxidase
ROS Reactive oxygen species
SOD Superoxide dismutase

REFERENCES

[1] Zalata AA, Christophe AB, Depuydt CE, Schoonjans F, Comhaire FH. White blood cells cause oxidative damage to the fatty acid composition of phospholipids of human spermatozoa. Int J Androl 1998;21:154—62.

[2] Sanocka D, Kurpisz M. Reactive oxygen species and sperm cells. Reprod Biol Endocrinol 2004;2:12.

[3] Makker K, Agarwal A, Sharma R. Oxidative stress & male infertility. Indian J Med Res 2009;129:357—67.

[4] Sies H. Strategies of antioxidant defense. Eur J Biochem 1993;215:213—9.

[5] Ufer C, Wang CC, Borchert A, Heydeck D, Kuhn H. Redox control in mammalian embryo development. Antioxid Redox Signal 2010;13:833—75.

[6] Pierce GB, Parchment RE, Lewellyn AL. Hydrogen peroxide as a mediator of programmed cell death in the blastocyst. Differentiation 1991;46:181—6.

[7] Suh JK, Poulsen LL, Ziegler DM, Robertus JD. Yeast flavin-containing monooxygenase generates oxidizing equivalents that control protein folding in the endoplasmic reticulum. Proc Natl Acad Sci U S A 1999;96(6):2687—91.

[8] Giustarini D, Dalle-Donne I, Colombo R, Milzani A, Rossi R. Is ascorbate able to reduce disulfide bridges? A cautionary note. Nitric Oxide 2008;19(3):252—8.

[9] Naviaux RK. Oxidative shielding or oxidative stress? J Pharmacol Exp Ther 2012;342:608—18.

[10] Sun JZ, Tang XL, Park SW, Qiu Y, Turrens JF, Bolli R. Evidence for an essential role of reactive oxygen species in the genesis of late preconditioning against myocardial stunning in conscious pigs. J Clin Invest 1996;97(2):562—76.

[11] Ristow M, Zarse K, Oberbach A, Kloting N, Birringer M, Kiehntopf M, et al. Antioxidants prevent health-promoting effects of physical exercise in humans. Proc Natl Acad Sci U S A 2009;106(21):8665—70.

[12] Tosic J, Walton A. Formation of hydrogen peroxide by spermatozoa and its inhibitory effect of respiration. Nature 1946;158:485.

[13] Gil-Guzman E, Ollero M, Lopez MC, Sharma RK, Alvarez JG, Thomas Jr AJ, et al. Differential production of reactive oxygen species by subsets of human spermatozoa at different stages of maturation. Hum Reprod 2001;16(9):1922—30.

[14] MacLeod J. The role of oxygen in the metabolism and motility of human spermatozoa. Am J Physiol 1943;138:512—8.

[15] Poulos A, Darin-Bennett A, White IG. The phospholipid-bound fatty acids and aldehydes of mammalian spermatozoa. Comp Biochem Physiol B 1973;46(3):541—9.

[16] Greco E, Iacobelli M, Rienzi L, Ubaldi F, Ferrero S, Tesarik J. Reduction of the incidence of sperm DNA fragmentation by oral antioxidant treatment. J Androl 2005;26(3):349—53.

[17] Menezo YJ, Hazout A, Panteix G, Robert F, Rollet J, Cohen-Bacrie P, et al. Antioxidants to reduce sperm DNA fragmentation: an unexpected adverse effect. Reprod Biomed Online 2007;14(4):418—21.

[18] Lee MA, Trucco GS, Bechtol KB, Wummer N, Kopf GS, et al. Capacitation and acrosome reactions in human spermatozoa monitored by a chlortetracycline fluorescence assay. Fertil Steril 1987;48:649—58.

[19] de Lamirande E, Harakat A, Gagnon C. Human sperm capacitation induced by biological fluids and progesterone, but not by NADH or NADPH, is associated with the production of superoxide anion. J Androl 1998;19(2):215—25.

[20] de Lamirande E, Tsai C, Harakat A, Gagnon C. Involvement of reactive oxygen species in human sperm acrosome reaction induced by A23187, lysophosphatidylcholine, and biological fluid ultrafiltrates. J Androl 1998;19(5):585—94.

[21] Halliwell B. The antioxidant paradox. Lancet 2000;355(9210):1179—80.

[22] Stephens NG, Parsons A, Schofield PM, Kelly F, Cheeseman K, Mitchinson MJ. Randomised controlled trial of vitamin E in patients with coronary disease: Cambridge Heart Antioxidant Study (CHAOS). Lancet 1996;347(9004):781—6.

[23] Dietary supplementation with n-3 polyunsaturated fatty acids and vitamin E after myocardial infarction: results of the GISSI-Prevenzione trial. Gruppo Italiano per lo Studio della Sopravvivenza nell'Infarto miocardico. Lancet 1999;354(9177):447—55.

[24] Tavilani H, Goodarzi MT, Doosti M, Vaisi-Raygani A, Hassanzadeh T, Salimi S, et al. Relationship between seminal antioxidant enzymes and the phospholipid and fatty acid composition of spermatozoa. Reprod Biomed Online 2008;16(5):649—56.

[25] Chen H, Chow PH, Cheng SK, Cheung AL, Cheng LY, O WS. Male genital tract antioxidant enzymes: their source, function in the female, and ability to preserve sperm DNA integrity in the golden hamster. J Androl 2003;24(5):704—11.

[26] Kobayashi T, Miyazaki T, Natori M, Nozawa S. Protective role of superoxide dismutase in human sperm motility: superoxide dismutase activity and lipid peroxide in human seminal plasma and spermatozoa. Hum Reprod 1991;6(7):987—91.

[27] Jeulin C, Soufir JC, Weber P, Laval-Martin D, Calvayrac R. Catalase activity in human spermatozoa and seminal plasma. Gamete Res 1989;24(2):185—96.

[28] Maser RL, Magenheimer BS, Calvet JP. Mouse plasma glutathione peroxidase. cDNA sequence analysis and renal proximal tubular expression and secretion. J Biol Chem 1994;269(43):27066—73.

[29] Schwaab V, Baud E, Ghyselinck N, Mattei MG, Dufaure JP, Drevet JR. Cloning of the mouse gene encoding plasma glutathione peroxidase: organization, sequence and chromosomal localization. Gene 1995;167(1—2):25—31.

[30] Fraga CG, Motchnik PA, Shigenaga MK, Helbock HJ, Jacob RA, Ames BN. Ascorbic acid protects against endogenous oxidative DNA damage in human sperm. Proc Natl Acad Sci U S A 1991;88(24):11003—6.

[31] Suleiman SA, Ali ME, Zaki ZM, el-Malik EM, Nasr MA. Lipid peroxidation and human sperm motility: protective role of vitamin E. J Androl 1996;17(5):530—7.

[32] Ursini F, Heim S, Kiess M, Maiorino M, Roveri A, Wissing J, et al. Dual function of the selenoprotein PHGPx during sperm maturation. Science 1999;285(5432):1393—6.

[33] Hekimoglu A, Kurcer Z, Aral F, Baba F, Sahna E, Atessahin A. Lycopene, an antioxidant carotenoid, attenuates testicular injury caused by ischemia/reperfusion in rats. Tohoku J Exp Med 2009;218(2):141—7.

[34] Ferreira AL, Yeum KJ, Liu C, Smith D, Krinsky NI, Wang XD, et al. Tissue distribution of lycopene in ferrets and rats after lycopene supplementation. J Nutr 2000;130(5):1256—60.

[35] Yoganathan T, Eskild W, Hansson V. Investigation of detoxification capacity of rat testicular germ cells and Sertoli cells. Free Radic Biol Med 1989;7(4):355—9.

[36] Bauche F, Fouchard MH, Jegou B. Antioxidant system in rat testicular cells. FEBS Lett 1994;349(3):392—6.

[37] Peltola V, Huhtaniemi I, Ahotupa M. Antioxidant enzyme activity in the maturing rat testis. J Androl 1992;13(5):450—5.

[38] Mendis-Handagama SM, Zirkin BR, Scallen TJ, Ewing LL. Studies on peroxisomes of the adult rat Leydig cell. J Androl 1990;11(3):270—8.

[39] Luo L, Chen H, Trush MA, Show MD, Anway MD, Zirkin BR. Aging and the brown Norway rat leydig cell antioxidant defense system. J Androl 2006;27(2):240—7.

[40] Zini A, Schlegel PN. Identification and characterization of antioxidant enzyme mRNAs in the rat epididymis. Int J Androl 1997;20(2):86—91.

[41] Perry AC, Jones R, Hall L. Isolation and characterization of a rat cDNA clone encoding a secreted superoxide dismutase reveals the epididymis to be a major site of its expression. Biochem J 1993;293(Pt 1):21—5.

[42] Vernet P, Faure J, Dufaure JP, Drevet JR. Tissue and developmental distribution, dependence upon testicular factors and attachment to spermatozoa of GPX5, a murine epididymis-specific glutathione peroxidase. Mol Reprod Dev 1997;47(1):87—98.

[43] Zini A, de Lamirande E, Gagnon C. Reactive oxygen species in semen of infertile patients: levels of superoxide dismutase- and catalase-like activities in seminal plasma and spermatozoa. Int J Androl 1993;16(3):183—8.

[44] Godeas C, Tramer F, Micali F, Soranzo M, Sandri G, Panfili E. Distribution and possible novel role of phospholipid hydroperoxide glutathione peroxidase in rat epididymal spermatozoa. Biol Reprod 1997;57(6):1502—8.

[45] Potts RJ, Notarianni LJ, Jefferies TM. Seminal plasma reduces exogenous oxidative damage to human sperm, determined by the measurement of DNA strand breaks and lipid peroxidation. Mutat Res 2000;447:249—56.

[46] Owen DH, Katz DF. A review of the physical and chemical properties of human semen and the formulation of a semen simulant. J Androl 2005;26:459—69.

[47] Alkan I, Simsek F, Haklar G, Kervancioglu E, Ozveri H, Yalcin S, et al. Reactive oxygen species production by the spermatozoa of patients with idiopathic infertility: relationship to seminal plasma antioxidants. J Urol 1997;157(1):140—3.

[48] Yeung CH, Cooper TG, De Geyter M, De Geyter C, Rolf C, Kamischke A, et al. Studies on the origin of redox enzymes in seminal plasma and their relationship with results of in-vitro fertilization. Mol Hum Reprod 1998;4(9):835—9.

[49] Lewis SE, Sterling ES, Young IS, Thompson W. Comparison of individual antioxidants of sperm and seminal plasma in fertile and infertile men. Fertil Steril 1997;67(1):142—7.

[50] Zhang H, Limphong P, Pieper J, Liu Q, Rodesch CK, Christians E, et al. Glutathione-dependent reductive stress triggers mitochondrial oxidation and cytotoxicity. FASEB J 2012;26(4):1442—51.

[51] Korge P, Calmettes G, Weiss JN. Increased reactive oxygen species production during reductive stress: the roles of mitochondrial glutathione and thioredoxin reductases. Biochim Biophys Acta 2015;1847:514—25.

[52] Aon MA, Cortassa S, O'Rourke B. Redox-optimized ROS balance: a unifying hypothesis. Biochim Biophys Acta 2010;1797(6—7):865—77.

[53] Zhang X, Min X, Li C, Benjamin IJ, Qian B, Zhang X, et al. Involvement of reductive stress in the cardiomyopathy in transgenic mice with cardiac-specific overexpression of heat shock protein 27. Hypertension 2010;55(6):1412—7.

[54] Rajasekaran NS, Connell P, Christians ES, Yan LJ, Taylor RP, Orosz A, et al. Human alpha B-crystallin mutation causes oxido-reductive stress and protein aggregation cardiomyopathy in mice. Cell 2007;130(3):427—39.

[55] Castagne V, Lefevre K, Natero R, Clarke PG, Bedker DA. An optimal redox status for the survival of axotomized ganglion cells in the developing retina. Neuroscience 1999;93:313—20.

[56] Mentor S, Fisher D. Aggressive antioxidant reductive stress impairs brain endothelial cell angiogenesis and blood brain barrier function. Curr Neurovasc Res 2017;14:71−81.

[57] Fisher D, Mentor S. Antioxidant-induced reductive stress has untoward consequences on the brain microvasculature. Neural Regen Res 2017;12:743−4.

[58] Jacob RA, Pianalto FS, Agee RE. Cellular ascorbate depletion in healthy men. J Nutr 1992;122(5):1111−8.

[59] Rolf C, Cooper TG, Yeung CH, Nieschlag E. Antioxidant treatment of patients with asthenozoospermia or moderate oligoasthenozoospermia with high-dose vitamin C and vitamin E: a randomized, placebo-controlled, double-blind study. Hum Reprod 1999;14(4):1028−33.

[60] Podmore ID, Griffiths HR, Herbert KE, Mistry N, Mistry P, Lunec J. Vitamin C exhibits pro-oxidant properties. Nature 1998;392(6676):559.

[61] Rehman A, Collis CS, Yang M, Kelly M, Diplock AT, Halliwell B, et al. The effects of iron and vitamin C co-supplementation on oxidative damage to DNA in healthy volunteers. Biochem Biophys Res Commun 1998;246(1):293−8.

[62] Kang SA, Jang YJ, Park H. In vivo dual effects of vitamin C on paraquat-induced lung damage: dependence on released metals from the damaged tissue. Free Radic Res 1998;28(1):93−107.

[63] Verma A, Kanwar KC. Human sperm motility and lipid peroxidation in different ascorbic acid concentrations: an in vitro analysis. Andrologia 1998;30(6):325−9.

Chapter 1.8

Physiological Role of Reactive Oxygen Species in Male Reproduction

Damayanthi Durairajanayagam

Universiti Teknologi MARA, Sungai Buloh, Selangor, Malaysia

INTRODUCTION

Free radicals are short-lived but highly reactive chemical intermediates that are formed during the stepwise enzymatic reduction of oxygen. They are made up of one or more electrons with unpaired valence electron(s) in the outer shell [1]. Two of the most common forms of active oxygen are the reactive oxygen species (ROS) and its subclass, the reactive nitrogen species (RNS). Both ROS and RNS are produced as normal by-products of various biological processes within the body [2]. In physiological amounts, they have an active involvement in the majority of normal functions of living organisms. However, excessive production of ROS causes the oxidation of lipids in cell membranes, carbohydrates, and amino acids in proteins as well as impairs nucleic acids [3].

In the male reproductive system, ROS plays a dual role. At minimal concentrations, it exerts a key physiological role in activating the intracellular signaling pathways involved in spermatozoa maturation and function. On the other hand, high levels of ROS exert a detrimental effect on semen quality and function, and this could subsequently lead to male infertility [4]. Male infertility affects 15 out of every 100 couples within the reproductive age group, with the male factor being the cause for half of these cases [5]. There is increasing evidence that oxidative stress is a chief causative factor that leads to male infertility [6,7]. It is the disruption of the delicate balance between ROS and antioxidants that results in a state of oxidative stress and consequently causes a significant impairment of spermatozoa.

Spermatozoa are particularly vulnerable to ROS-induced damage due to the fact that their plasma membranes consist of very large amounts of polyunsaturated fatty acids (PUFAs) [8]. When ROS attack PUFAs in the sperm cell membrane, a lipid peroxidation cascade is triggered. Second, spermatozoa, being almost devoid of cytoplasm, contain very low concentrations of scavenging enzymes [9]. Thus the sperm relies heavily on the antioxidant enzymes present in the seminal plasma to help protect the plasma membrane surrounding the acrosome and tail. Without the appropriate enzymes in the cytoplasm, spermatozoa lack the ability to repair the damage caused by the high levels of ROS [10].

Despite the detrimental effects of high ROS concentrations or oxidative stress on sperm functionality, low physiological levels of ROS bring about beneficial effects on the various processes involved in the development of the male germ cell. This chapter will discuss the physiological roles of ROS and its mechanism of action in regulating human sperm maturation and function.

REACTIVE OXYGEN SPECIES: ENDOGENOUS GENERATION AND SOURCES

ROS contain both radical and nonradical oxygen derivatives. Examples of radicals include superoxide anion (O_2^-), hydroxyl radical (OH^-), and peroxyl radical (HO_2^-), while hydrogen peroxide (H_2O_2) is a nonradical derivative [11] (Table 1).

There are two main sources through which normal human spermatozoa are able to generate ROS. The first occurs at the sperm plasma membrane through the nicotinamide adenine dinucleotide phosphate (NADPH) oxidase (NOX), while the

TABLE 1 Reactive Oxygen Species (ROS) and Reactive Nitrogen Species (RNS)

ROS	RNS
Radicals	
Hyperoxide/superoxide anion ($\cdot O_2^-$)	Nitric oxide ($\cdot NO$)
Hydroxyl radical ($\cdot OH$)	Nitrogen dioxide ($\cdot NO_2$)
Peroxyl radical ($RO_2\cdot$)	
Alkoxyl radical ($RO\cdot$)	
Hydroperoxyl ($HO_2\cdot$)	
Nonradicals	
Hydrogen peroxide (H_2O_2)	Peroxynitrite anion (NO_3^-)
Singlet oxygen ($^1O_2$)	Nitrous oxide (N_2O)
Ozone (O_3)	Peroxynitrous acid (HNO_3)
Hypochlorous acid ($HOCl$)	Nitroxyl anion (NO^-)
Hypobromus acid ($HOBr$)	Nitrous acid (HNO_2)

second occurs at the inner mitochondrial membrane through the nicotinamide adenine dinucleotide (NADH)-dependent oxidoreductase. The ROS contribution of the latter system is generally considered to be very low [12].

The primary ROS that is most abundantly generated in human spermatozoa is superoxide anion. It is a typical by-product of oxidative phosphorylation during cellular respiration in the mitochondria. Superoxide anion reacts with itself in a dismutation reaction to produce hydrogen peroxide and oxygen molecule, O_2. Superoxide anion can produce the hydroxyl radical through the metal-catalyzed Haber-Weiss reaction or the Fenton reaction, whereby ferrous ions act as reducing agents in the generation of the hydroxyl radical from hydrogen peroxide [11]. The highly reactive hydroxyl radical is responsible for the initiation of the lipid peroxidation cascade, which consequently leads to a detrimental loss of sperm function [13].

The main producers of ROS in human semen are the activated (peroxidase positive) leukocytes such as macrophages and polymorphonucleocytes, which are mainly released with prostatic and seminal vesicle secretions [14,15]. Activated leukocytes can cause a 100-fold increase in ROS production compared to the nonactivated form of leukocytes [16]. Among the factors that can activate leukocytes are infection and inflammation [17]. In order to fight infections, the NOX catalyzes the formation of free radicals through the hexose monophosphate shunt, which leads to the formation of NADPH. The NOX transfers electrons from NADPH to oxygen to produce superoxide anion [18].

Another significant source of excessive ROS production in semen is immature or damaged sperm with either abnormal head morphology or retention of cytoplasm [19]. During the normal sperm differentiation and maturation process, excess cytoplasm is extruded into a residual body. Failure of or defect in cytoplasmic extrusion results in the retention of excess residual cytoplasm in the abnormal sperm and the retention of excess of cytoplasmic enzymes such as glucose-6-phosphate dehydrogenase (G6PDH) and NOX [20]. These enzymes facilitate the intracellular availability of NADPH, which leads to the generation of ROS [21].

Excessive seminal ROS levels play an important role in the pathophysiology of male infertility. In the seminal plasma of infertile men, high seminal ROS levels were directly correlated with a high percentage of apoptosis [22]. Sperm DNA damage can take place as a direct consequence of oxidative stress (OS) or secondary to dysregulated apoptosis factors. High ROS levels are also associated with lipid peroxidation and the subsequent reduction in sperm motility [23].

REACTIVE NITROGEN SPECIES: ENDOGENOUS GENERATION AND SOURCES

RNS are nitrogen-containing compounds, examples of which include nitric oxide ($\cdot NO$), nitrous oxide (N_2O), peroxynitrite (NO_3^-), nitroxyl anion (NO^-), and peroxynitrous acid (HNO_3) (Table 1). The major RNS in human spermatozoa is nitric oxide. Sources of RNS in the male reproductive system are the penis, testes, epididymides, accessory glands (e.g., seminal vesicles, prostate gland), and seminal ejaculate [24].

Nitric oxide is generated in a redox-reaction between L-arginine and oxygen, which forms L-citrulline as a by-product. This reaction is initiated by NADPH and catalyzed by the enzyme nitric oxide synthase (NOS). Nitric oxide reacts with superoxide anion to form the highly toxic peroxynitrite anion [25]. The reaction between superoxide anion and nitric oxide occurs three times quicker compared to the dismutation of superoxide catalyzed by the enzyme superoxide dismutase (SOD). As nitric oxide concentration reaches the nanomolar range and approximate SOD concentration in the tissue, competition ensues between nitric oxide and SOD for the removal of superoxide anion by forming peroxynitrite [26].

Accumulation of RNS contributes to a state of nitrosative stress, which may exert pathological effects on the male reproductive system, possibly leading to a compromise in sperm function as well as its fertilizing ability [24]. Excess levels of nitric oxide have been implicated in lipid peroxidation of the PUFAs within the sperm plasma membrane [27], inhibition of steroidogenesis in testicular Leydig cells [28], and apoptosis of germ cells [29].

PHYSIOLOGICAL LEVELS OF REACTIVE OXYGEN SPECIES AND SPERM FUNCTION

Spermatogenesis and Sperm Maturation

Spermatogenesis involves an exceptionally complex sequence of cellular events that begins with the development of germ cells, spermatogonia, leading up to the production of the highly specialized male gamete, spermatozoa. The maturation process of spermatozoa involves highly organized physiological development along with morphological alterations leading up to sperm activation.

During spermatogenesis, the spermatogonia undergo mitosis either to provide a renewing stem cell population or to produce primary spermatocytes. Mitosis functions to proliferate and maintain a pool of spermatogonia cells, whose genetic contents are identical to its parent cell. Next, primary spermatocytes undergo meiosis I to form secondary spermatocytes, which then undergo meiosis II to produce spermatids that contain half the number of chromosomes compared to its parent cells. Throughout the entire meiotic phase, homologous chromosomes pair up, cross over, and exchange genetic material to produce an entirely new genome, ensuring genetic diversity [30].

Next spermiogenesis takes place where haploid spermatids undergo morphological changes to form highly specialized spermatozoa with remodeled and fully compacted chromatin. Human sperm go through eight different stages as it matures from spermatid to spermatozoa. Morphological changes noted include progressive condensation of the nuclear chromatin and inactivation of the genome, as well as formation of the axoneme, acrosome cap, and flagellum [31]. Toward the end of spermiogenesis, the surrounding Sertoli cells extrude and phagocytose most of the sperm cytoplasm, producing residual bodies [32]. The remnant portion of Sertoli cell cytoplasm becomes the cytoplasmic droplet present around the midpiece of the spermatozoa after spermiogenesis [20]. The lack of SPEM1 (spermatid maturation 1) protein, expressed exclusively in cytoplasm of elongating or elongated spermatids, leads to abnormal cytoplasm removal and deformation of late spermatids [33]. Along with the various steps that occur during sperm maturation, cytoplasmic extrusion is a critical step in attaining the sperm-zona binding capacity and sperm fertilization potential [34].

Following spermiogenesis, the mature but immotile spermatozoa travel from the Sertoli cell into the lumen of the seminiferous tubules. Spermatozoa then pass from the testis to the epididymis where posttesticular concentration, maturation, and temporary storage of spermatozoa take place. During the passage through the epididymis, spermatozoa attain their full maturity, ability to fertilize, and motility [35]. However, it is only in the postejaculatory phase that spermatozoa are able to move under their own control. During sperm maturation in the epididymis, sperm plasma membrane is altered based on removal, as well as addition and rearrangement of novel sperm surface proteins [36]. Not only does the spermatozoa undergo membrane, nuclear, and enzyme-related remodeling during its time in the epididymis, the signal transduction mechanism required for the subsequent capacitation and hyperactivation events are also put in place [36,37].

During the protamination of sperm chromatin, histones are initially replaced by transition proteins, and then subsequently by protamines [38]. Protamination facilitates the condensation of sperm chromatin, which helps protect the paternal genome from damage. Moreover, DNA compaction improves the sperm head volume and shape, thereby optimizing its hydrodynamics [39]. Approximately 85% of histones are substituted with protamines during the protamination process, while the remaining 15% are carried over by the mature spermatozoa [40]. Shortly after fertilization, the protamines in the sperm chromatin are replaced by histones from the oocyte. This decondensation of the sperm nucleus then leads to the formation of a male pronucleus [41].

The maturing spermatozoa travelling through the epididymis will undergo chromatin packaging to achieve chromatin stability, and these events are regulated by redox processes that concurrently maintain the structural maturation of the sperm cell as well as its protection against ROS-induced damage. An example of enzymes with dual effects is the glutathione peroxidase (GPX) family, which function either as thiol peroxidases or ROS scavengers [42]. Another example of thiol peroxidases is the peroxiredoxin enzymes. Peroxiredoxins function as hydroperoxide scavengers and are involved in the regulation of hydrogen peroxide and ROS-dependent signaling events [43].

By acting as oxidizing agents, physiological levels of ROS induce chromatin condensation, which improves its stability, thereby increasing the defense of the compacted DNA against physical or chemical damage [44]. Condensation of the sperm chromatin involves a profound and sequential reorganization of DNA-associated proteins. Protamines, which contain an abundance of cysteine residues, are phosphorylated immediately upon its synthesis. However upon binding to DNA, the majority of the phosphate groups are removed and the cysteine residues undergo oxidization. The disulfide bridges formed between the protamines bring adjacent DNA closer together, thereby condensing the sperm chromatin [38]. As spermatozoa move from the caput to caudal epididymis, strong disulfide bonds are formed between the cysteine residues of the protamines (by oxidation of the thiol groups of cysteine residues), which contribute to the stability of the chromatin [45].

The lumen of the mammalian epididymis contains significant quantities of hydrogen peroxide that participates in sulfoxidation of protamines required for sperm DNA compaction. The mammalian epididymis also contains several GPX (GPX1, GPX3, GPX4, and GPX5), which are localized in the epididymal epithelium and luminal compartment. The most abundant of these are the selenium-dependent GPX3 cytosolic enzyme, which is increasingly expressed from caput to cauda, and the selenium-independent GPX5, which is secreted only in the caput epithelium. Thus, GPX5 acts as disulfide isomerases in controlling the amount of luminal hydrogen peroxide available for optimal ROS-mediated sulfoxidation events while simultaneously acting as true hydrogen peroxide luminal scavengers in protecting maturing cauda epididymal spermatozoa from hydrogen peroxide-mediated DNA damage [42].

The GPX family of enzymes is involved in the oxidation of free thiols (reduced form), which leads to the formation of disulphide bridges (oxidized form). The GPX4 isoform, also known as phospholipid hydroperoxide glutathione peroxidase (PHGPX), is the only GPX isoform that can reduce phospholipid hydrogen peroxides. In spermatids, the nuclear form of PHGPX is involved in the cross-linking of protamine thiols, which is required for stabilization of sperm chromatin [46]. In the absence of the PHGPX enzyme, PHGPX-knockout mice were found to have weak formation of chromatin disulphide bonds and poor chromatin condensation, along with increased free thiol levels [47].

The sperm mitochondrial capsule encases the outer membrane of the mitochondria of mammalian spermatozoa. This selenium- and disulfide-enriched structure contains mainly PHGPX as well as the sperm mitochondrion-associated cysteine-rich protein (SMCP) and fragments of specific keratins [48]. In spermatids, PHGPX is an active, soluble peroxidase, but in mature spermatozoa, PHGPX becomes an enzymatically inactive, oxidatively cross-linked, insoluble protein in the mitochondrial capsule. As such, PHGPX acts as a structural protein that provides mechanical stability to the mitochondrial midpiece in the sperm [49].

The structural protection of the mitochondria is warranted as the mitochondria plays a critical role in cellular metabolism, regulation of ROS generation, and apoptosis. As an energy source for the differentiation and function of spermatozoa, sperm mitochondria serve as both a source and target of ROS [50]. In this capacity, PHGPX also confers protection of germ cells against oxidative damage [51] as well as regulates apoptotic signals [52].

The process of spermatogenesis requires a high amount of testosterone within the testis. Testosterone is produced by the Leydig cells, and its secretion is regulated by luteinizing hormone (LH). Besides LH, other hormones secreted from the anterior pituitary that play a role in spermatogenesis are the follicle stimulating hormone (FSH) and prolactin. FSH stimulates the Sertoli cells to develop and secrete nutrients and growth factors required by the germ cells for their normal development. Prolactin along with inhibin, which is secreted by the Sertoli cells, both take part in the regulation of normal sperm development [53]. The gonadotropin releasing hormone (GnRH) secreted by the hypothalamus stimulates LH and FSH action on the Leydig and Sertoli cells, respectively. Release of these hormones that are involved in testicular function is regulated via a feedback mechanism along the hypothalamic-pituitary-testicular axis. Hypothalamic GnRH coordinates the synthesis and secretion of both LH and FSH with the transcription and translation of the gonadotropin genes. GnRH secretion activates signaling cascades, which mobilize intracellular calcium and activate protein kinase C (PKC) isoforms and the mitogen-activated protein kinase (MAPK) family of second messengers in the gonadotropes of the anterior pituitary. In the nucleus, the MAPKs activate factors to increase immediate-early response genes, which are regulated either directly by ROS signaling or via ROS-mediated MAPK activation [54].

A major source of GnRH-induced intracellular ROS is the NOX/dual oxidase (DUOX) family. Inhibition of NOX/DUOX activity was found to suppress GnRH-stimulated FSH and LH secretion. Thus, ROS generated from NOX/DUOX is crucial for GnRH signaling in gonadotropes by linking the activation of PKC to downstream stimulation of MAPK signaling and gene expression [54]. Moreover, NOX-derived ROS were found to be involved in thyroid hormone biosynthesis [55], another hormone that has a role in male reproduction [56]. The presence of NOX isoforms have also been reported in the prostate and testis, and their actions in the latter are likely to be of importance in spermatogenesis and fertilization [55].

It is widely accepted that controlled amounts of ROS are essential for the specific oxidative processes involved in sperm development and maturation. The delicate balance between ROS and antioxidant strategies must be regulated precisely in order to maintain normal sperm physiology and protect from the adverse effects of excessive ROS on sperm development [36]. Perhaps the intake of high levels of antioxidants into a well-controlled redox homeostatic environment could end up eliminating too much ROS [57], which could inadvertently compromise certain critical steps in sperm physiology that necessitates a particular level of ROS for proper functioning.

In one study, males with two or more past in vitro fertilization or intracytoplasmic sperm injection failures were given a daily oral antioxidant regime comprising vitamins C and E, β-carotene, zinc, and selenium for 90 days to encompass a complete spermatogenesis cycle [58]. Among the antioxidants prescribed, vitamins C and E, and selenium exert a direct antioxidant effect by neutralizing existing ROS, while selenium and zinc are essential contributors to sperm DNA synthesis and protamine packaging [59]. Although ROS production and sperm DNA fragmentation was decreased, sperm nuclear decondensation was found to be increased, potentially mediated by the strong redox potential of vitamin C, which had disrupted the intermolecular disulphide linkages between protamines. Thus it seems that a certain amount of ROS is a requisite for maintaining the integrity of the disulfide cross-links to ensure proper DNA compaction [58]. The process of locking the disulphide bridges consists of a cascade of three oxidation/reduction processes. These processes are initiated by oxidation and lead to (1) peroxidation of sperm membrane lipids, (2) oxidization of glutathione to regenerate sperm membrane integrity, (3) oxidation of protamine cysteines, and (4) formation of disulphide bridges, along with reduction of oxidized glutathione and regeneration of reduced glutathione. It is therefore clear that a balance between pro-and antioxidants must be upheld to ensure proper compaction of sperm DNA as well as offer protection against oxidative damage [60].

The lack of cytoplasm in the spermatozoon limits its antioxidant contents and thereby its capacity to control ROS levels, which may leak into the cytoplasm from its highly dense mitochondria within the midpiece [61]. The seminal plasma, however, contains an abundance of different enzymatic and nonenzymatic antioxidants, which include SOD, catalase, GPX, vitamins C and E, and zinc. The seminal fluid is secreted by the seminal vesicles, prostate gland, and Cowper's gland and provides a medium for sperm sustenance and transport [30]. The antioxidants of the seminal fluid contribute greatly to male fertility by maintaining redox homeostasis [62].

Further studies on the role of physiological levels of ROS in spermatogenesis and that of the cellular systems that maintain ROS at physiological levels are required to fully understand the positive contribution of ROS on male fertility. However, such studies, whether in vivo or in vitro, has its own challenges. These include the inability as yet to study sperm development in vitro, inconsistencies present amid the highly divergent redox conditions in vivo compared to in vitro, and lack of genetic animal models to explicitly allocate distinct redox-dependent processes to the specific steps of spermatogenesis in vivo. Deeper knowledge regarding the molecular role of ROS and its regulatory mechanisms in spermatogenesis will be useful in anticipating high ROS-induced negative outcomes of gametogenesis and improving assisted reproduction techniques [63].

Capacitation, Hyperactivation, and Chemotaxis

Immediately upon ejaculation, human spermatozoa are incapable of progressive motility and fertilization. However, as it travels along the female reproductive tract, spermatozoa gain the ability to fertilize the oocyte through the critical processes of capacitation and hyperactivation. During capacitation, spermatozoa go through a series of biochemical changes and a complex cascade of molecular events that ultimately optimizes its fertilizing capacity. Hyperactivation occurs spontaneously and in a time-dependent manner with capacitation whereas the acrosome reaction occurs after the completion of capacitation. It is only the capacitated sperm that are capable of undergoing acrosome reaction and subsequently fertilization [64].

Capacitation also facilitates the development of a more vigorous, distinct motility pattern termed hyperactivation, which involves a low-frequency, high-amplitude, asymmetric flagellar movement with a nonlinear trajectory and significant lateral displacement of the sperm head resulting in propulsive movement. In contrast, nonhyperactivated sperm demonstrate a high-frequency, low-amplitude, symmetrical flagellar beat pattern and linear velocity that result in forward, progressive motion [65]. Therefore, hyperactivation equips the mature spermatozoa with adequate forward thrust necessary to drive the sperm head forward and through the cumulus cells to penetrate the zona pellucida surrounding the oocyte [66,67]. Hyperactivation helps ensure that only viable and mature sperm gain access to the oocyte and thus is a requisite for fertilization [62]. During hyperactivation, cellular responsiveness to chemotactic signaling increases in order to better orientate the sperm toward the oocyte [68].

During capacitation, spermatozoa undergo an intricate and timely sequence of modifications that involve ionic, metabolic, and membrane alterations as they pass through the female reproductive tract [69]. Molecular changes that occur during capacitation include the removal of cholesterol, entry of bicarbonate (HCO_3^-) and calcium (Ca^{2+}) ions, generation of ROS, increase in intracellular pH and cyclic adenosine monophosphate (cAMP) levels, protein phosphorylation (serine/threonine (Ser/Thr) and tyrosine (Tyr)), and hyperpolarization of the sperm membrane [66,70]. Capacitation also involves ROS-induced tyrosine phosphorylation of the sperm tail, which helps facilitate the switch in characteristic movement from forward progressive to propulsive motility in hyperactivated spermatozoa [67].

Phosphorylation/dephosphorylation of proteins is a form of posttranslational modification that commonly regulates protein activity by either adding or removing phosphate groups from Ser, Thr, or Tyr residues of protein moieties, which will then either activate or inactivate these proteins. The phosphorylation or dephosphorylation of these phosphoproteins is regulated by the counteracting activity of protein kinases and phosphatases, respectively [71]. Posttranslational modifications play an important role in sperm function as spermatozoa are incapable of synthesizing proteins [69].

The physiological role of ROS on potentiating capacitation has been elucidated over the years through extensive research. Exposure of spermatozoa to minimal levels of exogenous hydrogen peroxide initiates capacitation, and subsequently induces high rates of sperm—oocyte fusion. The initiation of capacitation was observed based on the spermatozoa's functional response (display of hyperactivated motility and its readiness to undergo acrosome reaction) to the divalent calcium ionophore, A23187. Not only does A23187 increase intracellular Ca^{2+} levels, it also enhances the rate of hydrogen peroxide production and increases tyrosine phosphorylation [72]. The presence of ROS induces phosphorylation and is a requisite for increasing the number of tyrosine phosphorylated (P-Tyr) proteins (molecular weight ~ 100 kDa) [73,74].

Human spermatozoa can generate ROS such as superoxide anion, which then spontaneously dismutate to hydrogen peroxide [75,76]. It is widely accepted that hydrogen peroxide plays a vital role in the process of capacitation while superoxide anion serves as an essential molecule for regulating hyperactivation [77,78]. Superoxide anion generated from an established biological inducer of hyperactivation (e.g., xanthine + xanthine oxidase + catalase) was demonstrated to trigger sperm hyperactivation and capacitation, but both these processes were inhibited by the addition of SOD [79,80]. Low concentrations of hydrogen peroxide were found to induce capacitation by activating adenylyl cyclase and causing an increase in cAMP levels, which then leads to protein kinase A (PKA)-dependent protein tyrosine phosphorylation. These effects of low dose hydrogen peroxide were comparable to that of bicarbonate, which is a known activator of soluble adenylyl cyclase in sperm [81].

As sperm capacitation is an oxidative process, it can apparently be induced exogenously using low concentrations of specific oxidants. Besides superoxide anion and hydrogen peroxide, low and controlled concentrations of nitric oxide have a significant role in sperm function. Nitric oxide produced by human sperm act as an intracellular signaling molecule in the capacitation and acrosome reaction. Low levels of nitric oxide induce capacitation in human sperm in vitro through mechanisms involving hydrogen peroxide [82]. Nitric oxide could either (1) directly react with hydrogen peroxide to generate singlet oxygen or (2) further oxidize to nitrosonium cation before reacting with hydrogen peroxide to form peroxynitrite anion. The resulting singlet oxygen or peroxynitrite anion from these reactions could then act on either membrane or cellular lipids/thiol-containing molecules, respectively. The highly reactive peroxynitrite anion could also decompose into nitrogen dioxide and hydroxyl radical [83]. However, since NOS activity was undetected in human sperm in this study, it was suggested that the sperm comes into contact with nitric oxide in the female reproductive tract where it then enhances the capacitation process [82].

In a later in vitro study, nitric oxide-releasing compounds were found to hasten the capacitation process in human sperm and stimulate tyrosine phosphorylation of sperm proteins. However, NOS inhibitors decreased the acrosome reaction [84]. In a subsequent study, it was reported that noncapacitating sperm produced low levels of nitric oxide, whereas capacitating sperm had a time-dependent increase of nitric oxide production. Nitric oxide acts as a cellular messenger by modulating the cAMP-PKA pathway involved in capacitation [85].

Early during the capacitation process, low levels of ROS are generated to trigger the phosphorylation cascade, which can be categorized into the early, middle, and late time points [69]. Within the first 30 min of the initiation of capacitation, ROS act as signaling molecules to carry out the early activation of the adenylyl cyclase-PKA pathway [86], leading to protein phosphorylation. This early phosphorylation of proteins with the arginine-X-X-Ser/Thr motif [87] is required to activate the late phosphorylation of tyrosine proteins, which takes place 2 h after capacitation had initially begun [88].

Tyrosine phosphorylation of the human sperm flagellar proteins is involved in the acquisition of hyperactive motility [89]. During capacitation, there is a significant increase in phosphorylation mainly in the principal piece of human sperm flagellum. The tyrosine phosphorylated proteins involved in capacitation are mainly the protein A-kinase anchoring proteins (AKAPs) (namely AKAP4 (also known as AKAP82), its precursor pro-AKAP4, and FSP95) [90] as well as calcium-binding and tyrosine phosphorylation-regulated protein (CABYR), which are found on the cytoskeletal fibrous sheath of human sperm flagellum. AKAPs act as scaffolds for the integration of cAMP and other signaling molecules such as protein kinases (e.g., PKA) [69] and protein phosphatases [91]. The cross-talk between tyrosine phosphorylation and Ca^{2+} in the signal transduction pathway is believed to involve CABYR [92].

Intracellular calcium signaling is the primary regulator of sperm flagellar beat and thus regulates sperm motility [93]. Cation channels of sperm (CatSper) are a Ca^{2+}-permeable channel that is expressed solely in the membrane of the sperm flagellum [94]. These channels are pH-activated and progesterone-sensitive in human spermatozoa [95]. Motility in human sperm is regulated by two independent but interlinked Ca^{2+} signaling pathways comprising (1) the activation of CatSper in the flagellum (by alkalinization or progesterone-induced), which increases intracellular calcium levels, and (2) the mobilization of stored Ca^{2+} at the sperm neck (via Ca^{2+}-induced Ca^{2+} release). Ca^{2+} signals generated from both these signaling mechanisms regulate different behaviors in human sperm: the release of stored Ca^{2+} strongly induces hyperactive motility while activation of CatSper enhances penetration into a viscous medium (mimicking the cervical mucus or cumulus matrix) [96]. Other stimuli that could induce a CatSper-dependent increase in intracellular Ca^{2+} levels include serum albumin, pH (intracellular alkalinization), cyclic nucleotides (cAMP and cyclic guanosine monophosphate (cGMP)), soluble adenylyl cyclase, and zona pellucida glycoprotein [64].

Albumin-induced removal of cholesterol is an essential trigger for capacitation and hyperactivation [97]. Bovine serum albumin (BSA) has been shown to induce capacitation in vitro by facilitating cholesterol efflux and increasing membrane fluidity in the presence of bicarbonate [98]. The removal of cholesterol also correlates with an increase in protein phosphorylation [99]. In human spermatozoa, BSA was found to induce capacitation by generating ROS (superoxide anion and nitric oxide) [100]. Molecularly, the removal of cholesterol can activate certain transporters (e.g., sodium (Na^+)/HCO_3^- cotransporter (NBC)) or ion channels (e.g., CatSper), which then regulates signaling pathways such as the cAMP-PKA pathway [101].

Sperm capacitation is mediated by an increase in cAMP content and subsequent activation of PKA. Exposure of human sperm to papaverine (a phosphodiesterase inhibitor) increased both cAMP content and PKA activity to markedly increase progesterone-induced intracellular Ca^{2+} levels. This suggested that progesterone-induced Ca^{2+} entry is upregulated by PKA activation [102]. It was later found that the regulation of capacitation by the PKA-dependent pathway is initiated by the influx of both Ca^{2+} and bicarbonate ions [103]. During sperm capacitation, protein tyrosine phosphorylation is dependent on PKA activity. The enzyme PKA acts by adding a phosphate to a target protein, thus modifying its structure and altering its activity. Exogenous addition of superoxide anion, hydrogen peroxide, and nitric oxide was found to trigger an immediate generation of cAMP in spermatozoa in vitro and subsequently cause PKA activation [69].

During capacitation, the activation of PKA depends primarily on cAMP produced by the bicarbonate-dependent soluble adenylyl cyclase [103]. Elevated Ca^{2+} levels along with ROS also lead to activation of adenylyl cyclase. Superoxide anion causes adenylyl cyclase activation by oxidizing a thiol group. Adenylyl cyclase activity increases the production of adenosine triphosphate-induced cAMP via the adenylyl cyclase/cAMP/PKA pathway. High cAMP levels then stimulate PKA activation causing Ser/Thr phosphorylation, which is involved in both the activation of protein tyrosine kinases (PTKs) and inhibition of protein tyrosine phosphatases (PTPs). Phosphatase enzymes catalyze the breakdown of cAMP and terminate its function. ROS on the other hand inhibit phosphatase activity, causing an increase in intracellular cAMP levels, which then stimulates protein phosphorylation. Hydrogen peroxide stimulates PTK activity and inhibits PTP activation, whereas superoxide anion directly stimulates tyrosine phosphorylation. Activation of PKA also stimulates the membrane-bound NOX, which is a crucial ROS-producing enzyme, to cause an increase in ROS levels [104].

Acrosome Reaction

Upon successfully undergoing and completing a series of biochemical and physiological processes during hyperactivation and capacitation, the spermatozoa is now ready for the next step of acrosome reaction, which occurs immediately after capacitation. Since sperm capacitation is a prerequisite for a normal acrosomal reaction and the subsequent fertilization event, only capacitated sperm will proceed to this stage. Hyperactivation, however, is not as necessary for acrosome reaction as it is for fertilization.

Acrosome reaction is a process of exocytosis involving the fusion of the outer acrosomal membrane with the plasma membrane of the sperm head. Next, fenestration and vesiculation of the fused membranes occur. This eventually leads to the dispersion of the acrosomal matrix. At this point, proteolytic enzymes are released (primarily acrosin and hyaluronidase), which then digest the cumulus oophorus and zona pellucida, creating an aperture to facilitate sperm movement across these layers. This process allows the spermatozoa to gain access to the oocyte for sperm—oocyte fusion to transpire [105].

The role of ROS in acrosome reaction is debatable. Moreover, there is no clear consensus as yet as to which ROS plays the major role in acrosome reaction. Based on past studies, hydrogen peroxide [72] and superoxide anion [106] have been suggested to be the oxygen radical involved in A23187-induced acrosome reaction. In one study, hydrogen peroxide was found to simulate the effects of A23187 and upregulate tyrosine phosphorylation of proteins. However, the source of hydrogen peroxide involved during the experiment could not be specified [72].

In another study, spermatozoa undergoing A23187-induced acrosome reaction were found to produce marked amounts of superoxide anion. Exogenously added superoxide anion was unable to induce acrosome reaction but altered the lipid membrane by causing the release of unesterified fatty acids from membrane phospholipids [107]. In an effort to clear up the discrepancy, a subsequent study used a variety of inducers of acrosome reaction, namely A23187 (a calcium ionophore), fetal cord serum ultrafiltrate (FCSu) and follicular fluid ultrafiltrate (FFu) (biological fluids), and a lipid-disturbing agent lysophosphatidylcholine to induce acrosome reaction in capacitated sperm only. This study demonstrated that low levels of both hydrogen peroxide and superoxide anion exert a significant effect on acrosome reaction [108].

It was also later demonstrated that human spermatozoa do have a detectable level of NOS activity, and that incubation with protein-enriched extracts of human follicular fluid increased NOS activity. The study also proposed that NO synthesized by human sperm may be involved in follicular fluid-induced acrosomal reaction [109]. During the acrosome reaction, NO possibly acts either by increasing prostaglandin E2 (PGE2) or via an increase in cGMP levels and protein kinase G activation [110].

Thus it seems that at low and controlled concentrations, ROS such as hydrogen peroxide, superoxide anion, and nitric oxide provide a stimulatory effect on acrosome reaction [108,110,111]. However, in comparison to the level of positive contribution of these ROS on capacitation, low levels of hydrogen peroxide have a very minimal effect on acrosome reaction [78,106]. Similarly, the effects of superoxide anion on acrosome reaction were reported to be even less pronounced compared to hydrogen peroxide [76,112]. One study looked into the effect of both low and high ROS levels on acrosin activity in human spermatozoa, but found that ROS did not seem to affect acrosin activity at the doses used [113].

During the functional maturation of sperm, the processes of capacitation and acrosome reaction occur very quickly one after another. The biochemistry of acrosome reaction seems to greatly overlap with that of capacitation. Both processes involve the influx of Ca^{2+} as well as increased levels of cAMP and PKA. However, the regulatory pathways of ROS in the acrosome reaction process are not as well described as that of the capacitation process (even though this also is not fully elucidated yet) [104]. Similarly, in the presence of low levels of ROS, both capacitation and acrosome reaction involve the tyrosine phosphorylation of the same proteins, particularly those with the molecular weights of 70, 76, 81, and 105 kDa. Thus it was suggested that ROS regulates capacitation and acrosome reaction via a common biochemical pathway that results in the tyrosine phosphorylation of similar proteins [108].

Besides protein phosphorylation, ROS also exerts a positive effect on selected molecules involved in the pathways of the acrosome reaction process, such as soluble adenylyl cyclase, PKC, and phospholipase A2 (PLA2) [114,115]. PLA2 is an enzyme that cleaves intact phosphoglycerolipids into free fatty acids and lysophospholipids [116]. PLA2 is activated in human spermatozoa in response to progesterone [117], which is an endogenous inducer of acrosome reaction. Progesterone secreted by cumulus cells act as a vital cofactor in this exocytosis event. The binding of agonists progesterone or zona pellucida glycoprotein-3 (ZP3) to sperm plasma membrane receptors activates signaling pathways involved in the acrosome reaction [118].

Phospholipase A2 along with guanosine triphosphate-binding proteins and Ca^{2+} are part of the signaling cascade leading to acrosome reaction in human sperm [119]. Increase in intracellular Ca^{2+} levels, along with activation of adenylate cyclase and phospholipase C, stimulate an increase in PLA2 activity. These changes are required for membrane fusion to occur [118,119]. During acrosome reaction, the fusion between outer acrosomal and plasma membranes results in the exposure of the inner acrosomal membrane. Activation of PLA2 increases the plasma membrane fluidity of the spermatozoa in preparation of sperm—oocyte fusion. Thus, PLA2 is involved in the regulation of acrosome reaction and subsequently in achieving a successful sperm—oocyte fusion [107,120]. ROS in the form of both superoxide anion and hydrogen peroxide are able to cause the activation of PLA2 [121].

Sperm—Oocyte Fusion

Following the acrosome reaction process, the spermatozoon is able to effectively penetrate the zona pellucida and reach the peri-vitelline space, where it will fuse with the oolemma. The fusion of spermatozoon and oocyte marks the end of a successful journey for the spermatozoon. At this stage, the sperm plasma membrane is very fluid due to the unusually high content of long chain PUFAs (mainly docosahexaenoic acid, 22:6). High membrane fluidity is beneficial during the membrane fusion events of fertilization. Sperm membrane fluidity is further enhanced by the activity of PLA2 [116]. ROS in the form of hydrogen peroxide, via the activation of tyrosine kinase, is able to activate PKC to then trigger an increase in PLA2 activity [120]. ROS also exert an inhibitory effect on PTPs, which will suppress dephosphorylation and therefore increase PLA2 activity [122].

Physiological levels of ROS contribute positively to the event of sperm−oocyte fusion. Low levels of ROS, in both hydrogen peroxide and superoxide anion forms, have been shown to increase sperm−oocyte fusion rates [72,123,124]. An increase in phosphorylation of tyrosine proteins is also associated with higher rates of fertilization [123]. This seems to indicate that the event of sperm−oocyte fusion correlates well with the processes of capacitation and acrosome reaction that take place before it [125]. A strong correlation exists between ROS levels within the physiological levels and the rate of sperm−oocyte fusion [1,123].

CONCLUSION

Spermatogenesis and the processes involved in sperm function are all subject to redox regulation. Therefore, maintenance of ROS levels within the physiological range is absolutely critical for proper sperm functioning and in ensuring the success of fertilization. ROS play an important role in certain oxidative processes during sperm development and maturation. ROS take part in signal transduction of biochemical cascades, probably through the oxidation of thiol groups of cysteine residues, which controls the activation of adenylyl cyclase that increases cAMP levels, which then leads to PKA-dependent protein tyrosine phosphorylation.

In the maturing epididymal spermatozoa, hydrogen peroxide mediates the sulfoxidation of protamines necessary for chromatin condensation that will improve chromatin stability and strengthen DNA integrity. Similarly, PHGPX and hydrogen peroxide induce the oxidation of free thiols to form disulphide bridges in the mitochondrial capsule, which provides mechanical stability to the mitochondria in the sperm midpiece. With regard to the endocrine regulation of spermatogenesis, ROS generated from NOX/DUOX is crucial for GnRH signaling in gonadotropes, which helps sustain the secretion of GnRH and subsequently LH and FSH.

Upon ejaculation, human sperm undergo the capacitation process in order to gain its fertilizing potential. Human spermatozoa are able to produce superoxide anion, hydrogen peroxide, and nitric oxide. At low and controlled levels, these ROS contribute positively toward sperm function with hydrogen peroxide playing a vital role in inducing capacitation while superoxide anion serves as an essential molecule in regulating hyperactivation. Similarly, superoxide anion and nitric oxide induce capacitation via the regulation of the same adenylyl cyclase/cAMP/PKA intracellular pathway to phosphorylate protein. While hydrogen peroxide induces PTK activity and inhibits phosphatase activity, superoxide anion directly stimulates tyrosine phosphorylation. Activation of PKA also stimulates a NOX-induced increase in ROS levels. ROS-mediated tyrosine phosphorylation is also required for the chemotaxis of capacitated sperm.

Low levels of hydrogen peroxide, superoxide anion, and nitric oxide provide a stimulatory effect on the acrosome reaction, which occurs immediately after capacitation. ROS stimulate soluble adenylyl cyclase, PKC, and PLA2 in the signaling cascade leading to acrosome reaction in human sperm. Increase in intracellular Ca^{2+} levels, along with activation of adenylate cyclase and phospholipase C, stimulate an increase in PLA2 activity. Both superoxide anion and hydrogen peroxide activate PLA2, which increases sperm plasma membrane fluidity in preparation of sperm−oocyte fusion.

Sperm−oocyte fusion correlates well with the earlier processes of capacitation and acrosome reaction. Via the activation of tyrosine kinase, hydrogen peroxide activates PKC and triggers increased PLA2 activity. ROS also inhibit PTPs, which decrease dephosphorylation to increase PLA2 activity. Increase in tyrosine phosphorylation induced by both hydrogen peroxide and superoxide anion results in higher rates of fertilization.

It is evident that a subtle balance between the formation and degradation of ROS must be sustained for the proper functioning and survival of spermatozoa. Despite current knowledge of the beneficial actions of ROS, further in-depth understanding of the actions of low and controlled amounts of ROS and the mechanisms through which they regulate human sperm function in vivo is still required. Additional clinical studies are warranted to determine the physiological range of ROS levels in both the fertile and sub- or infertile population, as this will be particularly helpful in the management of male reproductive health.

LIST OF ACRONYMS AND ABBREVIATIONS

A23187 divalent calcium ionophore
AKAP A-kinase anchoring protein
Arg arginine
ATP adenosine triphosphate
BSA bovine serum albumin
Ca^{2+} calcium ion
CABYR calcium-binding and tyrosine phosphorylation-regulated protein
cAMP cyclic adenosine monophosphate
cAMP-PKA cyclic adenosine monophosphate-protein kinase A
CatSper cation channels of sperm

cGMP cyclic guanosine monophosphate
DUOX dual oxidase
FCSu fetal cord serum ultrafiltrate
FFu follicular fluid ultrafiltrate
FSH follicle stimulating hormone
G6PDH glucose-6-phosphate dehydrogenase
GnRH gonadotropin releasing hormone
GPX glutathione peroxidases
GTP guanosine triphosphate
H$_2$O$_2$ hydrogen peroxide
HCO$_3$$^-$ bicarbonate
HNO$_3$ peroxynitrous acid
HO$_2$$^-$ peroxyl radical
ICSI intracytoplasmic sperm injection
IVF in vitro fertilization
kDa kilo Dalton
LH luteinizing hormone
LPC lysophosphatidylcholine
MAPK mitogen-activated protein kinase
N$_2$O nitrous oxide
NADH nicotinamide adenine dinucleotide
NADPH nicotinamide adenine dinucleotide phosphate
NBC sodium bicarbonate cotransporter
NO nitric oxide
NO$^-$ nitroxyl anion
NO$^\bullet$ nitric oxide
NO$_3$$^-$ peroxynitrite
NOS nitric oxide synthase
NOX NADPH oxidase
O$_2$$^-$ superoxide anion
O$_2$ oxygen molecule
OH$^-$ hydroxyl radical
PGE2 prostaglandin E2
PHGPX phospholipid hydrogen peroxide glutathione peroxidase
PKA protein kinase A
PKC protein kinase C
PLA2 phospholipase A2
PTK protein tyrosine kinase
PTP protein tyrosine phosphatase
P-Tyr tyrosine phosphorylated
PUFA polyunsaturated fatty acid
RNS reactive nitrogen species
ROS reactive oxygen species
Ser serine
SMCP sperm mitochondrion-associated cysteine-rich protein
SOD superoxide dismutase
Thr threonine
Tyr tyrosine
ZP3 zona pellucida glycoprotein-3

REFERENCES

[1] Griveau JF, Le Lannou D. Reactive oxygen species and human spermatozoa: physiology and pathology. Int J Androl April 1997;20(2):61–9. PMID: 9292315.

[2] Kothari S, Thompson A, Agarwal A, du Plessis SS. Free radicals: their beneficial and detrimental effects on sperm function. Indian J Exp Biol May 2010;48(5):425–35. 20795359.

[3] Agarwal A, Prabakaran SA. Mechanism, measurement, and prevention of oxidative stress in male reproductive physiology. Indian J Exp Biol November 2005;43(11):963–74. 16315393.

[4] Henkel RR. Leukocytes and oxidative stress: dilemma for sperm function and male fertility. Asian J Androl January 2011;13(1):43–52. PMCID: 3739401, 21076433.

[5] Sharlip ID, Jarow JP, Belker AM, Lipshultz LI, Sigman M, Thomas AJ, et al. Best practice policies for male infertility. Fertil Steril May 2002;77(5):873−82. 12009338.

[6] Aitken RJ, Smith TB, Jobling MS, Baker MA, De Iuliis GN. Oxidative stress and male reproductive health. Asian J Androl January−February 2014;16(1):31−8. PMCID: 3901879, 24369131.

[7] Agarwal A, Durairajanayagam D, Halabi J, Peng J, Vazquez-Levin M. Proteomics, oxidative stress and male infertility. Reprod Biomed Online July 2014;29(1):32−58. 24813754.

[8] Alvarez JG, Storey BT. Differential incorporation of fatty acids into and peroxidative loss of fatty acids from phospholipids of human spermatozoa. Mol Reprod Dev November 1995;42(3):334−46. PMID: 8579848.

[9] Aitken RJ, Roman SD. Antioxidant systems and oxidative stress in the testes. Adv Exp Med Biol 2008;636:154−71. 19856167.

[10] Agarwal A, Saleh RA, Bedaiwy MA. Role of reactive oxygen species in the pathophysiology of human reproduction. Fertil Steril April 2003;79(4):829−43. 12749418.

[11] Sharma RK, Agarwal A. Role of reactive oxygen species in male infertility. Urology December 1996;48(6):835−50. PMID: 8973665.

[12] Koppers AJ, De Iuliis GN, Finnie JM, McLaughlin EA, Aitken RJ. Significance of mitochondrial reactive oxygen species in the generation of oxidative stress in spermatozoa. J Clin Endocrinol Metabol August 2008;93(8):3199−207. 18492763.

[13] Ayala A, Munoz MF, Arguelles S. Lipid peroxidation: production, metabolism, and signaling mechanisms of malondialdehyde and 4-hydroxy-2-nonenal. Oxid Med Cell Longev 2014;2014:360438. PMCID: 4066722, 24999379.

[14] Whittington K, Ford WC. Relative contribution of leukocytes and of spermatozoa to reactive oxygen species production in human sperm suspensions. Int J Androl August 1999;22(4):229−35. 10442295.

[15] Saleh RA, Agarwal A, Kandirali E, Sharma RK, Thomas AJ, Nada EA, et al. Leukocytospermia is associated with increased reactive oxygen species production by human spermatozoa. Fertil Steril December 2002;78(6):1215−24. 12477515.

[16] Plante M, de Lamirande E, Gagnon C. Reactive oxygen species released by activated neutrophils, but not by deficient spermatozoa, are sufficient to affect normal sperm motility. Fertil Steril August 1994;62(2):387−93. PMID: 8034089.

[17] Potts JM, Pasqualotto FF. Seminal oxidative stress in patients with chronic prostatitis. Andrologia October 2003;35(5):304−8. 14535860.

[18] Babior BM. NADPH oxidase: an update. Blood March 01, 1999;93(5):1464−76. 10029572.

[19] Gil-Guzman E, Ollero M, Lopez MC, Sharma RK, Alvarez JG, Thomas Jr AJ, et al. Differential production of reactive oxygen species by subsets of human spermatozoa at different stages of maturation. Hum Reprod September 2001;16(9):1922−30. 11527899.

[20] Rengan AK, Agarwal A, van der Linde M, du Plessis SS. An investigation of excess residual cytoplasm in human spermatozoa and its distinction from the cytoplasmic droplet. Reprod Biol Endocrinol November 17, 2012;10:92. PMCID: 3551780, 23159014.

[21] Aitken RJ, Baker MA. Reactive oxygen species generation by human spermatozoa: a continuing enigma. Int J Androl August 2002;25(4):191−4. 12121567.

[22] Moustafa MH, Sharma RK, Thornton J, Mascha E, Abdel-Hafez MA, Thomas Jr AJ, et al. Relationship between ROS production, apoptosis and DNA denaturation in spermatozoa from patients examined for infertility. Hum Reprod January 2004;19(1):129−38. 14688171.

[23] Aitken RJ, Koppers AJ. Apoptosis and DNA damage in human spermatozoa. Asian J Androl January 2011;13(1):36−42. PMCID: 3739394, 20802502.

[24] Doshi SB, Khullar K, Sharma RK, Agarwal A. Role of reactive nitrogen species in male infertility. Reprod Biol Endocrinol December 15, 2012;10:109. PMCID: 3558381, 23241221.

[25] Herrero MB, Gagnon C. Nitric oxide: a novel mediator of sperm function. J Androl May−June 2001;22(3):349−56. 11330633.

[26] Wolin MS. Interactions of oxidants with vascular signaling systems. Arterioscler Thromb Vasc Biol June 2000;20(6):1430−42. 10845855.

[27] Zhang H, Zheng RL. Possible role of nitric oxide on fertile and asthenozoospermic infertile human sperm functions. Free Radic Res October 1996;25(4):347−54. PMID: 8889498.

[28] Rosselli M, Keller PJ, Dubey RK. Role of nitric oxide in the biology, physiology and pathophysiology of reproduction. Hum Reprod Update January−February 1998;4(1):3−24. PMID: 9622410.

[29] Lee NP, Cheng CY. Nitric oxide/nitric oxide synthase, spermatogenesis, and tight junction dynamics. Biol Reprod February 2004;70(2):267−76. 14522829.

[30] Durairajanayagam D, Rengan AK, Sharma RK, Agarwal A. Sperm biology from production to ejaculation. In: Schattman GL, Esteves SC, Agarwal A, editors. Unexplained infertility: pathophysiology, evaluation and treatment. New York, NY: Springer New York; 2015. p. 29−42.

[31] Holstein AF, Schulze W, Davidoff M. Understanding spermatogenesis is a prerequisite for treatment. Reprod Biol Endocrinol November 14, 2003;1:107. PMCID: 293421, 14617369.

[32] Huszar G, Patrizio P, Vigue L, Willets M, Wilker C, Adhoot D, et al. Cytoplasmic extrusion and the switch from creatine kinase B to M isoform are completed by the commencement of epididymal transport in human and stallion spermatozoa. J Androl January−February 1998;19(1):11−20. PMID: 9537287.

[33] Zheng H, Stratton CJ, Morozumi K, Jin J, Yanagimachi R, Yan W. Lack of Spem1 causes aberrant cytoplasm removal, sperm deformation, and male infertility. Proc Natl Acad Sci U S A April 17, 2007;104(16):6852−7. PMCID: 1871874, 17426145.

[34] Huszar G, Vigue L. Spermatogenesis-related change in the synthesis of the creatine kinase B-type and M-type isoforms in human spermatozoa. Mol Reprod Dev March 1990;25(3):258−62. PMID: 2331374.

[35] Aitken RJ, Vernet P. Maturation of redox regulatory mechanisms in the epididymis. J Reprod Fertil Suppl 1998;53:109−18. 10645271.

[36] Vernet P, Aitken RJ, Drevet JR. Antioxidant strategies in the epididymis. Mol Cell Endocrinol March 15, 2004;216(1−2):31−9. 15109742.

[37] Ford WC. Regulation of sperm function by reactive oxygen species. Hum Reprod Update September−October 2004;10(5):387−99. 15218008.

[38] Balhorn R. The protamine family of sperm nuclear proteins. Genome Biol 2007;8(9):227. PMCID: 2375014, 17903313.

[39] Champroux A, Torres-Carreira J, Gharagozloo P, Drevet JR, Kocer A. Mammalian sperm nuclear organization: resiliencies and vulnerabilities. Basic Clin Androl 2016;26:17. PMCID: 5175393, 28031843.

[40] Bench GS, Friz AM, Corzett MH, Morse DH, Balhorn R. DNA and total protamine masses in individual sperm from fertile mammalian subjects. Cytometry April 01, 1996;23(4):263−71. PMID: 8900468.

[41] Huret JL. Nuclear chromatin decondensation of human sperm: a review. Arch Androl 1986;16(2):97−109. PMID: 3527098.

[42] Noblanc A, Kocer A, Chabory E, Vernet P, Saez F, Cadet R, et al. Glutathione peroxidases at work on epididymal spermatozoa: an example of the dual effect of reactive oxygen species on mammalian male fertilizing ability. J Androl November−December 2011;32(6):641−50. 21441427.

[43] Rhee SG, Chae HZ, Kim K. Peroxiredoxins: a historical overview and speculative preview of novel mechanisms and emerging concepts in cell signaling. Free Radic Biol Med June 15, 2005;38(12):1543−52. 15917183.

[44] Rousseaux J, Rousseaux-Prevost R. Molecular localization of free thiols in human sperm chromatin. Biol Reprod May 1995;52(5):1066−72. PMID: 7626706.

[45] Noblanc A, Kocer A, Drevet JR. Recent knowledge concerning mammalian sperm chromatin organization and its potential weaknesses when facing oxidative challenge. Basic Clin Androl 2014;24:6. PMCID: 4715350, 26779341.

[46] Ursini F, Maiorino M, Brigelius-Flohe R, Aumann KD, Roveri A, Schomburg D, et al. Diversity of glutathione peroxidases. Meth Enzymol 1995;252:38−53. PMID: 7476373.

[47] Conrad M, Moreno SG, Sinowatz F, Ursini F, Kolle S, Roveri A, et al. The nuclear form of phospholipid hydroperoxide glutathione peroxidase is a protein thiol peroxidase contributing to sperm chromatin stability. Mol Cell Biol September 2005;25(17):7637−44. PMCID: 1190272, 16107710.

[48] Maiorino M, Roveri A, Benazzi L, Bosello V, Mauri P, Toppo S, et al. Functional interaction of phospholipid hydroperoxide glutathione peroxidase with sperm mitochondrion-associated cysteine-rich protein discloses the adjacent cysteine motif as a new substrate of the selenoperoxidase. J Biol Chem November 18, 2005;280(46):38395−402. 16159880.

[49] Ursini F, Heim S, Kiess M, Maiorino M, Roveri A, Wissing J, et al. Dual function of the selenoprotein PHGPx during sperm maturation. Science August 27, 1999;285(5432):1393−6. 10464096.

[50] Venkatesh S, Deecaraman M, Kumar R, Shamsi MB, Dada R. Role of reactive oxygen species in the pathogenesis of mitochondrial DNA (mtDNA) mutations in male infertility. Indian J Med Res February 2009;129(2):127−37. 19293438.

[51] Lenzi A, Gandini L, Picardo M, Tramer F, Sandri G, Panfili E. Lipoperoxidation damage of spermatozoa polyunsaturated fatty acids (PUFA): scavenger mechanisms and possible scavenger therapies. Front Biosci January 01, 2000;5:E1−15. 10702376.

[52] Nomura K, Imai H, Koumura T, Arai M, Nakagawa Y. Mitochondrial phospholipid hydroperoxide glutathione peroxidase suppresses apoptosis mediated by a mitochondrial death pathway. J Biol Chem October 08, 1999;274(41):29294−302. 10506188.

[53] Guyton AC, Hall JE. Textbook of medical physiology. 11th ed. Philadelphia: Elsevier Saunders; 2006. p. 1152.

[54] Kim T, Lawson MA. GnRH regulates gonadotropin gene expression through NADPH/dual oxidase-derived reactive oxygen species. Endocrinology June 2015;156(6):2185−99. PMCID: 4430611, 25849727.

[55] Bedard K, Krause KH. The NOX family of ROS-generating NADPH oxidases: physiology and pathophysiology. Physiol Rev January 2007;87(1):245−313. 17237347.

[56] Flood DE, Fernandino JI, Langlois VS. Thyroid hormones in male reproductive development: evidence for direct crosstalk between the androgen and thyroid hormone axes. Gen Comp Endocrinol October 01, 2013;192:2−14. 23524004.

[57] Gliszczynska-Swiglo A, Oszmianski J. Antioxidants and prooxidant activity of food components. In: Bartosz G, editor. Food oxidants and antioxidants: chemical, biological, and functional properties. Boca Raton: CRC Press; 2013. p. 375−432.

[58] Menezo YJ, Hazout A, Panteix G, Robert F, Rollet J, Cohen-Bacrie P, et al. Antioxidants to reduce sperm DNA fragmentation: an unexpected adverse effect. Reprod Biomed Online April 2007;14(4):418−21. 17425820.

[59] Tunc O, Thompson J, Tremellen K. Improvement in sperm DNA quality using an oral antioxidant therapy. Reprod Biomed Online 2009;18(6):761−8.

[60] Menezo Y, Entezami F, Lichtblau I, Belloc S, Cohen M, Dale B. Oxidative stress and fertility: incorrect assumptions and ineffective solutions? Zygote February 2014;22(1):80−90. 22784645.

[61] Pahune PP, Choudhari AR, Muley PA. The total antioxidant power of semen and its correlation with the fertility potential of human male subjects. J Clin Diagn Res June 2013;7(6):991−5. PMCID: 3708257, 23905087.

[62] Du Plessis SS, Harlev A, Mohamed MI, Habib E, Kothandaraman N, Cakar Z. Physiological role of reactive oxygen species (ROS) in the reproductive system. In: Agarwal A, Sharma RK, Gupta S, Harlev A, Du Plessis SS, Esteves SC, et al., editors. Oxidative stress in human reproduction. Switzerland: Springer International; 2017. p. 47−64.

[63] Conrad M, Ingold I, Buday K, Kobayashi S, Angeli JP. ROS, thiols and thiol-regulating systems in male gametogenesis. Biochim Biophys Acta August 2015;1850(8):1566−74. 25450170.

[64] Jin SK, Yang WX. Factors and pathways involved in capacitation: how are they regulated? Oncotarget January 10, 2017;8(2):3600−27. PMCID: 5356907, 27690295.

[65] Burkman LJ. Discrimination between nonhyperactivated and classical hyperactivated motility patterns in human spermatozoa using computerized analysis. Fertil Steril February 1991;55(2):363−71. PMID: 1991534.

[66] de Lamirande E, Leclerc P, Gagnon C. Capacitation as a regulatory event that primes spermatozoa for the acrosome reaction and fertilization. Mol Hum Reprod March 1997;3(3):175−94. PMID: 9237244.

[67] Aitken RJ, Curry BJ. Redox regulation of human sperm function: from the physiological control of sperm capacitation to the etiology of infertility and DNA damage in the germ line. Antioxidants Redox Signal February 01, 2011;14(3):367−81. 20522002.

[68] Eisenbach M. Mammalian sperm chemotaxis and its association with capacitation. Dev Genet 1999;25(2):87–94. 10440842.

[69] O'Flaherty C, de Lamirande E, Gagnon C. Positive role of reactive oxygen species in mammalian sperm capacitation: triggering and modulation of phosphorylation events. Free Radic Biol Med August 15, 2006;41(4):528–40. 16863985.

[70] Visconti PE, Westbrook VA, Chertihin O, Demarco I, Sleight S, Diekman AB. Novel signaling pathways involved in sperm acquisition of fertilizing capacity. J Reprod Immunol January 2002;53(1–2):133–50. 11730911.

[71] Naz RK, Rajesh PB. Role of tyrosine phosphorylation in sperm capacitation/acrosome reaction. Reprod Biol Endocrinol November 09, 2004;2:75. PMCID: 533862, 15535886.

[72] Aitken RJ, Paterson M, Fisher H, Buckingham DW, van Duin M. Redox regulation of tyrosine phosphorylation in human spermatozoa and its role in the control of human sperm function. J Cell Sci May 1995;108(Pt 5):2017–25. PMID: 7544800.

[73] Leclerc P, de Lamirande E, Gagnon C. Regulation of protein-tyrosine phosphorylation and human sperm capacitation by reactive oxygen derivatives. Free Radic Biol Med 1997;22(4):643–56. PMID: 9013127.

[74] Dona G, Fiore C, Tibaldi E, Frezzato F, Andrisani A, Ambrosini G, et al. Endogenous reactive oxygen species content and modulation of tyrosine phosphorylation during sperm capacitation. Int J Androl October 2011;34(5 Pt 1):411–9. 20738429.

[75] Aitken RJ, Clarkson JS. Cellular basis of defective sperm function and its association with the genesis of reactive oxygen species by human spermatozoa. J Reprod Fertil November 1987;81(2):459–69. PMID: 2828610.

[76] de Lamirande E, Gagnon C. Impact of reactive oxygen species on spermatozoa: a balancing act between beneficial and detrimental effects. Hum Reprod October 1995;10(Suppl. 1):15–21. PMID: 8592032.

[77] Griveau JF, Renard P, Le Lannou D. An in vitro promoting role for hydrogen peroxide in human sperm capacitation. Int J Androl December 1994;17(6):300–7. PMID: 7744509.

[78] de Lamirande E, Jiang H, Zini A, Kodama H, Gagnon C. Reactive oxygen species and sperm physiology. Rev Reprod January 1997;2(1):48–54. PMID: 9414465.

[79] de Lamirande E, Gagnon C. A positive role for the superoxide anion in triggering hyperactivation and capacitation of human spermatozoa. Int J Androl February 1993;16(1):21–5. PMID: 8385650.

[80] de Lamirande E, Gagnon C. Human sperm hyperactivation and capacitation as parts of an oxidative process. Free Radic Biol Med February 1993;14(2):157–66. PMID: 8381103.

[81] Rivlin J, Mendel J, Rubinstein S, Etkovitz N, Breitbart H. Role of hydrogen peroxide in sperm capacitation and acrosome reaction. Biol Reprod February 2004;70(2):518–22. 14561655.

[82] Zini A, De Lamirande E, Gagnon C. Low levels of nitric oxide promote human sperm capacitation in vitro. J Androl September–October 1995;16(5):424–31. PMID: 8575982.

[83] Stamler JS, Singel DJ, Loscalzo J. Biochemistry of nitric oxide and its redox-activated forms. Science December 18, 1992;258(5090):1898–902. PMID: 1281928.

[84] Herrero MB, de Lamirande E, Gagnon C. Nitric oxide regulates human sperm capacitation and protein-tyrosine phosphorylation in vitro. Biol Reprod September 1999;61(3):575–81. 10456831.

[85] Belen Herrero M, Chatterjee S, Lefievre L, de Lamirande E, Gagnon C. Nitric oxide interacts with the cAMP pathway to modulate capacitation of human spermatozoa. Free Radic Biol Med September 15, 2000;29(6):522–36. 11025196.

[86] Lefievre L, Jha KN, de Lamirande E, Visconti PE, Gagnon C. Activation of protein kinase A during human sperm capacitation and acrosome reaction. J Androl September–October 2002;23(5):709–16. 12185106.

[87] O'Flaherty C, de Lamirande E, Gagnon C. Phosphorylation of the Arginine-X-X-(Serine/Threonine) motif in human sperm proteins during capacitation: modulation and protein kinase A dependency. Mol Hum Reprod May 2004;10(5):355–63. 14997001.

[88] Leclerc P, de Lamirande E, Gagnon C. Cyclic adenosine 3′,5′monophosphate-dependent regulation of protein tyrosine phosphorylation in relation to human sperm capacitation and motility. Biol Reprod September 1996;55(3):684–92. PMID: 8862788.

[89] Nassar A, Mahony M, Morshedi M, Lin MH, Srisombut C, Oehninger S. Modulation of sperm tail protein tyrosine phosphorylation by pentoxifylline and its correlation with hyperactivated motility. Fertil Steril May 1999;71(5):919–23. 10231057.

[90] Carrera A, Moos J, Ning XP, Gerton GL, Tesarik J, Kopf GS, et al. Regulation of protein tyrosine phosphorylation in human sperm by a calcium/calmodulin-dependent mechanism: identification of A kinase anchor proteins as major substrates for tyrosine phosphorylation. Dev Biol November 25, 1996;180(1):284–96. PMID: 8948591.

[91] Rahamim Ben-Navi L, Almog T, Yao Z, Seger R, Naor Z. A-kinase anchoring protein 4 (AKAP4) is an ERK1/2 substrate and a switch molecule between cAMP/PKA and PKC/ERK1/2 in human spermatozoa. Sci Rep November 30, 2016;6:37922. PMCID: 5128789, 27901058.

[92] Naaby-Hansen S, Mandal A, Wolkowicz MJ, Sen B, Westbrook VA, Shetty J, et al. CABYR, a novel calcium-binding tyrosine phosphorylation-regulated fibrous sheath protein involved in capacitation. Dev Biol February 15, 2002;242(2):236–54. 11820818.

[93] Darszon A, Nishigaki T, Beltran C, Trevino CL. Calcium channels in the development, maturation, and function of spermatozoa. Physiol Rev October 2011;91(4):1305–55. 22013213.

[94] Lishko PV, Kirichok Y, Ren D, Navarro B, Chung JJ, Clapham DE. The control of male fertility by spermatozoan ion channels. Annu Rev Physiol 2012;74:453–75. PMCID: 3914660, 22017176.

[95] Brenker C, Goodwin N, Weyand I, Kashikar ND, Naruse M, Krahling M, et al. The CatSper channel: a polymodal chemosensor in human sperm. EMBO J April 04, 2012;31(7):1654–65. PMCID: 3321208, 22354039.

[96] Alasmari W, Costello S, Correia J, Oxenham SK, Morris J, Fernandes L, et al. Ca^{2+} signals generated by CatSper and Ca^{2+} stores regulate different behaviors in human sperm. J Biol Chem March 01, 2013;288(9):6248–58. PMCID: 3585060, 23344959.

[97] Noguchi T, Fujinoki M, Kitazawa M, Inaba N. Regulation of hyperactivation of hamster spermatozoa by progesterone. Reprod Med Biol 2008;7(2):63—74.

[98] Demarco IA, Espinosa F, Edwards J, Sosnik J, De La Vega-Beltran JL, Hockensmith JW, et al. Involvement of a Na+/HCO-3 cotransporter in mouse sperm capacitation. J Biol Chem February 28, 2003;278(9):7001—9. 12496293.

[99] Gadella BM, Harrison RA. The capacitating agent bicarbonate induces protein kinase A-dependent changes in phospholipid transbilayer behavior in the sperm plasma membrane. Development June 2000;127(11):2407—20. 10804182.

[100] de Lamirande E, Lamothe G. Reactive oxygen-induced reactive oxygen formation during human sperm capacitation. Free Radic Biol Med February 15, 2009;46(4):502—10. 19071212.

[101] Suzuki F, Yanagimachi R. Changes in the distribution of intramembranous particles and filipin-reactive membrane sterols during in vitro capacitation of golden hamster spermatozoa. Mol Reprod Dev 1989;23(3):335—47.

[102] Torres-Flores V, Hernandez-Rueda YL, Neri-Vidaurri Pdel C, Jimenez-Trejo F, Calderon-Salinas V, Molina-Guarneros JA, et al. Activation of protein kinase A stimulates the progesterone-induced calcium influx in human sperm exposed to the phosphodiesterase inhibitor papaverine. J Androl September—October 2008;29(5):549—57. 18497338.

[103] Ickowicz D, Finkelstein M, Breitbart H. Mechanism of sperm capacitation and the acrosome reaction: role of protein kinases. Asian J Androl November 2012;14(6):816—21. PMCID: 3720105, 23001443.

[104] Du Plessis SS, Agarwal A, Halabi J, Tvrda E. Contemporary evidence on the physiological role of reactive oxygen species in human sperm function. J Assist Reprod Genet April 2015;32(4):509—20. PMCID: 4380893, 25646893.

[105] de Lamirande E, O'Flaherty C. Sperm activation: role of reactive oxygen species and kinases. Biochim Biophys Acta January 2008;1784(1):106—15. 17920343.

[106] Griveau JF, Renard P, Le Lannou D. Superoxide anion production by human spermatozoa as a part of the ionophore-induced acrosome reaction process. Int J Androl April 1995;18(2):67—74. PMID: 7665212.

[107] Griveau JF, Dumont E, Renard P, Callegari JP, Le Lannou D. Reactive oxygen species, lipid peroxidation and enzymatic defence systems in human spermatozoa. J Reprod Fertil January 1995;103(1):17—26. PMID: 7707295.

[108] de Lamirande E, Tsai C, Harakat A, Gagnon C. Involvement of reactive oxygen species in human sperm acrosome reaction induced by A23187, lysophosphatidylcholine, and biological fluid ultrafiltrates. J Androl September—October 1998;19(5):585—94. PMID: 9796619.

[109] Revelli A, Soldati G, Costamagna C, Pellerey O, Aldieri E, Massobrio M, et al. Follicular fluid proteins stimulate nitric oxide (NO) synthesis in human sperm: a possible role for NO in acrosomal reaction. J Cell Physiol January 1999;178(1):85—92. PMID: 9886494.

[110] Herrero MB, de Lamirande E, Gagnon C. Nitric oxide is a signaling molecule in spermatozoa. Curr Pharmaceut Des 2003;9(5):419—25. 12570819.

[111] O'Flaherty CM, Beorlegui NB, Beconi MT. Reactive oxygen species requirements for bovine sperm capacitation and acrosome reaction. Theriogenology July 15, 1999;52(2):289—301. 10734395.

[112] de Lamirande E, Gagnon C. Capacitation-associated production of superoxide anion by human spermatozoa. Free Radic Biol Med March 1995;18(3):487—95. PMID: 9101239.

[113] Ichikawa T, Oeda T, Ohmori H, Schill WB. Reactive oxygen species influence the acrosome reaction but not acrosin activity in human spermatozoa. Int J Androl February 1999;22(1):37—42. 10068942.

[114] Gopalakrishna R, McNeill TH, Elhiani AA, Gundimeda U. Methods for studying oxidative regulation of protein kinase C. Meth Enzymol 2013;528:79—98. 23849860.

[115] Korbecki J, Baranowska-Bosiacka I, Gutowska I, Chlubek D. The effect of reactive oxygen species on the synthesis of prostanoids from arachidonic acid. J Physiol Pharmacol August 2013;64(4):409—21. 24101387.

[116] Flesch FM, Gadella BM. Dynamics of the mammalian sperm plasma membrane in the process of fertilization. Biochim Biophys Acta November 10, 2000;1469(3):197—235. 11063883.

[117] Baldi E, Falsetti C, Krausz C, Gervasi G, Carloni V, Casano R, et al. Stimulation of platelet-activating factor synthesis by progesterone and A23187 in human spermatozoa. Biochem J May 15, 1993;292(Pt 1):209—16. PMID: 8503848. PMCID: 1134290.

[118] Patrat C, Serres C, Jouannet P. The acrosome reaction in human spermatozoa. Biol Cell July 2000;92(3—4):255—66. 11043413.

[119] Dominguez L, Yunes RM, Fornes MW, Burgos M, Mayorga LS. Calcium and phospholipase A2 are both required for the acrosome reaction mediated by G-proteins stimulation in human spermatozoa. Mol Reprod Dev March 1999;52(3):297—302. 10206661.

[120] Goldman R, Ferber E, Zort U. Reactive oxygen species are involved in the activation of cellular phospholipase A2. FEBS Lett September 07, 1992;309(2):190—2. PMID: 1505682.

[121] Sawada M, Carlson JC. Rapid plasma membrane changes in superoxide radical formation, fluidity, and phospholipase A2 activity in the corpus luteum of the rat during induction of luteolysis. Endocrinology June 1991;128(6):2992—8. PMID: 1645257.

[122] Zor U, Ferber E, Gergely P, Szucs K, Dombradi V, Goldman R. Reactive oxygen species mediate phorbol ester-regulated tyrosine phosphorylation and phospholipase A2 activation: potentiation by vanadate. Biochem J November 01, 1993;295(Pt 3):879—88. PMID: 7694572. PMCID: 1134643.

[123] Aitken RJ. Molecular mechanisms regulating human sperm function. Mol Hum Reprod March 1997;3(3):169—73. PMID: 9237243.

[124] Aitken RJ, Buckingham DW, Irvine DS. The extragenomic action of progesterone on human spermatozoa: evidence for a ubiquitous response that is rapidly down-regulated. Endocrinology September 1996;137(9):3999—4009. PMID: 8756577.

[125] Oyeyipo IP, Skosana B, Du Plessis SS. Reactive oxygen species and male fertility: the physiological role. In: Ahmad SI, editor. Reactive oxygen species in biology and human health. CRC Press; 2016. p. 305—23.

Part II

Clinical Aspects

Chapter 2.1

Epidemiology of Oxidative Stress in Male Fertility

Michael Owyong and Ranjith Ramasamy
University of Miami Miller School of Medicine, Miami, FL, United States

INTRODUCTION

Reactive oxygen species (ROS) are oxidizing agents generated as by-products from the metabolism of oxygen. The formation of ROS in seminal plasma occurs at a cellular level within the plasma membrane and/or mitochondria. Due to an unpaired electron in their outer shell, ROS are highly reactive and capable of interacting with nucleic acids to induce base modifications and DNA fragmentation. Seminal oxidative stress occurs when the uncontrolled production of ROS exceeds the antioxidant capacity of the seminal plasma. However, the blood—testis barrier protects testicular spermatozoa from seminal oxidative stress. As a class, ROS comprise both radical and nonradical oxygen derivatives, as well as a subclass of nitrogen-containing compounds known as reactive nitrogen species. Reactive nitrogen species are responsible for the subtype of oxidative stress known as nitrosative stress. Seminal oxidative stress can occur secondary to unknown reasons, iatrogenic causes, or known medical conditions, or may originate from lifestyle factors or environmental toxicants (see Table 1).

IDIOPATHIC

No causal factor of infertility is found in at least 30% of infertile men [1]. However, even in cases of normozoospermic idiopathic male factor infertility, significantly higher levels of ROS are found when compared with fertile controls [2—4]. The lower levels of total antioxidant capacity found in this population further compound this state of oxidative stress [5].

IATROGENIC

Centrifugation

The preparation of sperm for use in assisted reproductive technologies requires centrifugation of human semen to separate the spermatozoa from the seminal plasma. Both the direct effect of centrifugation through mechanical damage of the sperm plasma membrane [6], as well as the indirect adverse effect caused by removing spermatozoa from protective antioxidants found within the seminal plasma [7], contribute to the increased formation of ROS and affect sperm viability [8].

Cryopreservation

Cryopreservation of human sperm is used to store retrieved spermatozoa before assisted reproduction and to preserve spermatozoa before undergoing chemotherapy, radiotherapy, or vasectomy. Despite its utility, cryopreservation impairs the integrity of the mitochondrial membrane leading to the release of ROS [9,10], as well as the integrity of the cell plasma membrane resulting in the loss of superoxide dismutase, an important peroxidative protectant enzyme [11,12].

TABLE 1 Changes in Semen Parameters Associated With Endogenous and Exogenous Sources of Reactive Oxygen Species

		Results
Idiopathic		No statistically significant changes in ejaculate volume, sperm concentration, motility, or vitality [4].
Iatrogenic	Centrifugation	Statistically significant increase in sperm motility and normal morphology.[a]
	Cryopreservation	Statistically significant decrease in sperm motility and vitality [9].
	Medications	Opioids associated with statistically significant decrease in sperm concentration, motility, and normal morphology [17].
		SSRIs associated with statistically significant decrease in sperm motility and normal morphology [20].
Lifestyle	Advanced paternal age	Statistically significant decrease in sperm concentration and motility [22].
	Dietary antioxidant intake	No statistically significant changes in sperm concentration, motility, or normal morphology [25].
	Smoking	Statistically significant decrease in sperm motility and normal morphology [28].
	Alcohol	Statistically significant decrease in sperm concentration, motility, and normal morphology [33].
	Obesity	Statistically significant decrease in sperm concentration, motility, normal morphology, and vitality [36].
	Psychological stress	Statistically significant decrease in sperm concentration, motility, and normal morphology [40].
Environmental	Air pollution	No statistically significant changes in ejaculate volume, sperm concentration, motility, or normal morphology [43].
	Pesticides	Statistically significant decrease in sperm motility and vitality, as well as an increase in pH [46].
	Plasticizers	Statistically significant decrease in sperm concentration, motility, and normal morphology [49].
	Heavy metals	Cadmium associated with statistically significant decrease in sperm concentration [52].
		Selenium associated with statistically significant increase in sperm concentration, motility, and viability [52].
	Non-ionizing radiation	Statistically significant decrease in sperm motility and vitality [55].
Infection	Genitourinary tract	Statistically significant decrease in sperm concentration [59].
	Systemic	HIV associated with leukocytospermia and statistically significant decrease in sperm motility [62].
		Hepatitis B virus associated with statistically significant decrease in ejaculate volume, sperm concentration, motility, normal morphology, and vitality, as well as a decrease in pH [64].
Autoimmune	Vasectomy reversal	Statistically significant decrease in sperm concentration and motility [67].
	Chronic nonbacterial prostatitis	No statistically significant changes in sperm concentration, motility, or normal morphology [72].
Testicular	Varicocele	Statistically significant decrease in sperm concentration [76].
	Torsion	Late surgical intervention with orchiectomy associated with statistically significant decrease in sperm concentration.[b]
	Cryptorchidism	Statistically significant decrease in sperm concentration, motility, normal morphology, and vitality [83].

Continued

TABLE 1 Changes in Semen Parameters Associated With Endogenous and Exogenous Sources of Reactive Oxygen Species—cont'd

		Results
Chronic disease	Diabetes	Statistically significant decrease in ejaculate volume [85].
	Chronic renal failure	Statistically significant decrease in sperm concentration and motility.[c]
	β-thalassemia	Statistically significant decrease in sperm motility [92].
	Thyroid dysfunction	Hypothyroidism associated with statistically significant decrease in sperm concentration, motility, and normal morphology.[d]
		Hyperthyroidism associated with statistically significant decrease in sperm motility.[e]
	Hyperhomocysteinemia	Statistically significant decrease in sperm motility [98].

[a]*Ghaleno LR, Valojerdi MR, Janzamin E, Chehrazi M, Sharbatoghli M, Yazdi RS. Evaluation of conventional semen parameters, intracellular reactive oxygen species, DNA fragmentation and dysfunction of mitochondrial membrane potential after semen preparation techniques: a flow cytometric study. Arch Gynecol Obstet 2014;289(1):173–80.*
[b]*Anderson MJ, Dunn JK, Lipshultz LI, Coburn M. Semen quality and endocrine parameters after acute testicular torsion. J Urol 1992;147(6):1545–50.*
[c]*Lehtihet M, Hylander B. Semen quality in men with chronic kidney disease and its correlation with chronic kidney disease stages. Andrologia 2015;47(10):1103–8.*
[d]*Nikoobakht MR, Aloosh M, Nikoobakht N, Mehrsay AR, Biniaz F, Karjalian MA. The role of hypothyroidism in male infertility and erectile dysfunction. Urol J 2012;9(1):405–9.*
[e]*Krassas GE, Pontikides N, Deligianni V, Miras K. A prospective controlled study of the impact of hyperthyroidism on reproductive function in males. J Clin Endocrinol Metab 2002;87(8):3667–71.*

Medications

Medications including cyclophosphamide, opioids, and selective serotonin reuptake inhibitors have been linked to seminal oxidative stress in animal and/or human studies.

Cyclophosphamide is a cytotoxic alkylating agent used as a component of drug regimens for chemotherapy, immunosuppression after organ transplantation, and for the treatment of nephrotic syndrome. Administration of cyclophosphamide in male adult rats induces a state of oxidative stress by decreasing testicular levels of superoxide dismutase, catalase, and glutathione [13], resulting in excessive lipid peroxidation as manifested by an increase in the levels of its end product, malondialdehyde [14,15].

Opioid analgesics are prescribed for treating moderate to severe pain. An estimated 3.8 million Americans aged 12 or older in 2015 reported the misuse of prescription pain relievers [16]. Consumption of opioids lowers the antioxidant activity of superoxide dismutase and catalase within seminal plasma [17]. Administration of tramadol in male adult rats results in the development of oxidative stress in testicular tissues by decreasing the levels of superoxide dismutase, catalase, and glutathione, while increasing serum malondialdehyde [18].

Selective serotonin reuptake inhibitors are prescribed for the treatment of depression, anxiety disorders, and for premature ejaculation. Patients receiving selective serotonin reuptake inhibitors have increased sperm DNA damage caused by the serotonin-mediated generation of ROS [19,20].

LIFESTYLE

Advanced Paternal Age

It was estimated that males aged 45–64 years would make up 25.9% of all males in the United States by 2015, while those aged 65 years and over would comprise another 13.3% [21]. Males aged 40 years and over exhibit higher levels of sperm oxidative DNA damage when compared to younger males [22]. Animal studies using the brown Norway rat also show that advanced age is associated with increased ROS production and decreased antioxidant enzymatic capacity within epididymal spermatozoa [23].

Dietary Antioxidant Intake

Dietary deficiencies of antioxidants such as vitamin C and vitamin E have been linked with sperm oxidative damage. It is worth noting that seminal levels of antioxidants are a better reflection of biological effect than reported levels of oral intake. However, oral intake of antioxidants, such as vitamin C, affects seminal concentrations within 1 month [24].

Vitamin C, or ascorbic acid, is an antioxidant commonly found in fruits (e.g., oranges and pineapple) and vegetables (e.g., broccoli and kale). Seminal levels of ascorbic acid are negatively correlated with the concentrations of an oxidized nucleoside, 8-OHdG, within sperm DNA of fertile men, to the extent that a 50% reduction in seminal ascorbic acid resulted in a 91% increase in 8-OHdG levels [24]. Vitamin E works synergistically with vitamin C, and as such, only studies investigating combinations of vitamin C and E have been published to date. Daily oral treatment with vitamins C and E results in a significant reduction in sperm DNA damage in infertile men when compared to placebo [25].

Smoking

Cigarettes are the most commonly used tobacco product among U.S. adults [26], and the prevalence of cigarette smoking in 2015 was higher among males and among adults aged 25−44 years [27]. Smoking results in a 48% increase in seminal leukocyte concentrations and a 107% increase in seminal levels of ROS [28], along with decreased levels of seminal plasma antioxidants such as vitamin C [29] and vitamin E [30].

Alcohol

In the world, alcohol consumption per person (15 years and older) equals an average of 6.2 L of pure alcohol per year, and in the United States, it is estimated that 10.7% of males have an alcohol use disorder [31]. No study to date has directly examined the link between alcohol intake and sperm oxidative damage. However, heavy alcohol users have a trend toward higher seminal leukocyte concentrations when compared with nonusers and after controlling for past sexually transmitted diseases and multiple substance exposures [32]. Infertile patients who drink two to three units of alcohol every day have significantly decreased sperm density, percent normal forms, and percent motile forms [33].

Obesity

From 2011 to 2014, the prevalence of obesity was 34.3% among U.S. males aged 20 and over [34]. Adipose tissue is known to be a major source of leptin, which enhances the production of proinflammatory cytokines and ROS [35]. Fertile obese men have significantly higher seminal ROS and sperm DNA fragmentation when compared with fertile normal-weight and overweight men [36]. In addition, the accumulation of adipose tissue within the groin region results in heating of the testicle, which has been linked with oxidative stress in mouse models [37].

Psychological Stress

About 31% of adult men in the United States reported feeling increasingly stressed in 2015, with younger adults reporting higher stress levels [38]. Psychological stress is linked to increased levels of seminal ROS mediated by elevated concentrations of nitric oxide [39], along with reduced levels of antioxidants such as glutathione [40].

ENVIRONMENTAL
Air Pollution

Approximately 38.9% of people in the United States live in counties where they are exposed to unhealthful levels of air pollution in the form of either ozone or particle pollution [41]. It is known that air pollutants are capable of generating ROS through the release of proinflammatory cytokines such as IL-8 and TNF-α [42]. Increased seasonal air pollution in the form of particulate matter, nitrogen oxides, and sulfur dioxide is significantly associated with increased sperm DNA damage, even after adjusting for variables such as tobacco and alcohol use [43].

Pesticides

The use of pesticides in the United States totaled over 1.1 billion pounds in 2012 with the majority being applied in the agricultural sector [44]. Farm workers and applicators have detectable urinary levels of organophosphate metabolites, which are associated with increased ROS and reduced glutathione levels [45]. This occupational exposure to organophosphate and carbamate pesticides is significantly correlated with increased sperm DNA fragmentation [46,47].

Plasticizers

Plasticizers, such as phthalates, are chemical additives used to increase the plasticity of materials and are found in a wide range of applications including bottles, bank cards, clothing, and medical devices. The presence of phthalate metabolites in the urine of infertile men is associated with increased sperm DNA damage [48]. Bisphenol A is a related compound used in the production of certain plastics. Urinary bisphenol A concentration in men from subfertile couples is associated with increased sperm DNA damage, even after adjusting for age, body mass index, and tobacco use [49].

Heavy Metals

In the United States, most lead exposures have been occupational such that the prevalence of elevated blood lead levels was 22.5 adults per 100,000 employed in 2012 with 91.5% of these adults being males [50]. Increased sperm DNA fragmentation is significantly associated with the level of occupational exposure to lead and is positively correlated with the percentage of sperm with excessive superoxide anion production [51]. Another heavy metal found in industrial workplaces is cadmium, which is capable of accumulating to detectable levels within seminal plasma and is significantly correlated with oxidative sperm DNA damage [52].

Non-ionizing Radiation

Mobile phones are now an integral part of daily life for millions of individuals, and about 96% of adult men in the United States reported owning a cell phone in 2016 [53]. However, mobile phones emit radiofrequency electromagnetic waves, a type of non-ionizing radiation. The increased use of mobile phones and the storage of these devices in pants pockets have prompted studies linking the radiation from mobile phones with seminal oxidative stress. It has been suggested that radiofrequency electromagnetic waves produce oxidative stress through the nicotinamide adenine dinucleotide oxidase-mediated formation of ROS [54]. In fact, semen samples from healthy and infertile patients exposed to cellular phone radiation show a significant increase in the level of ROS when compared to controls [55].

INFECTION

Genitourinary Tract

Approximately 20% of all urinary tract infections occur in men with an estimated lifetime prevalence of 13,689/100,000 men between 1988 and 1994 [56]. During urogenital infections, leukocytes are responsible for the generation of ROS [57]. Significantly increased levels of superoxide anions are found in patients with sperm cultures positive for bacteria, and this is correlated with increased white blood cell counts [58]. However, the elevated production of ROS during urogenital infections does not require leukocytospermia. Men with lower urinary tract symptoms and positive semen cultures for *Ureaplasma urealyticum* have significantly higher levels of ROS in the absence of leukocytospermia [59]. Even men with nonbacterial inflammation of the genital tract have elevated levels of ROS in their sperm [60].

Systemic

Chronic systemic infections with HIV and hepatitis B virus (HBV) have been linked with increased seminal oxidative stress.

In 2014, there were 722,244 males reported to be living in the United States with a diagnosed HIV infection [61]. In men, there is a significant association between HIV-seropositivity and leukocytospermia, which is a known cause of oxidative stress [62].

Between 2011 and 2012, there was an estimated prevalence of 847,000 people living in the United States with chronic HBV infection [63]. Men with HBV infection have significantly higher seminal plasma levels of malondialdehyde, a marker of oxidative stress, when compared to controls [64].

There has been interest in other chronic systemic infections, such as tuberculosis, leprosy, malaria, and Chagas disease, but no study to date has linked these diseases with seminal oxidative stress.

AUTOIMMUNE

Vasectomy Reversal

About 6% of men who receive a vasectomy eventually undergo a vasectomy reversal [65]. It is known that surgical disruption of the genital tract is a risk factor for the formation of antisperm antibodies and that pregnancy rates decline after primary vaso-vasotomy with longer interval since vasectomy [66]. Oxidative stress has been suggested as a possible mechanism. Both fertile and infertile men have significantly higher seminal levels of ROS when compared to controls after undergoing vasectomy reversal [67,68].

Chronic Nonbacterial Prostatitis

In the United States, prostatitis has an estimated overall prevalence of 9% [69]. It has been suggested that the etiology of chronic nonbacterial prostatitis (NIH category IIIB) is an autoimmune response to seminal or prostate antigens [70,71]. When compared to controls, men with chronic nonbacterial prostatitis have significantly higher seminal levels of ROS, irrespective of their leukocytospermia status [72,73].

TESTICULAR

Varicocele

The prevalence of varicoceles in healthy adult men is age-related and increases by approximately 10% for each decade of life, starting at 18% between ages 30 and 39 [74]. However, the incidence of varicoceles in men with secondary infertility is about 81% [75]. Seminal oxidative stress is believed to be the mechanism underlying varicocele-associated male infertility. Men with varicoceles have significantly higher seminal levels of ROS and decreased total antioxidant capacity levels [76,77], along with increased sperm DNA damage [78].

Testicular Torsion

The overall incidence of testicular torsion is estimated at 1.1 per 100,000 males, and at 2.9 per 100,000 males aged 24 and younger [79]. In cases of unilateral torsion, it is known that testicular ischemia-reperfusion injury induces oxidative stress that affects the ipsilateral testis [80]. Work on animal models show an increased recruitment of neutrophils and production of proinflammatory cytokines within the testis, along with significantly elevated levels of a lipid peroxidation end product when compared to controls, 4 h after torsion repair [81].

Cryptorchidism

The incidence of cryptorchidism at birth is 6.9% and is significantly higher in preterm than in full-term newborns: 30.1% and 3.4%, respectively [82]. Men with a history of cryptorchidism requiring orchiopexy have significantly higher levels of ROS and significantly increased sperm DNA damage when compared to controls [83].

CHRONIC DISEASE

Diabetes

About 15.5 million men aged 20 years or older in the United States have diabetes [84]. Men with diabetes have significantly higher levels of sperm DNA fragmentation when compared to controls [85]. Oxidative stress has been proposed as the underlying pathology, given that animal models of diabetes show a significant increase in seminal and testicular levels of ROS [86].

Chronic Kidney Disease

Chronic kidney disease has a prevalence of 13.5% among men in the United States [87]. In 2013, the reported incidence of end-stage renal disease was 117,162 cases with 88.2% of these cases requiring hemodialysis [87]. However, hemodialysis is ineffective in controlling the chronic state of inflammation and oxidative stress in uremia [88]. It is no surprise then that even men with end-stage renal disease on hemodialysis have significantly higher levels of lipid peroxidation by-products within their testes when compared to controls [89].

β-thalassemia

It is estimated that at least 5.2% of the world population carry a significant hemoglobin gene variant, including hemoglobin S, α-thalassemia, and β-thalassemia [90]. Patients with β-thalassemia are subjected to oxidative stress from having to receive regular blood transfusions, and have significantly higher serum levels of lipid peroxidation by-products [91]. In addition, men with transfusion-dependent β-thalassemia major have significantly higher seminal levels of a lipid peroxidation end product [92].

Thyroid Dysfunction

Within the U.S. population, hypothyroidism and hyperthyroidism have a prevalence of 4.6% and 1.3%, respectively [93]. Adult male rats with experimentally induced hypothyroidism have significantly increased testicular markers of lipid peroxidation when compared to controls [94]. Similarly, adult male rats with experimentally induced hyperthyroidism demonstrate a significant increase in testicular levels of a lipid peroxidation end product, along with a significant decrease in the activities of endogenous antioxidants when compared to controls [95].

Hyperhomocysteinemia

Elevated plasma levels of homocysteine are associated with several chronic diseases, including stroke, extracranial carotid artery stenosis, dementia, Alzheimer's disease, hip fracture, and congestive heart failure [96]. It has been suggested that homocysteine and its cyclic isomer, homocysteine thiolactone, promote oxidative stress [97] such that the addition of either homocysteine or homocysteine thiolactone to human spermatozoa significantly increases the generation of ROS [98].

CONCLUSION

This chapter provides an overview of the various causes of seminal oxidative stress. Iatrogenic causes include centrifugation, cryopreservation, and medications such as cyclophosphamide, opioids, and selective serotonin reuptake inhibitors. Lifestyle factors include age, diet, tobacco use, alcohol intake, obesity, and stress. Environmental toxicants include exposure to air pollution, pesticides, plasticizers, heavy metals, and non-ionizing radiation. Pathologies such as urinary tract infection, chronic nonbacterial prostatitis, varicocele, testicular torsion, and cryptorchidism are well-established causes of seminal oxidative stress. However, other causes such as diabetes, chronic kidney disease, β-thalassemia, thyroid dysfunction, and hyperhomocysteinemia are only now just becoming recognized as potential causes of seminal oxidative stress. This overview of the various causes that contribute to oxidative stress will help identify those with risk factors linked to male infertility. In addition, this overview will hopefully stimulate further research in less well-established causes of seminal oxidative stress, as well as in unique subtypes of oxidative stress, such as the nitrosative stress induced by peroxynitrite and other derivatives of nitric oxide.

LIST OF ACRONYMS AND ABBREVIATIONS

ROS Reactive oxygen species

REFERENCES

[1] Jungwirth A, Diemer T, Dohle G, Giwercman A, Kopa Z, Tournaye H, et al. Guidelines in male infertility. European Association of Urology 2013; 2014.

[2] Venkatesh S, Shamsi MB, Deka D, Saxena V, Kumar R, Dada R. Clinical implications of oxidative stress & sperm DNA damage in normozoospermic infertile men. Indian J Med Res 2011;134(3):396−8.

[3] Khodair H, Omran T. Evaluation of reactive oxygen species (ROS) and DNA integrity assessment in cases of idiopathic male infertility. Egypti J Dermatol Venerol 2013;33(2):51–5.

[4] Mayorga-Torres BJM, Cardona-Maya W, Cadavid Á, Camargo M. Evaluation of sperm functional parameters in normozoospermic infertile individuals. Actas Urol Esp 2013;37(4):221–7.

[5] Pasqualotto FF, Sharma RK, Kobayashi H, Nelson DR, Thomas Jr AJ, Agarwal A. Oxidative stress in normospermic men undergoing infertility evaluation. J Androl 2001;22(2):316–22.

[6] Aitken RJ, Clarkson JS. Significance of reactive oxygen species and antioxidants in defining the efficacy of sperm preparation techniques. J Androl 1988;9(6):367–76.

[7] Potts RJ, Notarianni LJ, Jefferies TM. Seminal plasma reduces exogenous oxidative damage to human sperm, determined by the measurement of DNA strand breaks and lipid peroxidation. Mutat Res Fund Mol Mech Mutagen 2000;447(2):249–56.

[8] Shekarriz M, DeWire DM, Thomas Jr AJ, Agarwal A. A method of human semen centrifugation to minimize the iatrogenic sperm injuries caused by reactive oxygen species. Eur Urol 1995;28(1):31–5.

[9] Wang AW, Zhang H, Ikemoto I, Anderson DJ, Loughlin KR. Reactive oxygen species generation by seminal cells during cryopreservation. Urology 1997;49(6):921–5.

[10] Saleh RA, Hcld AA. Oxidative stress and male infertility: from Research Bench to Clinical Practice. J Androl 2002;23(6):737–52.

[11] Lasso JL, Noiles EE, Alvarez JG, Storey BT. Mechanism of superoxide dismutase loss from human sperm cells during cryopreservation. J Androl 1994;15(3):255–65.

[12] Alvarez JG, Storey BT. Evidence that membrane stress contributes more than lipid peroxidation to sublethal cryodamage in cryopreserved human sperm: glycerol and other polyols as sole cryoprotectant. J Androl 1993;14(3).

[13] Abd El Tawab AM, Shahin NN, AbdelMohsen MM. Protective effect of Satureja montana extract on cyclophosphamide-induced testicular injury in rats. Chem Biol Interact 2014;224:196–205.

[14] Ghosh D, Das UB, Misro M. Protective role of alpha-tocopherol-succinate (provitamin-E) in cyclophosphamide induced testicular gametogenic and steroidogenic disorders: a correlative approach to oxidative stress. Free Radic Res 2002;36(11):1209–18.

[15] Das UB, Mallick M, Debnath JM, Ghosh D. Protective effect of ascorbic acid on cyclophosphamide- induced testicular gametogenic and androgenic disorders in male rats. Asian J Androl 2002;4(3):201–7.

[16] Quality CfBHSa. Key substance use and mental health indicators in the United States: Results from the 2015 National Survey on Drug Use and Health. 2016;HHS Publication No. SMA 16–4984(NSDUH Series H-51).

[17] Safarinejad MR, Asgari SA, Farshi A, Ghaedi G, Kolahi AA, Iravani S, et al. The effects of opiate consumption on serum reproductive hormone levels, sperm parameters, seminal plasma antioxidant capacity and sperm DNA integrity. Reprod Toxicol 2013;36:18–23.

[18] Ahmed MA, Kurkar A. Effects of opioid (tramadol) treatment on testicular functions in adult male rats: the role of nitric oxide and oxidative stress. Clin Exp Pharmacol Physiol 2014;41(4):317–23.

[19] Tanrikut C, Feldman AS, Altemus M, Paduch DA, Schlegel PN. Adverse effect of paroxetine on sperm. Fertil Steril 2010;94(3):1021–6.

[20] Safarinejad MR. Sperm DNA damage and semen quality impairment after treatment with selective serotonin reuptake inhibitors detected using semen analysis and sperm chromatin structure assay. J Urol 2008;180(5):2124–8.

[21] Mather M, Jacobsen LA, Pollard KM. Aging in the United States. Popul Bull 2015;70(2).

[22] Koh S-A, Sanders K, Burton P. Effect of male age on oxidative stress markers in human semen. J Reprod Biotechnol Fertil 2016;5. https://doi.org/10.1177/2058915816673242.

[23] Weir CP, Robaire B. Spermatozoa have decreased antioxidant enzymatic capacity and increased reactive oxygen species production during aging in the Brown Norway rat. J Androl 2007;28(2):229–40.

[24] Fraga CG, Motchnik PA, Shigenaga MK, Helbock HJ, Jacob RA, Ames BN. Ascorbic acid protects against endogenous oxidative DNA damage in human sperm. Proc Natl Acad Sci USA 1991;88(24):11003–6.

[25] Greco E, Iacobelli M, Rienzi L, Ubaldi F, Ferrero S, Tesarik J. Reduction of the incidence of sperm DNA fragmentation by oral antioxidant treatment. J Androl 2005;26(3):349–53.

[26] Hu SS. Tobacco product use among adults—United States, 2013–2014. MMWR Morb Mortal Wkly Rep 2016;65.

[27] Jamal A, Homa DM, O'Connor E, Babb SD, Caraballo RS, Singh T, et al. Current cigarette smoking among adults—United States, 2005–2014. MMWR Morb Mortal Wkly Rep 2015;64(44):1233–40.

[28] Saleh RA, Agarwal A, Sharma RK, Nelson DR, Thomas Jr AJ. Effect of cigarette smoking on levels of seminal oxidative stress in infertile men: a prospective study. Fertil Steril 2002;78(3):491–9.

[29] Mostafa T, Tawadrous G, Roaia MM, Amer MK, Kader RA, Aziz A. Effect of smoking on seminal plasma ascorbic acid in infertile and fertile males. Andrologia 2006;38(6):221–4.

[30] Fraga CG, Motchnik PA, Wyrobek AJ, Rempel DM, Ames BN. Smoking and low antioxidant levels increase oxidative damage to sperm DNA. Mutat Res 1996;351(2):199–203.

[31] Organization WH. Global status report on alcohol and health 2014. World Health Organization; 2014.

[32] Close CE, Roberts PL, Berger RE. Cigarettes, alcohol and marijuana are related to pyospermia in infertile men. J Urol 1990;144(4):900–3.

[33] Condorelli RA, Calogero AE, Vicari E, La Vignera S. Chronic consumption of alcohol and sperm parameters: our experience and the main evidences. Andrologia 2015;47(4):368–79.

[34] Ogden CL, Carroll MD, Fryar CD, Flegal KM. Prevalence of obesity among adults and youth: United States, 2011–2014. NCHS Data Brief 2015;219(219):1–8.

[35] Singer G, Granger DN. Inflammatory responses underlying the microvascular dysfunction associated with obesity and insulin resistance. Microcirculation 2007;14(4−5):375−87.

[36] Taha EA, Sayed SK, Gaber HD, Abdel Hafez HK, Ghandour N, Zahran A, et al. Does being overweight affect seminal variables in fertile men? Reprod Biomed Online 2016;33(6):703−8.

[37] Ishii T, Matsuki S, Iuchi Y, Okada F, Toyosaki S, Tomita Y, et al. Accelerated impairment of spermatogenic cells in SOD1-knockout mice under heat stress. Free Radic Res 2005;39(7):697−705.

[38] Association AP. Stress in America: the impact of discrimination. Stress in America™ Survey. 2016. Retrieved from: www.stressinamerica.org.

[39] Eskiocak S, Gozen AS, Taskiran A, Kilic AS, Eskiocak M, Gulen S. Effect of psychological stress on the L-arginine-nitric oxide pathway and semen quality. Braz J Med Biol Res 2006;39(5):581−8.

[40] Eskiocak S, Gozen AS, Yapar SB, Tavas F, Kilic AS, Eskiocak M. Glutathione and free sulphydryl content of seminal plasma in healthy medical students during and after exam stress. Hum Reprod (Oxf) 2005;20(9):2595−600.

[41] State of the Air 2017. American Lung Association.

[42] Gonzalez-Flecha B. Oxidant mechanisms in response to ambient air particles. Mol Aspect Med 2004;25(1−2):169−82.

[43] Rubes J, Selevan SG, Evenson DP, Zudova D, Vozdova M, Zudova Z, et al. Episodic air pollution is associated with increased DNA fragmentation in human sperm without other changes in semen quality. Hum Reprod (Oxf) 2005;20(10):2776−83.

[44] Atwood D, Paisley-Jones C. Pesticides industry sales and usage: 2008−2012 market estimates. Washington, DC: US Environmental Protection Agency; 2017.

[45] Muniz JF, McCauley L, Scherer J, Lasarev M, Koshy M, Kow YW, et al. Biomarkers of oxidative stress and DNA damage in agricultural workers: a pilot study. Toxicol Appl Pharmacol 2008;227(1):97−107.

[46] Miranda-Contreras L, Gomez-Perez R, Rojas G, Cruz I, Berrueta L, Salmen S, et al. Occupational exposure to organophosphate and carbamate pesticides affects sperm chromatin integrity and reproductive hormone levels among Venezuelan farm workers. J Occup Health 2013;55(3):195−203.

[47] Sanchez-Pena LC, Reyes BE, Lopez-Carrillo L, Recio R, Moran-Martinez J, Cebrian ME, et al. Organophosphorous pesticide exposure alters sperm chromatin structure in Mexican agricultural workers. Toxicol Appl Pharmacol 2004;196(1):108−13.

[48] Hauser R, Meeker JD, Singh NP, Silva MJ, Ryan L, Duty S, et al. DNA damage in human sperm is related to urinary levels of phthalate monoester and oxidative metabolites. Hum Reprod (Oxf) 2007;22(3):688−95.

[49] Meeker JD, Ehrlich S, Toth TL, Wright DL, Calafat AM, Trisini AT, et al. Semen quality and sperm DNA damage in relation to urinary bisphenol A among men from an infertility clinic. Reprod Toxicol 2010;30(4):532−9.

[50] Alarcon WA. Summary of notifiable noninfectious conditions and disease outbreaks: elevated blood lead levels among employed adults - United States, 1994−2012. MMWR Morb Mortal Wkly Rep 2015;62(54):52−75.

[51] Hsu PC, Chang HY, Guo YL, Liu YC, Shih TS. Effect of smoking on blood lead levels in workers and role of reactive oxygen species in lead-induced sperm chromatin DNA damage. Fertil Steril 2009;91(4):1096−103.

[52] Xu DX, Shen HM, Zhu QX, Chua L, Wang QN, Chia SE, et al. The associations among semen quality, oxidative DNA damage in human spermatozoa and concentrations of cadmium, lead and selenium in seminal plasma. Mutat Res 2003;534(1−2):155−63.

[53] Mobile fact sheet. Pew Research Center; 2016.

[54] Desai NR, Kesari KK, Agarwal A. Pathophysiology of cell phone radiation: oxidative stress and carcinogenesis with focus on male reproductive system. Reprod Biol Endocrinol 2009;7(1):114.

[55] Agarwal A, Desai NR, Makker K, Varghese A, Mouradi R, Sabanegh E, et al. Effects of radiofrequency electromagnetic waves (RF-EMW) from cellular phones on human ejaculated semen: an in vitro pilot study. Fertil Steril 2009;92(4):1318−25.

[56] Griebling TL. Urologic diseases in America project: trends in resource use for urinary tract infections in men. J Urol 2005;173(4):1288−94.

[57] Ochsendorf FR. Infections in the male genital tract and reactive oxygen species. Hum Reprod Update 1999;5(5):399−420.

[58] Mazzilli F, Rossi T, Marchesini M, Ronconi C, Dondero F. Superoxide anion in human semen related to seminal parameters and clinical aspects. Fertil Steril 1994;62(4):862−8.

[59] Potts JM, Sharma R, Pasqualotto F, Nelson D, Hall G, Agarwal A. Association of ureaplasma urealyticum with abnormal reactive oxygen species levels and absence of leukocytospermia. J Urol 2000;163(6):1775−8.

[60] D'Agata R, Vicari E, Moncada ML, Sidoti G, Calogero AE, Fornito MC, et al. Generation of reactive oxygen species in subgroups of infertile men. Int J Androl 1990;13(5):344−51.

[61] Centers for Disease Control and Prevention. Diagnoses of HIV infection in the United States and dependent areas, 2015. HIV Surveillance Report. 2016.

[62] Umapathy E, Simbini T, Chipata T, Mbizvo M. Sperm characteristics and accessory sex gland functions in HIV-infected men. Arch Androl 2001;46(2):153−8.

[63] Roberts H, Kruszon-Moran D, Ly KN, Hughes E, Iqbal K, Jiles RB, et al. Prevalence of chronic hepatitis B virus (HBV) infection in U.S. Households: National Health and Nutrition Examination Survey (NHANES), 1988−2012. Hepatology 2016;63(2):388−97.

[64] Qian L, Li Q, Li H. Effect of hepatitis B virus infection on sperm quality and oxidative stress state of the semen of infertile males. Am J Reprod Immunol 2016;76(3):183−5.

[65] Sandlow JI, Nagler HM. Vasectomy and vasectomy reversal: important issues. Preface. Urol Clin N AM 2009;36(3):xiii−xiv.

[66] Belker AM, Thomas Jr AJ, Fuchs EF, Konnak JW, Sharlip ID. Results of 1,469 microsurgical vasectomy reversals by the Vasovasostomy Study Group. J Urol 1991;145(3):505−11.

[67] Nandipati KC, Pasqualotto FF, Thomas Jr AJ, Agarwal A. Relationship of interleukin-6 with semen characteristics and oxidative stress in vasectomy reversal patients. Andrologia 2005;37(4):131–4.

[68] Kolettis PN, Sharma RK, Pasqualotto FF, Nelson D, Thomas Jr AJ, Agarwal A. Effect of seminal oxidative stress on fertility after vasectomy reversal. Fertil Steril 1999;71(2):249–55.

[69] Roberts RO, Lieber MM, Rhodes T, Girman CJ, Bostwick DG, Jacobsen SJ. Prevalence of a physician-assigned diagnosis of prostatitis: the Olmsted County Study of Urinary Symptoms and Health Status Among Men. Urology 1998;51(4):578–84.

[70] Batstone GR, Doble A, Gaston JS. Autoimmune T cell responses to seminal plasma in chronic pelvic pain syndrome (CPPS). Clin Exp Immunol 2002;128(2):302–7.

[71] Motrich RD, Maccioni M, Molina R, Tissera A, Olmedo J, Riera CM, et al. Reduced semen quality in chronic prostatitis patients that have cellular autoimmune response to prostate antigens. Hum Reprod (Oxf) 2005;20(9):2567–72.

[72] Pasqualotto FF, Sharma RK, Potts JM, Nelson DR, Thomas AJ, Agarwal A. Seminal oxidative stress in patients with chronic prostatitis. Urology 2000;55(6):881–5.

[73] Shahed AR, Shoskes DA. Oxidative stress in prostatic fluid of patients with chronic pelvic pain syndrome: correlation with gram positive bacterial growth and treatment response. J Androl 2000;21(5):669–75.

[74] Levinger U, Gornish M, Gat Y, Bachar GN. Is varicocele prevalence increasing with age? Andrologia 2007;39(3):77–80.

[75] Gorelick JI, Goldstein M. Loss of fertility in men with varicocele. Fertil Steril 1993;59(3):613–6.

[76] Hendin BN, Kolettis PN, Sharma RK, Thomas Jr AJ, Agarwal A. Varicocele is associated with elevated spermatozoal reactive oxygen species production and diminished seminal plasma antioxidant capacity. J Urol 1999;161(6):1831–4.

[77] Agarwal A, Prabakaran S, Allamaneni SS. Relationship between oxidative stress, varicocele and infertility: a meta-analysis. Reprod Biomed Online 2006;12(5):630–3.

[78] Saleh RA, Agarwal A, Sharma RK, Said TM, Sikka SC, Thomas Jr AJ. Evaluation of nuclear DNA damage in spermatozoa from infertile men with varicocele. Fertil Steril 2003;80(6):1431–6.

[79] Lee SM, Huh JS, Baek M, Yoo KH, Min GE, Lee HL, et al. A nationwide epidemiological study of testicular torsion in Korea. J Kor Med Sci 2014;29(12):1684–7.

[80] Filho DW, Torres MA, Bordin AL, Crezcynski-Pasa TB, Boveris A. Spermatic cord torsion, reactive oxygen and nitrogen species and ischemia-reperfusion injury. Mol Aspect Med 2004;25(1–2):199–210.

[81] Turner TT, Bang HJ, Lysiak JL. The molecular pathology of experimental testicular torsion suggests adjunct therapy to surgical repair. J Urol 2004;172(6 Pt 2):2574–8.

[82] Ghirri P, Ciulli C, Vuerich M, Cuttano A, Faraoni M, Guerrini L, et al. Incidence at birth and natural history of cryptorchidism: a study of 10,730 consecutive male infants. J Endocrinol Invest 2002;25(8):709–15.

[83] Smith R, Kaune H, Parodi D, Madariaga M, Morales I, Rios R, et al. Extent of sperm DNA damage in spermatozoa from men examined for infertility. Relationship with oxidative stress. Rev Med Chile 2007;135(3):279–86.

[84] Centers for Disease Control and Prevention. National diabetes statistics report: estimates of diabetes and its burden in the United States, 2014. Atlanta, GA: US Department of Health and Human Services; 2014.

[85] Agbaje IM, Rogers DA, McVicar CM, McClure N, Atkinson AB, Mallidis C, et al. Insulin dependant diabetes mellitus: implications for male reproductive function. Hum Reprod (Oxf) 2007;22(7):1871–7.

[86] Shrilatha B, Muralidhara. Occurrence of oxidative impairments, response of antioxidant defences and associated biochemical perturbations in male reproductive milieu in the Streptozotocin-diabetic rat. Int J Androl 2007;30(6):508–18.

[87] National Institutes of Health. Kidney disease statistics for the United States. Washington: NHI; 2016.

[88] Pupim LB, Himmelfarb J, McMonagle E, Shyr Y, Ikizler TA. Influence of initiation of maintenance hemodialysis on biomarkers of inflammation and oxidative stress. Kidney Int 2004;65(6):2371–9.

[89] Shiraishi K, Shimabukuro T, Naito K. Effects of hemodialysis on testicular volume and oxidative stress in humans. J Urol 2008;180(2):644–50.

[90] Modell B, Darlison M. Global epidemiology of haemoglobin disorders and derived service indicators. Bull World Health Orgn 2008;86(6):480–7.

[91] Livrea MA, Tesoriere L, Pintaudi AM, Calabrese A, Maggio A, Freisleben HJ, et al. Oxidative stress and antioxidant status in beta-thalassemia major: iron overload and depletion of lipid-soluble antioxidants. Blood 1996;88(9):3608–14.

[92] Carpino A, Tarantino P, Rago V, De Sanctis V, Siciliano L. Antioxidant capacity in seminal plasma of transfusion-dependent beta-thalassemic patients. Exp Clin Endocrinol Diabetes 2004;112(3):131–4.

[93] Hollowell JG, Staehling NW, Flanders WD, Hannon WH, Gunter EW, Spencer CA, et al. Serum TSH, T4, and thyroid antibodies in the United States Population (1988 to 1994): National Health and Nutrition Examination Survey (NHANES III). J Clin Endocrinol Metab 2002;87(2):489–99.

[94] Chattopadhyay S, Choudhury S, Roy A, Chainy GB, Samanta L. T3 fails to restore mitochondrial thiol redox status altered by experimental hypothyroidism in rat testis. Gen Comp Endocrinol 2010;169(1):39–47.

[95] Asker ME, Hassan WA, El-Kashlan AM. Experimentally induced hyperthyroidism influences oxidant and antioxidant status and impairs male gonadal functions in adult rats. Andrologia 2015;47(6):644–54.

[96] Selhub J. The many facets of hyperhomocysteinemia: studies from the Framingham cohorts. J Nutr 2006;136(6 Suppl.). 1726s–1730s.

[97] Sibrian-Vazquez M, Escobedo JO, Lim S, Samoei GK, Strongin RM. Homocystamides promote free-radical and oxidative damage to proteins. Proc Natl Acad Sci USA 2010;107(2):551–4.

[98] Aitken RJ, Flanagan HM, Connaughton H, Whiting S, Hedges A, Baker MA. Involvement of homocysteine, homocysteine thiolactone, and par-aoxonase type 1 (PON-1) in the etiology of defective human sperm function. Andrology 2016;4(2):345–60.

Chapter 2.2

Role of Oxidative Stress in the Etiology of Male Infertility and the Potential Therapeutic Value of Antioxidants

R. John Aitken[1], Geoffrey N. De Iuliis[1] and Joel R. Drevet[2]

[1]The University of Newcastle (UoN), University drive, Callaghan, NSW, Australia; [2]Université Clermont Auvergne (UCA), Clermont-Ferrand, France

INTRODUCTION

Male infertility is a relatively common complaint that is thought to affect approximately 1 in 20 of the male population [1]. Despite its prevalence, there has been relatively little attention paid to the underlying etiology of this condition, particularly in an era where intracytoplasmic sperm injection (ICSI) dominates the therapeutic landscape and all that is required of a male partner is a single spermatozoon. From the little work that has been done in the area it is widely appreciated that male infertility is not normally a question of sperm number but rather the functional competence of the spermatozoa. Detailed analyses of sperm function within the infertile population using carefully designed bioassays have demonstrated failures in motility and all the key elements of conception including sperm–zona recognition, acrosomal exocytosis, and sperm–oocyte fusion [2,3]. Some of these bioassays were even shown to be predictive of ultimate fertility in long-term prospective studies of spontaneous conception rates in untreated couples suffering from idiopathic infertility [4]. However, such assays were too time consuming and difficult to standardize to render them of practical value in a routine diagnostic context. For this reason, research was initiated on elucidating the underlying mechanisms responsible for the defective sperm function underpinning so much human infertility. It was in this context that Aitken and Clarkson [5] published a key article demonstrating that the spermatozoa of infertile males are characterized by oxidative stress triggered by the excessive generation of reactive oxygen species (ROS).

The capacity of spermatozoa to generate high levels of reactive oxygen species had been known since the 1940s when Tosic and Walton [6] published their classic paper in *Nature* demonstrating the capacity of bovine spermatozoa to generate ROS when exposed to high levels of aromatic amino acids as a consequence of intrinsic L-amino acid oxidase activity. Mann and colleagues at the University of Cambridge added to this foundation by demonstrating the vulnerability of spermatozoa to oxidative stress as a consequence of lipid peroxidation reactions involving the polyunsaturated fatty acids that abound in the plasma membranes of these cells [7]. The capacity of mammalian spermatozoa to generate ROS was subsequently confirmed in a series of landmark papers by Storey and colleagues, who highlighted the potential contribution of sperm mitochondria to hydrogen peroxide generation [8]. They also emphasized the particularly important role that superoxide dismutase (SOD) plays in maintaining redox homoeostasis in spermatozoa by converting superoxide anion to hydrogen peroxide, which then leaves the cell or is inactivated by glutathione peroxidase [9]. In addition, this group and others pointed to the inherent vulnerability of spermatozoa to oxidative attack because of two additional major factors. First, spermatozoa are largely devoid of cytoplasm in which to house the antioxidant enzymes that protect most somatic cells from oxidative stress; moreover, what cytoplasmic space is available is concentrated in the midpiece of the cell, leaving the plasma membrane overlying the sperm head and tail exposed to the risk of peroxidative damage [10]. Second, the ability of glutathione peroxidase to metabolize the hydrogen peroxide generated as a consequence of SOD activity, while dynamically active, is limited by the capacity of spermatozoa to generate nicotinamide adenine dinucleotide phosphate (NADPH) via the hexose monophosphate shunt [9,11].

SUMMARY OF CURRENT UNDERSTANDING IN RELATION TO HUMAN SPERMATOZOA

In the 30 years that have elapsed since the original discovery of ROS generation by human spermatozoa, what have we learned? Well, we now know that oxidative stress is a contributory factor in a majority of male infertility subjects whether their condition is idiopathic in origin [12] or associated with inflammation [13], oligozoospermia [14], asthenozoospermia [15], varicocele [16,17], or a variety of health and lifestyle factors such as obesity, poor nutrition, heat stress, smoking, or alcohol abuse [18]. We also know that a majority of the ROS that damage spermatozoa emanate from the mitochondria, with ROS release on the matrix side of the mitochondrial membrane at complex 1 being particularly damaging [19]. We have also become aware that mitochondrial ROS generation by human spermatozoa involves a self-perpetuating cycle of activity whereby free radical attack leads to the induction of lipid peroxidation chain reactions that culminate in the generation of cytotoxic lipid aldehydes such as 4-hydroxynonenal (4-HNE). The latter then form covalent adducts with proteins in the mitochondrial electron transport chain disrupting the flow of electrons and stimulating the generation of yet more ROS to continue the cycle [20].

In addition to mitochondria, we now know that there are various other potential sources of ROS in human spermatozoa including L-amino acid oxidases [21], NADPH oxidases [22] and excessive lipoxygenase activity [23]. However, the specific contribution that any of these nonmitochondrial pathways makes to the overall level of oxidative stress experienced by human spermatozoa is still unresolved [24]. Furthermore, while retention of excess residual cytoplasm has been implicated in the origins of oxidative stress in spermatozoa, the precise nature of this relationship is still subject to speculation. A reasonable hypothesis is that the presence of excess cytoplasm enhances the capacity of human spermatozoa to generate increased levels of NADPH as a consequence of the increased availability of glucose-6-phosphate dehydrogenase [25,26]. This NADPH might then enhance the activity of NADPH oxidases in human spermatozoa generating superoxide that is then converted to hydrogen peroxide as a consequence of the concomitant superabundance of SOD [26]. While plausible, the evidence linking high levels of ROS generation with the retention of excess residual cytoplasm is currently entirely circumstantial. What is certain is that the oxidative stress experienced by these cells impacts all aspects of sperm function as well as the integrity of the DNA in the sperm nucleus. Our current understanding of the molecular mechanisms underpinning these negative impacts on sperm quality and function are summarized below.

OXIDATIVE STRESS AND ITS IMPACT ON SPERM CELL STRUCTURES AND FUNCTIONS

Sperm movement was one of the first elements of sperm function to be negatively correlated with ROS and oxidative stress. The primary cause of the loss of motility is undoubtedly the damage done to the sperm plasma membrane as a consequence of the induction of lipid peroxidation reactions targeting the integrity of polyunsaturated fatty acids in the sperm plasma membrane [7,27]. In addition, lipid aldehydes like 4-HNE generated as a consequence of lipid peroxidation can form adducts with proteins such as dynein heavy chain that are essential for movement [28,29]. Moreover, lipid aldehydes generated as a result of lipid peroxidation are known to bind to paraoxonase 1 (PON-1); one of its main biochemical functions is to remove the toxic homocysteine cyclic congener, homocysteine thiolactone from spermatozoa. As a consequence of PON-1 inhibition, there is an increased availability of homocysteine thiolactone within the spermatozoa that interacts with the epsilon-amino group of lysine residues on sperm proteins, triggering a raft of significant biological changes in these cells that ultimately compromise sperm motility, including the promotion of mitochondrial ROS generation and suppression of protein carboxymethylation in the sperm tail [30].

Sperm–Zona Recognition

The ability of capacitated spermatozoa to bind to the zona pellucida is one of the key events in conception and the point in fertilization where sperm function is frequently compromised [3]. The vulnerability of this process has been recognized for some time and ultimately led to development of the hemi-zona assay as a means of quantifying deficiencies in this aspect of sperm function. In this bioassay, the two matching hemi-zona halves are used to effect a controlled comparison of binding from a fertile control versus a test sample. The power of this assay in predicting the outcome of intrauterine insemination and in vitro fertilization (IVF) therapies has been well described [31]. However, until recently, the biochemical basis of this defect remained a mystery. Through the use of an advanced mass spectrometry platform it has been found that the loss of zona-binding capacity is associated with reduced expression or loss of a molecular chaperone, HSPA2 [32]. This molecule normally exists as a complex with two other molecules, SPAM1, a hyaluronidase, and arylsulfatase A (ARSA), a zona-binding protein. In noncapacitated spermatozoa SPAM 1 is heavily expressed on the sperm surface to facilitate passage of these cells through the extracellular matrix presented by the female tract and contact with the egg; by contrast, ARSA is internalized or masked from view by some alternative mechanism. However, as spermatozoa capacitate and gain the ability to bind to the zona pellucida, SPAM1 is progressively withdrawn from the sperm surface to be replaced by ARSA. This dynamic pattern of ARSA expression is mediated by HSPA2. In the latter's absence, the spermatozoa of infertile males cannot express ARSA on the sperm surface and so never realize their latent ability to recognize the surface of the egg [32].

In light of these data, we might reasonably ask why HSPA2 expression is so compromised in the defective spermatozoa generated by infertile patients. In addressing this question, it was discovered that the loss of HSPA2 from the sperm proteome is another aspect of infertility induced by oxidative stress. Lipid aldehydes generated during lipid peroxidation bind to HSPA2 during the early stages of spermiogenesis and target this protein for ubiquitination and destruction in the proteasome [33]. In addition, alkylation of this molecular chaperone by 4-HNE causes the former to dissociate from its keeper protein, BAG6, further enhancing the instability of HSPA2 and compromising its ability to mediate sperm–zona recognition [34].

Sperm–Oocyte Fusion

The ability of human spermatozoa to acrosome react and generate a fusogenic equatorial segment capable of initiating fusion with the vitelline membrane of the oocyte is also notoriously sensitive to oxidative stress [25]. The underlying mechanisms presumably involve the induction of lipid peroxidation in the sperm plasma membrane and a consequential loss of membrane fluidity, fusability, and function. Whether proteins that are intimately involved in sperm–oocyte fusion such as IZUMO (which must become translocated to the equatorial segment following the acrosome reaction in order to interact with its receptor on the egg, JUNO) [35] are vulnerable to oxidative attack or alkylation by lipid aldehydes generated as a consequence of oxidative stress has not yet been investigated.

SPERM NUCLEAR OXIDATIVE STRESS AND ITS DEVELOPMENTAL IMPACT

Sperm Nuclear and DNA Damage

The plasma membrane is not the only subcellular sperm structure vulnerable to oxidative attack in spermatozoa; the nuclear compartment and the DNA in both the sperm nucleus and mitochondria are also susceptible in this regard. Oxidative damage at the sperm nuclear level has a range of outcomes. First, oxidative alterations may promote nuclear decondensation and DNA fragmentation. Nuclear DNA is, to a large extent, protected from oxidative damage because it has been condensed to the point of crystallization as a consequence of the remodeling of sperm chromatin that occurs during spermiogenesis. During this process, around 85% of human sperm histones are removed and replaced by small, basic, arginine-rich proteins known as protamines. These molecules, because of their net positive charge, are able to neutralize the negative charges carried by the phosphate groups in the DNA backbone and by overcoming the electrostatic repulsion between adjacent DNA strands, are able to effect the high level of DNA compaction typical of the sperm nucleus. The DNA in the sperm mitochondria is not packaged in this manner and as a result is more vulnerable to oxidative attack [36]. This matters little in terms of fundamental biology because the paternal mitochondria are destroyed following fertilization in order to make way for the maternal mitochondrial lineage. However, the increased vulnerability of mitochondrial DNA to oxidative attack does offer opportunities for monitoring oxidative DNA damage in the germ line in a diagnostic context [37].

It is not totally clear to anyone at this stage whether sperm DNA oxidation and sperm DNA fragmentation are tightly correlated. Clearly, sperm DNA fragmentation, to some extent, has an oxidative origin since high concentration of ROS (especially hydrogen peroxide) has the ability to cause single and double strand breaks (SSB, DSB) in most cell types with the sperm unable to escape this problem. However, the absence of sperm DNA fragmentation should not be translated into absence of DNA oxidative alterations, as it is often done. This was clearly emphasized in several mouse models of posttesticular oxidative stress in which high levels of DNA oxidation were recorded in caudal epididymal sperm without any sign of increased DNA fragmentation [38–40]. Only a mild level of decondensation and/or an increased susceptibility to sperm nuclear decondensation were reported in these models, when caudal sperm were challenged with a reducing agent [40]. Thus sperm DNA/nuclear oxidation and sperm DNA fragmentation are two conditions that should be considered separately to avoid misleading diagnoses. On the contrary, sperm nuclear condensation and sperm nuclear oxidation are rather well-associated phenomena. This is due to the fact that part of the final state of nuclear compaction is achieved during epididymal maturation through oxidative processes.

It is now clear that during epididymal maturation a large number of thiol groups found on the cysteine-rich protamines are turned into disulfide-bridges making intra- and interprotamine bounds. These events contribute to further condense the sperm nucleus and to lock it into its compacted state. Disulfide bridging of sperm protamines is permitted by the presence of a well-controlled luminal concentration of hydrogen peroxide in the epididymis [41] as well as disulfide isomerase-like enzymes in the sperm nucleus [39]. This finely regulated process can be challenged by factors either systemic or local, which may end up in ROS generation as reported earlier. Thus there is a fragile equilibrium between physiological oxidation that will allow an optimal sperm nuclear compaction and detrimental sperm nuclear oxidation. Excessive ROS generation by mature spermatozoa, besides affecting sperm membranes and amplifying ROS production, may transiently increase sperm nuclear condensation but then will rapidly promote spontaneous DNA fragmentation that will result in sperm nuclear decondensation and the increased oxidative damage of DNA and chromatin-associated proteins.

Because of the high level of compaction of sperm nuclear DNA and its haploid state, there is no transcription in mature spermatozoa. In addition, after spermiogenesis most of the sperm cytosol and its organelles have disappeared, impeding translation and any DNA repair mechanisms. Should the mature sperm nucleus be damaged, it will be carried into the oocyte upon fertilization. The oocyte will then have to attempt to correct all sperm DNA defects. Regarding sperm DNA oxidative alterations such as the common 8-oxodG residue, resulting from oxidative attack of the sensitive guanine base, Smith et al. [42] have shown that only the first step of the BER (base excision repair) pathway is at work in mature spermatozoa. The second enzymatic step of the BER pathway that will cut the oxidized base and replace it with a new guanine will occur in the oocyte cytosol upon decondensation of the sperm nucleus. Consequently, sperm DNA oxidation may yield paternal DNA fragmentation during the oocyte repair process after fertilization.

Despite the compaction of nuclear DNA into densely packed doughnut-like structures known as toroids (wrapping up 50–100 kb of DNA), there are still areas of the nuclear genome that are always vulnerable to oxidative attack. These correspond to the less dense genomic regions still organized in nucleosomes (where only 146 bp of DNA is associated per histone octamer). In the mouse nucleus, it was shown that persistent histone-bound DNA regions fall in two categories [43]. First, nucleosomes were found at nonregular intervals in the protamine-embedded DNA regions. Second, nucleosomes and consequently histone-rich DNA regions, were also found enriched in the small DNA linker strands that run between adjacent toroids. Interestingly, these DNA linkers were shown to be attached to the sperm nuclear matrix, anchoring the chromosomes at the sperm head periphery and at the base of the sperm head [40]. The peripheral location of these nucleosomal sperm nuclear domains and their less-condensed nature make them particularly prone to DNA oxidative damage [40]. In addition, because of the manner in which sperm chromosomes are packaged into the sperm head, some chromosomes possess interlinker regions that are more vulnerable to damage than others [36,40].

Quantitatively, DNA base oxidation is not a minor problem. In mouse models we have generated, the level of epididymal luminal oxidative stress is rather low [39,40]. Nevertheless, the number of oxidized regions on mouse chromosomes is considerable. Within more than 15,000 DNA regions (mean 400 bp-long) were found significantly oxidized, among which 1000 were heavily oxidized [36]. A theoretical calculation estimates that in a model of mild sperm DNA oxidative damage, approximately 1 million guanine residues will be oxidized and will have to be replaced by the oocyte BER pathway. Moreover, that is only the visible tip of the iceberg given guanine is the most sensitive base to oxidation but it is not the only base affected; indeed, all the other bases may suffer oxidative damage. This high number of base replacement puts heavy pressure on the oocyte repair machinery that then increases the possibility of mistakes or inability to repair at all. In the absence of 8-OHdG repair, an increased risk of de novo $G \rightarrow T$ transversion mutations (following Hoogsteen base pairing between 8-oxoG with adenine) in the embryonic cells and their transmission in the progeny will occur. These may have a tremendous impact on the developmental program as well as on the health of the offspring Fig. 1.

Oxidative Alterations of the Sperm Nucleus and Epigenetic Information

Besides the DNA, there are reasons to suspect that protein and RNA constituents of the sperm nucleus may also be affected by oxidation, thereby altering the epigenetic information carried by the paternal nucleus. Oxidation of protamines does not appear to be a significant problem because these proteins will be removed from the paternal nucleus after fertilization. On the other hand, oxidative alteration of those regions of sperm DNA still complexed within nucleosomes will switch on an oocyte BER pathway that may not replace the appropriate histone/histone variants in these oxidized paternal nucleosomes. It is therefore not difficult to imagine that changes in the paternal nucleosome composition (the so-called histone code) may result in subtle modifications in the expression of nearby genes in the developing embryo.

Another obvious example where sperm nuclear oxidative alterations may influence the expression of epigenetic information lies within the different chemical modifications of the methyl-cytosine (meC) classical imprinting mark. Right after fertilization there is a particular round of demethylation concerning mainly the paternal nucleus [44]. Demethylation

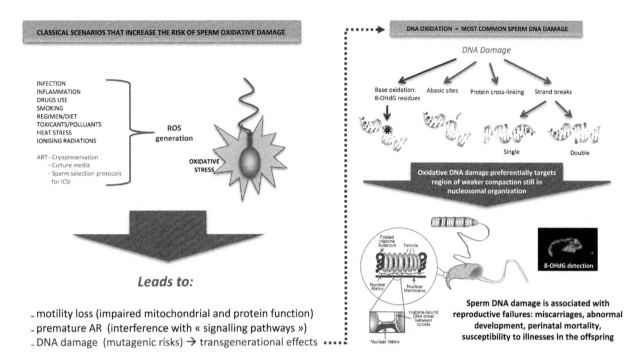

FIGURE 1 Examples of classical triggers that can lead to an oxidative stress environment for spermatozoa, whether pathophysiological or not. The exposure of spermatozoa to even low levels of reactive oxygen species may lead to a state of oxidative stress, amplified by the sperm cell themselves, which ultimately impairs sperm structures and function. The right side of the figure focuses on the various expressions of oxidative DNA damage that may then result. The architecture of the sperm nucleus yields regions that are more susceptible to oxidative alteration because of localized areas of poorer DNA compaction. Together these factors highlight the origins of increasing risks of complications associated with damaged (or insufficiently repaired) paternal DNA after fertilization.

starts with the oxidation of the meC into a hydroxyl methyl—cytosine residue (hmC) through the action of the ten eleven tranlocation (TET) enzyme machinery. HmC will subsequently be turned into formyl methyl-cytosine (fmC), carboxy methyl-cytosine (camC), then finally into cytosine [45]. Posttesticular oxidative alterations of mature sperm may therefore generate excessive hmC representation, possibly modifying the kinetics and the landscape of paternal DNA demethylation. This is expected since the oxidative deamination of 5-methylcytosine generates thymine and is responsible for GC → AT transition mutations following the formation of a glycol intermediate. The involvement of oxidative stress in CpG mutagenesis within the male germ line may then have a profound effect on the expression of paternally imprinted genes later on during development.

It was reported that the contribution of the spermatozoon to the embryo is not limited to the paternal DNA. Spermatozoa also incorporate a complex pool of short and long ncRNAs that have been assigned regulatory functions and constitute another form of paternal epigenetic inheritance. In 2016, two research groups reported that spermatozoa from males under particular environmental conditions such as an imbalanced diet or a behavioral stress show different sperm ncRNA loads that are responsible for the transmission in the progeny of the father phenotype [46,47]. Current unpublished studies suggest that posttesticular (i.e., epididymal) exposure to oxidative conditions changes the sperm ncRNA profile, potentially affecting embryonic development.

The developmental consequences of such oxidative DNA damage, in terms of the health and well-being of the offspring, is an extremely important question still awaiting resolution. In this context, it is significant that when spermatozoa are exposed to increasing levels of oxidative stress, DNA fragmentation occurs before spermatozoa lose their capacity for fertilization [48]. As a result, it is perfectly possible for a spermatozoon suffering from high levels of oxidative DNA damage to fertilize an oocyte and disrupt normal embryonic development. We see the consequences of this mechanism in action in the elevated cancer rates observed in the progeny of men who smoke heavily [49]. Unfortunately, we may see yet more examples of this association as the consequences of unrestricted ICSI use become apparent. Already, we are seeing evidence for an increased miscarriage rate being associated with ICSI, but not IVF [50]. The risk that we shall see further repercussions, as the fetuses that manage to develop to term mature into adults, should give cause for reflection.

THERAPEUTIC VALUE OF ANTIOXIDANT TREATMENTS

Key biomolecular processes that dictate sperm function, ranging from normal motility to an intact paternal genome, are susceptible to oxidative damage [7]. If spermatozoa are exposed to exogenous sources of ROS, or indeed induced to produce elevated endogenous levels, the biochemical damages that result, including lipid peroxidation, protein, and DNA damage, all attribute to loss of sperm function. Given the level of scientific and clinical importance now attributed to defective sperm function, there is an urgent need to further understand the underlying pathophysiology of this condition and develop appropriate forms of treatment. As such, the proposal of using antioxidants to combat the production of ROS or to intercept these species before biomolecule damage can ensue has been a long-held ambition [51]. While evidence exists to suggest that this approach is capable of delivering a therapeutic impact in animal models [52–55], definitive demonstration of antioxidant efficacy in a clinical context has not yet been achieved.

What Are Antioxidants?

If we investigate the chemical properties of an antioxidant, we identify that these molecules are simply chemicals that can participate in redox reactions, typically acting as electron donors or reducing agents and/or breaking down reactive molecules to relatively inert products. Antioxidant ability can be attained through donating an electron to the reactive oxidant (e.g., a ROS, the focus of this chapter), therefore suppressing further oxidative processes [56]. However, the term "antioxidant" perhaps has much wider connotations and complexity. The efficiency of direct redox chemistry or electron transfer is not always the defining feature of a recognized antioxidant and inhibitors of prooxidant enzymes such as NADPH-oxidases and lipoxygenases, modulation of signaling cascades or inflammatory responses that lead to oxidative stress and cofactors for antioxidant enzymes, which all result in reducing ROS levels, can be classed as antioxidants. Similarly, specialized molecules such as metal chelators, which have no particular redox activity but aid in reducing oxidative stress by selectively binding free Fenton metals such as $Cu^{(II)}$ and $Fe^{(III)}$, which otherwise propagate the production of superoxide and the hydroxyl radical, can be considered to have antioxidant properties. It should also be noted that because antioxidants are generally redox active molecules, given an appropriate environment, they can easily function in a prooxidant manner [57,58]. Appreciation of the diversity of compounds under the antioxidant umbrella and a comprehension of their role in moderating ROS are therefore critical considerations in designing rational antioxidant therapies.

Antioxidants can be categorized into two main groups, enzymes and small molecules. Enzymes that function to prevent or buffer ROS species production including several that are present in the male reproductive tract, such as catalase, the peroxiredoxins, SOD, and glutathione peroxidases, clearly have key roles in maintaining sperm quality and function [53]. The investigation of these entities as therapeutic supplements is largely restricted to culture or cell storage media, particularly in the context of cryopreservation [59,60]. Small molecule antioxidants also have major roles in providing a buffer against oxidative stress in the male reproductive tract and for the oral implementation of antioxidant therapeutics, are better suited to this role. The most well-known small molecule antioxidants include vitamins A, C, E, and the B complex, glutathione, pantothenic acid, coenzyme Q10, and carnitine derivatives as well as cofactors or micronutrients such as zinc and selenium. Some are chain-breaking antioxidants (vitamin E), quenching radicals generated during the lipid peroxidation process while some provide resources for endogenous antioxidant proteins (Se, vitamin B complex). These small molecular mass antioxidants can also be further subdivided into water-soluble and fat-soluble compounds. This physical property in part dictates retention time in the body; for example, fat-soluble antioxidants such as vitamin E (α-tocopherol) will partition to lipid-rich systems and have the potential to accumulate in fat stores or lipid bilayers. On the other hand, water-soluble compounds such as vitamin C (ascorbic acid) are quickly excreted through the urine following ingestion. Although the physical properties of antioxidant factors help us understand their role in the body or cell, an antioxidant must ultimately have the capacity to reduce concentrations of ROS or limit the biomolecule damage ROS would otherwise inflict.

Why Antioxidants?

As summarized in the section, "Oxidative Stress and Its Impact on Sperm Cell Structures and Functions," the origins of oxidative stress in the male germ line, while largely mitochondrial, can arise through numerous other influences including extrinsic influences. The specific cellular damages induced by these stressors can be equally as diverse. Given that spermatozoa discharge most of their cytoplasm as mature cells, they are therefore deficient in antioxidant enzymes, instead depending on the antioxidant properties of the extracellular environment provided by the male reproductive tract [61,62].

Magnifying the significance of this deficiency, there is abundant substrate (particularly polyunsaturated fatty acids) to propagating oxidative stress. The disruption of sperm function is a well-established consequence of oxidative stress as described in the section, "Sperm Nuclear Oxidative Stress and Its Developmental Impact." While the fundamental, molecular origins or triggers for excess ROS production in the male reproductive tract are still under investigation, it is timely to investigate the use of antioxidants in a therapeutic context. For the application of antioxidants in vitro for assisted reproduction, it is important to engineer incubation media that are supplemented with optimized antioxidants for spermatozoa. While some leading compounds have been successful in this context, including polyphenols like genistein [63,64], particularly for cryostorage, not all antioxidant molecules provide protection for spermatozoa and, in fact, several can induce ROS production [65].

The overriding negative health impacts of sperm oxidative stress lie in the damage to the sperm genome as this damage can lead to poor outcomes during pregnancy and also for offspring. While this DNA damage alone does not preclude a spermatozoon from participating in natural fertilization, the oxidative stress that leads to such damage may also impair sperm function, leading to loss of motility, disruption of oocyte-binding, and an induction of apoptosis-like processes. We could hypothesize that the frailty of the mature spermatozoon under oxidative insult is an adaptive design element that eliminates participation of a potentially promutagenic paternal genome from contributing to the next generation. Such considerations also raise concerns around assisted conception techniques such as ICSI, which may involve the fertilization of oocytes that nature, in its wisdom, would have excluded from this process. We therefore have a responsibility to verify that the therapeutic strategies that restore sperm parameters such as motility must also successfully protect against sperm DNA damage. In this context, it is encouraging that there is some preliminary evidence to suggest that antioxidants improve sperm DNA integrity [66].

Designing Antioxidant Therapeutics

The complex pathways of ROS production in spermatozoa, the types of reactive species produced, propagation of oxidative stress, and the biochemical consequences that lead to a loss of sperm function, are all important points to consider. All should be assimilated into the rational design of an antioxidant therapeutic, if the goal is to achieve the restoration of sperm function that leads to normal fertility, a good pregnancy outcome, and healthy offspring. Despite the undoubted complexity of the task, work already undertaken [67] and systematic investigations underway [54] suggest that the development of an optimized antioxidant formulation for clinical use in the context of male reproductive health is a feasible objective.

A classic pairing of antioxidants is the hydrophobic α-tocopherol molecule with ascorbic acid. Alone, α-tocopherol (known as vitamin E) partitions in the sperm plasma membrane and is able to lower lipid peroxidation [5,19] by intercepting ROS and lipid peroxides within the membrane structure. This well-studied phenomenon has shown to have therapeutic benefit [68–71] in a range of applications including sperm cryopreservation. The water-soluble ascorbic acid (known as vitamin C) can be rapidly absorbed by the gut (if orally administered) and can transiently accumulate in the cytoplasm of cells. As α-tocopherol becomes oxidized in the membranes under a state of oxidative stress, ascorbic acid can act as a direct reducing agent [72], hence regenerating reduced α-tocopherol and therefore antioxidant capacity in the cell membranes. This facilitates their synergistic partnership. Ascorbic acid, like most water-soluble antioxidant compounds, exhibits limited diffusion into the cell; however, selective uptake of ascorbate through membrane transporters accounts for the bulk of intracellular levels [73]. This simple example of an antioxidant formulation illustrates how the physical properties of antioxidant candidates can dictate their localization within biological systems and thus their ultimate efficacy. Therefore, matching antioxidant partition coefficients and other physical properties with suitable antioxidant power is an important consideration in the development of effective formulations.

Our group has investigated the antioxidant potential of polyphenols [65], flavonoids [65], and thiol molecules [74] for spermatozoa in vitro. The aim is to target ROS production and to neutralize reactive aldehyde products that result from lipid peroxidation cascades. Thiols such as penicillamine functioned as anticipated, neutralizing the ability of reactive aldehydes such as 4-HNE to alkylate and damage sperm proteins, but were unable to stop mitochondrial ROS production. Molecules such as resveratrol and genistein were confirmed to provide some therapeutic benefit, nonetheless, a range of polyphenol compounds including gallate compounds that are abundant in green tea revealed a prooxidant activity in vitro. Polyphenol compounds are well characterized to be potent antioxidant molecules [75], however the variety of structures that this class of reagent encapsulates is vast, representing an equally extensive range of chemical properties. Indeed, we found that the polyphenol epigallocatechin gallate depleted free thiols and glutathione leading to cellular ROS generation. Similar prooxidant responses were observed by other polyphenol compounds as they may act as substrates for quinone oxidoreductases in the sperm. An additional group of the polyphenols possessed hydrophobic or amphipathic properties, giving them the ability to intercalate into, and presumably disrupt, lipid bilayer structures in the sperm. The log P value quantifying this property was strongly correlated with the loss of mitochondrial membrane potential, which in turn, was correlated with hallmarks of ROS production and oxidative stress. This indicates that while these polyphenols may act as electron donors, their ability to perturb the redox state of the cell through alternative mechanisms can lead to the stimulation of ROS production and adverse functional consequences for the spermatozoa. Lipid peroxidation of the unsaturated fatty acids content in the sperm plasma membrane has a key role to play in the etiology of sperm pathology. Thus, lipid soluble antioxidants will be an important aspect of male infertility therapy. Moreover, recent enzyme targets of interest such as ALOX15 in sperm [23] provide scope to include additional nonantioxidant inhibitors within a carefully constructed antioxidant formulation. Also, worthy of note here is that therapeutics should minimize interference with physiological ROS signaling, responsible for initiating sperm processes such as capacitation, especially in the context of assisted reproduction.

For the infertile man suffering symptoms of oxidative stress in his gametes, a number of questions still remain. What is the origin of this stress? Is it localized only to the reproductive tract or do some patients suffer from systemic oxidative stress? The answer to these questions will also have wider implications for the formulation of antioxidant therapeutics. Regardless of these complexities, to assess the effectiveness of therapeutic agents, incorporation of robust sperm oxidative stress measurement is surely required. Showing measurable declines in oxidative markers as a result of treatment that further correlate with gain in sperm function is clearly an important component of studying antioxidant therapeutics for male infertility. Echoing the call from several recent reviews [56,76] well-designed clinical studies that also feature the sensitive measurement of oxidative stress markers and DNA integrity, as well as sperm functional assays, are now required to make significant headway toward alleviating the oxidative origins of male factor infertility.

REFERENCES

[1] McLachlan RI, de Kretser DM. Male infertility: the case for continued research. Med J Aust 2001;174:116–7.

[2] Irvine DS, Aitken RJ. Predictive value of in-vitro sperm function tests in the context of an AID service. Hum Reprod 1986;1:539–45.

[3] Liu DY, Baker HW. High frequency of defective sperm-zona pellucida interaction in oligozoospermic infertile men. Hum Reprod 2004;19:228–33.

[4] Aitken RJ, Irvine DS, Wu FC. Prospective analysis of sperm-oocyte fusion and reactive oxygen species generation as criteria for the diagnosis of infertility. Am J Obstet Gynecol 1991;164:542–51.

[5] Aitken RJ, Clarkson JS, Fishel S. Generation of reactive oxygen species, lipid peroxidation, and human sperm function. Biol Reprod 1989;41(1):183–97.

[6] Tosic J, Walton A. Formation of hydrogen peroxide by spermatozoa and its inhibitory effect on respiration. Nature 1946;158:485.

[7] Jones R, Mann T, Sherins RJ. Peroxidative breakdown of phospholipids in human spermatozoa: spermicidal effects of fatty acid peroxides and protective action of seminal plasma. Fertil Steril 1979;31:531–7.

[8] Holland MK, Storey BT. Oxygen metabolism of mammalian spermatozoa. Generation of hydrogen peroxide by rabbit epididymal spermatozoa. Biochem J 1981;198:273–80.

[9] Storey BT. Biochemistry of the induction and prevention of lipoperoxidative damage in human spermatozoa. Mol Hum Reprod 1997;3:203–13.

[10] Gomez E, Buckingham DW, Brindle J, Lanzafame F, Irvine DS,Aitken RJ. Development of an image analysis system to monitor the retention of residual cytoplasm by human spermatozoa: correlation with biochemical markers of the cytoplasmic space, oxidative stress, and sperm function. J Androl 1996;17:276–87.

[11] Williams AC, Ford WC. Functional significance of the pentose phosphate pathway and glutathione reductase in the antioxidant defenses of human sperm. Biol Reprod 2004;71:1309–16.

[12] Mayorga-Torres BJ, Camargo M, Cadavid ÁP, du Plessis SS, Cardona Maya WD. Are oxidative stress markers associated with unexplained male infertility? Andrologia 2017;49 [Epub ahead of print].

[13] Kullisaar T, Türk S, Kilk K, Ausmees K, Punab M, Mändar R. Increased levels of hydrogen peroxide and nitric oxide in male partners of infertile couples. Andrology 2013;1:850–8.

[14] Aitken RJ, Clarkson JS, Hargreave TB, Irvine DS, Wu FC. Analysis of the relationship between defective sperm function and the generation of reactive oxygen species in cases of oligozoospermia. J Androl 1989;10:214–20.

[15] Abasalt HC, Gholamali JS, Maryam GC. Lipid peroxidation and large-scale deletions of mitochondrial DNA in asthenoteratozoospermic patients. Indian J Biochem Biophys 2013;50:492–9.

[16] Mostafa T, Anis TH, El-Nashar A, Imam H, Othman IA. Varicocelectomy reduces reactive oxygen species levels and increases antioxidant activity of seminal plasma from infertile men with varicocele. Int J Androl 2001;24:261–5.

[17] Du Plessis SS, Agarwal A, Halabi J, Tvrda E. Contemporary evidence on the physiological role of reactive oxygen species in human sperm function. J Assist Reprod Genet 2015;32:509–20.

[18] Opuwari CS, Henkel RR. An update on oxidative damage to spermatozoa and oocytes. Biomed Res Int 2016;2016:9540142. https://doi.org/10.1155/2016/9540142 [Epub 2016 Jan 28].

[19] Koppers AJ, De Iuliis GN, Finnie JM, McLaughlin EA, Aitken RJ. Significance of mitochondrial reactive oxygen species in the generation of oxidative stress in spermatozoa. J Clin Endocrinol Metab 2008;93:3199−207.

[20] Aitken RJ, Whiting S, De Iuliis GN, McClymont S, Mitchell LA, Baker MA. Electrophilic aldehydes generated by sperm metabolism activate mitochondrial reactive oxygen species generation and apoptosis by targeting succinate dehydrogenase. J Biol Chem 2012;287:33048−60.

[21] Houston B, Curry B,Aitken RJ. Human spermatozoa possess an IL4I1 l-amino acid oxidase with a potential role in sperm function. Reproduction 2015;149:587−96.

[22] Musset B, Clark RA, DeCoursey TE, Petheo GL, Geiszt M, Chen Y, et al. NOX5 in human spermatozoa: expression, function, and regulation. J Biol Chem 2012;287:9376−88.

[23] Bromfield EG, Mihalas BP, Dun MD, Aitken RJ, McLaughlin EA, Walters JL, Nixon B. Inhibition of arachidonate 15-lipoxygenase prevents 4-hydroxynonenal-induced protein damage in male germ cells. Biol Reprod 2017;96:598−609.

[24] Aitken RJ, Ryan AL, Curry BJ, Baker MA. Multiple forms of redox activity in populations of human spermatozoa. Mol Hum Reprod 2003;9:645−61.

[25] Aitken RJ. A free radical theory of male infertility. Reprod Fertil Dev 1994;6:19−23.

[26] Aitken RJ, Buckingham DW, Carreras A, Irvine DS. Superoxide dismutase in human sperm suspensions: relationship with cellular composition, oxidative stress, and sperm function. Free Radic Biol Med 1996;21:495−504.

[27] Alvarez JG, Touchstone JC, Blasco L, Storey BT. Spontaneous lipid peroxidation and production of hydrogen peroxide and superoxide in human spermatozoa. Superoxide dismutase as major enzyme protectant against oxygen toxicity. J Androl 1987;8:338−48.

[28] Baker MA, Weinberg A, Hetherington L, Villaverde AI, Velkov T, Baell J, et al. Defining the mechanisms by which the reactive oxygen species by-product, 4-hydroxynonenal, affects human sperm cell function. Biol Reprod 2015;92:108.

[29] Moazamian R, Polhemus A, Connaughton H, Fraser B, Whiting S, Gharagozloo P, et al. Oxidative stress and human spermatozoa: diagnostic and functional significance of aldehydes generated as a result of lipid peroxidation. Mol Hum Reprod 2015;21:502−15.

[30] Aitken RJ, Flanagan HM, Connaughton H, Whiting S, Hedges A, Baker MA. Involvement of homocysteine, homocysteine thiolactone, and paraoxonase type 1 (PON-1) in the etiology of defective human sperm function. Andrology 2016;4:345−60.

[31] Oehninger S, Morshedi M, Franken D. The hemizona assay for assessment of sperm function. Meth Mol Biol 2013;927:91−102.

[32] Redgrove KA, Anderson AL, McLaughlin EA, O'Bryan MK, Aitken RJ, Nixon B. Investigation of the mechanisms by which the molecular chaperone HSPA2 regulates the expression of sperm surface receptors involved in human sperm-oocyte recognition. Mol Hum Reprod 2013;19(3):120−35.

[33] Bromfield EG, Aitken RJ, McLaughlin EA, Nixon B. Proteolytic degradation of heat shock protein A2 occurs in response to oxidative stress in male germ cells of the mouse. Mol Hum Reprod 2017;23:91−105.

[34] Bromfield E, Aitken RJ, Nixon B. Novel characterization of the HSPA2-stabilizing protein BAG6 in human spermatozoa. Mol Hum Reprod 2015;21:755−69.

[35] Aydin H, Sultana A, Li S, Thavalingam A, Lee JE. Molecular architecture of the human sperm IZUMO1 and egg JUNO fertilization complex. Nature 2016;534:562−5.

[36] Kocer A, Henry-Berger J, Noblanc A, Champroux A, Pogorelcnik R, Guiton R, et al. Oxidative DNA damage in mouse sperm chromosomes: size matters. Free Radic Biol Med 2015;89:993−1002.

[37] Sawyer DE, Mercer BG, Wiklendt AM, Aitken RJ. Quantitative analysis of gene-specific DNA damage in human spermatozoa. Mutat Res 2003;529:21−34.

[38] Conrad M, Moreno SG, Sinowatz F, Ursini F, Kölle S, Roveri A, et al. The nuclear form of phospholipid hydroperoxide glutathione peroxidase is a protein thiol peroxidase contributing to sperm chromatin stability. Mol Cell Biol 2005;25(17):7637−44.

[39] Chabory E, Damon C, Lenoir A, Kauselmann G, Kern H, Zevnik B, et al. Epididymis seleno-independent glutathione peroxidase 5 maintains sperm DNA integrity in mice. J Clin Invest 2009;119(7):2074−85.

[40] Noblanc A, Damon-Soubeyrand C, Karrich B, Henry-Berger J, Cadet R, Saez F, et al. DNA oxidative damage in mammalian spermatozoa: where and why is the male nucleus affected? Free Radic Biol Med 2013;65:719−23.

[41] Drevet JR. The antioxidant glutathione peroxidase family and spermatozoa: a complex story. Mol Cell Endocrinol 2006;250(1−2):70−9.

[42] Smith TB, De Iuliis GN, Lord T, Aitken RJ. The senescence-accelerated mouse prone 8 as a model for oxidative stress and impaired DNA repair in the male germ line. Reproduction 2013;146(3):253−62.

[43] Ward WS. Function of sperm chromatin structural elements in fertilization and development. Mol Hum Reprod 2010;16:30−6.

[44] McLay DW, Clarke HJ. Remodelling the paternal chromatin at fertilization in mammals. Reproduction 2003;125(5):625−33.

[45] Wu X, Zhang Y. TET-mediated active DNA demethylation: mechanism, function and beyond. Nat Rev Genet 2017. https://doi.org/10.1038/nrg.2017.33.

[46] Sharma U, Conine CC, Shea JM, Boskovic A, Derr AG, Bing XY, et al. Biogenesis and function of tRNA fragments during sperm maturation and fertilization in mammals. Science 2016;351(6271):391−6.

[47] Chen Q, Yan W, Duan E. Epigenetic inheritance of acquired traits through sperm RNAs and sperm RNA modifications. Nat Rev Genet 2016;17(12):733−43.

[48] Aitken RJ, Gordon E, Harkiss D, Twigg JP, Milne P, Jennings Z, et al. Relative impact of oxidative stress on the functional competence and genomic integrity of human spermatozoa. Biol Reprod 1998;59:1037−46.

[49] Lee KM, Ward MH, Han S, Ahn HS, Kang HJ, Choi HS, et al. Paternal smoking, genetic polymorphisms in CYP1A1 and childhood leukemia risk. Leuk Res 2009;33:250−8.

[50] Zhao J, Zhang Q, Wang Y, Li Y. Whether sperm deoxyribonucleic acid fragmentation has an effect on pregnancy and miscarriage after in vitro fertilization/intracytoplasmic sperm injection: a systematic review and meta-analysis. Fertil Steril 2014;102:998−1005.

[51] Vernet P, Aitken RJ, Drevet JR. Antioxidant strategies in the epididymis. Mol Cell Endocrinol 2004;216:31−9.

[52] Agarwal A, Majzoub A. Role of antioxidants in assisted reproductive techniques. World J Mens Health 2017;35.

[53] Gharagozloo P, Aitken RJ. The role of sperm oxidative stress in male infertility and the significance of oral antioxidant therapy. Hum Reprod 2011;26:1628−40.

[54] Gharagozloo P, Gutierrez-Adan A, Champroux A, Noblanc A, Kocer A, Calle J, et al. A novel antioxidant formulation designed to treat male infertility associated with oxidative stress: promising preclinical evidence from animal models. Hum Reprod 2016;31:252−62.

[55] Ross C, Morriss A, Khairy M, Khalaf Y, Braude P, Coomarasamy A, et al. A systematic review of the effect of oral antioxidants on male infertility. Reprod Biomed Online 2010;20:711−23.

[56] Walczak-Jedrzejowska R, Wolski JK, Slowikowska-Hilczer J. The role of oxidative stress and antioxidants in male fertility. Central Eur J Urol 2013;66(1):60−7.

[57] Eghbaliferiz S, Iranshahi M. Prooxidant activity of polyphenols, flavonoids, anthocyanins and carotenoids: updated review of mechanisms and catalyzing metals. Phytother Res 2016;30:1379−91.

[58] Gurer-Orhan H, Suzen S. Melatonin, its metabolites and its synthetic analogs as multi-faceted compounds: antioxidant, prooxidant and inhibitor of bioactivation reactions. Curr Med Chem 2015;22:490−9.

[59] Buffone MG, Calamera JC, Brigo-Olmedo S, de Vincentiis S, Calamera MM, Storey BT, et al. Superoxide dismutase content in sperm correlates with motility recovery after thawing of cryopreserved human spermatozoa. Fertil Steril 2012;97:293−8.

[60] Moubasher AE, El Din AM, Ali ME, El-sherif WT, Gaber HD. Catalase improves motility, vitality and DNA integrity of cryopreserved human spermatozoa. Andrologia 2013;45:135−9.

[61] Aitken RJ, Curry BJ. Redox regulation of human sperm function: from the physiological control of sperm capacitation to the etiology of infertility and DNA damage in the germ line. Antioxidants Redox Signal 2011;14:367−81.

[62] Rhemrev JP, van Overveld FW, Haenen GR, Teerlink T, Bast A, Vermeiden JP. Quantification of the nonenzymatic fast and slow TRAP in a postaddition assay in human seminal plasma and the antioxidant contributions of various seminal compounds. J Androl 2000;21:913−20.

[63] Martinez-Soto JC, de DiosHourcade J, Gutierrez-Adan A, Landeras JL, Gadea J. Effect of genistein supplementation of thawing medium on characteristics of frozen human spermatozoa. Asian J Androl 2010;12:431−41.

[64] Thomson LK, Fleming SD, Aitken RJ, De Iuliis GN, Zieschang JA, Clark AM. Cryopreservation-induced human sperm DNA damage is predominantly mediated by oxidative stress rather than apoptosis. Hum Reprod 2009;24:2061−70.

[65] Aitken RJ, Muscio L, Whiting S, Connaughton HS, Fraser BA, Nixon B, et al. Analysis of the effects of polyphenols on human spermatozoa reveals unexpected impacts on mitochondrial membrane potential, oxidative stress and DNA integrity; implications for assisted reproductive technology. Biochem Pharmacol 2016;121:78−96.

[66] Ahmadi S, Bashiri R, Ghadiri-Anari A, Nadjarzadeh A. Antioxidant supplements and semen parameters: an evidence based review. Int J Reprod Biomed 2016;14:729−36.

[67] Tremellen K, Miari G, Froiland D, Thompson J. A randomised control trial examining the effect of an antioxidant (Menevit) on pregnancy outcome during IVF-ICSI treatment. Aust N Z J Obstet Gynaecol 2007;47:216−21.

[68] Gual-Frau J, Abad C, Amengual MJ, Hannaoui N, Checa MA, Ribas-Maynou J, et al. Oral antioxidant treatment partly improves integrity of human sperm DNA in infertile grade I varicocele patients. Hum Fertil 2015;18:225−9.

[69] Keskes-Ammar L, Feki-Chakroun N, Rebai T, Sahnoun Z, Ghozzi H, Hammami S, et al. Sperm oxidative stress and the effect of an oral vitamin E and selenium supplement on semen quality in infertile men. Arch Androl 2003;49:83−94.

[70] Suleiman SA, Ali ME, Zaki ZM, el-Malik EM, Nasr MA. Lipid peroxidation and human sperm motility: protective role of vitamin E. J Androl 1996;17:530−7.

[71] Taylor K, Roberts P, Sanders K, Burton P. Effect of antioxidant supplementation of cryopreservation medium on post-thaw integrity of human spermatozoa. Reprod Biomed Online 2009;18:184−9.

[72] Machlin LJ, Bendich A. Free radical tissue damage: protective role of antioxidant nutrients. FASEB J 1987;1:441−5.

[73] Wilson JX. Regulation of vitamin C transport. Annu Rev Nutr 2005;25:105−25.

[74] Aitken RJ, Gibb Z, Mitchell LA, Lambourne SR, Connaughton HS, De Iuliis GN. Sperm motility is lost in vitro as a consequence of mitochondrial free radical production and the generation of electrophilic aldehydes but can be significantly rescued by the presence of nucleophilic thiols. Biol Reprod 2012;87:110. https://doi.org/10.1095/biolreprod.112.102020.

[75] Krupkova O, Ferguson SJ, Wuertz-Kozak K. Stability of (−)-epigallocatechin gallate and its activity in liquid formulations and delivery systems. J Nutr Biochem 2016;37:1−12.

[76] Agarwal A, Durairajanayagam D, du Plessis SS. Utility of antioxidants during assisted reproductive techniques: an evidence based review. Reprod Biol Endocrinol 2014;12:112.

Chapter 2.3

Male Genital Tract Infections and Leukocytospermia

Shu-Jian Chen and Gerhard Haidl
Rheinische Friedrich-Wilhelms University, Bonn, Germany

DEFINITION

Presently, the diagnosis of leukocytospermia is given in a semen sample with the number of WBC/mL $\geq 1 \times 10^6$ by the World Health Organization (WHO) [1]. In order to obtain reliable results, it is mandatory to perform routine semen analysis strictly according to the WHO guidelines [1] and to count peroxidase-positive round cells, although practicing physicians working in infertility clinics raise concerns regarding the clinical usefulness of the WHO cut-off value in predicting detrimental effects of leukocytospermia on sperm functions and male infertility. However, the setting of WBC numbers in semen sample $\geq 1 \times 10^6$/mL as reference parameter of leukocytospermia remains a cornerstone in the investigation of male infertility. Nevertheless, leukocytospermia represents a marker of male genital tract infection/inflammation (MGTI), including epididymo-orchitis, epididymitis, prostatitis/vesiculitis, and urethritis, which is generally the consequence of ascending infections of pathogens transmitted by sexual activity or by urological pathogens [2].

ETIOLOGY AND PHYSIOPATHOLOGY

Infection and inflammation of the genital urinary tract are responsible for 13%−15% of couples with fertility disturbances [3,4]. Most of the inflammatory disorders within the male genital tract are caused by infectious pathogens, in which *Chlamydia trachomatis* is the most typical. Other common microorganisms identified by previous studies are gonococcus, *Escherichia coli*, *Proteus mirabilis*, *Streptococcus faecalis*, and pseudomonas [2]. If there is no evidence of infection, the inflammation may originate from environmental and lifestyle factors such as smoking, and harmful professional exposure as well [5]. Since there are possibilities of microbiological contamination, it is important to note, even if the culture of some microorganisms from ejaculates shows positive results indicating an infection. Therefore, good laboratory practices by properly preparing the ejaculate with avoidance of contaminations should always be the goal.

Leukocytes are present in the male genital tract, even in healthy, fertile individuals with no infection. In case of infection and/or inflammation of the male genital tract induced by intrinsic and extrinsic factors, the numbers of peroxidase-positive leukocytes are increasing. These leukocytes are then also activated and infiltrate infected organs. Activated leukocytes physiologically produce up to 1000× more reactive oxygen species (ROS) than ROS-producing spermatozoa [6,7]. Despite the fact that physiologically low levels of ROS, either produced by leukocytes or the male germ cells themselves, play an essential role in normal spermatogenesis and fertilization, excessive production of ROS in infections and inflammation, as well as cellular defense mechanisms, exert detrimental effects [6].

Many in-depth investigations have revealed that high amounts of ROS attack the sperm plasma membrane, which is particularly susceptible to oxidative stress, and initiate a process called lipid peroxidation. Ultimately, this will damage plasma membranes and decrease the fluidity of both sperm plasma and organelle membranes resulting in loss of membrane function. Consequently, sperm functions such as acrosome reaction or the ability to fuse with the oolemma will be compromised [6,8]. Besides the damage caused by elevated ROS production in MGTI, various proinflammatory cytokines and chemokines (e.g., IL-6, IL-8, IL-18, TNF-α) secreted by leukocytes trigger chemoattraction of even more leukocytes to the inflammatory sites, following recruitment and activation of neutrophils to phagocytosis and pathogen clearance [9−11].

Oxidants, Antioxidants, and Impact of the Oxidative Status in Male Reproduction. https://doi.org/10.1016/B978-0-12-812501-4.00011-0

CLINICAL AND LABORATORY FINDINGS

Careful history takings and physical examination could provide important information regarding the status and progression of MGTI. Clinical findings of one or repeated episodes of urinary urgency, pollakiuria, and/or dysuria indicate acute urinary infections or inflammation. Occasionally, patients may complain of painful ejaculatory sensations. These symptoms could relieve spontaneously or disappear after an adequate treatment with antibiotics. Yet the physical examination of the patient should pay more attention to palpation of any swelling or nodularity of the epididymis and vas deferens as well as the scrotal content. In concert with other tests including rectal examination, prostate massage, ultrasound, and general blood, urine, and semen analysis will provide more relevant information for the diagnosis of MGTI [2]. On the other hand, chronic orchitis and epididymo-orchitis due to local or systemic infection as well as noninfectious etiological factors may be asymptomatic and could therefore be neglected. However, spermatogenesis of these patients may be significantly reduced [12].

As a routine work-up in an andrological clinic, semen analysis plays a pivotal role in diagnosing MGTI and then predicting the fertility potential of these patients. According to WHO criteria, more than 1×10^6 peroxidase-positive cells per mL ejaculate are considered leukocytospermia [1]. As a consensus-based reference value, this WHO cutoff, with regard to its clinical significance and the impact of leukocytospermia on male fertility, has been challenged in several reports [9,13−16]. On the one hand, it must be stated that in an ejaculate only a minor proportion of leukocytes may originate from the epididymis and testis, whereas approximately 95% of total semen volume consists of prostatic and seminal vesicle secretions. Experimental and clinical studies have revealed that epididymitis/epididymo-orchitis exert more detrimental effects on semen quality and fertility than infections/inflammations at the site of prostate and seminal vesicles [7,9] since sperm are exposed much longer to leukocytes, microorganisms, and cellular and humoral inflammatory components in the testis and epididymis. Therefore, despite the fact that leukocytospermia implies an infectious condition in different reproductive organs, the impact of leukocytes on male fertility and the subsequent therapeutic options could be controversial [9].

On the other hand, previous studies have suggested that the WHO-defined threshold of 1×10^6 WBC/mL for leukocytospermia may be too high. According to Agarwal et al. [13], even lower numbers of leukocytes may be a significant risk for male fertility and would require treatment. Punab et al. [16] drew similar conclusions by demonstrating that, based on receiver operating characteristic curve analysis, the WHO-defined WBC cutoff point has very low sensitivity for discriminating between patients with and without significant bacteriospermia. These authors advocated a cutoff of 0.2×10^6 WBC/mL since it would be more optimal as a lower threshold for leukocytospermia.

Finally, the present WHO manual [1] recommends counting peroxidase-positive round cells as leukocytes using a phase-contrast microscope at ×400 magnification when performing semen analysis [1]. However, the overall number of seminal leukocytes determined using the peroxidase technique could not reflect their type or status of functional activity. As we know, the major proportion of leukocytes in semen are polymorphonuclear granulocytes (also called neutrophils). Other types of seminal leukocytes, such as macrophages, T lymphocytes, and mast cells, cannot be detected cytochemically by their peroxidase content. Not only neutrophils, but also macrophage and mast cells are able to damage spermatozoa by secreting proteases and producing ROS, subsequently triggering DNA fragmentation and apoptosis [9,15,17]. Considering these methodological drawbacks, Fathy et al. [9] compared a novel flow cytometric approach (fluorescence-activated cell sorting; FACS) using CD18 as pan-leukocyte marker with the WHO-recommended peroxidase method. The overall results obtained by these two methods showed a highly significant correlation ($r = 0.9$, $P < .001$, $n = 47$). However, seminal FACS analysis could identify patients positive for MGTI, which would have been missed by using the WHO-recommended peroxidase method. In addition, variation of macrophages (CD18+/HLA-Dr+/CD66abce−) and neutrophils (CD18+/HLA-Dr−/CD66abce+) in leukocytes could be demonstrated to reveal the state of leukocyte infiltration in individual semen samples [9]. Most interestingly, macrophages that are preferentially producing IL-1β, TNF-α, and IL-6 in chronic male genital tract inflammation were also detected [9]. Hence, FACS could potentially represent a diagnostic milestone in identifying the elaborate profile of seminal leukocytes.

Based on work of our group as well as other groups, we suggest a revision in diagnostic criteria and definition of MGTI, with special emphasis on an optimal cutoff of leukocytospermia and more information from subpopulations of seminal leukocytes including their functional impact. Furthermore, in the diagnostic work-up of our group, apart from counting seminal leukocytes by conventional peroxidase technique, levels of ROS >500 relative light units/sec/10^6 sperm (referred to as RLU/s) and seminal IL-6 concentrations >30 pg/mL are supplementary indicators of MGTI.

TREATMENT

Generally accepted therapeutic guidelines for MGTI and/or leukocytospermia are not yet available. Based on current best evidence, the therapeutic approaches for these disturbances are antibiotics and antioxidants [18]. Depending on the localization of MGTI, treatment with proper antibiotics should be given. A previous metaanalysis showed that sperm parameters, such as sperm concentration, motility, and morphology, improved after using broad-spectrum antibiotics in patients with leukocytospermia. However, as the most important end points for the antibiotic treatment, the pregnancy rate or adverse events were not reported [19].

Various antioxidant supplements, mainly a combination of multivitamins and minerals (amino acid chelated), coenzyme Q10, have also presented favorable effects in protecting spermatozoa from exogenous oxidants in several in vitro studies [20,21]. Contrary, due to a lack of well-designed randomized controlled trials (RCTs) in human studies, strong evidence of these antioxidants improving leukocytospermia in vivo have not yet been provided [18,22]. Nevertheless, regular exercise training and refraining from smoking and alcohol consumption could be recommended as adjunct lifestyle approaches to MGTI and/or leukocytospermia [5,23].

CONCLUSIONS

Male genital tract infections have been considered an important factor causing male infertility. Besides physical examination, leukocyte detection in semen plays an essential role in evaluating MGTI. The threshold setting of more than 1×10^6 leukocytes per mL in defining MGTI is still under debate; however, it presents an approximate value for physicians and is very helpful for diagnosis of MGTI in current clinical practice. Although most published reports stressed the detrimental effects of ROS mainly deriving from semen leukocytes, physiological levels of leukocytes and ROS have beneficial effects in male fertilization. Treatment of MGTI rely not only on proper antibiotics, but also antioxidants, whereas antioxidant administration should be based on combined evaluation of seminal leukocytes, ROS levels, oxidative status, and seminal total antioxidant capacity levels. Well-designed RCTs in evaluating therapeutic approaches for MGTI are needed urgently.

REFERENCES

[1] World Health Organization. WHO laboratory manual for the examination of human semen and semen-cervical mucus interaction. 5th ed. Cambridge: Cambridge University Press; 2010.

[2] Schill WB, Comhaire FH, Hargreave TB. Andrology for the clinician. In: Infection/inflammation of the accessory sex glands. Springer Berlin Heidelberg; 2006.

[3] Henkel R, Maass G, Jung A, Haidl G, Schill WB, Schuppe HC. Age-related changes in seminal polymorphonuclear elastase in men with asymptomatic inflammation of the genital tract. Asian J Androl 2007;9:299—304.

[4] Nieschlag E, Behre HM. Andrology. In: Male reproductive Health and dysfunction. Berlin: Springer; 2000.

[5] Pasqualotto FF, Umezu FM, Salvador M, Borges Jr E, Sobreiro BP, Pasqualotto EB. Effect of cigarette smoking on antioxidant levels and presence of leukocytospermia in infertile men: a prospective study. Fertil Steril 2008;90:278—83.

[6] Henkel RR. Leukocytes and oxidative stress: dilemma for sperm function and male fertility. Asian J Androl 2011;13:43—52.

[7] Wolff H. The biologic significance of white blood cells in semen. Fertil Steril 1995;63:1143—57.

[8] Chen SJ, Allam JP, Duan YG, Haidl G. Influence of reactive oxygen species on human sperm functions and fertilizing capacity including therapeutical approaches. Arch Gynecol Obstet 2013;288:191—9.

[9] Fathy A, Chen SJ, Novak N, Schuppe HC, Haidl G, Allam JP. Differential leucocyte detection by flow cytometry improves the diagnosis of genital tract inflammation and identifies macrophages as proinflammatory cytokine-producing cells in human semen. Andrologia 2014;46:1004—12.

[10] Lotti F, Maggi M. Interleukin 8 and the male genital tract. J Reprod Immunol 2003;100:54—65.

[11] Matalliotakis IM, Cakmak H, Fragouli Y, Kourtis A, Arici A, Huszar G. Increased IL-18 levels in seminal plasma of infertile men with genital tract infections. Am J Reprod Immunol 2006;55:428—33.

[12] Schuppe HC, Meinhardt A, Allam JP, Bergmann M, Weidner W, Haidl G. Chronic orchitis: a neglected cause of male infertility? Andrologia 2008;40:84—91.

[13] Agarwal A, Mulgund A, Alshahrani S, Assidi M, Abuzenadah AM, Sharma R, Sabanegh E. Reprod Biol Endocrinol 2014;12:126.

[14] Haidl G. New WHO-reference limits-revolution or storm in a teapot? Asian J Androl 2011;13:208—11.

[15] Henkel R, Kierspel E, Stalf T, Mehnert C, Menkveld R, Tinneberg HR, Schill WB, Kruger TF. Effect of reactive oxygen species produced by spermatozoa and leukocytes on sperm functions in non-leukocytospermic patients. Fertil Steril 2005;83:635—42.

[16] Punab M, Lõivukene K, Kermes K, Mändar R. The limit of leucocytospermia from the microbiological viewpoint. Andrologia 2003;35:271—8.

[17] Haidl F, Haidl G, Oltermann I, Allam JP. Seminal parameters of chronic male genital inflammation are associated with disturbed sperm DNA integrity. Andrologia 2015;47:464—9.

[18] Jung JH, Kim MH, Kim J, Baik SK, Koh SB, Park HJ, Seo JT. Treatment of leukocytospermia in male infertility: a systematic review. World J Mens Health 2016;34:165−72.

[19] Skau PA, Folstad I. Do bacterial infections cause reduced ejaculate quality? A meta-analysis of antibiotic treatment of male infertility. Behav Ecol 2003;14:40−7.

[20] Barbato V, Talevi R, Braun S, Merolla A, Sudhakaran S, Longobardi S, Gualtieri R. Supplementation of sperm media with zinc, D-aspartate and co-enzyme Q10 protects bull sperm against exogenous oxidative stress and improves their ability to support embryo development. Zygote 2017;25:168−75.

[21] Zalata A, Elhanbly S, Abdalla H, Serria MS, Aziz A, El-Dakrooy SA, El-Bakary AA, Mostafa T. In vitro study of cypermethrin on human spermatozoa and the possible protective role of vitamins C and E. Andrologia 2014;46:1141−7.

[22] Piomboni P, Gambera L, Serafini F, Campanella G, Morgante G, De Leo V. Sperm quality improvement after natural anti-oxidant treatment of asthenoteratospermic men with leukocytospermia. Asian J Androl 2008;10:201−6.

[23] Maleki BH, Tartibian B. High-intensity exercise training for improving reproductive function in infertile patients: a randomized controlled trial. J Obstet Gynaecol Can 2017;39:545−58.

FURTHER READING

[1] Erel CT, Sentürk LM, Demir F, Irez T, Ertüngealp E. Antibiotic therapy in men with leukocytospermia. Int J Fertil Women's Med 1997;42:206−10.

[2] Pajovic B, Pajovic L, Vukovic M. Effectiveness of antibiotic treatment in infertile patients with sterile leukocytospermia induced by tobacco use. Syst Biol Reprod Med 2017;8:1−6.

[3] Weidner W, Pilatz A, Diemer T, Schuppe HC, Rusz A, Wagenlehner F. Male urogenital infections: impact of infection and inflammation on ejaculate parameters. World J Urol 2013;31:717−23.

Chapter 2.4

Varicocele

Nicholas N. Tadros[1] and Edmund Sabanegh, Jr. [2]

[1]Southern Illinois University, Springfield, IL, United States; [2]Cleveland Clinic Foundation, Cleveland, OH, United States

INTRODUCTION

Scrotal varicoceles, defined as abnormally dilated scrotal veins, are thought to be the most common attributable cause of infertility in the male, especially in cases where the man has conceived previously (secondary infertility) [1]. In the largest population study on varicoceles to date, the World Health Organization found varicoceles in 11.7% of the men with normal semen parameters [2], but up to 42% of men with primary infertility [3] and up to 81% of men [4] with secondary infertility. While the pathophysiology of infertility in the setting of a varicocele is likely multifactorial, many share a common pathway through the creation of reactive oxygen species (ROS) and resultant oxidative stress.

ANATOMY

Varicoceles develop from structural abnormalities of the veins draining blood from the testis. The venous drainage of the testis is variable but classically starts in the scrotum as the pampiniform plexus and eventually drains into a single testicular (internal spermatic) vein. This vein then drains into the renal vein on the left, or the inferior vena cava (IVC) on the right. The pampiniform plexus can also drain into the vein associated with the vas deferens, which eventually drains into the inferior epigastric vein via the cremasteric veins.

Varicoceles likely result when there is too much back pressure in this drainage system, which can be caused by a few mechanisms. The left testicular vein is 8–10 cm longer than the right and inserts into the left renal vein at approximately a 90-degree angle. This increases turbulent flow and back pressure compared to the right testicular vein, which inserts more obliquely into the low pressure IVC at a more oblique angle. These factors are responsible for the substantially lower incidence of clinically significant right-sided varicoceles (1%–2%) [2]. Large unilateral right-sided varicoceles can suggest the possibility of venous obstruction caused by retroperitoneal tumors and may require further workup. Other contributing factors to varicocele formation are incompetent (acquired or congenital) or absent (congenital) venous valves in the testicular veins that allow retrograde reflux of blood that increases pressure and eventually causes venous dilation [5].

DIAGNOSIS

While there are excellent imaging studies that can diagnose varicoceles, the most clinically relevant diagnostic tool remains the physical examination. It is important that patients are examined in the standing and supine positions. Laterality is important as isolated right-sided varicoceles may indicate other significant pathology as previously described. A grade is usually assigned to the varicocele based on physical examination findings:

- Subclinical: Not palpable or visible at rest or during Valsalva maneuver but seen on scrotal ultrasound
- Grade I (small): palpable only during the Valsalva maneuver
- Grade II (moderate): palpated without Valsalva maneuver
- Grade III (large): visible through the scrotal skin and classically described as feeling like a "bag of worms"

This unvalidated grading scheme has made outcomes research difficult. Hargreave and Liakatas compared the examination findings between two experienced physicians and found grade discordance in 26% of patients [6].

Due to this variability in physical exam findings and the high prevalence of varicoceles in male infertility, physicians have utilized imaging modalities on occasion to assist with diagnosis.

Ultrasound

Scrotal ultrasound has the advantage of being noninvasive as well as free from ionizing radiation. It can diagnose other scrotal pathology and provide more accurate testicular size measurements. Ultrasound can detect nonpalpable varicoceles with a >94% sensitivity and specificity [7]. Because these subclinical varicoceles are not thought to worsen oxidative stress or fertility, routine ultrasound use for varicocele screening is not recommended nor is the treatment of subclinical varicoceles. Its use may be required in special cases such as large body habitus or equivocal physical examination findings. It is important that the radiologist and ultrasonographer measure the size of the veins with and without Valsalva in addition to just commenting on the presence or absence of a varicocele. Diagnostic criteria for ultrasound diagnosis demonstrates reversal of venous blood flow with Valsalva and/or spermatic vein diameter >3 mm [8].

Other Diagnostic Modalities

Venography of the testicular veins can be used for both diagnosis and treatment of varicoceles. Venography is the most sensitive imaging modality, with nearly 100% sensitivity. Unfortunately, its clinical utility is limited since up to 70% of patients without a clinical varicocele are found to have reflux during venography [9,10]. Venography is also used for percutaneous treatments such as sclerotherapy and embolization.

VARICOCELES AND MALE INFERTILITY

Semen Characteristics

In the original World Health Organization (WHO) study, the 9034 men with infertility demonstrated lower sperm concentration and motility compared to the fertile control group [2]. Since that time, the WHO reference ranges and evaluation methods for semen analysis have changed three times (1992, 1999, 2010). Using the most recent WHO, 5th edition, reference ranges (2010), a metaanalysis of 10 studies showed the semen of men with varicoceles have a reduced sperm count, decreased motility, and abnormal morphology. The semen volume remained within normal limits in these patients [11].

Pathophysiology

While varicocele formation is usually the result of anatomic or functional inadequacy of the drainage system, there are multiple mechanisms that actually impair spermatogenesis in this setting. The leading theory postulates that poor venous drainage disrupts the countercurrent exchange of heat from the spermatic cord causing a relative hyperthermia of the scrotum that then affects both testes [12]. The cellular processes of the testis are exquisitely sensitive to increased temperature, and hyperthermia causes reductions in testosterone synthesis by Leydig cells, injury to germinal cell membranes, altered protein metabolism, and reduced Sertoli cell function [13]. When a varicocele is ligated, scrotal temperature returns to normal [14].

The impaired venous drainage causes hypoxia, poor clearance of gonadotoxins, and elevated levels of oxidative stress including increases in mitochondrial, plasma membrane, cytoplasmic, and peroxisomal ROS production [15]. Another cause of increased oxidative stress is an increased level of catecholamines (specifically norepinephrine) in refluxing venous blood. This elevated level of norepinephrine causes constriction of the intratesticular blood vessels and decreased arterial perfusion leading to hypoxia and increased ROS production [16].

The level of oxidative stress seems to correlate with varicocele grade [17]. This has been reproduced in multiple other studies that have shown an increase in other oxidative stress metabolites including seminal malondialdehyde, nitric oxide (NO), superoxide dismutase, glutathione peroxidase, and ascorbic acid [18–21]. Two of these studies [18,20] have shown seminal antioxidant levels were inversely correlated with varicocele grade as well. Taken together these studies indicate that the grade of varicocele may predict the severity of oxidative stress.

However, given the high incidence of varicoceles in fertile men, it is postulated that different intrinsic susceptibility to the previous processes must exist among men with varicoceles to explain the variability in effects on fertility [22]. In fact, Cocuzza et al. found that levels of ROS are not correlated with varicocele grade or testis volume in *fertile* men [23].

MECHANISMS OF REACTIVE OXYGEN SPECIES PRODUCTION

Scrotal Hyperthermia

Scrotal thermoregulation serves to counteract the large amount of heat produced during spermatogenesis. This is why optimal spermatogenesis occurs at a temperature approximately $2-4°C$ below normal body temperature. On the other hand, oogenesis in the ovaries of women does not have such temperature constraints since it occurs inside the body. Well-vascularized thin scrotal skin, numerous sweat glands, and absence of subcutaneous fat help to facilitate heat exchange within the scrotum [24]. Varicoceles increase scrotal temperature by interfering with the vascular countercurrent exchange mechanism [25]. In vitro studies have shown a direct relationship between temperature and the release of ROS. An early study of rabbit and mouse spermatozoa showed a linear rate of spontaneous lipid peroxidation, an index of oxidative stress, as measured by the formation of malonaldehyde as the temperature increased from $34°C$ to $40°C$ [26]. Not all human reproductive cells exhibit the same vulnerability to heat either. Spermatogonia B, spermatocytes, and early spermatids are much more susceptible to heat stress then spermatogonia A, Sertoli, and Leydig cells [27,28]. Increased temperature does not explain ROS generation in varicoceles entirely though since most men with varicoceles have increased scrotal temperature, but the majority of these men are fertile [29,30].

Renal and Adrenal Metabolites

Research in the 1960s and 1970s advanced the theory that varicoceles cause testicular exposure to more toxic hormones and their metabolites due to reflux [31]. Many of these studies focused on the elevated levels of cortisol and renin in the dilated veins of the scrotum [32]. Further research identified elevated levels of norepinephrine and prostaglandins E and F within the spermatic vein [33,34]. These metabolites are thought to contribute to testicular hypoxia, which will be discussed in greater detail later. Following the discovery of adrenomedullin, a potent vasodilator originally found in pheochromocytomas, there has been renewed interest in the reflux theory. Ozbek et al. found that in men with varicocele, adrenomedullin levels within the internal spermatic vein were significantly higher than that in the brachial vein [35]. They postulated that these increased levels were from retrograde flow of venous blood from the adrenal gland and kidney, which can cause vasodilation and disrupt the countercurrent heat exchange system.

Hypoperfusion and Hypoxia

Hypoperfusion of the testis (and resulting ischemia) can occur in the presence of varicoceles when the venous pressure exceeds arterial pressure and does not allow for adequate blood flow through the testis. This leads to tissue hypoxia and a buildup of ischemic-related proteins. Gat et al. identified histologic signs of ischemic damage within the testes of men with varicocele including germ-cell degeneration, Leydig cell atrophy, and fibrotic thickening of the basement membranes of seminiferous tubules [36]. This causes ischemia activation and release of many ROS and other inflammatory factors that cause increased oxidative stress. Hypoxia will also drive the cells to primary glycolysis with increased production of toxic by-products such as lactate, though there are conflicting results as to whether or not these metabolites caused sperm damage and infertility [37−39].

Hypoxia can lead to an increase in cytokine expression in testicular tissues such as IL-1 [40] and IL-6 [41]. Both IL-1 and IL-6 are proinflammatory cytokines that cause increased ROS generation and oxidative stress [42] as well as the accumulation of inflammatory cells in the semen, which likely leads to leukospermia and further oxidative damage [43].

MOLECULAR MECHANISMS

All of these processes lead to increased oxidative stress in the presence of a varicocele, though there are many cellular mechanisms that cause this spermatotoxic environment. These include generation of NO, xanthine dehydrogenase, insufficient heat shock proteins (HSPs), and production of ROS by mitochondria, among other pathways.

Nitric Oxide Production

NO has many useful functions. Along with its role in vascular smooth muscle, it is important in sperm motility and function when present at physiologic levels [44]. But in excess, NO can actually *decrease* sperm motility and cause sperm toxicity [45]. NO is synthesized from L-arginine by nitric oxide synthase (NOS). This is present as one of three types: inducible NOS (iNOS), endothelial NOS (eNOS), and neuronal NOS (nNOS). The latter two (eNOS and nNOS) produce small amounts of NO necessary for normal function. iNOS on the other hand can produce much larger amounts of NO that is metabolically active for longer time periods and is the likely culprit in NO-mediated sperm dysfunction in men with varicoceles. In fact, iNOS knockout mice have increased testicular volume, sperm concentration, and resistance to heat-induced cell death [46]. NOS is found in many cells of the reproductive system including Sertoli cells, Leydig cells, premature spermatocytes, and early spermatids. It is also found in high concentrations in cells undergoing apoptosis [47]. Higher NO concentrations have been measured in the Leydig cells of varicocele patients compared to normal controls [48] and increased iNOS expression in testicular biopsy samples from men with grade II or III varicocele than in those with grade I varicocele or healthy controls [49]. In this setting, increased temperature is thought to upregulate iNOS. Guo and colleagues subjected cynomolgus monkeys to short exposure of increased heat over 2 days to test this hypothesis. They found that increased iNOS expression in testicular germ cells and Sertoli cells. On day 28, iNOS expression in germ cells was similar to that of their controls, but higher levels of iNOS expression were still detectable in the Sertoli cells. This was thought to be due to the high iNOS apoptotic germ cells undergoing phagocytosis [27]. In the rest of the body, NO serves as a potent vasodilator, and the scrotum is no exception. Increased NO release may also serve as a reaction to the increased venous stasis and hypoxic conditions that a varicocele creates. This increased NO production can then cause more sperm damage.

Regardless of how NO is produced in the setting of a varicocele, it has a similar mechanism of action to create oxidative stress. NO readily diffuses into the cells and reacts with superoxide anions to produce oxidative metabolites such as peroxynitrite and peroxynitrous acid [50]. NO can also decrease the levels of glutathione reductase (recycler of reduced glutathione, a natural antioxidant from its oxidized form), which can further worsen the redox balance [51]. Given this knowledge, researchers have used NOS inhibitors in varicocele rat models in an attempt to prevent NO mediated damage. Abbasi et al. showed that aminoguanidine, an inducible NO synthase inhibitor, improved sperm count, motility, morphology, vitality, and DNA fragmentation when given to rats with varicocele [52,53].

Reactive Oxygen Species Production by Mitochondria

Mitochondria produce adenosine triphosphate (ATP) from products of the citric acid cycle, fatty acid oxidation, and amino acid oxidation. At the inner membrane, electrons from nicotinamide adenine dinucleotide (NADH) and $FADH_2$ (reduced form of flavin adenine dinucleotide) pass through the electron transport chain to oxygen, which is then reduced to water. This process comprises an enzymatic series of electron donors and acceptors. Each electron donor will pass electrons to a more electronegative acceptor until electrons are passed to oxygen, the terminal electron acceptor in the chain. This complex cycle is carried out by multiple mitochondrial redox carries named complex I—IV. This passage of electrons releases energy, which is eventually used to generate a proton gradient across the mitochondrial membrane, which is stored as potential energy. A small percentage of electrons do not complete all the steps in the electron transport chain and instead will directly bond to oxygen (primarily from the leak of electrons from complex I and III), resulting in the formation of ROS, specifically the free-radical superoxide. Hypoxia and heat stress can directly activate complex III of the electron transport chain, which will increase ROS release [54]. Tan et al. showed that complex I and IV activity is reduced when exposed to heat stress in hepatic cells. This promotes more electron leaks from complex III with the formation of superoxide [55]. Increased NO production (as discussed earlier) can nitrosylate complexes I and IV causing decreased activity as well, which will also promote excessive release of ROS by complex III.

As a protective mechanism against heat- and hypoxia-induced oxidative stress, testis germ cells can activate mitochondrial uncoupling proteins (UCPs) [56]. These proteins function to transfer protons from the intermembrane space to the matrix of the mitochondria and decrease ROS production by decreasing the availability of protons for ATP generation. These UCPs require coenzyme Q, a cofactor that facilitates proton transfer across membranes [57]. Unfortunately, spermatic coenzyme Q is reduced in men with varicoceles [58], which in turn will decrease UCP effects and increase ROS generation. Ferramosca et al. compared 40 men with and without varicoceles. Oxidative stress was observed in the serum and seminal fluid of the varicocele patients. They showed a 59% increase in serum reactive oxygen metabolites and a threefold increase in the level of sperm lipid peroxides. They also found DNA fragmentation to be doubled in the varicocele cohort and observed a 27% decrease in mitochondrial respiratory activity in comparison to the control group [59].

Heat Shock Proteins

HSPs regulate translation, transcription, and signal transduction on a regular basis within the cell. When the cell is exposed to hypoxic or heat stress, HSP expression and transcription is increased. These proteins help facilitate the correction of protein misfolding and denaturation, which can eventually lead to cell apoptosis. Multiple studies have evaluated HSPA2 mRNA in men with varicocele [39,60,61]. Each of these studies found a decrease in HSPA2 mRNA in the semen of oligospermic men with varicocele when compared to men without varicocele. Yesilli et al. [39] studied the HSPA2 protein expression in semen of 56 men with varicocele and 25 men without varicocele. They also had data on 26 men in the varicocele group who underwent microsurgical subinguinal varicocelectomy. They found that the mean sperm HSPA2 activity was significantly lower in the varicocele group than in the control group. But even more interesting, they found that sperm HSPA2 activity increased significantly after varicocelectomy compared to their preoperative levels. Other studies have shown an *increase* in HSPA4 expression in men with varicocele and oligospermia, so further research is needed to determine the exact role of these proteins in men with varicocele [62].

Heme Oxygenase

Heme oxygenase (HO) is an enzyme that catalyzes the degradation of heme, which produces biliverdin, ferrous iron, and carbon monoxide [63]. Its enzymatic activity is most apparent in the spleen, where it is part of erythrocyte breakdown; and in bruises, where it is the cause of the changing skin color. There are two main isoforms of the enzyme, and heme oxygenase 1 (HO-1) is an inducible isoform upregulated in oxidative stress and hypoxia [64]. Heme oxygenase 2 (HO-2) does not exhibit stress-related upregulation. In the rat, HO-2 is found in germ cells, spermatocytes, and round spermatids [65], while HO-1 is found in small amounts in macrophages, and Sertoli and Leydig cells. During oxidative stress, Leydig cells upregulate HO-1 expression, which leads to increased apoptosis of premeiotic germ cells [66]. The antioxidant effects of HO-1 come from the degradation of heme, a known stimulator of ROS production, as well as the ROS scavenging properties of the breakdown products, biliverdin and bilirubin [67,68]. While the majority of these studies have been performed in animal models, Aziz et al. studied the seminal 1 plasma HO enzyme activity in oligoastheno-teratozoospermia (OAT) men with varicoceles. They found that seminal HO enzyme activity decreased significantly in OAT cases compared with controls. Seminal plasma HO in OAT cases associated with varicocele decreased significantly compared with OAT cases without varicocele and healthy controls. They concluded that varicoceles have a negative impact on HO activity, and improved semen parameters after varicocele ligation may be due in part to improved heme oxidase activity [69].

Xanthine Oxidase

In its dehydrogenated form, this protein normally catalyzes the conversion of xanthine to hypoxanthine and uric acid. In hypoxic conditions, its disulfide bond is oxidized or it undergoes proteolysis to be converted to xanthine oxidase [70,71]. These two forms differ only in the fact that the oxidative form creates a superoxide and hydrogen peroxide during the conversion of xanthine. Xanthine oxidase is found in low amounts in spermatogonia, spermatocytes, and spermatids but is highly expressed in spermatozoa [72,73]. In varicocele patients, xanthine oxidase activity was increased $7\times$ in the endothelial cells of the spermatic veins compared to the peripheral vein control, but no studies directly evaluate the xanthine oxidase activity in the semen of men with varicoceles. In the aforementioned mitochondrial reactions, adenosine diphosphate buildup is a result of NO inhibiting ATP production. This can also lead to an increased accumulation of xanthine oxidase substrates, which then increase the enzyme's activity and thus the production of ROS [74].

Epididymal Damage

The epididymis is composed of metabolically active principal cells that have the ability to generate ROS and produce antioxidants. Experimental varicocele models have shown microscopic and ultrastructural changes in the epididymis in rats with varicoceles compared to controls [75]. These changes include reduction in weight of the left epididymis and in the tubular diameter of the caput region [76]. Degeneration of the epididymal epithelium and edema of the interstitial tissue is noted in rats with varicoceles, and the carnitine (an antioxidant) contents and the alpha-glucosidase activity in the caput, corpus, and cauda epididymis is lower than in controls [77]. Ischemia is one of the main contributors to these findings and its damage is not just limited to the testis.

TREATMENT OF VARICOCELE-RELATED OXIDATIVE STRESS

Measurement of Oxidative Stress

Multiple studies have compared fertile and infertile men with and without varicoceles in different combinations. When compared to men with idiopathic male infertility, men with infertility and varicoceles had increased levels of NO, superoxide dismutase, and other ROS [78–80]. Their total antioxidant capacity (TAC) is also lower compared to infertile and fertile men without varicoceles [81]. Unfortunately, not all studies have found the same results as some have noted *higher* levels of TAC and some antioxidants in infertile men with varicoceles [82,83]. This may be due to an inability for the antioxidants to adequately neutralize ROS despite the presence of the appropriate reductants [84]. Even fertile men with varicoceles appear to have higher levels of oxidative stress than their fertile counterparts without varicoceles [20,85,86]. There is no consensus on why these men just exhibit higher oxidative stress without infertility but it is likely due to other genetic predispositions that have not been elucidated yet.

Varicocele Repair

Varicocele repair can be performed with a number of techniques including percutaneous and surgical methods. The first percutaneous treatment of a varicocele was described in 1978 when Lima and colleagues used hypertonic glucose and ethanolamine oleate to sclerose the testicular vein [87]. Due to recurrence rates as high as 11% [88] and lower initial success rates, percutaneous embolization is not considered to be the gold standard for initial varicocele treatment although it does retain a role in treatment of postsurgical recurrence [13,89]. Many surgical techniques have been used to ligate varicoceles including retroperitoneal (Palomo), laparoscopic, inguinal, and subinguinal techniques. Each has their pros and cons regarding success rates, recurrence, and postoperative complications. A review of over 5000 patients across 33 studies found that microscopic assisted inguinal and subinguinal varicocelectomy resulted in better outcomes than the other techniques across multiple parameters including pregnancy rates, recurrence, and complications [90].

Given the important role that oxidative stress plays in varicocele pathology, many studies have also examined the change in oxidative stress and ROS production before and after varicocele repair. Varicocele ligation has been shown to decrease multiple markers of oxidative stress including 8-OHdG (8-hydroxy-2′-deoxyguanosine), NO, and superoxide dismutase [79,91]. Sperm HSPA2 activity has also been shown to increase after varicocele ligation compared to the preoperative values [39]. Not only are ROS decreased after varicocele repair, but antioxidants and TAC can increase after varicocele treatment. Cervellione et al. found an increase in TAC 1 year after varicocelectomy in 11 adolescents [92]. In another study, 31 men with varicocele (before and after varicocele ligation) and 31 fertile controls had their oxidative stress index (OSI), total oxidant capacity (TOC), TAC, superoxide dismutase, and glutathione measured in peripheral and internal spermatic vein blood. TOC and OSI were significantly higher in the varicocele group and higher in the spermatic vein compared to median cubital vein [93]. Postoperatively, TOC and OSI were reduced to the levels of that seen in the fertile controls. A similar study found that levels of NO and malondialdehyde decreased significantly in the seminal plasma and peripheral and spermatic vein blood after varicocelectomy [94]. Unfortunately, some studies have shown that even though varicocelectomy can decrease ROS levels substantially, levels may not return to that of fertile men [95]. Other studies have found an increase in antioxidants such as ascorbate [91,96], selenium, and zinc [97]. Two conflicting studies have evaluated the levels of vitamin E after varicocele repair. One study compared pre- and postvaricocelectomy vitamin E levels and found that they returned to normal levels after surgery [97]. The other study found that vitamin E levels actually decreased after varicocele repair [96]. Given that vitamin E levels are very dependent on dietary intake, it is difficult to draw definitive conclusions from these studies. Treatment with these antioxidants will be discussed in greater detail later.

Semen Analysis and Pregnancy Outcomes

The ultimate outcomes of varicocele repair (improved semen analysis and pregnancy rate) are the topic of much debate due to variable diagnostic criteria, follow-up, and outcomes reporting. A Cochrane review looked at 10 randomized controlled studies comparing varicocele repair with no treatment and found an odds ratio for pregnancy of 1.47 with a 95% confidence interval of 1.05–2.05. Given the low quality of evidence and the wide confidence interval, the authors concluded that the results are inconclusive [98]. This metaanalysis has been criticized for including studies in which the majority of patients had normal semen analysis and subclinical varicoceles. There have been many other studies that show improved semen parameters and pregnancy rates after varicocelectomy [99]. Multiple studies have shown an improvement in semen parameters after varicocelectomy in infertile men with clinical varicoceles. A metaanalysis of 17 studies by Agarwal et al. found that men with clinical varicoceles and abnormal pretreatment semen parameters had a mean increase in sperm concentration of 9.7 million/mL, motility increase of 9.9%, and strict sperm morphology improvement of 3% after varicocelectomy [1]. Large varicoceles seem to exert a greater negative effect on semen parameters than smaller ones and larger varicoceles also show a larger improvement in parameters after varicocelectomy. Steckel et al. showed that the fertility index (sperm count × motility%) of men with grade 3 varicoceles improved to a greater degree (128%) than men with grade 1 (27%) or grade 2 (21%) varicoceles after varicocelectomy [100]. Similarly, repair of bilateral varicoceles improved outcomes compared to unilateral varicocele repair [101].

Many large retrospective studies have found a 30%–50% pregnancy rate after varicocelectomy [102–104] with pregnancy usually occurring an average of 8 months after surgery [105]. A metaanalysis of five studies from 1988 to 2002 comparing varicocelectomy versus no treatment found the pregnancy odds ratio to be 2.87 in favor of the treatment group. The overall pregnancy rate varied significantly between studies though, from 20% to 60% [106]. A well-designed prospective randomized trial by Madgar et al. randomized 45 men to retroperitoneal varicocele ligation or no treatment. Pregnancy rates were six times higher in the intervention group compared to the control group (10%). Even more convincingly, the control group then underwent varicocelectomy after 1 year in the study and their pregnancy rates increased by fourfold postprocedure [107]. The most recent prospective, randomized controlled trial comparing pregnancy rates in patients who underwent microscopic subinguinal varicocelectomy versus no treatment found that spontaneous pregnancy was achieved in 32.9% of the couples in the varicocelectomy arm versus only 13.9% in the control arm within the first year [108].

Treatment With Antioxidants

Oral antioxidants either alone or in combination with varicocelectomy are commonly recommended by male infertility specialists though there are few studies addressing the treatment of varicocele-induced oxidative stress with antioxidant supplementation. One study evaluated oligozoospermic infertile men with and without varicocele treated with a 6-month course of oral antioxidants (L-carnitine and acetyl-L-carnitine) and an antiinflammatory (cinnoxicam), just the antioxidants, or placebo. They found that men with low-grade varicocele and idiopathic OAT responded better to the combination of antioxidants and antiinflammatories than those who were prescribed placebo or just antioxidants. The combination group had significantly improved semen parameters. This group also had improved pregnancy rates (38%) compared to the antioxidant group (21.8%) and the placebo group (1.7%) [109]. Animal studies have shown that rats with varicoceles treated with aminoguanidine (an NOS inhibitor) had improved semen parameters [52] and reduced DNA fragmentation [53]. Another study using rats with varicoceles found a decrease in ROS production after treatment with vitamin E [110]. These human and animal studies seem to point to the fact that antioxidants can improve varicocele-induced oxidative stress, though only varicocele repair can potentially stop the cause of the oxidative stress. Paradiso Galatioto et al. evaluated the effects of antioxidants in men who were 6 months postretrograde embolization of their varicocele but had persistent oligospermia (5–20 million/ml) [111]. The 22 men who were placed on antioxidants (N-acetylcysteine; vitamins C, E, and A; thiamine; riboflavin; zinc; and others) had a statistically significant increase in sperm count but no improvement in motility and morphology. Their logistic regression analysis showed that a man treated with antioxidant therapy was 20 times more likely to have a normal sperm count compared to the untreated group. Unfortunately, there was no difference in pregnancy rates between the two groups.

CONCLUSIONS

Varicocele-induced oxidative stress is a complex process involving multiple physiologic and cellular mechanisms. The testis, epididymis, and even the mitochondria of the spermatozoa all play a role in regulating the fine balance between oxidant and antioxidant levels. Varicoceles cause testicular hypoxia, ischemia, and oxidative stress through reflux of toxic metabolites and scrotal hyperthermia. This in turn creates ROS and downregulates antioxidant defense mechanisms. These pathways have not been fully elucidated and are an area of continued research. Varicocelectomy has been shown to decrease oxidative stress and increase antioxidant concentration and capacity. This is likely one of the main factors in improved semen parameters and pregnancy rates seen in men after varicocele repair.

REFERENCES

[1] Agarwal A, Deepinder F, Cocuzza M, Agarwal R, Short RA, Sabanegh E, et al. Efficacy of varicocelectomy in improving semen parameters: new meta-analytical approach. Urology 2007;70(3):532–8.

[2] Organization WH. The influence of varicocele on parameters of fertility in a large group of men presenting to infertility clinics. Fertil Steril 1992;57(6):1289–93.

[3] Nagler H, Luntz R, Martinis F. Varicocele. In: Lipshultz L, Howards S, editors. Infertility in the male. 3rd ed. St. Louis: Mosby Year Book; 1997. p. 336–59.

[4] Gorelick JI, Goldstein M. Loss of fertility in men with varicocele. Fertil Steril 1993;59(3):613–6.

[5] Braedel HU, Steffens J, Ziegler M, Polsky MS, Platt ML. A possible ontogenic etiology for idiopathic left varicocele. J Urol 1994;151(1):62–6.

[6] Hargreave TB, Liakatas J. Physical examination for varicocele. Br J Urol 1991;67(3):328.

[7] Trum JW, Gubler FM, Laan R, van der Veen F. The value of palpation, varicoscreen contact thermography and colour Doppler ultrasound in the diagnosis of varicocele. Hum Reprod 1996;11(6):1232–5.

[8] Meacham RB, Townsend RR, Rademacher D, Drose JA. The incidence of varicoceles in the general population when evaluated by physical examination, gray scale sonography and color Doppler sonography. J Urol 1994;151(6):1535–8.

[9] Ahlberg NE, Bartley O, Chidekel N, Fritjofsson A. Phlebography in varicocele scroti. Acta Radiol Diagn 1966;4(5):517–28.

[10] Narayan P, Gonzales R, Amplatz K. Varicocele and male subfertility. In: Presented at the American Fertility Society, Houston; March 1980.

[11] Agarwal A, Sharma R, Harlev A, Esteves SC. Effect of varicocele on semen characteristics according to the new 2010 World Health Organization criteria: a systematic review and meta-analysis. Asian J Androl 2016;18:163–70.

[12] Goldstein M, Eid JF. Elevation of intratesticular and scrotal skin surface temperature in men with varicocele. J Urol 1989;142(3):743–5.

[13] Khera M, Lipshultz LI. Evolving approach to the varicocele. Urol Clin North Am 2008;35(2):183–9. viii.

[14] Wright EJ, Young GP, Goldstein M. Reduction in testicular temperature after varicocelectomy in infertile men. Urology 1997;50(2):257–9.

[15] Agarwal A, Hamada A, Esteves SC. Insight into oxidative stress in varicocele-associated male infertility: part 1. Nat Rev Urol 2012;9(12):678–90.

[16] Chakraborty J, Hikim AP, Jhunjhunwala JS. Stagnation of blood in the microcirculatory vessels in the testes of men with varicocele. J Androl 1985;6(2):117–26.

[17] Allamaneni SSR, Naughton CK, Sharma RK, Thomas AJ, Agarwal A. Increased seminal reactive oxygen species levels in patients with varicoceles correlate with varicocele grade but not with testis size. Fertil Steril 2004;82(6):1684–6.

[18] Abd-Elmoaty MA, Saleh R, Sharma R, Agarwal A. Increased levels of oxidants and reduced antioxidants in semen of infertile men with varicocele. Fertil Steril 2010;94(4):1531–4.

[19] Blumer CG, Restelli AE, Del Giudice PT, Fraietta R, Bertolla RP, Cedenho AP. Effect of varicocele on sperm function and semen oxidative stress. Biol Reprod 2009;81(Suppl. 1):471.

[20] Mostafa T, Anis T, Imam H, El-Nashar AR, Osman IA. Seminal reactive oxygen species-antioxidant relationship in fertile males with and without varicocele. Andrologia 2009;41(2):125–9.

[21] Ishikawa T, Fujioka H, Ishimura T, Takenaka A, Fujisawa M. Increased testicular 8-hydroxy-2′-deoxyguanosine in patients with varicocele. BJU Int 2007;100(4):863–6.

[22] Miyaoka R, Esteves SC. A critical appraisal on the role of varicocele in male infertility. Adv Urol 2012;2012:597495.

[23] Cocuzza M, Athayde KS, Agarwal A, Pagani R, Sikka SC, Lucon AM, et al. Impact of clinical varicocele and testis size on seminal reactive oxygen species levels in a fertile population: a prospective controlled study. Fertil Steril 2008;90(4):1103–8.

[24] Skandhan KP, Rajahariprasad A. The process of spermatogenesis liberates significant heat and the scrotum has a role in body thermoregulation. Med Hypotheses 2007;68(2):303–7.

[25] Merla A, Ledda A, Di Donato L, Di Luzio S, Romani GL. Use of infrared functional imaging to detect impaired thermoregulatory control in men with asymptomatic varicocele. Fertil Steril 2002;78(1):199–200.

[26] Alvarez JG, Storey BT. Spontaneous lipid peroxidation in rabbit and mouse epididymal spermatozoa: dependence of rate on temperature and oxygen concentration. Biol Reprod 1985;32(2):342–51.

[27] Guo J, Jia Y, Tao S-X, Li Y-C, Zhang X-S, Hu Z-Y, et al. Expression of nitric oxide synthase during germ cell apoptosis in testis of cynomolgus monkey after testosterone and heat treatment. J Androl 2009;30(2):190–9.

[28] Hadziselimovic F, Herzog B. The importance of both an early orchidopexy and germ cell maturation for fertility. Lancet 2001;358(9288):1156–7.

[29] Shiraishi K, Takihara H, Naito K. Testicular volume, scrotal temperature, and oxidative stress in fertile men with left varicocele. Fertil Steril 2009;91(4):1388–91.

[30] Salisz JA, Kass EJ, Steinert BW. The significance of elevated scrotal temperature in an adolescent with a varicocele. Adv Exp Med Biol 1991;286:245–51.

[31] MacLeod J. Seminal cytology in the presence of varicocele. Fertil Steril 1965;16(6):735–57.

[32] Lindholmer C, Thulin L, Eliasson R. Concentrations of cortisol and renin in the internal spermatic vein of men with varicocele. Andrologie 1973;5(1):21–2.

[33] Cohen MS, Plaine L, Brown JS. The role of internal spermatic vein plasma catecholamine determinations in subfertile men with varicoceles. Fertil Steril 1975;26(12):1243–9.

[34] Ito H, Fuse H, Minagawa H, Kawamura K, Murakami M, Shimazaki J. Internal spermatic vein prostaglandins in varicocele patients. Fertil Steril 1982;37(2):218–22.

[35] Ozbek E, Yurekli M, Soylu A, Davarci M, Balbay MD. The role of adrenomedullin in varicocele and impotence. BJU Int 2000;86(6):694–8.

[36] Gat Y, Zukerman Z, Chakraborty J, Gornish M. Varicocele, hypoxia and male infertility. Fluid Mechanics analysis of the impaired testicular venous drainage system. Hum Reprod 2005;20(9):2614−9.

[37] Girgis SM, El-Rahman Y, Awad H, Eisa I, Younan N, Mittawy B, et al. Lactate and pyruvate levels in the testicular vein of subfertile males with varicocele as a test for the theory of underlying hypoxia. Andrologia 1981;13(1):16−9.

[38] Buonaguidi A, Grasso M, Lania C, Castelli M, Francesca F, Rigatti P. Experience with the determination of LDH-X in seminal plasma as diagnostic and prognostic factor in varicocele. Arch Esp Urol 1992;46(1):35−9.

[39] Yeşilli C, Mungan G, Seçkiner I, Akduman B, Açikgöz S, Altan K, et al. Effect of varicocelectomy on sperm creatine kinase, HspA2 chaperone protein (creatine kinase-M type), LDH, LDH-X, and lipid peroxidation product levels in infertile men with varicocele. Urology 2005;66(3):610−5.

[40] Sahin Z, Celik-Ozenci C, Akkoyunlu G, Korgun ET, Acar N, Erdogru T, et al. Increased expression of interleukin-1α and interleukin-1β is associated with experimental varicocele. Fertil Steril 2006;85:1265−75.

[41] Nallella KP, Allamaneni SSR, Pasqualotto FF, Sharma RK, Thomas AJ, Agarwal A. Relationship of interleukin-6 with semen characteristics and oxidative stress in patients with varicocele. Urology 2004;64(5):1010−3.

[42] Moretti E, Cosci I, Spreafico A, Serchi T, Cuppone AM, Collodel G. Semen characteristics and inflammatory mediators in infertile men with different clinical diagnoses. Int J Androl 2009;32(6):637−46.

[43] Tortolero I, Duarte Ojeda JM, Pamplona Casamayor M, Alvarez González E, Arata-Bellabarba G, Regadera J, et al. The effect of seminal leukocytes on semen quality in subfertile males with and without varicocele. Arch Esp Urol 2004;57(9):921−8.

[44] Wu T-P, Huang B-M, Tsai H-C, Lui M-C, Liu M-Y. Effects of nitric oxide on human spermatozoa activity, fertilization and mouse embryonic development. Arch Androl 2004;50(3):173−9.

[45] Rosselli M, Dubey RK, Imthurn B, Macas E, Keller PJ. Effects of nitric oxide on human spermatozoa: evidence that nitric oxide decreases sperm motility and induces sperm toxicity. Hum Reprod 1995;10(7):1786−90.

[46] Lue Y, Sinha Hikim AP, Wang C, Leung A, Swerdloff RS. Functional role of inducible nitric oxide synthase in the induction of male germ cell apoptosis, regulation of sperm number, and determination of testes size: evidence from null mutant mice. Endocrinology 2003;144(7):3092−100.

[47] Zini A, O'Bryan MK, Magid MS, Schlegel PN. Immunohistochemical localization of endothelial nitric oxide synthase in human testis, epididymis, and vas deferens suggests a possible role for nitric oxide in spermatogenesis, sperm maturation, and programmed cell death. Biol Reprod 1996;55(5):935−41.

[48] Santoro G, Romeo C, Impellizzeri P, Ientile R, Cutroneo G, Trimarchi F, et al. Nitric oxide synthase patterns in normal and varicocele testis in adolescents. BJU Int 2001;88(9):967−73.

[49] Shiraishi K, Naito K. Nitric oxide produced in the testis is involved in dilatation of the internal spermatic vein that compromises spermatogenesis in infertile men with varicocele. BJU Int 2007;99(5):1086−90.

[50] Jourd'heuil D, Jourd'heuil FL, Kutchukian PS, Musah RA, Wink DA, Grisham MB. Reaction of superoxide and nitric oxide with peroxynitrite. Implications for peroxynitrite-mediated oxidation reactions in vivo. J Biol Chem 2001;276(31):28799−805.

[51] Beltrán B, Orsi A, Clementi E, Moncada S. Oxidative stress and S-nitrosylation of proteins in cells. Br J Pharmacol 2000;129(5):953−60.

[52] Abbasi M, Alizadeh R, Abolhassani F, Amidi F, Hassanzadeh G, Ejtemaei Mehr S, et al. Aminoguanidine improves epididymal sperm parameters in varicocelized rats. Urol Int 2011;86(3):302−6.

[53] Abbasi M, Alizadeh R, Abolhassani F, Amidi F, Ragerdi KI, Fazelipour S, et al. Effect of aminoguanidine in sperm DNA fragmentation in varicocelized rats: role of nitric oxide. Reprod Sci 2011;18(6):545−50.

[54] Abele D, Heise K, Pörtner HO, Puntarulo S. Temperature-dependence of mitochondrial function and production of reactive oxygen species in the intertidal mud clam *Mya arenaria*. J Exp Biol 2002;205(Pt 13):1831−41.

[55] Tan G-Y, Yang L, Fu Y-Q, Feng J-H, Zhang M-H. Effects of different acute high ambient temperatures on function of hepatic mitochondrial respiration, antioxidative enzymes, and oxidative injury in broiler chickens. Poult Sci 2010;89(1):115−22.

[56] Zhang K, Shang Y, Liao S, Zhang W, Nian H, Liu Y, et al. Uncoupling protein 2 protects testicular germ cells from hyperthermia-induced apoptosis. Biochem Biophys Res Commun 2007;360(2):327−32.

[57] Echtay KS, Winkler E, Frischmuth K, Klingenberg M. Uncoupling proteins 2 and 3 are highly active H(+) transporters and highly nucleotide sensitive when activated by coenzyme Q (ubiquinone). Proc Natl Acad Sci U S A 2001;98(4):1416−21.

[58] Mancini A, Conte G, Milardi D, De Marinis L, Littarru GP. Relationship between sperm cell ubiquinone and seminal parameters in subjects with and without varicocele. Andrologia 1998;30(1):1−4.

[59] Ferramosca A, Albani D, Coppola L, Zara V. Varicocele negatively affects sperm mitochondrial respiration. Urology 2015;86(4):735−9.

[60] Lima SB, Cenedeze MA, Bertolla RP, Filho PAH, Oehninger S, Cedenho AP. Expression of the HSPA2 gene in ejaculated spermatozoa from adolescents with and without varicocele. Fertil Steril 2006;86(6):1659−63.

[61] Esfahani MHN, Abbasi H, Mirhosseini Z, Ghasemi N, Razavi S, Tavalaee M, et al. Can altered expression of HSPA2 in varicocele patients lead to abnormal spermatogenesis? Int J Fertil Steril 2010;4(3).

[62] Ferlin A, Speltra E, Patassini C, Pati MA, Garolla A, Caretta N, et al. Heat shock protein and heat shock factor expression in sperm: relation to oligozoospermia and varicocele. J Urol 2010;183(3):1248−52.

[63] Kikuchi G, Yoshida T, Noguchi M. Heme oxygenase and heme degradation. Biochem Biophys Res Commun 2005;338(1):558−67.

[64] Shibahara S, Sato M, Muller RM, Yoshida T. Structural organization of the human heme oxygenase gene and the function of its promoter. Eur J Biochem 1989;179(3):557−63.

[65] Ewing JF, Maines MD. Distribution of constitutive (HO-2) and heat-inducible (HO-1) heme oxygenase isozymes in rat testes: HO-2 displays stage-specific expression in germ cells. Endocrinology 1995;136(5):2294−302.

[66] Ozawa N, Goda N, Makino N, Yamaguchi T, Yoshimura Y, Suematsu M. Leydig cell-derived heme oxygenase-1 regulates apoptosis of premeiotic germ cells in response to stress. J Clin Invest 2002;109(4):457—67.

[67] Lin QS, Weis S, Yang G, Zhuang T, Abate A, Dennery PA. Catalytic inactive heme oxygenase-1 protein regulates its own expression in oxidative stress. Free Radic Biol Med 2008;44(5):847—55.

[68] Maines MD. The heme oxygenase system and its functions in the brain. Cell Mol Biol (Noisy-le-grand) 2000;46(3):573—85.

[69] Abdel Aziz MT, Mostafa T, Atta H, Kamal O, Kamel M, Hosni H, et al. Heme oxygenase enzyme activity in seminal plasma of oligoastheno-teratozoospermic males with varicocele. Andrologia 2010;42(4):236—41.

[70] McKelvey TG, Höllwarth ME, Granger DN, Engerson TD, Landler U, Jones HP. Mechanisms of conversion of xanthine dehydrogenase to xanthine oxidase in ischemic rat liver and kidney. Am J Physiol 1988;254(5 Pt 1):G753—60.

[71] Skibba JL, Stadnicka A, Kalbfleisch JH, Powers RH. Effects of hyperthermia on xanthine oxidase activity and glutathione levels in the perfused rat liver. J Biochem Toxicol 1989;4(2):119—25.

[72] Kawaguchi S, Fukuda J, Kumagai J, Shimizu Y, Kawamura K, Tanaka T. Expression of xanthine oxidase in testicular cells. Akita J Med 2009;36:99—105.

[73] Yaman O, Soygür T, Yilmaz E, Elgün S, Keskineğe A, Göğüş O. The significance of testicular reactive oxygen species on testicular histology in infertile patients. Int Urol Nephrol 1999;31(3):395—9.

[74] Mitropoulos D, Deliconstantinos G, Zervas A, Villiotou V, Dimopoulos C, Stavrides J. Nitric oxide synthase and xanthine oxidase activities in the spermatic vein of patients with varicocele: a potential role for nitric oxide and peroxynitrite in sperm dysfunction. J Urol 1996;156(6):1952—8.

[75] Mahmoud SA, Zahran NM. Electron microscopic study of the left caput epididymal epithelium of adult albino rats in an experimental left varicocele model. Egypt J Histol 2011;34(3):483—95.

[76] Ozturk U, Kefeli M, Asci R, Akpolat I, Buyukalpelli R, Sarikaya S. The effects of experimental left varicocele on the epididymis. Syst Biol Reprod Med 2008;54(4—5):177—84.

[77] Zhang Q-Y, Qiu S-D, Ma X-N, Yu H-M, Wu Y-W. Effect of experimental varicocele on structure and function of epididymis in adolescent rats. Asian J Androl 2003;5(2):108—12.

[78] Mehraban D, Ansari M, Keyhan H, Sedighi Gilani M, Naderi G, Esfehani F. Comparison of nitric oxide concentration in seminal fluid between infertile patients with and without varicocele and normal fertile men. Urol J 2005;2(2):106—10.

[79] Sakamoto Y, Ishikawa T, Kondo Y, Yamaguchi K, Fujisawa M. The assessment of oxidative stress in infertile patients with varicocele. BJU Int 2008;101(12):1547—52.

[80] Xu Y, Xu Q-Y, Yang B-H, Zhu X-M, Peng Y-F. [Relationship of nitric oxide and nitric oxide synthase with varicocele infertility]. Zhonghua Nan ke Xue 2008;14(5):414—7.

[81] Saleh RA, Agarwal A, Sharma RK, Said TM, Sikka SC, Thomas AJ. Evaluation of nuclear DNA damage in spermatozoa from infertile men with varicocele. Fertil Steril 2003;80(6):1431—6.

[82] Meucci E, Milardi D, Mordente A, Martorana GE, Giacchi E, De Marinis L, et al. Total antioxidant capacity in patients with varicoceles. Fertil Steril 2003;79:1577—83.

[83] Mancini A, Milardi D, Bianchi A, Festa R, Silvestrini A, De Marinis L, et al. Increased total antioxidant capacity in seminal plasma of varicocele patients: a multivariate analysis. Arch Androl 2007;53(1):37—42.

[84] Hamada A, Esteves SC, Agarwal A. Insight into oxidative stress in varicocele-associated male infertility: part 2. Nat Rev Urol 2013;10(1):26—37.

[85] Hendin BN, Kolettis PN, Sharma RK, Thomas AJ, Agarwal A. Varicocele is associated with elevated spermatozoal reactive oxygen species production and diminished seminal plasma antioxidant capacity. J Urol 1999;161(6):1831—4.

[86] Pasqualotto FF, Sundaram A, Sharma RK, Borges E, Pasqualotto EB, Agarwal A. Semen quality and oxidative stress scores in fertile and infertile patients with varicocele. Fertil Steril 2008;89(3):602—7.

[87] Lima SS, Castro MP, Costa OF. A new method for the treatment of varicocele. Andrologia 1978;10(2):103—6.

[88] Kaufman SL, Kadir S, Barth KH, Smyth JW, Walsh PC, White RI. Mechanisms of recurrent varicocele after balloon occlusion or surgical ligation of the internal spermatic vein. Radiology 1983;147(2):435—40.

[89] Punekar SV, Prem AR, Ridhorkar VR, Deshmukh HL, Kelkar AR. Post-surgical recurrent varicocele: efficacy of internal spermatic venography and steel-coil embolization. Br J Urol 1996;77(1):124—8.

[90] Diegidio P, Jhaveri JK, Ghannam S, Pinkhasov R, Shabsigh R, Fisch H. Review of current varicocelectomy techniques and their outcomes. BJU Int 2011;108(7):1157—72.

[91] Chen S-S, Huang WJ, Chang LS, Wei Y-H. Attenuation of oxidative stress after varicocelectomy in subfertile patients with varicocele. J Urol 2008;179(2):639—42.

[92] Cervellione RM, Cervato G, Zampieri N, Corroppolo M, Camoglio F, Canoglio F, et al. Effect of varicocelectomy on the plasma oxidative stress parameters. J Pediatr Surg 2006;41(2):403—6.

[93] Altintas R, Ediz C, Celik H, Camtosun A, Tasdemir C, Tanbek K, et al. The effect of varicocoelectomy on the relationship of oxidative stress in peripheral and internal spermatic vein with semen parameters. Andrology 2016;4(3):442—6.

[94] Kiziler AR, Aydemir B, Guzel S, Yazici CM, Gulyasar T, Malkoc E, et al. Comparison of before and after varicocelectomy levels of trace elements, nitric oxide, asymmetric dimethylarginine and malondialdehyde in the seminal plasma and peripheral and spermatic veins. Biol Trace Elem Res 2015;167(2):172—8.

[95] Khera M, Najari BB, Alukal JP, Mohamed O, Grober ED, Lipshultz LI. The effect of varicocele repair on semen reactive oxygen species activity in infertile men. Fertil Steril 2007;88:S387—8.

[96] Mostafa T, Anis TH, El-Nashar A, Imam H, Othman IA. Varicocelectomy reduces reactive oxygen species levels and increases antioxidant activity of seminal plasma from infertile men with varicocele. Int J Androl 2001;24(5):261−5.

[97] Hurtado de Catalfo GE, Ranieri-Casilla A, Marra FA, de Alaniz MJT, Marra CA. Oxidative stress biomarkers and hormonal profile in human patients undergoing varicocelectomy. Int J Androl 2007;30(6):519−30.

[98] Kroese AC, de Lange NM, Collins J, Evers JL. Surgery or embolization for varicoceles in subfertile men. Cochrane Database Syst Rev 2012;10.

[99] Jungwirth A, Giwercman A, Tournaye H, Diemer T, Kopa Z, Dohle G, et al. European Association of Urology guidelines on male infertility: the 2012 update. Eur Urol 2012;62(2):324−32.

[100] Steckel J, Dicker AP, Goldstein M. Relationship between varicocele size and response to varicocelectomy. J Urol 1993;149(4):769−71.

[101] Richardson I, Grotas AB, Nagler HM. Outcomes of varicocelectomy treatment: an updated critical analysis. Urol Clin North Am 2008;35(2):191−209. viii.

[102] Abdulmaaboud MR, Shokeir AA, Farage Y, Abd El-Rahman A, El-Rakhawy MM, Mutabagani H. Treatment of varicocele: a comparative study of conventional open surgery, percutaneous retrograde sclerotherapy, and laparoscopy. Urology 1998;52(2):294−300.

[103] Segenreich E, Israilov S, Shmuele J, Niv E, Baniel J, Livne P. Evaluation of the relationship between semen parameters, pregnancy rate of wives of infertile men with varicocele, and gonadotropin-releasing hormone test before and after varicocelectomy. Urology 1998;52(5):853−7.

[104] Perimenis P, Markou S, Gyftopoulos K, Athanasopoulos A, Barbalias G. Effect of subinguinal varicocelectomy on sperm parameters and pregnancy rate: a two−group study. Eur Urol 2001;39(3):322−5.

[105] Pryor JL, Howards SS. Varicocele. Urol Clin North Am 1987;14(3):499−513.

[106] Marmar JL, Agarwal A, Prabakaran S, Agarwal R, Short RA, Benoff S, et al. Reassessing the value of varicocelectomy as a treatment for male subfertility with a new meta-analysis. Fertil Steril 2007;88(3):639−48.

[107] Madgar I, Weissenberg R, Lunenfeld B, Karasik A, Goldwasser B. Controlled trial of high spermatic vein ligation for varicocele in infertile men. Fertil Steril 1995;63(1):120−4.

[108] Abdel-Meguid TA, Al-Sayyad A, Tayib A, Farsi HM. Does varicocele repair improve male infertility? An evidence-based perspective from a randomized, controlled trial. Eur Urol 2011;59(3):455−61.

[109] Cavallini G, Ferraretti AP, Gianaroli L, Biagiotti G, Vitali G. Cinnoxicam and L-carnitine/acetyl-L-carnitine treatment for idiopathic and varicocele-associated oligoasthenospermia. J Androl 2004;25(5):761−70. discussion 71−72.

[110] Cam K, Simsek F, Yuksel M, Turkeri L, Turker L, Haklar G, et al. The role of reactive oxygen species and apoptosis in the pathogenesis of varicocele in a rat model and efficiency of vitamin E treatment. Int J Androl 2004;27(4):228−33.

[111] Paradiso Galatioto G, Gravina GL, Angelozzi G, Sacchetti A, Innominato PF, Pace G, et al. May antioxidant therapy improve sperm parameters of men with persistent oligospermia after retrograde embolization for varicocele? World J Urol 2008;26(1):97−102.

Chapter 2.5

Malnutrition and Obesity

Kristian Leisegang

School of Natural Medicine, University of the Western Cape, Bellville, South Africa

INTRODUCTION

Malnutrition, meaning *bad nutrition*, is an umbrella term for poor nutritional intake and refers either to excess consumption (overnutrition) or inadequate consumption or absorption of one or more nutrients (undernutrition) [1]. Malnutrition is therefore a state in which the physical function of an individual is impaired to the point where he or she can no longer maintain adequate bodily performance such as growth, pregnancy, physical work, and reduced disease susceptibility [1].

The nutritional status of a person is directly related to life expectancy, morbidity, and mortality, and influences the course of disease as well as optimal patient management strategies in community and hospital settings [2]. As a closely related concept, the body mass index (BMI) is also associated with longevity and quality of life, with an excessive or reduced BMI being correlated with an increase in morbidity and mortality (Table 1) [3]. There is a clear association between nutritional status, BMI, and male reproductive potential, where the BMI correlated to male fertility potential on a J-shaped curve with an increasing risk for poor semen analysis in both underweight individuals and overweight and obese individuals is observed (Fig. 1) [4].

Malnutrition and micronutrient deficiencies (MNDs) are associated with increased oxidative stress (OS) systemically as well as in the male reproductive tract. This increased OS has been hypothesized to underlie infertility in malnourished males, although there are few studies related to undernutrition and male infertility and associated mechanisms [5]. Malnutrition is a chronic disease of global pandemic proportions, developing from the interaction of genetic, environmental, socioeconomic, and psychological (behavioral) factors, mediated by complex metabolic cellular and molecular mediators [1,6,7].

The BMI (Table 1) is used to classify the potential impact of malnutrition and morbidity and mortality risk [8−10]. Undernourishment is often associated with unintended weight loss, being underweight (BMI < 18.5 kg/m^2), acute or chronic diseases, and/or eating difficulties, whereas overnourishment is associated with weight gain and obesity (BMI > 30 kg/m^2) (Table 1) [11].

TABLE 1 Body Mass Index Categories and Risk of Co-Morbidities

BMI	Classification	Risk of Co-Morbidities	Consequences
<18.5	Underweight (Undernourished)	Increased	Immunodeficiency related infectious disease and malignancies
18.5−24.9	Normal Weight	Low	N/A
25.0−29.9	Overweight	Mild	Non-Communicable Chronic Diseases (e.g. CVD; T2DM; malignancies; degenerative disease)
30.0−34.9	Class I Obesity	Moderate	
35.0−39.9	Class II Obesity	Severe	
>40	Class III Obesity	Very Severe	

Oxidants, Antioxidants, and Impact of the Oxidative Status in Male Reproduction. https://doi.org/10.1016/B978-0-12-812501-4.00013-4

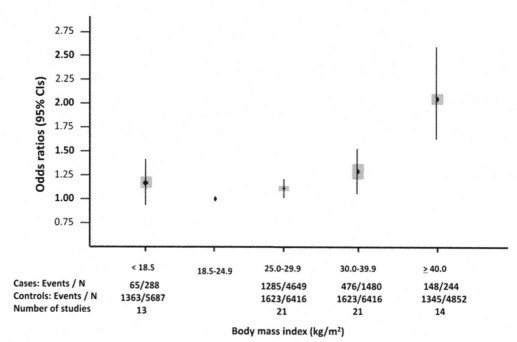

	< 18.5	18.5-24.9	25.0-29.9	30.0-39.9	≥ 40.0
Cases: Events / N	65/288		1285/4649	476/1480	148/244
Controls: Events / N	1363/5687		1623/6416	1623/6416	1345/4852
Number of studies	13		21	21	14

FIGURE 1 The association between BMI and abnormal oligozoospermia or azoospermia according to categories of BMI. This has been adapted from the meta-analysis study conducted by Sermondade and colleagues [4].

KEY NUTRIENTS ASSOCIATED WITH MALE REPRODUCTION AND INFERTILITY

Semen contains approximately 1%–5% spermatozoa, with the seminal fluid deriving predominantly from seminal vesicles (65%–70%) and prostate (25%–30%). Seminal fluid contains numerous proteins, amino acids, fructose, and micronutrients including vitamins and minerals [12]. This supplies nutrition and protection to the spermatozoa in the acidic, viscous, and immune-protected female reproductive tract [12]. Although there is significant variation in semen nutrients and sperm parameters, an overview of the mean concentrations of important nutrients in human semen is provided in Table 2 [12].

The amino acid concentration in semen is significantly higher than plasma, and increases exponentially in the hours following ejaculation, particularly glutamic acid [13]. Prostate fluid provides proteolytic enzymes, citric acid, acid phosphates, lipids, and zinc [12]. Amines such as spermine, spermidine, and putrescine are responsible for the smell and flavor of semen. Metal binding proteins, including transferrin, lactoferrin, haptoglobin, hemopexin, metallothionein, ceruloplasmin, ferritin, albumin, and myoglobin, are also important nutrients in semen for antioxidant defenses [14]. The seminal vesicles further supply amino acids, citrate, enzymes, phosphorylcholine, prostaglandins, proteins, and vitamin C [12].

The reproductive potential in males is determined by a wide array of genetic and environmental factors, of which nutritional status is an important component [15]. Trace elements for antioxidant defenses include iron, copper, selenium, zinc, calcium, and manganese. These act as components of antioxidant enzymes or transport proteins, which participate in mediating antioxidant reactions of ceruloplasmin, superoxide dismutase (SOD), glutathione peroxidase (GPx), and catalase (CAT). Both deficiency, and in some cases also excess, of these trace elements may contribute to OS in mammalian tissues [16].

Calcium is closely related to sperm motility, acrosome reaction, and fertilization [12]. Zinc protects sperm against bacteria, prevents chromosome damage, and is also important in testicular development and sperm maturation [17]. Zinc and copper have essential roles in antioxidant defenses such as cofactors for SOD1 (CuZn-SOD), while manganese is a critical cofactor in SOD2 (Mn-SOD) [14]. Increased seminal zinc and copper levels are positively associated with improved sperm parameters, as well as reduced OS and improved immune function locally and systemically [18]. Deficiency of trace metals, particularly selenium and zinc, may play an important role in impaired antioxidant defenses [19].

Selenium in semen is important for selenium-dependent GPx, and semen appears to have the highest concentration of selenium in male biological tissues [14]. Seminal manganese may positively influence the non-enzymatic antioxidant systems [20]. Iron is important in spermatogenesis, particularly in roles associated with DNA synthesis, electron transport, cellular respiration, and proliferation. Alongside copper, iron is further associated with critical redox reactions regulating

TABLE 2 Important Nutrients in the Composition of Human Semen [12]

Category	Nutrient	Concentration (mg/mL)
Proteins	Total protein	±50.4
	Albumin	±15.5
Sugars	Fructose	±2.72
	Glucose	±1.02
Ions (Minerals)	Sodium	±3.00
	Calcium	±2.76
	Chloride	±1.42
	Potassium	±1.09
	Zinc	±0.16
	Magnesium	±0.11
	Copper	—
	Selenium	—
Other nutrients	Citrate	±5.28
	Lactic acid	±0.62
	Urea	±0.45
	L-Carnitine	±0.05

OS via Haber−Weiss and/or Fenton reactions [21]. Furthermore, iron is potentially detrimental to male reproductive potential, as increased iron in the seminal fluid may negatively affect sperm motility, and correlates with OS and inflammatory cytokines [22]. This is further supported when investigating total ion levels of median micronutrient concentrations in human semen, consisting of calcium, magnesium, zinc, copper, iron, and selenium. Patients with higher total ion levels suggest correlation with increased OS and reduced antioxidant defense with increased proinflammatory cytokines [23]. Therefore, although these minerals are essential in male and female reproduction and fertility, some of these become toxic in higher concentrations, particularly iron and copper, which can induce excessive OS when in toxic concentrations [21]. Additionally, there are numerous nutrients in semen that act primarily as antioxidants and free radical scavengers to neutralize excessive reactive oxygen species (ROS) including SOD, glutathione, thioredoxin, vitamin A and other β-carotenes, vitamin C, vitamin E, folate, zinc, selenium, carnitine, taurine, tryptophan, and spermine [24].

Carotenoids are a group of phytochemicals responsible for different colors of foods, and have important roles in maintaining good health and prevention of numerous chronic diseases. Many of these molecules contribute to dietary vitamin A, a fat-soluble antioxidant. Vitamin C is a water-soluble antioxidant found in high concentrations in semen. Acting as a cofactor in hydroxylation processes, vitamin C is utilized in collagen and proteoglycan synthesis and components of the extracellular matrix alongside vitamin E [17]. Vitamin E is fat-soluble antioxidant that neutralizes free radical damage of lipid-rich cellular membranes, and also improves function of other antioxidants and inhibits excessive ROS production from the spermatozoa [17]. All folates are metabolically active forms of folic acid, a group of water-soluble B vitamins involved in one carbon metabolism. This is critical in DNA synthesis and epigenetic regulation of genetic expressions via formation of purine and pyrimidine, remethylation of homocysteine into methionine and S-adenosylmethionine [25]. This includes a critical role in spermatogenesis and sperm quality [25]. In addition, vitamin B12 (cobalamin) is associated with increased sperm count, enhanced motility, and reduced DNA damage in spermatozoa [25]. The beneficial effects of vitamin B12 on semen quality may be due to increased functionality of reproductive organs, decreased homocysteine toxicity, reduced amounts of generated nitric oxide, decreased levels of oxidative damage to sperm, reduced amount of energy produced by spermatozoa, decreased inflammation-induced semen impairment, and control of nuclear factor-κB activation [26].

L-Carnitine (3-aminobutyric acid) is considered a semi-vitamin, as it is an essential substance required for human function [17]. This nutrient is involved in mitochondrial metabolic activities via transportation of acetyl and acyl groups across the inner membrane, mobilization of long chain free fatty acids (FFAs) for oxidative phosphorylation, and also acting as an antioxidant and protecting spermatozoa against ROS. Seminal carnitine and acetyl-carnitine are considered markers for semen quality and possibly epididymis function, as carnitine is found in higher concentrations in the epididymis [27,28]. Total carnitine is reduced in many infertile male patients [29]. Coenzyme Q10 (CoQ10), also known as ubiquinone when fully oxidized, is a fat-soluble vitamin-like antioxidant molecule that is a critical component of the respiratory chain. This is predominantly produced endogenously through at least 12 genes, and dietary sources predominantly from high metabolic organ meats such as heart, liver, and muscle [30]. Low levels of CoQ10 in seminal plasma are associated with reduced sperm parameters, which may be via OS [31].

HUMAN ADIPOSE TISSUE

Adipose tissue is categorized into brown adipose tissue (BAT) and white adipose tissue (WAT) [32,33]. WAT comprises of adipocytes, preadipocytes, fibroblasts, macrophages, and lymphocytes, and is known to synthesize and secrete a variety of adipocyte-derived proteins that actively participate in various metabolic, endocrine, immune, and neurological regulatory activities (via endocrine, paracrine, and autocrine pathways). Significant examples of these proteins include leptin, adiponectin, resistin, platelet activating inhibitor 1, visfatin, omentin, apelin, and adipsin, as well as inflammatory (e.g., tumor necrosis factor-alpha [TNFα], IL-1, IL-6, and IL-8) and immune regulating (e.g., IL-4 and IL-10) cytokines. Adipocyte-derived hormones and cytokines are generally termed adipokines. WAT is therefore an important regulatory organ similar to any endocrine organ, and adipocyte dysfunction due to excessive or reduced total and proportional fat ratios is closely associated with various comorbidities and reduced life expectancy [32,33].

WAT is heterogonous and can be classified into subcutaneous adipose tissue (SAT) and visceral adipose tissue (VAT) with distinct phenotypic expressions associated with an increased BMI [32,33]. SAT is generally considered to be protective against features associated with obesity and related comorbidities [34]. This is due to various phenotypic differences in energy metabolism within this tissue when accumulating in excess. SAT is also generally observed in increasing proportions in females compared to males on a genetic and endocrine (particularly estrogen) basis, and may be partly responsible for the increased risk of obesity to males [3]. Furthermore, the inability to convert excess carbohydrates to lipids for storage in subcutaneous tissue is thought to be a prominent mechanism in the lower risk associated with increased SAT [34].

Increased body fat percentage, specifically VAT, generally results in an altered secretion pattern of adipokines and other adipose tissue—derived proteins, and results in adipocyte dysfunction. These modifications have been found to play a significant role in obesity related comorbidities, particularly related to chronic inflammation, OS, insulin resistance, and induction of apoptosis, which contributes to the development of clinical risk factors such as dyslipidemia, hypertension, and hyperglycemia [32—35]. This so-called lipotoxicity is generally a cause of cellular injury and tissue dysfunction in numerous systems [7].

UNDERNUTRITION AND UNDERWEIGHT MALES

Being underweight according to the BMI (<18.5 kg/m^2) reflects a state of malnutrition [10]. However, this does not reflect total energy stores. With loss of adipose tissue, lean body mass becomes an increasingly main source of energy reserves resulting in muscle atrophy and tissue wasting [10]. Macronutrient undernutrition is sometimes termed protein-energy malnutrition (PEM), with kwashiorkor and marasmus being two major forms of PEM observed in developing societies, and increasingly in hospitals and in chronically ill children in developed societies [36]. Undernutrition with macro- and/or micronutrient deficiencies are a major public health concern globally that required further attention for optimal growth and development, physically, neurologically, and cognitively, as well as for the development and function of the reproductive system [1,37]. Malnutrition is therefore a major public health threat and socioeconomic burden, and undernutrition often passes unnoticed, untreated, or ignored [8].

Diagnosis is important in the clinical management of underweight individuals, and clinical presentation depends on the specific nutrients or total energy that is absent from the diet [8]. Diagnostic criteria for undernutrition include the Malnutrition Universal Screening Tool, Nutritional Risk Screening 2002 (NRS202), and the European Society for Clinical Nutrition and Metabolism criteria [8]. These are stratified with various definitions and criteria cut-off considerations involving BMI, recent weight loss, and presence of acute or chronic disease [8].

When measured in the lower BMI range, patients have an increasing risk of death mainly due to susceptibility to infectious diseases and organ dysfunctions (particular respiratory diseases), with undernutrition being the leading cause of immunodeficiency [3,10,38]. Medical associations of chronic undernutrition include various cancers, gastrointestinal diseases, and lung diseases [10]. Severe, acute, or chronic deficiency of dietary nutrients leads to increased OS, with depleted antioxidant status (e.g., SOD, vitamin E, and zinc) and systemic inflammation involving increased production of superoxide, hydroxyl radicals, and hydrogen peroxide [19].

Furthermore, underweight men tend to have lower sperm concentrations than normal weight men and are at risk of infertility (Fig. 1) [4,15,39]. It is known that chronic undernutrition is associated with increased OS in the male reproductive tract with increased lipid peroxidation and protein carbonylation [37]. Furthermore, chronic macronutrient malnutrition in the fetal-to-prepuberty phase is associated with changes in the development of the testicular structure and poor spermatogenesis in adult life [40]. Nutritional under- and/or overnourishment in the parents prior to fertilization and during fetal life also negatively impact endocrine, metabolic, adiposity, immune regulation, and reproductive outcomes in the progeny [41]. Thus clinical consideration of macro- and/or micronutrient deficiencies is critical in the evaluation of male patients for fertility potential.

OBESITY: CLINICAL DEFINITION, RISK FACTORS, AND EPIDEMIOLOGY

Obesity can be defined as a condition in which excess body fat has accumulated to a degree in which health may be adversely affected [6,9]. However, the impact of excess fat accumulation on health outcomes is modified by the distribution of fat in the body. The associated health consequences vary considerably between obese individuals [6,9]. Obesity is a multifactorial and complex pathophysiological syndrome mediated by OS, inflammation, insulin resistance, hyperleptinemia, adipose tissue hypoxia and in males, hypogonadism (Fig. 2) [2,35,42]. The risk of developing non-communicable chronic disease impacting morbidity and mortality, particularly cardiovascular disease (CVD), type-2 diabetes mellitus (T2DM), and various cancers, rises exponentially with increasing adiposity [3,6,9].

Obesity is now of pandemic proportions, with an estimated 1.4 billion adults with a BMI above that considered as an optimal healthy weight (BMI > 25), and this includes over 200 million men [43]. Globally, the prevalence of adults described as being overweight or obese has increased from 28% to 36% in men (29%–38% in women) from 1980 to 2013. This may be as high as >50% of the adult population living in South Asia and Latin America [44].

Genetic predisposition is associated with obesity risk, which includes the significant ethnic variation in risk presentations, and males are at more risk than females [6,45,46]. Aging is also a significant risk factor. Aging and obesity share many common phenotypic changes associated with chronic disease complications, including OS [47]. Multifactorial environmental risk factors for obesity includes nutritional status, physical activity, socioeconomic factors, psychological factors, and other important but less reported risks such as quantity and quality of sleep [6,9]. In a modern Westernized

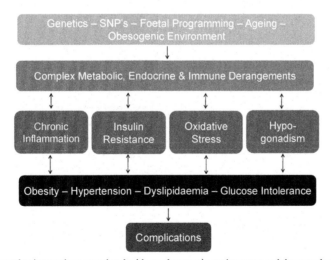

FIGURE 2 An illustration of the complex interactions associated with an obesogenic environment and the complex interactions between the underlying mediators and co-morbidities associated with obesity. These factors include oxidative stress, chronic inflammation, insulin resistance and, in males, hypogonadism, which are associated with various deleterious complications including metabolic syndrome, type 2 diabetes mellitus, cardiovascular disease, various cancers and neurodegernative diseases.

society, the abundance of an excess supply of energy-dense food and an increasingly sedentary lifestyle is closely associated with the obesity epidemic [6]. The pathophysiology of obesity is further mediated by complex underlying metabolic cellular and molecular mediators [7]. Although the underlying causes and mechanisms remain complex, the shift of populations to a more "obesogenic" environment can be described as an underlying phenomenon associated with the obesity pandemic.

CLINICAL ASSESSMENT OF ADIPOSITY AND FAT DISTRIBUTION

The BMI is a standard measure to define different weight categories and reflects the potential risk of comorbidities and mortality [6,9]. Table 1 shows the weight classifications with a simplistic relationship between BMI and the risk of co-morbidity. Obesity is therefore defined clinically as a BMI of over 30 kg/m^2 [9]. Although considered age- and gender-independent, interpretation of BMI grading in relation to risk may differ for different populations [9].

The use of this tool can be limiting, as BMI does not differentiate between lean muscle mass and adipose tissue mass, nor is the distribution of any excess adipose tissues considered (e.g., SAT vs. VAT distribution). Furthermore, complications of obesity are not only associated with fat mass distribution, but also the size of adipocytes within adipose tissues [10]. Metabolic derangements and risks of comorbidities associated with excess body fat are related specifically to excessive visceral (abdominal) fat [10,48]. Dollo et al. provide detailed insight into body composition phenotypes and related health risks in metabolic susceptibility to obesity and metabolic syndrome across ethnic groups [10]. BMI has high specificity but low sensitivity to identify adiposity, and may fail to identify half the population with excess body fat [49]. A measure of body fat percentage and/or fat distribution is important in calculating the risk of obesity comorbidities in a clinical setting [9].

Body fat percentage can be determined using a formula that includes BMI, gender, and age [49]. Although not generally accepted as a definition for obesity, many authorities have associated obesity with >25% body fat in males and >30% in females. Conversely, techniques that accurately measure body fat such as hydrostatic weighing, isotope dilution, or bioelectrical impedance analysis are rarely used in clinical practice [49].

Waist circumference (WC) has also been increasingly utilized to assess obesity risk, reflecting intra-abdominal fat with or without the inclusion of hip circumference, or more recently, the height. WC is associated with visceral (abdominal) adiposity. The cut-off thresholds for WC vary with gender and ethnicity, and in males ranges from 88 to 94 cm, with upper limits of >104 cm previously suggested in males. A limited summary of WC cut-off recommendations for males is provided in Table 3 [46]. WC correlates and has a stronger association with the development of obesity-associated metabolic risks and well-defined comorbidities than BMI alone [46]. It is important to be certain that an increased WC is due to VAT deposits and not subcutaneous fat, which is only possible with CT or MRI technology [50]. The waist-to-hip ratio (WHR) recommendations currently define risk cut-off values of >0.9 for males, and a waist-to-height ratio of >0.5 [51].

TABLE 3 A Summary of the Current Criteria for the Clinical Diagnosis of Metabolic Syndrome in Asian, Caucasian, and Sub-Saharan African Males

Criteria	Categorical Cut-Off Points
Waist circumference	Sub-Saharan African ≥ 94 cm; Caucasian ≥ 94 cm; Asian ≥ 90 cm;
Blood pressure (or relevant medication)	Systolic ≥ 130 mmHg and/or diastolic ≥ 85 mmHg
Fasting triglycerides (or relevant medication)	>1.70 mmol/L
HDL cholesterol (or relevant medication)	<1.00 mmol/L
Fasting glucose (or relevant medication)	>5.5 mmol/L

Categorical cut of values for waist circumference vary based on ethnic background. Waist circumference and HDL-cholesterol have different cut-off values in females. *HDL*, high-density lipoprotein.

PATHOPHYSIOLOGICAL DERANGEMENTS OF OBESITY: THE METABOLIC SYNDROME

An increase in the prevalence of obesity is associated with rising levels of hypertension, dyslipidemia, and hyperglycemia, which are complex and interrelated phenotypic changes statistically associated with CVD and T2DM risks [52]. The metabolic syndrome (MetS) is defined as a collection of numerous metabolic risk factors that tend to cluster together, resulting in an increased risk for CVD, T2DM, and various cancers [46]. The common features that cluster together include central (abdominal) obesity, hypertension, dyslipidemia (particularly low high-density lipoprotein [HDL]-cholesterol), and glucose intolerance (Table 3) [52,53].

MetS can present with different phenotypic expressions according to different components in each individual, and has therefore proven difficult (and even controversial), to define and diagnose [46]. Currently, the generally accepted diagnostic criteria include meeting any three of five central criteria: increased WC, hypertension, reduced HDL cholesterol, increased triglycerides, or hyperglycemia (Table 3) [46].

These diagnostic expressions appear to be linked together by complex and poorly understood pathophysiological mechanisms that are not part of the diagnostic criteria, but mediate the underlying derangements of obesity and MetS. This includes, but is not limited to, insulin resistance (hyperinsulinemia), leptin resistance (hyperleptinemia), low-grade chronic inflammation, OS, and an increased sympathetic nervous system tone [50,52,53]. In males, obesity and MetS is further associated with hypogonadism and numerous risks for reproductive dysfunction and reduced fertility potential [53,54], and require clinical evaluation and consideration in patient management in general, as well as in male reproductive and infertility assessment.

OBESITY, METABOLIC SYNDROME, AND MALE REPRODUCTION OUTCOMES

In a chapter entitled "The health disadvantages of excessive weight" in his *Canon of Medicine*, Avicenna (1593) wrote "this [obese] human [man] has a cold temperament; this is why he is infertile, unable to impregnate [woman] and has low semen" [55]. The impact of BMI on sperm parameters has been investigated recently, with over 10,000 articles published on the subject [4]. Although results have been inconsistent and inconclusive [4,54,56,58,59], the data appear to implicate obesity as negatively impacting male reproductive potential via poor semen quality, semen parameters, and poor spermatogenesis, in addition to hormonal (e.g., hypogonadism) and physical (e.g., increased testicular heat) derangements [39,54,57]. Furthermore, both obesity and male factor infertility have coincidently been increasing in incidence globally over the last few decades [56].

Results from studies investigating whether obesity negatively affects semen quality have been inconsistent, with some indicating a negative relationship while others not finding similar relationships [4,54,56,58,60,61]. Although there is still variable evidence to show negatively modulated sperm parameters in obese men, a disproportionately large number of men seeking infertility treatment are reportedly obese [54]. Further lines of evidence suggest that paternal obesity is associated with reduced live birth rates, particularly following assisted reproductive technology [62] and impaired offspring metabolic and reproductive health [57]. Transgenerational epigenetic inheritance further suggests that molecular changes in sperm that arise from obesity-related impaired spermatogenesis (e.g., modified sperm RNA levels, DNA methylation, protamination, and histone acetylation) can negatively impact the development of offspring [43]. Interestingly, infertile males, independent of BMI, with abnormal semen parameters have an increased risk of all-cause mortality, suggesting a common mechanism between fertility potential, health and wellness, and risk of morbidity and mortality in males [63]. These common mechanisms include systemic inflammation, OS, and dysfunctional DNA repair mechanisms [63]. MetS, as a diagnostic criterion that may be independent of obesity, as well as its diagnostic components (Table 3), have also been suggested to be associated with poor semen quality [53,64−66].

Obesity further impacts endocrine regulation, providing a basis for poor semen quality. Hormonal changes in obesity directly relevant to male reproduction include reduced serum total testosterone, free testosterone, sex hormone binding globulin (SHBG) and progesterone, and increased serum estrogen, insulin (insulin resistance), leptin, follicular stimulating hormone (FSH), luteinizing hormone (LH), and prolactin [63,66,67] (Table 4). Lower serum testosterone in nonobese men (lower quartile), including those with asymptomatic androgen deficiency, also increases the risk of developing obesity, MetS, and T2DM [67], and clinical administration of testosterone can improve many of the characteristics associated with these metabolic derangements [68].

There are additional physical mechanisms that have been implicated in obesity-related male infertility. These include erectile dysfunction and increased scrotal temperature due to excessive adiposity in the groin regions [54,57]. Thus, the relationship between obesity and male infertility is multifactorial and complex [56], and calls for a better understanding of the underlying mechanisms that result in abnormal sperm function in obese men [54,56,57].

TABLE 4 Associate Endocrine, Immune, and Oxidative Stress Markers in Obese Males

Category	Marker	Direction of Potential Change
Endocrine changes	Total testosterone	↓
	Free testosterone	↓
	SHBG	↓
	Progesterone	↓
	Estrogen	↑
	Gonadotropins	↑
	Prolactin	↑
	Insulin	↑
Adipokine changes	Adiponectin	↓
	Resistin	↑
	Platelet activating inhibitor-1	↑
	Angiotensin II	↑
Immune changes	Hs-CRP	↑
	Tumor necrosis factor-alpha	↑
	Interleukin 1-beta	↑
	Interleukin 2	↓
	Interleukin 6	↑
	Interleukin 8	↑
	Interleukin 10	↓
	Interferon gamma	↑
	Leptin	↑
Oxidative stress markers	Total antioxidant capacity	↓
	Malondialdehyde	↑
	Oxidized low density lipoprotein	↑
	F2 isoprostanes (F2-IsoP)	↑
	8-iso-Prostaglandin F2a (8-iso-PGF2a)	↑
	Protein carbonylation	↑
	Cu–Zn-SOD	↓
	Mn-SOD	↓
	Catalase	↓
	Glutathione peroxidase	↓
Micronutrients	Vitamins A, B1, B9, B12, C, D, E	↓
	Selenium	↓
	Zinc	↓
	Iron	↓

CRP, C-reactive protein; *SHBG*, sex hormone binding globulin; *SOD*, superoxide dismutase.

OBESITY AND MICRONUTRIENT DEFICIENCIES

Micronutrients are essential for normal and optimal human physiology at molecular and cellular levels [69]. There is a widespread global MND that still exists in various parts of the world, affecting over 2 billion people. MNDs mostly affect pregnant females and children under 5 years of age, with iron, iodine, folate, vitamin A, and zinc being the most common MNDs globally [69]. MNDs significantly influence day-to-day physiological functions and performance, including behavior, emotional state, and intellectual and physical activity [70]. Although food security and access to quality food is a cause in many geographical and socioeconomic locations (undernutrition), modern agriculture methods, and the processing of high-energy foods for widespread and cheap consumption, have led to a reduction in micronutrient content [69]. Additionally, malabsorption syndromes need to be considered in patients presenting with micro- and/or macronutrient deficiencies [69].

Although often defined as a disease due to nutritional excess, obesity is conversely associated with high levels of MND, due in part to high energy foods being generally micronutrient-poor [71–73]. This may also be due to increased metabolic demands in obesity [70]. Examples of obesity-related MNDs include vitamins A, B1, B6, B9, B12, C, D, and E, as well as biotin, iron, zinc, and selenium [69,71–73]. In terms of prevalence in obese individuals, the most common deficiencies include vitamin D (90%), selenium (58%), vitamin C (45%), zinc (30%), and vitamin B1 (29%) [69]. Establishment of an MND can be assessed using biomarkers, dietary intake records, or nonspecific clinical indicators (e.g., anemia, failure-to-thrive, obesity). However, there are generally no clear, specific, and reliable biomarkers or related cut-off values for many of the MNDs, and these biomarkers are affected by acute phase response in acute or chronic inflammatory diseases [69].

OBESITY, OXIDATIVE STRESS, AND THE MALE REPRODUCTIVE SYSTEM

Various lines of evidence suggest the pathogenesis of visceral obesity and comorbidities are also mediated by OS [7,74]. Physiologically, the regulatory functions of ROS include the generation by nicotinamide adenine dinucleotide phosphate (NADPH) complexes that activate signal-transducing systems in cellular responses to insulin and TNFα [42]. Increased adipose tissue, particularly VAT, is known to undergo changes such as OS, inflammation, and hypoxia [35]. Alterations in these systems can further contribute to excessive systemic OS, resulting in alterations of genetic phenotypic expressions and dysfunction of signaling pathways. In turn, these alterations further exacerbate chronic inflammation, as OS is known to induce low-grade inflammation. OS further stimulates lipogenesis, contributing further to adiposity, and a self-perpetuating cycle can exist within this context (Fig. 2) [42].

Systemic OS in this context is associated with superoxide generation, oxidative phosphorylation, glyceraldehyde auto-oxidation, protein kinase C (PKC) activation, and polyol and hexosamine pathways [74]. As with many of the complex molecular mediators of obesity, increased VAT can specifically induce local and systemic OS, and conversely OS can induce adipocyte dysfunction and lipotoxicity (altered pattern of adipokine secretion and recruitment of proinflammatory lymphocytes and macrophages, which further induces OS) [75]. In contrast, markers of antioxidant defenses are reduced in obese patients, which further induces as OS phenotype [76]. Although further research is required, contribution to OS in obesity and MetS can be due to hyperglycemia, dyslipidemia, hyperleptinemia, chronic inflammation, and other phenomenon such as endothelial cell dysfunction and mitochondrial dysfunction [7,48].

Genetic predisposition to obesity includes single nucleotide polymorphisms (SNPs) in numerous antioxidant defense systems. Limited studies have indicated that genotypic variants in genes including GPX1, CAT, PON1, PRDX3, SOD2, and PPARγ predispose individuals to obesity and related phenotypic changes including OS, insulin resistance, and inflammation through reduced antioxidant capacity (Fig. 2) [42].

Dietary intake of fats and carbohydrates also contribute to systemic OS, specifically FFAs [77]. Increased caloric intake (high-energy diets) increases NADPH oxidase activation and generates ROS, alongside a reduction in antioxidant defenses such as SOD, CAT, and glutathione, inducing OS [78]. FFAs are further known to generate increased mitochondrial hydrogen peroxide due to saturation of the electron transport chain [77]. High energy diets are associated with dysfunctional testicular metabolism and markers of OS including increased testicular lactate and reduced testicular alanine content; increased testicular creatine content and glycine metabolism is favored for energy production [79]. High energy diets disrupt tightly regulated testicular metabolism leading to inefficient energy supply to germ cells, spermatogenesis dysfunction, sperm defects, mitochondrial dysfunction in testicular tissues, and an increase in ROS and OS [80].

Typically, inflammation and OS occur in a close relationship together, and both of these phenomena have been well established in malnutrition and MetS patients [53]. Increased VAT results in an altered secretion pattern of adipokines from adipocytes themselves and adipose tissue–associated macrophages and T-lymphocyte influx. These have a significant role in multiple metabolic and inflammatory responses in human physiology and pathology, with a corresponding enhanced basal inflammatory and OS state [33,81]. Inflammation associated with obesity and MetS is characterized by a dominant Th1-lymphocyte and M1 macrophage shift, with reduced Th2-lymphocyte, T-regulatory (Treg) lymphocytes, and M2-macrophage activity [82]. This immune dysregulation is associated with related cytokine increase in peripheral blood, mediating numerous associated phenomenon including insulin resistance and OS [32,52]. Demonstrated clinically by a subtle and detrimental increase in serum C-reactive protein (CRP), obesity and MetS is associated with increased serum inflammatory cytokines, particularly TNFα, IL1β, IL6, and IL8, and reduced immune regulating cytokines such as IL-4 and IL-10. CRP correlates with this innate immune response and OS, in obese patients, and is important in the clinical assessment. These proinflammatory cytokines are well demonstrated stimulators for the excess production of ROS, and other modulators upregulate adipocyte NADPH oxidase activity, which comprises a major molecular pathway for ROS production in these cells [7]. Further research on immune modulation in the male reproductive tract, and even epididymal fat, is required.

ROS in the male reproductive tract and ejaculate also derive from seminal leukocytes and play significant defensive and destructive roles in infections, inflammation, and cellular defense. It is suggested that increased cytokines associated with adiposity can exert toxic effects on spermatozoa via ROS [83,84]. Although it can be hypothesized that MetS-related phenomena, such as inflammation and OS, may mediate damage to spermatozoa mitochondria and DNA integrity, the mechanisms of these relationships require further investigation [85].

There is evidence suggesting that obesity is associated with increased seminal ROS and male reproductive tract inflammation, although this is limited [86,87]. Furthermore, hyperinsulinemia and hyperleptinemia in obese males is associated with increased seminal insulin and leptin concentrations [61]. These markers of reproductive tract inflammation on OS are observed in the absence of local infections, and thought to be partially generated via local macrophage and other leukocyte activation [85]. Systemic inflammatory and OS changes and markers in the serum, including antioxidant status, appear closely correlated [88]. Proinflammatory cytokines, particularly TNFα, IL1β, IL6, and IL8, are known to modulate both OS and antioxidant status, with increased concentrations correlating positively with ROS and OS in seminal fluid [47]. High levels of OS in the male reproductive tract and seminal fluid, associated with sperm lipid peroxidation of the polyunsaturated fatty acids in the spermatozoa membrane and DNA damage, has been extensively implicated in male factor infertility [83]. The limited evidence suggesting a direct relationship between systemic and local inflammation and OS in the setting of obesity and MetS may have direct detrimental effects on semen quality, spermatogenesis, and spermatozoal function [86]. Furthermore, male reproductive OS and associated inflammation is involved in the pathogenesis of various sexual dysfunction, most notably, erectile dysfunction, as well as prostate pathologies including benign prostatic hyperplasia and prostate cancer, of which obesity and aging are significant risk factors [47]. Further studies to elicit these mechanisms are required.

Insulin, leptin, inflammatory cytokines, and OS are all proposed to directly modulate Leydig cell steroidogenesis, with all of these phenomena associated with an increase in serum in males with MetS [53]. It has been demonstrated that Leydig cell mitochondrial membrane potential (MMP), adenosine triphosphate (ATP) synthesis, and mitochondrial calcium concentrations are all required for steroidogenesis, and that this is a key control point for steroidogenesis [89]. These mechanisms may be disrupted by OS, known to inhibit both ovarian and testicular steroidogenesis, most notably, the initial step of cholesterol transfer into Leydig cell mitochondria [89,90]. ROS disrupt various stages of steroidogenesis, including mitochondrial function and MMP, ATP synthesis by the mitochondria, and steroidogenic acute regulatory protein (StAR) transcription [89].

Therefore, in the setting of chronic inflammation and OS associated with obesity and MetS, these mechanisms provide an important role in both the etiology and propagation of MetS in males, negatively influencing reproductive potential and overall health and well-being. It is therefore warranted to investigate blood and seminal fluid for inflammatory and OS markers in males that present with unexplained infertility, poor sperm analysis, or hypogonadism [88].

NUTRITION, WEIGHT MANAGEMENT PROGRAMS, AND MALE REPRODUCTIVE OUTCOMES

Natural weight loss should be the cornerstone of obese males presenting with reproductive or sexual dysfunction following assessment for relevant underlying causes. This can be achieved primarily through appropriate quantity and quality of nutritional intake and regular exercise [91]. The aim of therapy would be to correct underlying metabolic, immune, and endocrine dysfunction via objective clinical assessment, correct any possible nutritional deficiencies, and improve OS. In underweight males, appropriate diagnosis of undernutrition and specific deficiencies must be identified for appropriate management. However, the optimal diet for fertility in males is yet to be established [92].

Data from observational and human interventional studies suggest that consumption of multiple nutrients rather than a single dietary component is beneficial in reducing obesity and its associated pathologies [48]. Dietary consumption of foods rich in monounsaturated fatty acids, omega-3 polyunsaturated fatty acids, antioxidants, micronutrients, phytochemicals, and probiotics has been found to be helpful in maintaining body weight and reducing the incidence of metabolic diseases [93]. Similar dietary intake of antioxidant-rich foods, particularly those found in the Mediterranean diet, are also associated with better fertility outcomes. These include diets rich in β-carotenes; folate; vitamins C, D, and E; selenium; zinc; and lycopene [94,95].

Studies have shown that the Mediterranean, or "Prudent," dietary patterns, which are characterized by high intakes of fruits and vegetables, fish, and whole grains, are associated with higher semen quality across a BMI range [95,96]. Adherence to the Mediterranean diet has been shown to improve semen parameters in males, and those with least adherence have increased risk of reduced sperm concentration and motility [97]. Additionally, fish, shellfish, and seafood are associated positively with sperm quality parameters [94,95]. However, causality has not been demonstrated for these findings.

The so-called Westernized diets are detrimentally associated with semen quality. This includes diets rich in energy-dense and nutrient-poor foods, processed meats, soy foods, potatoes, dairy products including cheese, coffee (caffeine), alcohol, and sugar-added foods and beverages [95]. Food with phytoestrogens or compounds that have estrogenic activity should be avoided, with the major example being soy products due to the isoflavones. Others may include walnuts, cereals, legumes, and berries, among others [92]. These dietary habits in males are further associated with decreased chance of fertilization rates in their partners [95].

It is further recommended that nutritional consideration in males should include the elimination of foods rich in natural or synthetic endocrine disruptors, particularly environmental estrogens and estrogen receptor ligands and antiandrogens [98]. The majority of dairy products are from pregnant cows and are high in estrogen, progesterone, insulin, and insulin-like growth factors [98]. Consumption of these products is associated with reduced male fertility potential and decreased testosterone levels [98]. Environmental pesticides are also associated with poor semen quality, low testosterone, and reduced fertility potential [99−101]. Consumption of fruit and vegetables with high pesticide residues from agricultural processing may mitigate any beneficial effects in sperm quality, whereas consumption of fruits and vegetables with low pesticide residues have been correlated with better sperm analysis in males [100,101]. Pesticides such as organophosphates, organochlorine, and bipyridyl herbicide can impair spermatogenesis by inducing OS [102]. Others mechanisms associated with pesticide contamination include endocrine disruptors (e.g., organophosphates, pyrethroids) or alkylating the chromatin structure of sperm cells (e.g., organophosphates, 2,4-dichlorophenoxyacetic acid) [15]. Other chemicals associated with nutritional intake that negatively affect sperm parameters include bisphenol A (BPA), dioxins, and phthalates, alongside heavy metals in the food supply, or via food preparation, such as mercury, lead, aluminum, and so on [15]. There is therefore an argument to recommend more organic, unprocessed, and varied dietary options in these patients.

It is interesting to note that low-calorie diets for obese individuals may further aggravate MNDs associated with obesity. MNDs may not be corrected by a protein-rich formula diet containing vitamins and minerals based on current recommended dietary intakes and micronutrient levels remain low or become even lower. This may be due to increased demand and unbalanced dispersal of lipophilic compounds in the body [70]. Caloric restriction is well known to be associated with reducing systemic OS, reducing the risk of aging and related comorbidities as well as obesity and associated comorbidities, and extends the maximum life span in all mammals [103]. However, this must be performed appropriately without leading to further nutrient deficiencies. Caloric restriction can improve maximum life span via reduction of body fat, delayed age-related neuroendocrine and immunological changes (similar to those of obesity), increasing DNA repair capacity in all tissues, modification of gene expressions, enhanced apoptosis capabilities, reduced body temperature and metabolic rate, and improvement in OS and related systemic markers [103]. Bariatric surgery is associated with improved weight management; however, the overall impact on male fertility of this approach is still required as this is associated with numerous MNDs [91].

Exercise is a cornerstone of weight management, and an appropriate amount of regular exercise can be beneficial for male reproductive parameters [104]. Recommendations should be a minimum of 1 h of moderate intensity exercise three to five times per week [15]. Consistent physical training reduces OS markers and inflammatory markers in obese patients [104] and diet combined with exercise in obese male rats has been shown to increase sperm quality and reduce sperm OS [105,106]. Endurance training is associated with reduced OS and adiposity in rats fed high-fat diets with metabolic derangements, and improved endogenous antioxidant defenses including SOD, glutathione S-transferase, glutathione, and CAT [78]. Exercise training may further improve inflammation and OS in obesity due to immunomodulation, through macrophage phenotypic switching (M1 to M2) and prevention of leukocyte infiltration into adipose tissue [107]. It should be cautioned, however, as with antioxidant therapy, that excessive or extreme exercise or sport participation in males may negatively affect sperm parameters and even DNA integrity of spermatozoa [108].

NUTRITIONAL SUPPLEMENTATION AND ANTIOXIDANTS

Around 30%–80% of male subfertility cases may be due to excessive OS in the male reproductive tract [109]. The majority of foods and drugs available for male infertility, particularly in complementary and alternative medicine (CAM), are composed of various antioxidants with various levels of evidence that suggest an important therapeutic role [110]. Cellular antioxidants can be enzymatic (such as SOD, catalase, and glutathione peroxidase) or nonenzymatic (such as glutathione; thiols; vitamins A, E, and C; some metals; and phytonutrients such as flavonoids, polyphenols, and iso-flavones). The role of these antioxidants is to prevent ROS concentrations reaching too high levels above the physiological needs [111]. Many of these antioxidants can be acquired through the diet or oral supplementation as therapeutic inter-vention, as deficiencies in seminal plasma and dietary habits associated with these antioxidants have been associated with poor semen quality [112].

Antioxidants commonly used for male subfertility treatment include single or combination vitamins, minerals, and other compounds including carotenoids; vitamins C, D, and E; selenium; zinc; magnesium; carnitine; and CoQ10 [109]. It is thought that oral supplementation with antioxidants may improve sperm quality by reducing OS [109]. Consumption of antioxidants and micronutrients are associated with reduced sperm DNA damage and thus less risk of developing failed conception, pregnancy-related complications, and genetically defective offspring. Besides, intake of vitamins C and E, selenium, zinc, folic acid, N-acetyl cysteine, L-carnitine, and coenzyme Q10 have also been suggested to improve sperm parameters like motility, viability, and morphology along with boosting better fertilization potential and pregnancy out-comes in infertile men [113].

Supplementation of antioxidant micronutrients and vitamins is suggested to positively influence male reproductive impact of obesity and MetS, and improving sperm parameters and fertility potential as well as systemic endocrine and immune markers (e.g., improving insulin sensitivity and testosterone levels, and reducing inflammation and OS) even in the absence of no significant changes to BMI, WC, or adiposity [114]. Furthermore, in males taking antioxidants during assisted reproduction, there is a fourfold increase in live birth rates [115]. Further investigation with randomized, controlled, clinical trials is needed to confirm the safety and efficacy of antioxidant supplementation in the medical management and treatment of male infertility [115].

Nutritional supplementation, particularly with various antioxidants, has shown benefit as single agents or in combi-nation in male fertility. However, oversupplementation is detrimental and toxic to spermatozoa, and consideration of factors influencing fertility beyond nutritional status should be considered in the assessment and management plan. Ideally, demonstration of the oxidative status in the male reproductive tract and serum in patients is warranted prior to the recommendation of supplementation of trace nutrients and antioxidants [116]. However, antioxidants are widely available and inexpensive when compared to other fertility treatments and many men are already using these to improve their fertility.

In metal overload, especially metals such as iron and copper, N-acetyl cysteine (NAC) has been generally used as an antioxidant in this context [31]. NAC is suggested to module OS by decreasing ROS production in health complications resulting from metal toxicity [31]. Further supplementation for metal toxicity can include vitamin E, manganese, zinc, catechins from green tea, or curcuminoids [31].

Increasingly, there is an interest in the use of phytochemical compounds as medicinal alternatives due to their lack of toxicity and the relative ease and cost of production [47]. These antioxidant-rich phytotherapeutic extracts are rich in flavonoids, polyphenols, and catechin compounds for example, and require further investigation for the benefits to aging and age-related reproductive decline in males [47]. Herbs with significant antioxidant activity that have been well studied for benefit in obesity and associated comorbidities, as well as evidence of benefit for infertile males, includes epi-gallocatechin gallate from green tea [117], white tea [118], curcuminoids (turmeric extract) [119], and resveratrol (grape seed extracts) [120,121]. Additional phytotherapeutic agents may be useful for reproductive dysfunction and hypo-gonadism in obese males with increased OS, including *Panax ginseng* and other ginseng spp., *Eurycoma longifolia*, and *Tribulus terrestris*, among many others [122].

CONCLUSION

Nutritional status influences male reproductive systems, with genetics, lifestyle, and environmental factors further modulating this. Undernourishment and overnourishment are associated with underweight and overweight/obese males, respectively, reduced sperm parameters, and increased risk of comorbidities and mortality. These associations are partly mediated by OS and inflammation, with a decrease in various important antioxidants and increased production of ROS. A clinical investigation into lifestyle factors, such as nutritional intake and exercise, should be done and nutritional deficiencies corrected. Further consideration of therapeutic intervention with various single or combination antioxidants is warranted. Supplementation of antioxidants and phytonutrients must be used with caution, as further investigations are required to determine most appropriate nutrients, efficacy, safety, and dosage of antioxidant approaches. Antioxidants, alongside appropriate lifestyle changes and avoidance of environmental risks where possible, may offer an important strategy to improve fertility outcomes in malnourished and obese males, and potentially prevent the impact of excessive OS on disease development in the reproductive tract as well as globally. However, more research is required in malnourished males to fully understand the mechanisms and the best treatment options in different subgroups.

GLOSSARY

Adipokine Cytokine secreted by adipocytes.

Cytokine Any of a number of protein secreted by cells of the immune system that has an effect on other cells.

Dyslipidemia Abnormally elevated cholesterol or fats (lipids) in the blood.

Fenton reaction A complex and capable reaction of generating both hydroxyl radicals and higher oxidation states of iron; a source of oxidative stress.

Macronutrient Nutrient required in large amounts, including carbohydrates, proteins, and fats.

Malnutrition A condition that results from eating a diet in which nutrients are either not enough or are too much such that the diet causes health problems. It may involve calories, protein, carbohydrates, vitamins, or minerals.

Micronutrient A chemical element or substance required in trace amounts for the normal growth and development of living organisms.

Mineral A chemical element required as an essential nutrient to perform functions necessary for life.

Factor-κB Protein complex that controls transcription of DNA, cytokine production, and cell survival.

Haber−Weiss reaction Generates hydroxyl radicals from hydrogen peroxide and superoxide.

Insulin resistance A resistance to the effects of the hormone insulin, resulting in increasing blood sugar and numerous metabolic derangements.

Lipotoxicity A syndrome that results from the accumulation of lipid intermediates in nonadipose tissue, leading to cellular dysfunction and death.

Vitamin An organic compound and a vital nutrient that an organism requires in limited amounts.

LIST OF ACRONYMS AND ABBREVIATIONS

ATP Adenosine triphosphate
BAT Brown adipose tissue
BPA Bisphenol A
BMI Body mass index
CAT Catalase
CoQ10 Coenzyme Q10
CRP C-reactive protein
CVD Cardiovascular disease
DF DNA fragmentation
DNA Deoxyribonucleic acid
ECGC Epigallocatechin gallate
ESPEN European Society for Clinical Nutrition and Metabolism
FFA Free fatty acid
FSH Follicular stimulating hormone
GPx Glutathione peroxidase
HDL High-density lipoprotein
IL Interleukin
LDL Low-density lipoprotein
LH Luteinizing hormone
MetS Metabolic syndrome
MMP Mitochondrial membrane potential
MND Micronutrient deficiencies
MUST Malnutrition Universal Screening Tool
NAC N-acetyl-cysteine
NADPH Nicotinamide adenine dinucleotide phosphate
NRS202 Nutritional Risk Screening 2002
OS Oxidative stress
PEM Protein-energy malnutrition

PKC Protein kinase C
ROS Reactive oxygen species
PON Paraoxonase
PPARy Peroxisome proliferator-activated receptor-gamma
PRDX Peroxide reductase
SHBG Sex hormone binding globulin
SAT Subcutaneous adipose tissue
SNP Single nucleotide polymorphism
SOD Superoxide dismutase
StAR Steroidogenic acute regulatory protein
T2DM Type-2 diabetes mellitus
Treg Regulatory T-lymphocyte (Fox3P+)
TNFα Tumor necrosis factor-alpha
VAT Visceral adipose tissue
WAT White adipose tissue
WC Waist circumference
WHR Waist-to-hip ratio
WHO World Health Organization

REFERENCES

[1] Bain LA, Awah PK, Geraldine N, Kindong NP, Sigal Y, Bernard N, et al. Malnutrition in Sub-Saharan Africa: burden, causes and prospects. Pan Afr Med J 2013;6(15):120.

[2] Hull HR, Thornton J, Wang J, Pierson Jr RN, Kaleem Z, Pi-Sunyer X, et al. Fat-free mass index: changes and race/ethnic differences in adulthood. Int J Obes 2010;35(1):121–7.

[3] Whitlock G, Lewington S, Sherliker P, Clarke R, Emberson J, Halsey J, et al. Prospective Studies Collaboration. Body-mass index and cause-specific mortality in 900,000 adults: collaborative analyses of 57 prospective studies. Lancet 2009;373:1083–96.

[4] Sermondade N, Faure C, Fezeu L, Shayeb AG, Bonde JP, Jensen TK, et al. BMI in relation to sperm count: an updated systematic review and collaborative meta-analysis. Hum Reprod Update 2013;19(3):221–31.

[5] Alhashem F, Alkhateeb M, Sakr H, Alshahrani M, Alsunaidi M, Elrefaey H, et al. Exercise protects against obesity induced semen abnormalities via downregulating stem cellfactor, upregulating Ghrelin and normalizing oxidative stress. EXCLI J 2014;26(13):551–72.

[6] Haslam DW, James WP. Obesity. Lancet 2005;366:1197–209.

[7] Fernández-Sánchez A, Madrigal-Santillán E, Bautista M, Esquivel-Soto J, Morales-González A, Esquivel-Chirino C, et al. Inflammation, oxidative stress, and obesity. Int J Mol Sci 2011;12(5):3117–32.

[8] Poulia KA, Klek S, Doundoulakis I, Bouras E, Karayiannis D, Baschali A, Passakiotou M, Chourdakis M. The two most popular malnutrition screening tools in the light of the new ESPEN consensus definition of the diagnostic criteria for malnutrition. Clin Nutr 2017;36(4):1130–5.

[9] World Health Organisation. Obesity: preventing and managing the global epidemic: report of a WHO consultation. 2000.

[10] Dulloo AG, Jacquet J, Solinas G, Montani JP, Schutz Y. Body composition phenotypes in pathways to obesity and the metabolic syndrome. Int J Obes 2010;34(Suppl. 2):S4–17.

[11] Westergren A, Lindholm C, Axelsson C, Ulander K. Prevalence of eating difficulties and malnutrition among persons within hospital care and special accommodations. J Nutr Health Aging 2008;12(1):39–43.

[12] Owen DH, Katz DF. A review of the physical and chemical properties of human semen and the formulation of a semen simulant. J Androl 2005;26(4):459–69.

[13] Frohlich JU, Nissen HP, Heinze I, Schirren C, Kreysel HW. Free amino acid composition of human seminal plasma in different andrological diagnoses. Andrologia 1980;12:162–6.

[14] Surai PF, Fisinin VI. Selenium in pig nutrition and reproduction: boars and semen quality—a review. Asian-Australas J Anim Sci 2015;28(5):730–46.

[15] Sharma R, Biedenharn KR, Fedor JM, Agarwal A. Lifestyle factors and reproductive health: taking control of your fertility. Reprod Biol Endocrinol 2013;11:66.

[16] Magálová T. The antioxidant defense system and trace elements. Bratisl Lek Listy 1994;95(12):562–5.

[17] Ahmadi S, Bashiri R, Ghadiri-Anari A, Nadjarzadeh A. Antioxidant supplements and semen parameters: an evidence based review. Int J Reprod Biomed (Yazd) 2016;14(12):729–36.

[18] Kasperczyk A, Dobrakowski M, Czuba ZP, Kapka-Skrzypczak L, Kasperczyk S. Environmental exposure to zinc and copper influences sperm quality in fertile males. Ann Agric Environ Med 2016;23(1):138–43.

[19] Ghone RA, Suryakar AN, Kulhalli PM, Bhagat SS, Padalkar RK, Karnik AC, et al. A study of oxidative stress biomarkers and effect of oral antioxidant supplementation in severe acute malnutrition. J Clin Diagn Res 2013;7(10):2146–8.

[20] Kasperczyk A, Dobrakowski M, Zalejska-Fiolka J, Horak S, Birkner E. Magnesium and selected parameters of the non-enzymatic antioxidant and immune systems and oxidative stress intensity in the seminal plasma of fertile males. Magnes Res 2015;28(1):14–22.

[21] Tvrda E, Peer R, Sikka SC, Agarwal A. Iron and copper in male reproduction: a double-edged sword. J Assist Reprod Genet 2015;32(1):3—16.

[22] Kasperczyk A, Dobrakowski M, Czuba ZP, Kapka-Skrzypczak L, Kasperczyk S. Influence of iron on sperm motility and selected oxidative stress parameters in fertile males - a pilot study. Ann Agric Environ Med 2016;23(2):292—6.

[23] Kasperczyk A, Dobrakowski M, Horak S, Zalejska-Fiolka J, Birkner E. The influence of macro and trace elements on sperm quality. J Trace Elem Med Biol 2015;30:153—9.

[24] Talevi R, Barbato V, Fiorentino I, Braun S, Longobardi S, Gualtieri R. Protective effects of in vitro treatment with zinc, d-aspartate and coenzyme q10 on human sperm motility, lipid peroxidation and DNA fragmentation. Reprod Biol Endocrinol 2013;11:81.

[25] Wong WY, Thomas CM, Merkus JM, Zielhuis GA, Steegers-Theunissen RP. Male factor subfertility: possible causes and the impact of nutritional factors. Fertil Steril 2000;73(3):435—42.

[26] Banihani SA. Vitamin B12 and semen quality. Biomolecules 2017;7(2):E42.

[27] De Rosa M, Boggia B, Amalfi B, Zarrilli S, Vita A, Colao A, Lombardi G. Correlation between seminal carnitine and functional spermatozoal characteristics in men with semen dysfunction of various origins. Drugs R D 2005;6(1):1—9.

[28] Nagata M, Suzuki T. L-carnitine partially improves metabolic syndrome symptoms but does not reverse perturbed sperm function or infertility in high fat diet induced obese mice. M J Nutr 2017;2(1):013.

[29] Gürbüz B, Yalti S, Fiçicioğlu C, Zehir K. Relationship between semen quality and seminal plasma total carnitine in infertile men. J Obstet Gynaecol 2003;23(6):653—6.

[30] Lafuente R, González-Comadrán M, Solà I, López G, Brassesco M, Carreras R, et al. Coenzyme Q10 and male infertility: a meta-analysis. J Assist Reprod Genet 2013;30(9):1147—56.

[31] Nadjarzadeh A, Shidfar F, Amirjannati N, Vafa MR, Motevalian SA, Gohari MR, et al. Effect of coenzyme Q10 supplementation on antioxidant enzymes activity and oxidative stress of seminal plasma: a double-blind randomised clinical trial. Andrologia 2014;46(2):177—83.

[32] Wozniac SE, Gee LL, Wachtel M, Frezza EE. Adipose tissue: the new endocrine organ? Dig Dis Sci 2009;54(9):1847—56.

[33] Juge-Aubry CE, Henrichot E, Meier CA. Adipose tissue: a regulator of inflammation. J Clin Endocrinol 2005;19(4):547—66.

[34] Kwon H, Pessin JE. Adipokines mediate inflammation and insulin resistance. Front Endocrinol 2013;4:71.

[35] Trayhurn P. Hypoxia and adipose tissue function and dysfunction in obesity. Physiol Rev 2013;93:1—21.

[36] Hendricks KM, Duggan C, Gallagher L, Carlin AC, Richardson DS, Collier SB, et al. Malnutrition in hospitalized pediatric patients. Current prevalence. Arch Pediatr Adolesc Med 1995;149(10):1118—22.

[37] Muzi-Filho H, Bezerra CGP, Souza AM, Boldrini LC, Takiya CM, Oliveira FL, et al. Undernutrition affects cell survival, oxidative stress, Ca^{2+} handling and signaling pathways in vas deferens, crippling reproductive capacity. PLoS One 2013;8(7):e69682.

[38] Katona P, Katona-Apte J. The interaction between nutrition and infection. Clin Infect Dis 2008;46:1582—8.

[39] Luque EM, Tissera A, Gaggino MP, Molina RI, Mangeaud A, Vincenti LM, et al. Body mass index and human sperm quality: neither one extreme nor the other. Reprod Fertil Dev December 18, 2015;29. https://doi.org/10.1071/RD15351 [Epub ahead of print].

[40] Genovese P, Núñez ME, Pombo C, Bielli A. Undernutrition during foetal and post-natal life affects testicular structure and reduces the number of Sertoli cells in the adult rat. Reprod Domest Anim 2010;45:233—6.

[41] Alzamendi A, Zubiría G, Moreno G, Portales A, Spinedi E, Giovambattista A. High risk of metabolic and adipose tissue dysfunctions in adult male progeny, due to prenatal and adulthood malnutrition induced by fructose rich diet. Nutrients 2016;8(3):178.

[42] Rupérez AI, Gil A, Aguilera CM. Genetics of oxidative stress in obesity. Int J Mol Sci 2014;15(2):3118—44.

[43] Davidson LM, Millar K, Jones C, Fatum M, Coward K. Deleterious effects of obesity upon the hormonal and molecular mechanisms controlling spermatogenesis and male fertility. Hum Fertil 2015;18(3):184—93.

[44] Ng M, Fleming T, Robinson M, Thomson B, Graetz N, Margono C, et al. Global, regional, and national prevalence of overweight and obesity in children and adults during 1980—2013: a systematic analysis for the Global Burden of Disease Study 2013. Lancet 2014;384:766—81.

[45] Meldrum DR, Morris MA, Gambone JC. Obesity pandemic: causes, consequences, and solutions-but do we have the will? Fertil Steril 2017;107(4):833—9.

[46] Alberti KG, Eckel RH, Grundy SM, Zimmet PZ, Cleeman JI, Donato KA, et al. Harmonizing the metabolic syndrome: a joint interim statement of the International Diabetes Federation Task Force on Epidemiology and Prevention; National Heart, Lung, and Blood Institute; American Heart Association; World Heart Federation; International Atherosclerosis Society; and International Association for the Study of Obesity. Circulation 2009;120:1640—5.

[47] Leisegang K, Henkel R, Agarwal A. Redox regulation of fertility in aging male and the role of antioxidants: a savior or stressor. Curr Pharm Des May 2, 2017;23 [Epub ahead of print].

[48] Manna P, Jain SK. Obesity, oxidative stress, adipose tissue dysfunction, and the associated health risks: causes and therapeutic strategies. Metab Syndr Relat Disord 2015;13(10):423—44.

[49] Okorodudu DO, Jumean FM, Montori VM, Romero-Corral A, Somers VK, Erwin PJ, et al. Diagnostic performance of body mass index to identify obesity as defined by body adiposity: a systematic review and meta-analysis. Int J Obes 2010;34:791—9.

[50] Eckel RH, Grundy SM, Zimmet PZ. The metabolic syndrome. Lancet 2005;365(9468):1415—28.

[51] Almeda-Valdes P, Aguilar-Salinas CA, Uribe M, Canizales-Quinteros S, Méndez-Sánchez N. Impact of anthropometric cut-off values in determining the prevalence of metabolic alterations. Eur J Clin Invest 2016;46(11):940—6.

[52] Huang PL. A comprehensive definition for metabolic syndrome. DMM 2009;2:231—7.

[53] Kasturi SS, Tannir J, Brannigan R. The metabolic syndrome and male infertility. J Androl 2008;29:251—9.

[54] du Plessis SS, Cabler S, McAlister DA, Sabanegh E, Agarwal A. The effect of obesity on sperm disorders and male infertility. Nat Rev Urol 2010;7:153−61.

[55] Avicenna. The disadvantages of excessive weight. In: Avicenna, editor. The canon of medicine, book IV: diseases involving more than one member; the Cosmetic art. . Rome: Medical Press; 1593. p. 173−4.

[56] Hammoud AO, Gibson M, Peterson CM, Meikle W, Carrell DT. Impact of male obesity on infertility: a critical review of the current literature. Fertil Steril 2008;90(4):897−904.

[57] Palmer NO, Bakos HW, Fullston T, Lane M. Impact of obesity on male fertility, sperm function and molecular composition. Spermatogenesis 2012;2(4):253−63.

[58] MacDonald AA, Herbison GP, Showell M, Farquhar CM. The impact of body mass index on semen parameters and reproductive hormones in human males: a systematic review with meta-analysis. Hum Reprod Update 2010;16(3):293−311.

[59] Eisenberg ML, Kim S, Chen Z, Sundaram R, Schisterman EF, Buck Louis GM. The relationship between male BMI and waist circumference on semen quality: data from the LIFE study. Hum Reprod 2014;29(2):193−200.

[60] Bandel I, Bungum M, Richtoff J, Malm J, Axelsson J, Pedersen HS, et al. No association between body mass index and sperm DNA integrity. Hum Reprod 2015;30(7):1704−13.

[61] Leisegang K, Bouic PJD, Menkveld R, Henkel RR. Body weight is associated with increased seminal insulin and leptin: a novel link between infertility? Reprod Biol Endocrinol 2014;12:34.

[62] Bakos HW, Henshaw RC, Mitchell M, Lane M. Paternal body mass index is associated with decreased blastocyst development and reduced live birth rates following assisted reproductive technology. Fertil Steril 2011;95(5):1700−4.

[63] Eisenberg ML, Li S, Behr B, Cullen MR, Galusha D, Lamb DJ, Lipshultz LI. Semen quality, infertility and mortality in the USA. Hum Reprod 2014;29(7):1567−74.

[64] Lotti F, Corona G, Degli Innocenti S, Filimberti E, Scognamiglio V, Vignozzi L, et al. Seminal, ultrasound and psychobiological parameters correlate with metabolic syndrome in male members of infertile couples. Andrology 2013;1(2):229−39.

[65] Lotti F, Corona G, Vignozzi L, Rossi M, Maseroli E, Cipriani S, et al. Metabolic syndrome and prostate abnormalities in male subjects of infertile couples. Asian J Androl 2014;16(2):295−304.

[66] Leisegang K, Udodong A, Bouic PJ, Henkel RR. Effect of the metabolic syndrome on male reproductive function: a case-controlled pilot study. Andrologia 2014;46(2):167−76.

[67] Pasquali R. Obesity and androgens: facts and perspectives. Fertil Steril 2006;85(5):1319−40.

[68] Saad F, Gooren L. The role of testosterone in the metabolic syndrome: a review. J Steroid Biochem Mol Biol 2009;114(1−2):40−3.

[69] Bailey RL, West Jr KP, Black RE. The epidemiology of global micronutrient deficiencies. Ann Nutr Metab 2015;66(2):22−33.

[70] Damms-Machado A, Weser G, Bischoff SC. Micronutrient deficiency in obese subjects undergoing low calorie diet. Nutr J 2012;1(11):34.

[71] Kaidar-Person O, Person B, Szomstein S, Rosenthal RJ. Nutritional deficiencies in morbidly obese patients: a new form of malnutrition? Part A: vitamins. Obes Surg 2008;18(7):870−6.

[72] Kaidar-Person O, Person B, Szomstein S, Rosenthal RJ. Nutritional deficiencies in morbidly obese patients: a new form of malnutrition? Part B: minerals. Obes Surg 2008;18(8):1028−34.

[73] Via M. The malnutrition of obesity: micronutrient deficiencies that promote diabetes. ISRN Endocrinol 2012;2012:103472.

[74] Savini I, Catani MV, Evangelista D, Gasperi V, Avigliano L. Obesity associated oxidative stress: Strategies finalized to improve redox state. Int J Mol Sci 2013;14:10497−538.

[75] Esposito K, Ciotola M, Giugliano D. Oxidative stress in the metabolic syndrome. J Endocrinol Invest 2006;29:791−5.

[76] Chrysohoou C, Panagiotakos DB, Pitsavos C, Skoumas I, Papademetriou L, Economou M, et al. The implication of obesity on total antioxidant capacity apparently healthy men and women: the ATTICA study. Nutr Metab Cardiovasc Dis 2007;17:590−7.

[77] Anderson EJ, Lustig ME, Boyle KE, Woodlief TL, Kane DA, Lin CT, et al. Mitochondrial H_2O_2 emission and cellular redox state link excess fat intake to insulin resistance in both rodents and humans. J Clin Invest 2009;119(3):573−81.

[78] Emami SR, Jafari M, Haghshenas R, Ravasi A. Impact of eight weeks endurance training on biochemical parameters and obesity-induced oxidative stress in high fat diet-fed rats. J Exerc Nutr Biochem 2016;20(1):29−35.

[79] Rato L, Alves MG, Dias TR, Lopes G, Cavaco JE, Socorro S, Oliveira PF. High-energy diets may induce a pre-diabetic state altering testicular glycolytic metabolic profile and male reproductive parameters. Andrology 2013;1(3):495−504.

[80] Rato L, Alves MG, Cavaco JE, Oliveira PF. High-energy diets: a threat for male fertility? Obes Rev 2014;15(12):996−1007.

[81] Kintscher U, Hartge M, Hess K, Foryst-Ludwig A, Clemenz M, Wabitsch M, et al. T-lymphocyte infiltration in visceral adipose tissue: a primary event in adipose tissue inflammation and the development of obesity-mediated insulin resistance. Arterioscler Thromb Vasc Biol 2008;28(7):1304−10.

[82] Lumeng CN. Innate immune activation in obesity. Mol Aspects Med 2013;34(1):12−29.

[83] Henkel R. The impact of oxidants on sperm function. Andrologia 2005;37(6):205−6.

[84] Henkel RR. Leukocytes and oxidative stress: dilemma for sperm function and male fertility. Asian J Androl 2011;13(1):43−52.

[85] Tilg H, Moschen AR. Adipocytokines: mediators linking adipose tissue, inflammation and immunity. Nat Rev Immunol 2006;6:772−83.

[86] Leisegang K, Bouic PJ, Henkel RR. Metabolic syndrome is associated with increased seminal inflammatory cytokines and reproductive dysfunction in a case-controlled male cohort. Am J Reprod Immunol 2016;76(2):155−63.

[87] Rosety I, Elosegui S, Pery MT, Fornieles G, Rosety JM, Díaz AJ, et al. Association between abdominal obesity and seminal oxidative damage in adults with metabolic syndrome. Rev Med Chil 2014;142(6):732−7.

[88] Benedetti S, Tagliamonte MC, Catalani S, Primiterra M, Canestrari F, De Stefani S, et al. Differences in blood and semen oxidative status in fertile and infertile men, and their relationship with sperm quality. Reprod Biomed Online 2012;25(3):300—6.

[89] Hales DB, Allen JA, Shankara T, Janus P, Buck S, Diemer T, et al. Mitochondrial function in Leydig cell steroidogenesis. Ann N Y Acad Sci 2005;1061:120—34.

[90] Midzak AS, Chen H, Aon MA, Papadopoulos V, Zirkin BR. ATP synthesis, mitochondrial function, and steroid biosynthesis in rodent primary and tumor Leydig cells. Biol Reprod 2011;84(5):976—85.

[91] Kasum M, Anić-Jurica S, Čehić E, Klepac-Pulanić T, Juras J, Žužul K. Influence of male obesity on fertility. Acta Clin Croat 2016;55(2):301—8.

[92] Collins GG, Rossi BV. The impact of lifestyle modifications, diet, and vitamin supplementation on natural fertility. Fertil Res Pract 2015;1:11.

[93] Gonzalez-Castejon M, Rodriguez-Casado A. Dietary phytochemicals and their potential effects on obesity: a review. Pharmacol Res 2011;64:438—55.

[94] Gaskins AJ, Colaci DS, Mendiola J, Swan SH, Chavarro JE. Dietary patterns and semen quality in young men. Hum Reprod 2012;27(10):2899—907.

[95] Salas-Huetos A, Bulló M, Salas-Salvadó J. Dietary patterns, foods and nutrients in male fertility parameters and fecundability: a systematic review of observational studies. Hum Reprod Update 2017;10:1—19.

[96] Cutillas-Tolín A, Minguez-Alarcon L, Mendiola J, Lopez-Espin JJ, Jorgensen N, Navarrete-Munoz EM, et al. Mediterranean and Western dietary patterns are related to markers of testicular function among healthy men. Hum Reprod 2015;30:2945—55.

[97] Karayiannis D, Kontogianni MD, Mendorou C, Douka L, Mastrominas M, Yiannakouris N. Association between adherence to the Mediterranean diet and semen quality parameters in male partners of couples attempting fertility. Hum Reprod 2017;32(1):215—22.

[98] Afeiche M, Williams PL, Mendiola J, Gaskins AJ, Jørgensen N, Swan SH, et al. Dairy food intake in relation to semen quality and reproductive hormone levels among physically active young men. Hum Reprod 2013;28(8):2265—75.

[99] Rozati R, Reddy PP, Reddanna P, Mujtaba R. Role of environmental estrogens in the deterioration of male factor fertility. Fertil Steril 2002;78:1187—94.

[100] Chiu YH, Afeiche MC, Gaskins AJ, Williams PL, Petrozza JC, Tanrikut C, et al. Fruit and vegetable intake and their pesticide residues in relation to semen quality among men from a fertility clinic. Hum Reprod 2015;30(6):1342—51.

[101] Chiu Y-H, Gaskins AJ, Williams PL, Mendiola J, Jørgensen N, Levine H, et al. Intake of fruits and vegetables with low-to-moderate pesticide residues is positively associated with semen-quality parameters among young healthy men. J Nutr 2016;146(5):1084—92.

[102] Abdollahi M, Ranjbar A, Shadnia S, Nikfar S, Rezaie A. Pesticides and oxidative stress: a review. Med Sci Monit 2004;10:RA141—R147.

[103] Sohal RS, Weindruch R. Oxidative stress, caloric restriction, and aging. Science 1996;273(5271):59—63.

[104] Oh S, Tanaka K, Warabi E, Shoda J. Exercise reduces inflammation and oxidative stress in obesity-related liver diseases. Med Sci Sports Exerc 2013;45:2214—22.

[105] Palmer NO, Bakos HW, Owens JA, Setchell BP, Lane M. Diet and exercise in an obese mouse fed a high-fat diet improve metabolic health and reverse perturbed sperm function. Am J Physiol Endocrinol Metab 2012;302:E768—80.

[106] de Farias JM, Bom KF, Tromm CB, Luciano TF, Marques SO, Tuon T, Silva LA, Lira FS, de Souza CT, Pinho RA. Effect of physical training on the adipose tissue of diet-induced obesity mice: interaction between reactive oxygen species and lipolysis. Horm Metab Res 2013;45(3):190—6.

[107] Kawanishi N, Yano H, Yokogawa Y, Suzuki K. Exercise training inhibits inflammation in adipose tissue via both suppression of macrophage infiltration and acceleration of phenotypic switching from M1 to M2 macrophages in high-fat-diet-induced obese mice. Exerc Immunol Rev 2010;16:105—18.

[108] Vaamonde D, Algar-Santacruz C, Abbasi A, García-Manso JM. Sperm DNA fragmentation as a result of ultra-endurance exercise training in male athletes. Andrologia March 15, 2017;50. https://doi.org/10.1111/and.12793 [Epub ahead of print].

[109] Showell MG, Mackenzie-Proctor R, Brown J, Yazdani A, Stankiewicz MT, Hart RJ. Antioxidants for male subfertility. Cochrane Database Syst Rev 2014;12:CD007411.

[110] Urman B, Oktem O. Food and drug supplements to improve fertility outcomes. Semin Reprod Med 2014;32(4):245—52.

[111] Seifried HE, Anderson DE, Fisher EI, Milner JA. A review of the interaction among dietary antioxidants and reactive oxygen species. J Nutr Biochem 2007;18(9):567—79.

[112] Vujkovic M, de Vries JH, Dohle GR, Bonsel GJ, Lindemans J, Macklon NS, et al. Associations between dietary patterns and semen quality in men undergoing IVF/ICSI treatment. Hum Reprod 2009;24(6):1304—12.

[113] Agarwal A, Nallella KP, Allamaneni SS, Said TM. Role of antioxidants in treatment of male infertility: an overview of the literature. Reprod Biomed Online 2004;8:616—27.

[114] Montanino Oliva M, Minutolo E, Lippa A, Iaconianni P, Vaiarelli A. Effect of myoinositol and antioxidants on sperm quality in men with metabolic syndrome. Int J Endocrinol 2016;2016:1674950.

[115] Mora-Esteves C, Shin D. Nutrient supplementation: improving male fertility fourfold. Semin Reprod Med 2013;31(4):293—300.

[116] Delimaris I, Piperakis SM. The importance of nutritional factors on human male fertility: a toxicological approach. J Transl Toxicol 2014;1(1):52—9.

[117] Mosbah R, Yousef MI, Mantovani A. Nicotine-induced reproductive toxicity, oxidative damage, histological changes and haematotoxicity in male rats: the protective effects of green tea extract. Exp Toxicol Pathol 2015;67(3):253—9.

[118] Oliveira PF, Tomás GD, Dias TR, Martins AD, Rato L, Alves MG, et al. White tea consumption restores sperm quality in prediabetic rats preventing testicular oxidative damage. Reprod Biomed Online 2015;31(4):544—56.

[119] Zhang L, Diao RY, Duan YG, Yi TH, Cai ZM. In vitro antioxidant effect of curcumin on human sperm quality in leucocytospermia. Andrologia 2017;49. https://doi.org/10.1111/and.12760 [Epub ahead of print].

[120] Eleawa SM, Alkhateeb MA, Alhashem FH, Bin-Jaliah I, Sakr HF, Elrefaey HM, Elkarib AO, Alessa RM, Haidara MA, Shatoor AS, Khalil MA. Resveratrol reverses cadmium chloride-induced testicular damage and subfertility by downregulating p53 and Bax and upregulating gonadotropins and Bcl-2 gene expression. J Reprod Dev 2014;60(2):115—27 [Epub 2014 Feb 1].

[121] Cui X, Jing X, Wu X, Yan M. Protective effect of resveratrol on spermatozoa function in male infertility induced by excess weight and obesity. Mol Med Rep 2016;14(5):4659—65.

[122] Ho CC, Tan HM. Rise of herbal and traditional medicine in erectile dysfunction management. Curr Urol Rep 2011;12(6):470—8.

Chapter 2.6

Role of Reactive Oxygen Species in Diabetes-Induced Male Reproductive Dysfunction

Luís Rato[1], Pedro F. Oliveira[2], Mário Sousa[2], Branca M. Silva[3] and Marco G. Alves[2]

[1](CICS-UBI) Health Sciences Research Centre, University of Beira Interior, Covilhã, Portugal; [2]Institute of Biomedical Sciences Abel Salazar, University of Porto, Porto, Portugal; [3]University of Beira Interior, Covilhã, Portugal

INTRODUCTION

The incidence of diabetes mellitus (DM) is increasing in modern societies and is now considered one of the most threatening public health problems [1,2]. At the beginning of this millennium, nearly 171 million people suffered from DM [1]. Unfortunately, according to the most recent statistics, this number will continue to rise, reaching more than 400 million of individuals with DM by 2030 [1]. Nonetheless, these projections can be underestimated as there is a large number of individuals unaware they have DM, due to poor or nonexistent diagnosis [1]. In fact, negligent behaviors associated with the lifestyle, such as overconsumption of high-energy foods and physical inactivity, greatly contribute to the increased prevalence of DM [3]. Though this disease is associated with aging, in recent years the average age at diagnosis is dropping. Thus the number of young men with diabetes is increasing, and their reproductive health may be compromised at a very early age [4]. The increased incidence of DM has been closely associated with falling birth rates [5] among diabetic individuals, in part due to reduced male sexual performance [6] and also due to the significant molecular changes occurring in the testis. One of the most important events mediating those effects is the oxidative environment, particularly in reproductive organs [7].

Hyperglycemia is a hallmark of DM, and glucose acts as a prooxidant molecule since overproduction of reactive oxygen species (ROS) may occur during its metabolism. In fact, high levels of glucose-derived pyruvate increase the flux of nicotinamide adenine dinucleotide (NADH) and flavin adenine dinucleotide into the electron transport chain (ETC) and consequently the voltage gradient across the mitochondrial membrane. This may hamper electron transfer, causing electron leakage and thus the production of ROS. Overproduction of ROS stimulated by hyperglycemia has been recognized as a major cause of male subfertility/infertility [8].

Spermatozoa are highly susceptible to oxidative injuries since they are practically devoid of ROS-scavenging enzymes and dependent on the existing antioxidant protection in the male reproductive tract [9]. ROS easily oxidize lipids and proteins and DNA. Notably, sperm from men with diabetes exhibit high levels of oxidized DNA, thus illustrating the association between DM and DNA damage [10,11]. Clinical and particularly animal studies have allowed unveiling the molecular mechanisms responsible for the reproductive dysfunctions induced by DM [12–14]. However, this is still an overlooked topic that should deserve more attention. Several efforts have been made in the search for a strategy to improve the deleterious effects of oxidative stress (OS) in testis promoted by DM [15]. In this regard, the use of specific antioxidants seems to be a promising strategy [10,16]. In this chapter we give a critical appraisal of the recent knowledge on diabetes-induced OS in the testicular environment and how high levels of ROS induced by DM have an impact on male fertility.

CURRENT KNOWLEDGE ON THE EFFECTS OF DIABETES MELLITUS IN MALE FERTILITY

DM is a complex disease showing several stages of development [17]. The increased blood glucose levels in the body result from defects in insulin secretion and/or insulin action [18]. In addition, remarkable alterations in lipid and protein metabolism [18] also occur causing several systemic complications [19]. The majority of DM cases have been classified as type-1 diabetes mellitus (T1DM) or type-2 diabetes mellitus (T2DM). While T1DM accounts for only 5%−10% of those individuals diagnosed with diabetes and is characterized by insulin deficiency [18], the predominant form of DM is T2DM, accounting for almost 90%−95% of all cases [18]. T2DM is characterized by increased production of insulin where the body develops resistance to its action [18]. The high incidence of DM, particularly among young men, has significantly contributed to the high prevalence rate of subfertility (more than 50%) in men with diabetes [20]. Consequently, it is also associated with decline of male reproductive health and the low fertility rates reported in modern societies [5].

Decreased libido and erectile dysfunction (ED) [6] have been identified as major characteristics of DM in male reproductive performance. The microvascular lesions induced by DM in the penile tissue is a cause for ED, and this accounts for nearly 50%−75% of diabetic individuals [21]. Retrograde ejaculation may also occur in some cases [22]. Apart from these conditions, the most remarkable effects of DM on male fertility develop almost subtly. Indeed, even these subtle changes in the molecular pathways governing reproductive events produce significant alterations that ultimately end in infertility. Deciphering these hidden effects is perhaps one of the major challenges that we are facing, and certainly, this will stimulate the debate and future research on the topic.

A well-known effect of DM on male reproductive health is the disruption of the reproductive axis [23]. Insulin dysfunction disrupts normal reproductive function since this hormone is crucial for the function of hypothalamus−pituitary−testicular (HPT) axis [24]. Insulin directly regulates the secretion of gonadotropins from the anterior pituitary due to its specific receptors located in the hypothalamus-pituitary complex [25]. Under normal physiological conditions, the hypothalamus releases gonadotropin-releasing hormone (GnRH) pulses stimulating the secretion of both luteinizing hormone (LH) and follicle-stimulating hormone (FSH) via the anterior pituitary. FSH and LH act on Sertoli cells (SCs) and Leydig cells (LCs), respectively, to stimulate spermatogenesis. Nevertheless, the secretion of both gonadotropins [26] is significantly reduced according to the degree of DM severity, which in some cases may result in testosterone deficiency [27].

Ding and collaborators [28] reported that men with diabetes had significantly lower serum testosterone levels as compared with healthy men. Besides endocrine alterations, structural changes in the seminiferous epithelium also occur, even during the early stages of DM (Table 1). Analysis of testicular biopsies from diabetic men showed a disrupted blood−testis barrier with several morphological changes including depleted germ cells in the seminiferous tubules, SC vacuolization, and thickness of seminiferous tubule wall [29]. The maintenance of the blood−testis barrier is assured by differentiated SCs and by several protein complexes [30]. DM induces SC degeneration and redistribution of key proteins such as occludin, involved in the formation of the blood−testis barrier [31], leading to a dysfunctional blood−testis barrier and spermatogenesis arrest.

Additionally, alterations in sperm parameters such as semen volume, sperm count, motility, and morphology have also been found in men with diabetes [32]. Nevertheless, there is still some controversy regarding sperm quality in men with diabetes. For example, earlier studies have shown declined sperm quality in young males with T1DM due to lower sperm count and significant decreases in sperm motility and morphology [33]. Other reports have also evaluated sperm motility in patients with T1DM but did not observe any correlations between sperm motility and age, the age of onset of DM, and duration of disease [34−36]. In this study, several parameters related to sperm motility, such as track speed, path velocity, progressive velocity, and lateral head displacement, were not altered. On the other hand, other parameters such as linearity and linear index that analyze the straightness of swimming were significantly increased in men with diabetes [34]. Taking into account such evidence, some mechanisms were hypothesized to explain the reduction in spermatozoa motility. These may include increased oxidative status [4], autoimmune disorder with the development of antisperm antibodies, and/or neuropathy, which may alter seminal vesicle function [37].

The knowledge on spermatozoa quality in patients with T1DM is very scanty and the majority of studies have limited the analysis to conventional sperm parameters [23]. Recently, La Vignera and collaborators [38] evaluated the effect of T1DM on both conventional and biofunctional sperm parameters. T1DM individuals exhibited a higher number of deletions in sperm mitochondrial DNA (mtDNA) compared with healthy men [38]. This led to the hypothesis that declined sperm motility observed in men with T1DM results in part from mitochondrial dysfunction (Table 1). Until now, this was the only study exploring the integrity of sperm mitochondrial DNA in men with T1DM.

Studies from animal models revealed that the effects of DM go far beyond the testicular milieu and diabetes induced in rats by intraperitoneal streptozotocin administration have altered sex behavior and diminished reproductive organ weight

TABLE 1 Summary of the Main Studies Reporting Reproductive Defects Induced by Different Stages of Diabetes Mellitus

Models	Type of Diabetes	Reproductive Effects	References
Animal Studies			
Akita mouse	T1DM	↓ Testis weight, seminiferous tubules diameter, and ↓ fertility	[98]
		Disruption of HPT axis	[99]
BB rat		↓ Testis weight	[100]
		↓ Serum T	
		Disruption of seminiferous tubules	
		↓ Sperm production	
GK rat	T2DM	↓ Sperm production	[101]
HED rat	Prediabetes	↑ Sperm abnormal morphology	[58]
STZ rat	Prediabetes	↓ Sperm motility and viability	[84]
	T1DM	↓ Testis weight	[26,80]
		Disruption of epididymis	[40]
		↓ LH, FSH, and T serum levels	[26,39,80]
		↓ Sperm production	[39,40]
		↓ Sperm counts and motility	[26,39,41,80,101]
		Erectile dysfunction	[21]
		Ejaculation dysfunction	[39,80]
		↓ Fertility	[41,80]
	T2DM	↓ Sperm motility and viability ↑ Sperm abnormal morphology	[52]
ALX rat	T2DM	Disruption of HPT axis, Disruption of seminiferous tubules, ↓ Number of Leydig and Sertoli cells, and spermatogonia	[102]
Clinical Studies			
T1DM		Disruption of seminiferous tubules	[29]
		Depletion of germ cells and Sertoli-cell vacuolization	[29]
		Erectile dysfunction	[21,103]
		Ejaculation dysfunction	[22,104]
		↓ Semen volume	[32,103]
		↓ Sperm counts, motility, and morphology	[32,33,103]
		↓ Sperm progressive motility, ↓ sperm mitochondrial function, and epididymal postejaculatory dysfunction	[38]
		↑ Sperm DNA fragmentation	[4,105]
T2DM		Erectile dysfunction	[106]
		↓ Semen volume	[4,35]
		↓ Sperm motility, ↑ sperm DNA fragmentation	[35]

BB rat, biobreeding genetic rodent model; *FSH*, follicle-stimulation hormone; *GK rats*, Goto-Kakizaki genetic rodent model; *HED rat*, high-energy diet rodent model; *HPT*, hypothalamus-pituitary testicular; *LH*, luteinizing hormone; *STZ rat*, streptozotocin-induced rodent model; *ALX rat*, alloxan-induced rodent model; *T*, testosterone; *T1DM*, type 1 diabetes mellitus; *T2DM*, type 2 diabetes mellitus; ↑, increase; ↓, decrease.

and testicular and epididymal sperm content [39]. DM causes regression of the epididymis, leading to decreased weight in caput, corpus, and caudal regions [39]. Furthermore, structural changes in the caput, corpus, and caudal epididymis resulted in epididymal lumen depleted from spermatozoa [40]. However, administration of exogenous insulin prevented some of these deleterious effects, but only in certain epididymal regions [40]. Kim and Moley [41] studied the quality of sperm from diabetic male mice and its capacity to fertilize the oocyte. They concluded that DM decreased sperm concentration and motility and may cause male subfertility by altering steroidogenesis [41]. Furthermore, it was also demonstrated that DM impairs the preimplantation of mouse embryos recovered from diabetic animals, and it was also observed that the growth of embryos was significantly arrested in diabetic animals compared with the embryos from normal animals [42].

An alternative to the assessment of conventional sperm parameters is the evaluation of the integrity of sperm nuclear DNA (nDNA) and mtDNA, which serves as a predictor of male fertility [15,43]. A study with both patients with T1DM and T2DM reported that they present a higher level of damage in sperm nDNA and mtDNA as compared to the control individuals, though semen parameters were normal [4]. This is an important finding since the relationship between sperm genomic integrity and male reproductive potential [43] help explain why men apparently exhibiting normal semen parameters remain subfertile.

DIABETES MELLITUS, OXIDATIVE STRESS, AND TESTICULAR METABOLISM

Diabetes is characterized by systemic prooxidative state [44] and OS is extremely deleterious to most systems of the body. It occurs when the production of ROS overwhelm the limited antioxidant capacity of the cells. ROS are generated from the reduction of O_2 or by oxidation of H_2O to yield products such as superoxide anion, hydrogen peroxide, and hydroxyl radical. Low amounts of ROS are required for normal physiological sperm function, specifically for maturation-related events [45], whereas excessive ROS levels are often correlated with reduced male fertility [46]. Hyperglycemia enhances OS and increases ROS formation, thereby altering the redox state of the cells. Several mechanisms contribute to this, such as an increased polyol pathway flux, increased intracellular formation of advanced glycation end products (AGEs), activation of protein kinase C, and an overproduction of superoxide in the mitochondria [8]. This is particularly relevant at testicular level due to a high variety of several biomolecules such as lipids and proteins, and DNA damage, which makes it a vulnerable target for ROS.

The endogenous sources of ROS in human spermatozoa are (1) the nicotinamide adenine dinucleotide phosphate (NADPH) oxidase system occurring at sperm plasma membrane or (2) through the NADH-dependent oxidoreductase (diaphorase) system in mitochondria. However, ROS can be generated by leukocytes present in semen and throughout the male reproductive tract [47]. These cells play a key role in infection, inflammation, and cell defense. Infiltrating phagocytic leukocytes are capable of producing up to 1000 times more ROS than spermatozoa [47]. Under normal conditions 1 mL of semen contains 1×10^6 leukocytes. However, according to the World Health Organization criteria, when the number of leukocytes is higher than 1×10^6/mL of semen leukocytospermia occurs [48]. DM is associated with inflammation in the male reproductive tract and accessory glands [49]. As a result activated leukocytes infiltrate and release high amounts of ROS, which decrease sperm quality by stimulating the oxidation of DNA and lipids [50]. It is noteworthy that the degree of OS is an excess of ROS in relation to the antioxidants present in the seminal plasma. If the amount of antioxidants is too low for a certain number of leukocytes, this also leads to OS [50].

Apart from the induced oxidative status, DM is one of the major health concerns for all professionals working in reproductive medicine/biology since it is capable of disrupting male fertility at multiple levels [51,52]. The hormonal fluctuations induced by DM, especially in testosterone levels, compromise spermatogenesis by directly disrupting the function of mature SCs [53]. These cells are responsible for the maintenance of spermatogenesis, metabolize several substrates, and generate the energy metabolites necessary for germ cells. Among these, lactate is the preferential energy source for developing germ cells [54]. It was observed that SCs metabolically adapt to testosterone deficiency induced by progressive stages of DM (prediabetes and T2DM) with the more pronounced effects being parallel with the lowest testosterone levels [53]. At the initial stage of DM, SCs did not take up glucose as efficiently as those cells exposed to T2DM-like conditions [53]. Instead, these cells preferentially consume pyruvate, probably due to a mechanism that is dependent on the expression and/or activity of glucose transporters, especially glucose transporter 3 (GLUT3), which is sensitive to insulin action [55]. Second, neither glucose nor pyruvate taken up by SCs were efficiently converted into lactate [52,53,56], thus suggesting that under DM conditions part of glucose is redirected to alternative pathways as glycogen synthesis. In fact, SCs express all molecular machinery involved in the metabolism of glycogen, but Rato and collaborators [52] have elaborated on the relevance of glycogen in the metabolic cooperation occurring within the seminiferous epithelium under diabetic conditions. Indeed, preliminary evidence shows that T2DM animals accumulate the glycogen precursor, uridine-diphosphate glucose, in testes [57].

A recent study from our group evaluated the impact of prediabetes induced by consumption of high-energy diets on testicular glucose metabolism and concluded that such metabolic changes were associated with a decline in the reproductive parameters [58]. Indeed, prediabetic animals exhibited a significant expression of glucose transporters 1 (GLUT1) and GLUT3, as well as an increase in the activity of phosphofructokinase, thus supporting the hypothesis of glycolytic pathway stimulation. This was reflected in the high lactate content, promoted by the increased expression of proteins associated with the production of that metabolite, specifically lactate dehydrogenase (LDH) and the monocarboxylate transporter 4 (MCT4) [58]. Nevertheless, enhanced glucose metabolism was associated with a prooxidative testicular environment, since the antioxidant capacity of prediabetic rats testis was decreased, while the oxidation of lipids and proteins in that tissue were increased [59]. This illustrates that even in the initial steps of DM, testicular oxidative damages occur at significant rates [58]. There are key players involved in the control of the molecular mechanisms responsible for prediabetes-induced OS [60], such as peroxisome proliferator-activated receptor gamma coactivator 1-α (PGC1-α) and sirtuin 3 (SIRT3). PGC1-α and SIRT3 are nuclear-encoded proteins crucial for mitochondrial function and the maintenance of antioxidant defense system [60]. Even though PGC-1α is involved in the induction of ROS-detoxifying enzymes and synergistically interacts with SIRT3 inducing the expression of antioxidant defenses [60], sperm quality was seriously compromised due to a substantial decrease in the percentage of motile and viable sperm, whereas the number of sperm with abnormal morphology was increased. The impact of DM on male reproductive potential has been a matter of great discussion and the previous data provide compelling evidence that metabolic changes may lead to a decline in sperm quality that may be accountable for the decline in the reproductive health of men with diabetes (Fig. 1).

IMPACT OF REACTIVE OXYGEN SPECIES ON MALE FERTILITY: FROM SPERMATOGENESIS TO SPERM MATURATION

The formation of spermatozoa is a continuous process with high-energy demands in which the high rates of mitochondrial oxygen consumption by different testicular cells result in increased production of ROS. During diabetes, the disruption of the lipid metabolism [61] leads to an accumulation of fatty acids. As more fats are available, the rate of β-oxidation increases in response to the high fatty acid content [62]. However, testicular mitochondria may not be able to oxidize all fatty acids [59]. This energy overload leads to mitochondrial stress, disrupting the normal functioning of testicular ETC, thus prefiguring mitochondrial dysfunction and concomitant formation of ROS [59].

ROS overproduction is generally associated with male infertility due to the significant damages induced in testicular tissue, which in some cases are irreversible [63,64]. Diabetes also increases germ cells and SCs apoptosis [65]. Stage VII−IX tubules showed increased levels of 8-hydrodeoxyguanosine [65]. However, it must be considered that moderate levels of ROS are of paramount importance in the regulation of several key reproductive events, such as capacitation, acrosome reaction, and fusion with the female gamete [66]. ROS at moderate levels are required for the self-renewal of tissues and regulate several cellular activities, including proliferation, differentiation, and genomic stability of embryonic stem cells [67]. ROS drive the self-renewal of germ line stem cells (GSC) [68] as reported by Morimoto and collaborators [68], who exposed GSC to α-lipoic acid, an ROS scavenger, and observed that GSC did not proliferate. Though the underlying mechanisms were not completely shown, it was proposed that proliferation of GSC is mediated by signaling pathway of rat sarcoma (RAS) protein [69]. RAS is essential for the self-renewal of spermatogonial stem cells (SSCs) and its activation enables long-term self-renewal of cultured spermatogonia, probably via phosphoinositide 3-kinase-AKT and mitogen-activated protein kinase pathways [69]. However, increased levels of ROS inhibited proliferation of H-RAS-transfected GSC [69], thus illustrating that ROS act downstream of RAS signaling.

Interestingly, GSC positively respond to increasing concentrations of H_2O_2 ranging from 30 to 100 μM, and the growth promoted by the action of H_2O_2 in the self-renewal of SSC could be stimulated by p38 MAPK and c-jun N-terminal kinase in a different manner [68]. Nonetheless, uncontrolled ROS production results in oxidative damages and influences the development of germ cells by restricting cell differentiation. Even within seminiferous epithelium germ cells are permanently exposed to endogenous ROS produced by testicular cells or those coming from the peripheral circulation. Furthermore, germ cells exhibit a high percentage of fatty acids in the plasma membrane and become a preferential target for ROS under stress conditions.

Although it is argued that DM-induced OS is extremely deleterious for the viability of germ cells, its vulnerability to the effects of ROS varies according to the developing stage [70]. Spermatozoa are highly sensitive to ROS damages [71] while spermatogonia are apparently more tolerant [72]. Previous studies in mice showed that heat-induced testicular OS

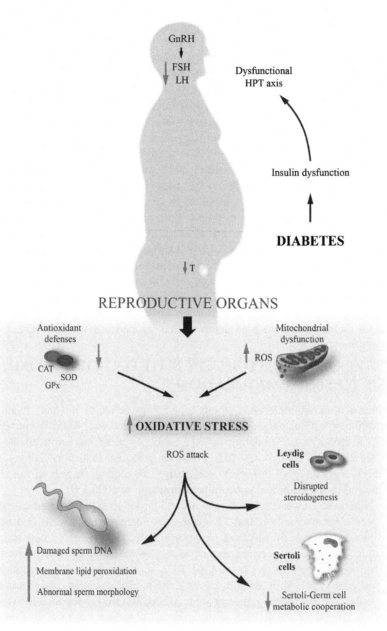

FIGURE 1 Oxidative stress occurs when there is an imbalance between antioxidants and reactive oxygen species. Diabetes predisposes for an increased oxidative environment, specifically in reproductive organs. ROS can easily target proteins, lipids, and DNA, as well as sperm plasma membrane. Consequently, sperm integrity and sperm membrane-related events will be compromised. Altogether the effects of ROS on testis ultimately compromise sperm quality leading to decreased reproductive performance and male infertility. *CAT*, catalase; *FSH*, follicle-stimulating hormone; *GnRH*, gonadotropin-releasing hormone; *GPx*, glutathione peroxidase; *LH*, luteinizing hormone; *ROS*, reactive oxygen species; *SOD*, superoxide dismutase; *T*, testosterone.

increased the number of apoptotic late-type germ cells, while the number of apoptotic spermatogonia was practically negligible [73]. Such evidence clearly illustrates the higher susceptibility of later stage germ cells to ROS compared to those lying in the unprotected side of the seminiferous epithelium. Why and how this happens needs to be fully addressed, but we cannot discard the role of protective factors expressed by spermatogonia. These cells exhibit high levels of copper/zinc superoxide dismutase, while spermatocytes and other differentiated germ cells exhibit a weak expression of copper/zinc superoxide dismutase [74], and therefore are unable to counteract the insults from both endogenous and exogenous ROS.

During spermatogenesis, germ cells lose most of their cytoplasm; however, there are inherent errors during this process and in dysfunctional germ cells, when the major part of cytoplasm is not extruded it leads to an excess of residual cytoplasm (ERC). Retention of residual cytoplasm has been positively correlated with ROS generation by spermatozoa, since the ERC activates the NADPH system, bringing about an excess of electrons that can contribute to overproduction of ROS [75]. The high production of ROS is related to the increased expression and activity of glucose-6-phosphate dehydrogenase, which fuels the generation of NADPH through the pentose phosphate pathway. Hence, this ERC may help unveil the missing link between poor sperm quality and increased ROS generation.

The role of ROS goes far beyond the seminiferous epithelium. After leaving the lumen of seminiferous tubules, spermatozoa proceed through the rete testis, efferent ducts, and begin their journey toward the epididymis where they undergo several modifications to acquire motility and fertilizing ability. At this stage, spermatozoa are completely dependent on the ROS levels and the activity of antioxidant enzymes. Previous studies have reported that DM increases the OS in the epididymal tissue, contributing to increased DNA fragmentation [10]. In fact, high levels of 8-hydrodeoxyguanosine in the semen of individuals with DM were correlated with the levels of nitrite/nitrate [11]. Significant damage during sperm epididymal transit may compromise downstream processes since sperm maturation continues throughout female reproductive tract, where spermatozoa become capacitated.

During capacitation, sperm motility changes from a progressive state to a highly energetic one where the continuous production of moderate levels of ROS is essential [76]. ROS and reactive nitrogen species oxidize cholesterol and facilitate sterol efflux from the sperm plasma membrane contributing to the membrane fluidity [77]. Combination of superoxide anion and nitric oxide forms peroxynitrite ($ONOO^-$) to allow the production of oxysterol, a cytotoxic species that oxidizes low-density lipoproteins. Oxysterol helps to remove cholesterol from the lipid bilayer, inhibits tyrosine phosphate and increases the production of $3',5'$-cyclic adenosine monophosphate (cAMP) [78], which is essential for the normal occurrence of capacitation. It is interesting to note the duality of ROS effects, since on the one hand low levels enhance sperm functionality, whereas an exacerbated production leads to peroxidation of lipids in the sperm membrane causing declined fluidity and therefore sperm dysfunction [79]. Decreased membrane functionality impedes the ability to undergo acrosomal exocytose and therefore sperm–oocyte fusion [80].

POSSIBLE ROLE OF ANTIOXIDANTS IN THE TREATMENT OF DIABETES-INDUCED MALE INFERTILITY

The incidence of DM is increasing in young men, particularly in developed societies [2,81]. DM together with other metabolic diseases has been considered a major factor for the marked decline of male fertility in recent decades. It is possible that in the coming years the number of individuals suffering from subfertility or even infertility associated with DM will considerably increase. For this reason, it becomes necessary to find new strategies that may help to improve the reproductive health of males with DM. Antioxidants have been considered a valuable strategy to counteract the deleterious effects that DM exerts on male fertility. Several natural compounds, often present in daily consumed plant-based foods and beverages, have been recognized for their ability to regulate male reproductive function [82]. White tea (*Camellia sinensis* L.) is one of the most common beverages consumed in the world and has a huge potential interest for male reproductive health [56]. It is rich in phenolic compounds and shows potent antioxidant activity with ameliorating properties relatively to DM. It was previously demonstrated that white tea prevents hyperglycemia by enhancing insulin activity and may prevent damage to pancreatic β-cells [83]. Such health-promoting effects have been also observed in male reproductive dysfunction associated with DM. Oliveira and collaborators [84] observed that the administration of white tea in prediabetic rats not only improved sperm motility, but also reversed the number of viable sperm to normal levels. The antioxidant activity of white tea was able to reduce testicular oxidative environment and associated organs, thus improving reproductive parameters. Still, the underlying mechanisms need to be fully clarified. It is possible that the presence of biologically active constituents of white tea, especially catechins, plays a key role in the management of DM-induced male infertility.

Based on this premise Dias and collaborators [85] used white tea as media supplement for the preservation of spermatozoa at room temperature and found an improvement in sperm viability [86]. These studies suggest that some usually consumed natural products may be valuable to counteract male reproductive dysfunctions. In the same way, resveratrol also shares a high antioxidant potential. Resveratrol can be found in the skin of grapes, blueberries, raspberries, and mulberries, and wine and has strong antioxidant properties [87]. Compelling evidence show that resveratrol improved the adverse effects of insulin resistance to male fertility [88,89]. DM-induced decrease in testes weight was recovered after 18 weeks of treatment with 400 mg/kg day^{-1} of resveratrol. The treatment also mitigated DM-induced sperm alterations by enhancing antioxidant defenses. The strong antioxidant capacity of resveratrol has also led to the use of this substance as an additive for postthaw bull sperm media [90].

The supplementation of the semen extender with resveratrol improved sperm motility and mitochondrial activity, contributing to an attenuated oxidative environment that often leads to lipid and DNA damage. Others compounds with antioxidant properties have also been used as a strategy to ameliorate the detrimental effects of DM on sperm parameters, as is the case of vitamin C [91]. Rosuvastatin is a member of statin family with antioxidant and antiinflammatory properties, and it was observed that diabetic animals treated with Rosuvastatin had increased sperm count and sperm motility possibly by suppressing the OS and apoptotic pathways in testicular tissue [92]. Scutellarin is a flavone glycoside isolated from *Erigeron breviscapus* and is also able to counteract the adverse effects of DM by decreasing lipid peroxidation and ROS levels in both testicular and epididymal tissues [93].

Relevant information regarding the use of antioxidants in the management of DM-induced reproductive dysfunctions is shown in Table 2. It must be taken into account that most of the available data focus on clinical reproductive parameters,

TABLE 2 Main Findings of the Most Recent Studies Exploring the Effects of Antioxidants in In Vivo and In Vitro Diabetic Animal Models

Natural Products	Cells/Tissue	Metabolic Effects	Oxidative Parameters	Reproductive Effects	References
Caffeine [5 µM]	Sertoli cells	↑ LDH activity ↑ lactate production	↑ Protein oxidation	nd	[56]
Caffeine [50 µM]	Sertoli cells	↑ LDH activity ↑ lactate content	na	nd	
White Tea [0.5 mg/mL]	Sertoli cells	↑ LDH activity ↑ lactate content	nd	nd	[107]
Melatonin [1 mM]	Sertoli cells	↓ LDH activity ↓ LDH expression ↓ Lactate content	nd	nd	[97]
EGCG [50 µM]	Sertoli cells	↑ Glucose and pyruvate consumption	↓ Mitochondrial membrane potential ↓ Lipid and protein oxidation	nd	[94]
White tea	Testis	↑ GLUTs expression	↑ Antioxidant capacity ↓ Lipid and protein oxidation	↑ Sperm motility ↑ Sperm viability	[84]
	Epididymis	↓ Lactate content	nd	↑ Sperm motility ↑ Sperm viability	[108]
Resveratrol	Testis	nd	↑ CAT activity ↑ SOD activity ↑ Glutathione levels	nd	[109]
Gum arabic	Testis	nd	↑ CAT activity ↑ SOD activity ↑ GPx	nd	[110]
Royal jelly	Testis	nd	↑ Antioxidant capacity ↑ CAT activity	Improvement of seminiferous tubular structure	[111]
Vitamin C	Epididymis	nd	nd	↑ Sperm motility ↑ Sperm viability	[91]
Rosuvastatin	nd	nd	↑ SOD activity ↑ Glutathione levels ↓ MDA	↑ Sperm count ↑ Sperm motility	[92]
Scutellarin	Testis	nd	↓ MDA ↓ ROS	nd	[93]
	Epididymis	nd	↓ MDA ↓ ROS	nd	

CAT, catalase; *GLUTs*, glucose transporters; *LDH*, lactate dehydrogenase; *MDA*, malondialdehyde; *na.*, not altered; *nd*, not determined; *ROS*, reactive oxygen species; *SOD*, superoxide dismutase; *EGCG*, Epigallocatechin-3-gallate.

while the molecular mechanisms underlying testicular oxidative improvement have been neglected. This issue has been overlooked but deserves special attention since some antioxidants improve testicular OS by altering the metabolic rates of testicular cells. For instance, tea constituents have received considerable attention since they can be used as dietary supplements to modulate spermatogenesis by altering the metabolic cooperation between SCs and germ cells. When the metabolic cooperation between SCs and germ cells is disrupted, fertility problems arise. Human SCs (hSCs) exposed to caffeine, a main tea constituent, led to increased production of lactate and alanine, and these alterations were associated with an improved oxidative profile [85] (Table 2). This was one of the first studies showing that tea constituents alone control testicular metabolic and oxidative profile.

Epigallocatechin-3-gallate (EGCG) represents nearly 50%−80% of all catechins in white tea. Our group also found that hSCs exposed to pharmacological concentrations of EGCG (50 μM) suffer a metabolic reprogramming [94], so that the high glucose and pyruvate uptake sustains lactate production (Table 2). Those metabolic changes were associated with a decrease in mitochondrial membrane potential, which could compromise energy production. In this context it is noteworthy that pharmacological levels of EGCG were associated with decreased lipid and protein oxidation, illustrating the protective role of this compound against ROS [94].

Another compound that has been available on the market and is used as a supplement, mainly as sleep aids, is melatonin. Increased evidence showed the beneficial effects of melatonin on male fertility due to its antioxidant properties [95] and the capacity to interact with the reproductive axis [96]. Furthermore, the role of melatonin in the regulation of glucose metabolism and the presence of its specific receptors on testicular tissue, particularly in SCs, has been highlighted [97], suggesting that this hormone may act as a regulator of SC metabolism. Melatonin-exposed SCs increased the expression of GLUT1 protein levels leading to a higher consumption of glucose [97]. This was not reflected in high amounts of lactate, probably due to a significant decrease in the expression and activity of LDH. These findings illustrate that melatonin regulates SC metabolism, and thus may affect spermatogenesis. Interestingly, melatonin cooperates with insulin in the regulation of glucose homeostasis, since SCs exposed to insulin plus melatonin favored lactate production and maintained the protein levels of glycolysis-related enzymes and transporters when compared with SCs cultured in insulin-only or melatonin-only conditions [97]. These data suggest a synergistic effect between insulin and melatonin in the control of spermatogenesis by enhancing the nutritional support of spermatogenesis by SCs.

CONCLUSION

Under normal circumstances, the male reproductive system has a controlled balance between ROS production and antioxidant activity. Low levels of ROS are required to ensure optimal sperm function necessary for fertilization and embryo development, but excessive amounts lead to lipid peroxidation and DNA damage, ultimately compromising sperm function and causing infertility. Diabetes has been correlated with increased levels of ROS and DNA damage in sperm as a main factor for the alterations in the male fertility potential. Thus it is essential to search for a strategy that may help to improve male reproductive potential, particularly in modern societies where lifestyle factors have significantly contributed to the decline in male fertility associated with metabolic diseases. In addition, this fact shows no tendency to improve in the years to come. Treatment based on antioxidants has arisen as a promising strategy to manage male infertility mainly through the control of the testicular metabolism. However, it is imperative to decipher the puzzle of testicular OS induced by DM to unveil the molecular mechanisms that can serve as a target for therapeutic intervention.

LIST OF ACRONYMS AND ABBREVIATIONS

cAMP $3',5'$-cyclic adenosine monophosphate
DM Diabetes mellitus
DNA Deoxyribonucleic acid
ED Erectile dysfunction
EGCG Epigallocatechin-3-gallate
ERC Excess of residual cytoplasm
ETC Electron transport chain
FSH Follicle-stimulating hormone
GLUT1 Glucose transporter 1
GLUT3 Glucose transporter 3
GnRH Gonadotropin-releasing hormone
GSC Germ line stem cells
HPT Hypothalamus−pituitary−testicular

hSC Human Sertoli cell
LC Leydig cell
LDH Lactate dehydrogenase
LH Luteinizing hormone
MCT4 Monocarboxylate transporter 4
mtDNA Mitochondrial DNA
NADH Nicotinamide adenine nucleotide
NADPH Nicotinamide adenine dinucleotide phosphate
nDNA Nuclear DNA
ONOO⁻ Peroxynitrite
OS Oxidative stress
PGC1-α Peroxisome proliferator-activated receptor gamma coactivator 1 α
RNA Ribonucleic acid
ROS Reactive oxygen species
SC Sertoli cell
SIRT3 Sirtuin 3
SSC Spermatogonial stem cell
T1DM Type 1 diabetes mellitus
T2DM Type 2 diabetes mellitus
UDP Uridine diphosphate

ACKNOWLEDGMENTS

This work was supported by the "Fundação para a Ciência e a Tecnologia" — FCT, cofunded by Fundo Europeu de Desenvolvimento Regional — FEDER via Programa Operacional Factores de Competitividade COMPETE/QREN to UMIB (Pest OE/SAU/UI0215/2014); POCI — COMPETE 2020 — Operational Programme Competitiveness and Internationalisation in Axis I. Strengthening research, technological development, and innovation (Project No. 007491) and National Funds by FCT — Foundation for Science and Technology (Project UID/Multi/00709); PF Oliveira (PTDC/BBB-BQB/1368/2014 and IFCT2015), MG Alves (PTDC/BIM-MET/4712/2014 and IFCT2015), L Rato was funded by Santander-Totta/University of Beira Interior (BIPD/ICI—CICS-BST-UBI).

REFERENCES

[1] World Health Organization, International Diabetes Federation. Definition and diagnosis of diabetes mellitus and intermediate hyperglycaemia: report of a WHO/IDF consultation. 2006.
[2] International Diabetes Federation. IDF diabetes atlas. 7th ed. Brussels: International Diabetes Federation; 2015.
[3] Wild S, Roglic G, Green A, et al. Global prevalence of diabetes: estimates for the year 2000 and projections for 2030. Diabetes Care 2004;27(5):1047—53.
[4] Agbaje IM, Rogers DA, McVicar CM, et al. Insulin dependant diabetes mellitus: implications for male reproductive function. Hum Reprod 2007;22(7):1871—7.
[5] Hamilton BE, Hoyert DL, Martin JA, et al. Annual summary of vital statistics: 2010—2011. Pediatrics 2013;131(3):548—58.
[6] Fedele D. Therapy Insight: sexual and bladder dysfunction associated with diabetes mellitus. Nat Clin Pract Urol 2005;2(6):282—90. quiz 309.
[7] Tabak O, Gelisgen R, Erman H, et al. Oxidative lipid, protein, and DNA damage as oxidative stress markers in vascular complications of diabetes mellitus. Clin Investig Med 2011;34(3):E163—71.
[8] Brownlee M. Biochemistry and molecular cell biology of diabetic complications. Nature 2001;414(6865):813—20.
[9] Sakkas D, Alvarez JG. Sperm DNA fragmentation: mechanisms of origin, impact on reproductive outcome, and analysis. Fertil Steril 2010;93(4):1027—36.
[10] Shrilatha B, Muralidhara. Early oxidative stress in testis and epididymal sperm in streptozotocin-induced diabetic mice: its progression and genotoxic consequences. Reprod Toxicol 2007;23(4):578—87.
[11] Amiri I, Karimi J, Piri H, et al. Association between nitric oxide and 8-hydroxydeoxyguanosine levels in semen of diabetic men. Syst Biol Reprod Med 2011;57(6):292—5.
[12] Aitken RJ, De Iuliis GN, Finnie JM, et al. Analysis of the relationships between oxidative stress, DNA damage and sperm vitality in a patient population: development of diagnostic criteria. Hum Reprod 2010;25(10):2415—26.
[13] Aitken RJ, Gibb Z, Baker MA, et al. Causes and consequences of oxidative stress in spermatozoa. Reprod Fertil Dev 2016;28(2):1—10.
[14] Kodama H, Yamaguchi R, Fukuda J, et al. Increased oxidative deoxyribonucleic acid damage in the spermatozoa of infertile male patients. Fertil Steril 1997;68(3):519—24.
[15] Agarwal A, Said TM. Role of sperm chromatin abnormalities and DNA damage in male infertility. Hum Reprod Update 2003;9(4):331—45.
[16] Dias TR, Alves MG, Casal S, et al. The single and synergistic effects of the major tea components caffeine, epigallocatechin-3-gallate and L-theanine on rat sperm viability. Food Funct 2016;7(3):1301—5.

[17] Weir GC, Bonner-Weir S. Five stages of evolving beta-cell dysfunction during progression to diabetes. Diabetes 2004;53(Suppl. 3):S16—21.

[18] American Diabetes Association. 2. Classification and diagnosis of diabetes. Diabetes Care 2017;40(Suppl. 1):S11—24.

[19] Joseph J, Koka M, Aronow WS. Prevalence of moderate and severe renal insufficiency in older persons with hypertension, diabetes mellitus, coronary artery disease, peripheral arterial disease, ischemic stroke, or congestive heart failure in an academic nursing home. J Am Med Dir Assoc 2008;9(4):257—9.

[20] La Vignera S, Calogero AE, Condorelli R, et al. Andrological characterization of the patient with diabetes mellitus. Minerva Endocrinol 2009;34(1):1—9.

[21] De Young L, Yu D, Bateman RM, Brock GB. Oxidative stress and antioxidant therapy: their impact in diabetes-associated erectile dysfunction. J Androl 2004;25(5):830—6.

[22] Ellenberg M, Weber H. Retrograde ejaculation in diabetic neuropathy. Ann Intern Med 1966;65(6):1237—46.

[23] La Vignera S, Condorelli R, Vicari E, et al. Diabetes mellitus and sperm parameters. J Androl 2012;33(2):145—53.

[24] Schoeller EL, Albanna G, Frolova AI, Moley KH. Insulin rescues impaired spermatogenesis via the hypothalamic-pituitary-gonadal axis in Akita diabetic mice and restores male fertility. Diabetes 2012;61(7):1869—78.

[25] Havrankova J, Schmechel D, Roth J, Brownstein M. Identification of insulin in rat brain. Proc Natl Acad Sci U S A 1978;75(11):5737—41.

[26] Seethalakshmi L, Menon M, Diamond D. The effect of streptozotocin-induced diabetes on the neuroendocrine-male reproductive tract axis of the adult rat. J Urol 1987;138(1):190—4.

[27] Pitteloud N, Hardin M, Dwyer AA, et al. Increasing insulin resistance is associated with a decrease in Leydig cell testosterone secretion in men. J Clin Endocrinol Metabol 2005;90(5):2636—41.

[28] Ding EL, Song Y, Malik VS, Liu S. Sex differences of endogenous sex hormones and risk of type 2 diabetes: a systematic review and meta-analysis. J Am Med Assoc 2006;295(11):1288—99.

[29] Cameron DF, Murray FT, Drylie DD. Interstitial compartment pathology and spermatogenic disruption in testes from impotent diabetic men. Anat Rec 1985;213(1):53—62.

[30] Cheng CY, Wong EW, Yan HH, Mruk DD. Regulation of spermatogenesis in the microenvironment of the seminiferous epithelium: new insights and advances. Mol Cell Endocrinol 2010;315(1—2):49—56.

[31] Ricci G, Catizone A, Esposito R, et al. Diabetic rat testes: morphological and functional alterations. Andrologia 2009;41(6):361—8.

[32] Padron RS, Dambay A, Suarez R, Mas J. Semen analyses in adolescent diabetic patients. Acta Diabetol Lat 1984;21(2):115—21.

[33] Bartak V, Josifko M, Horackova M. Juvenile diabetes and human sperm quality. Int J Fertil 1975;20(1):30—2.

[34] Niven MJ, Hitman GA, Badenoch DF. A study of spermatozoal motility in type 1 diabetes mellitus. Diabet Med 1995;12(10):921—4.

[35] Ali ST, Shaikh RN, Siddiqi NA, Siddiqi PQ. Semen analysis in insulin-dependent/non-insulin-dependent diabetic men with/without neuropathy. Arch Androl 1993;30(1):47—54.

[36] Ranganathan P, Mahran AM, Hallak J, Agarwal A. Sperm cryopreservation for men with nonmalignant, systemic diseases: a descriptive study. J Androl 2002;23(1):71—5.

[37] La Vignera S, Condorelli RA, Vicari E, et al. Seminal vesicles and diabetic neuropathy: ultrasound evaluation in patients with couple infertility and different levels of glycaemic control. Asian J Androl 2011;13(6):872—6.

[38] La Vignera S, Condorelli RA, Di Mauro M, et al. Reproductive function in male patients with type 1 diabetes mellitus. Andrology 2015;3(6):1082—7.

[39] Hassan AA, Hassouna MM, Taketo T, et al. The effect of diabetes on sexual behavior and reproductive tract function in male rats. J Urol 1993;149(1):148—54.

[40] Soudamani S, Malini T, Balasubramanian K. Effects of streptozotocin-diabetes and insulin replacement on the epididymis of prepubertal rats: histological and histomorphometric studies. Endocr Res 2005;31(2):81—98.

[41] Kim ST, Moley KH. Paternal effect on embryo quality in diabetic mice is related to poor sperm quality and associated with decreased glucose transporter expression. Reproduction 2008;136(3):313—22.

[42] Moley KH, Vaughn WK, DeCherney AH, Diamond MP. Effect of diabetes mellitus on mouse pre-implantation embryo development. J Reprod Fertil 1991;93(2):325—32.

[43] Sergerie M, Laforest G, Bujan L, et al. Sperm DNA fragmentation: threshold value in male fertility. Hum Reprod 2005;20(12):3446—51.

[44] Baynes JW. Role of oxidative stress in development of complications in diabetes. Diabetes 1991;40(4):405—12.

[45] Pourova J, Kottova M, Voprsalova M, Pour M. Reactive oxygen and nitrogen species in normal physiological processes. Acta Physiol 2010;198(1):15—35.

[46] Saalu LC. The incriminating role of reactive oxygen species in idiopathic male infertility: an evidence based evaluation. Pakistan J Biol Sci 2010;13(9):413—22.

[47] Ochsendorf FR. Infections in the male genital tract and reactive oxygen species. Hum Reprod Update 1999;5(5):399—420.

[48] Organization WH. WHO laboratory manual for the examination and processing of human semen. 5th ed. WHO Press; 2010.

[49] La Vignera S, Di Mauro M, Condorelli R, et al. Diabetes worsens spermatic oxidative "stress" associated with the inflammation of male accessory sex glands. Clin Ter 2009;160(5):363—6.

[50] Henkel RR. Leukocytes and oxidative stress: dilemma for sperm function and male fertility. Asian J Androl 2011;13(1):43—52.

[51] Corona G, Monami M, Rastrelli G, et al. Type 2 diabetes mellitus and testosterone: a meta-analysis study. Int J Androl 2011;34(6 Pt 1):528—40.

[52] Rato L, Alves MG, Dias TR, et al. Testicular metabolic reprogramming in neonatal streptozotocin-induced type 2 diabetic rats impairs glycolytic flux and promotes glycogen synthesis. J Diab Res 2015;2015:13.

[53] Rato L, Alves MG, Duarte AI, et al. Testosterone deficiency induced by progressive stages of diabetes mellitus impairs glucose metabolism and favors glycogenesis in mature rat Sertoli cells. Int J Biochem Cell Biol 2015;66:1—10.

[54] Boussouar F, Benahmed M. Lactate and energy metabolism in male germ cells. Trends Endocrinol Metabol 2004;15(7):345—50.

[55] Oliveira PF, Alves MG, Rato L, et al. Effect of insulin deprivation on metabolism and metabolism-associated gene transcript levels of in vitro cultured human Sertoli cells. Biochim Biophys Acta Gen Subj 2012;1820(2):84—9.

[56] Dias TR, Alves MG, Bernardino RL, et al. Dose-dependent effects of caffeine in human Sertoli cells metabolism and oxidative profile: relevance for male fertility. Toxicology 2015;328:12—20.

[57] Spiro MJ. Effect of diabetes on the sugar nucleotides in several tissues of the rat. Diabetologia 1984;26(1):70—5.

[58] Rato L, Alves MG, Dias TR, et al. High-energy diets may induce a pre-diabetic state altering testicular glycolytic metabolic profile and male reproductive parameters. Andrology 2013;1(3):495—504.

[59] Rato L, Duarte AI, Tomas GD, et al. Pre-diabetes alters testicular PGC-1alpha/SIRT3 axis modulating mitochondrial bioenergetics and oxidative stress. Biochim Biophys Acta Bioenerg 2014;1837(3):335—44.

[60] Kong X, Wang R, Xue Y, et al. Sirtuin 3, a new target of PGC-1α, plays an important role in the suppression of ROS and mitochondrial biogenesis. PLoS One 2010;5(7):e11707.

[61] Jensen B. Rat testicular lipids and dietary isomeric fatty acids in essential fatty acid deficiency. Lipids 1976;11(3):179—88.

[62] Chanseaume E, Tardy AL, Salles J, et al. Chronological approach of diet-induced alterations in muscle mitochondrial functions in rats. Obesity (Silver Spring) 2007;15(1):50—9.

[63] Villegas J, Kehr K, Soto L, et al. Reactive oxygen species induce reversible capacitation in human spermatozoa. Andrologia 2003;35(4):227—32.

[64] Guthrie HD, Welch GR. Effects of reactive oxygen species on sperm function. Theriogenology 2012;78(8):1700—8.

[65] Kilarkaje N, Al-Hussaini H, Al-Bader MM. Diabetes-induced DNA damage and apoptosis are associated with poly (ADP ribose) polymerase 1 inhibition in the rat testis. Eur J Pharmacol 2014;737:29—40.

[66] Shi Y, Buffenstein R, Pulliam DA, Van Remmen H. Comparative studies of oxidative stress and mitochondrial function in aging. Integr Comp Biol 2010;50(5):869—79.

[67] Li TS, Marban E. Physiological levels of reactive oxygen species are required to maintain genomic stability in stem cells. Stem Cell 2010;28(7):1178—85.

[68] Morimoto H, Iwata K, Ogonuki N, et al. ROS are required for mouse spermatogonial stem cell self-renewal. Cell Stem Cell 2013;12(6):774—86.

[69] Lee J, Kanatsu-Shinohara M, Morimoto H, et al. Genetic reconstruction of mouse spermatogonial stem cell self-renewal in vitro by Ras-cyclin D2 activation. Cell Stem Cell 2009;5(1):76—86.

[70] Arikawe A, Daramola A, Odofin A, Obika L. Alloxan-induced and insulin-resistant diabetes mellitus affect semen parameters and impair spermatogenesis in male rats. Afr J Reprod Health 2006;10(3):106—13.

[71] Aitken RJ, Clarkson JS. Cellular basis of defective sperm function and its association with the genesis of reactive oxygen species by human spermatozoa. J Reprod Fertil 1987;81(2):459—69.

[72] Celino FT, Yamaguchi S, Miura C, et al. Tolerance of spermatogonia to oxidative stress is due to high levels of Zn and Cu/Zn superoxide dismutase. PLoS One 2011;6(2):e16938.

[73] Paul C, Teng S, Saunders PT. A single, mild, transient scrotal heat stress causes hypoxia and oxidative stress in mouse testes, which induces germ cell death. Biol Reprod 2009;80(5):913—9.

[74] Nonogaki T, Noda Y, Narimoto K, et al. Localization of CuZn-superoxide dismutase in the human male genital organs. Hum Reprod 1992;7(1):81—5.

[75] Rengan AK, Agarwal A, van der Linde M, du Plessis SS. An investigation of excess residual cytoplasm in human spermatozoa and its distinction from the cytoplasmic droplet. Reprod Biol Endocrinol 2012;10:92.

[76] Agarwal A, Virk G, Ong C, du Plessis SS. Effect of oxidative stress on male reproduction. World J Mens Health 2014;32(1):1—17.

[77] Brouwers JF, Boerke A, Silva PF, et al. Mass spectrometric detection of cholesterol oxidation in bovine sperm. Biol Reprod 2011;85(1):128—36.

[78] Aitken RJ. The capacitation-apoptosis highway: oxysterols and mammalian sperm function. Biol Reprod 2011;85(1):9—12.

[79] Oliveira H, Spano M, Santos C, Pereira Mde L. Lead chloride affects sperm motility and acrosome reaction in mice: lead affects mice sperm motility and acrosome reaction. Cell Biol Toxicol 2009;25(4):341—53.

[80] Scarano WR, Messias AG, Oliva SU, et al. Sexual behaviour, sperm quantity and quality after short-term streptozotocin-induced hyperglycaemia in rats. Int J Androl 2006;29(4):482—8.

[81] Shaw JE, Sicree RA, Zimmet PZ. Global estimates of the prevalence of diabetes for 2010 and 2030. Diabetes Res Clin Pract 2010;87(1):4—14.

[82] Dias TR, Alves MG, Oliveira PF, Silva BM. Natural products as modulators of spermatogenesis: the search for a male contraceptive. Curr Mol Pharmacol 2014;7(2):154—66.

[83] Anderson RA, Polansky MM. Tea enhances insulin activity. J Agric Food Chem 2002;50(24):7182—6.

[84] Oliveira PF, Tomas GD, Dias TR, et al. White tea consumption restores sperm quality in prediabetic rats preventing testicular oxidative damage. Reprod Biomed Online 2015;31(4):544—56.

[85] Dias TR, Alves MG, Tomas GD, et al. White tea as a promising antioxidant medium additive for sperm storage at room temperature: a comparative study with green tea. J Agric Food Chem 2014;62(3):608—17.

[86] Dias TR, Alves MG, Oliveira PF, Silva BM. Natural products as modulators of spermatogenesis: the search for a male contraceptive. Curr Mol Pharmacol 2014;7(2):154—66.

[87] Gülçin I. Antioxidant properties of resveratrol: a structure—activity insight. Innovat Food Sci Emerg Technol 2010;11(1):210—8.

[88] Bakos HW, Mitchell M, Setchell BP, Lane M. The effect of paternal diet-induced obesity on sperm function and fertilization in a mouse model. Int J Androl 2011;34(5 Pt 1):402−10.

[89] Wang HJ, Wang Q, Lv ZM, et al. Resveratrol appears to protect against oxidative stress and steroidogenesis collapse in mice fed high-calorie and high-cholesterol diet. Andrologia 2015;47(1):59−65.

[90] Bucak MN, Ataman MB, Baspinar N, et al. Lycopene and resveratrol improve post-thaw bull sperm parameters: sperm motility, mitochondrial activity and DNA integrity. Andrologia 2015;47(5):545−52.

[91] Talebi AR, Mangoli E, Nahangi H, et al. Vitamin C attenuates detrimental effects of diabetes mellitus on sperm parameters, chromatin quality and rate of apoptosis in mice. Eur J Obstet Gynecol Reprod Biol 2014;181:32−6.

[92] Heeba GH, Hamza AA. Rosuvastatin ameliorates diabetes-induced reproductive damage via suppression of oxidative stress, inflammatory and apoptotic pathways in male rats. Life Sci 2015;141:13−9.

[93] Long L, Wang J, Lu X, et al. Protective effects of scutellarin on type II diabetes mellitus-induced testicular damages related to reactive oxygen species/Bcl-2/Bax and reactive oxygen species/microcirculation/staving pathway in diabetic rat. J Diab Res 2015:2015.

[94] Dias TR, Alves MG, Silva J, et al. Implications of epigallocatechin-3-gallate in cultured human Sertoli cells glycolytic and oxidative profile. Toxicol Vitro 2017;41.

[95] Cruz MH, Leal CL, da Cruz JF, et al. Role of melatonin on production and preservation of gametes and embryos: a brief review. Anim Reprod Sci 2014;145(3−4):150−60.

[96] Barrett P, Bolborea M. Molecular pathways involved in seasonal body weight and reproductive responses governed by melatonin. J Pineal Res 2012;52(4):376−88.

[97] Rocha CS, Martins AD, Rato L, et al. Melatonin alters the glycolytic profile of Sertoli cells: implications for male fertility. Mol Hum Reprod 2014;20.

[98] Maresch CC, Stute DC, Ludlow H, et al. Hyperglycemia is associated with reduced testicular function and activin dysregulation in the Ins2 Akita$^{+/-}$ mouse model of type 1 diabetes. Mol Cell Endocrinol 2017;446:91−101.

[99] Schoeller EL, Chi M, Drury A, et al. Leptin monotherapy rescues spermatogenesis in male Akita type 1 diabetic mice. Endocrinology 2014;155(8):2781−6.

[100] Cameron DF, Rountree J, Schultz RE, et al. Sustained hyperglycemia results in testicular dysfunction and reduced fertility potential in BBWOR diabetic rats. Am J Physiol 1990;259(6 Pt 1):E881−9.

[101] Amaral S, Moreno AJ, Santos MS, et al. Effects of hyperglycemia on sperm and testicular cells of Goto-Kakizaki and streptozotocin-treated rat models for diabetes. Theriogenology 2006;66(9):2056−67.

[102] Jelodar G, Khaksar Z, Pourahmadi M. Endocrine profile and testicular histomorphometry in adult rat offspring of diabetic mothers. J Physiol Sci 2009;59(5):377−82.

[103] Bartak V. Sperm quality in adult diabetic men. Int J Fertil 1979;24(4):226−32.

[104] Greene LF, Kelalis PP. Retrograde ejaculation of semen dueto diabetic neuropathy. J Urol 1967;98(6):696.

[105] Mallidis C, Agbaje IM, Rogers DA, et al. Advanced glycation end products accumulate in the reproductive tract of men with diabetes. Int J Androl 2009;32(4):295−305.

[106] Schoeffling K, Federlin K, Ditschuneit H, Pfeiffer EF. Disorders of sexual function in male diabetics. Diabetes 1963;12:519−27.

[107] Martins AD, Alves MG, Bernardino RL, et al. Effect of white tea (*Camellia sinensis* (L.)) extract in the glycolytic profile of Sertoli cell. Eur J Nutr 2014;53(6):1383−91.

[108] Dias TR, Alves MG, Rato L, et al. White tea intake prevents prediabetes-induced metabolic dysfunctions in testis and epididymis preserving sperm quality. J Nutr Biochem 2016;37:83−93.

[109] Faid I, Al-Hussaini H, Kilarkaje N. Resveratrol alleviates diabetes-induced testicular dysfunction by inhibiting oxidative stress and c-Jun N-terminal kinase signaling in rats. Toxicol Appl Pharmacol 2015;289.

[110] Fedail JS, Ahmed AA, Musa HH, et al. Gum arabic improves semen quality and oxidative stress capacity in alloxan induced diabetes rats. Asian Pacific J Reprod 2016;5(5):434−41.

[111] Ghanbari E, Nejati V, Khazaei M. Antioxidant and protective effects of Royal jelly on histopathological changes in testis of diabetic rats. Int J Reprod Biomed (Yazd) 2016;14(8):519−26.

Chapter 2.7

Thyroid Dysfunction and Testicular Redox Status: An Intriguing Association

Dipak Kumar Sahoo[1], Srikanta Jena[2] and Gagan B.N. Chainy[a,3]

[1]Iowa State University, Ames, IA, United States; [2]Ravenshaw University, Cuttack, Odisha, India; [3]Utkal University, Bhubaneswar, Odisha, India

INTRODUCTION

Infertility is a growing concern as globally, an estimated 48.5 million couples (15%) are affected by it [1,2]. The chief source of infertility is due to biological reasons, and psychological and emotional causes represent only 10% of the cases. Male infertility remains a hidden reproductive health disorder; still it contributes to more than half of all cases of childlessness worldwide [3]. Males are found to be merely accountable for 20%–30% of infertility cases that contribute up to 50% of overall cases. Furthermore, it has been revealed that the distribution of infertility due to male factors ranges from 20% to 70% and the global rates of male infertility range from 2.5% to 12%. While infertility rate is highest in Africa and Eastern Europe, at least 30 million men worldwide are infertile, estimated using the Sharlip factor [2].

Male fertility markers have been identified, studied, and evaluated extensively in order to comprehend the underlying molecular mechanisms that can lead to subfertility or infertility and also to permit precise diagnosis and design of therapeutic protocols. Changed thyroid status is recognized to unfavorably affect many organs and tissues in mammals. Nonetheless, for many years, the influence of thyroid disorders on male fertility remained debatable. The earlier reports showed that adult testes are metabolically insensitive to thyroid hormones (THs) as studied in thyroxine-injected rats [4]. The report of low concentrations of triiodothyronine nuclear binding sites in the adult organ [5] with inadequate available clinical data led to the general opinion that the testis was unresponsive to THs. However, various subsequent studies revealed the vital role TH plays in testicular development and male reproduction. Several studies also clearly demonstrated the association of TH with abnormal sexual function and male infertility, including for the functional development of the reproductive tract [6–9]. Moreover, the impact of altered TH status on male reproduction has been studied extensively in human subjects and animal models; the studies have mostly disclosed that altered thyroid function resulted in decreased sexual activity and fertility [10–12]. This chapter briefly represents a simplified picture of the current developments of our understanding regarding the role of the TH on testicular physiology, oxidative status, and fertility in general.

THYROID HORMONE AND ITS MODE OF ACTION

THs play a pivotal role in development, differentiation, growth, and metabolic homeostasis of virtually all tissues in vertebrates [13] via interacting with several signaling pathways. The signaling pathway for TH is complex and precisely regulated depending upon the organs because of the tissue-specific expression of TH transporters, presence of multiple TH receptor isoforms, and their cellular localization regulating the expression of TH receptor target genes, various TH response elements, distinct heterodimeric partners, and interactions with corepressors and coactivators [14,15]. Additionally, thyroid signals are also involved in cross-talk with other signaling pathways [14].

Under the regulation of the hypothalamic-pituitary axis, TH is secreted from the thyroid gland and it is synthesized in follicles of thyroid gland through iodination of tyrosine residues in the glycoprotein thyroglobulin (Fig. 1). Hypothalamus

---

a Present Address: Department of Biochemistry, North-Eastern Hill University, Shillong, Meghalaya 793022, India.

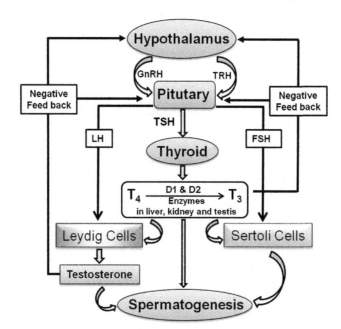

FIGURE 1 Diagrammatic representation of interaction between hypothalamus pituitary gonadal (HPG) and hypothalamus pituitary thyroid (HPT) axis and their roles in testicular development and spermatogenesis. *D1*, 5′-deiodinase type 1; *D2*, 5′-deiodinase type 2; *FSH*, follicle stimulating hormone; *GnRH*, gonadotropin-releasing hormone; *LH*, luteinizing hormone; *TRH*, thyroid releasing hormone; *TSH*, thyroid stimulating hormone; *T3*, triiodothyronine; *T4*, thyroxine. *The figure is modified from Rajender, S., Monicaz, M.G., Walterz, L., Agarwall, A. Thyroid, spermatogenesis, and male infertility. Front Biosci June 1, 2011, 3:843–55.*

secretes thyroid releasing hormone (TRH), which acts upon the pituitary gland, binding to G protein-coupled TRH-receptors on the thyrotropes, resulting in a rise in intracellular cyclic adenosine monophosphate and subsequent thyrotropin (thyroid stimulating hormone; TSH) release [16]. In response to feedback from circulating TH, the anterior pituitary secretes TSH that acts directly on the TSH receptor expressed on the membrane of thyroid follicular cells (Fig. 1). TSH controls iodide uptake mediated by the sodium/iodide symporter, followed by a series of steps needed for normal TH synthesis and secretion [14]. The thyroid gland secretes two iodine-containing hormones, triiodothyronine (T3) and thyroxine (T4). The prohormone T4 is activated to the active form T3 before regulating a wide range of genes [17]. The set point association between the level of serum T4 and T3 is stable for an individual, whereas it differs significantly among individuals and such variability in set point in the population indicates genetic effect involving one or more genes in the TH pathway [18].

The action of TH is manifested predominantly through a member of the superfamily of hormone-responsive nuclear transcription factors known as TH receptors (TRs) with more or less similar structures and mechanism of action [14]. The three functional receptor isoforms that bind T3 are TRα1, TRβ1, and TRβ2 [19]. The TRα gene encodes one T3-binding TRα1 and two splicing variants (TRα2 and TRα3). These two splicing variants vary from TRα1 in the length and amino acid sequences in the C-terminal region, beginning at amino acid 370, and without T3-binding activity [15]. The expression of the two TR genes, TRα and TRβ, differ depending upon the nature of the organ [14]. The TRβ1 isoform is mainly expressed in the liver and is known to facilitate the majority of the effects of T3 in this tissue [19]. The mechanism of action of TH is more or less similar in almost all types of cells and tissues. In general, binding of TH to TR promotes formation of TH and TR complex (TH-TR), which binds to the thyroid response element (TRE) present on the DNA and thereby regulates expression of genes in the presence of several activators, coactivators, and corepressors [14]. Liganded nuclear receptors associate with coactivators to enhance gene transcription, while nuclear receptors in the unliganded state bind to corepressors to promote gene repression. Both TRα and TRβ undergo posttranslational alteration by sumoylation, which is crucial for positive and negative gene regulation by TH. The nuclear TR has a zinc finger motif DNA binding domain and a COOH-terminal domain that enables ligand interactions together with binding of coactivators and co-repressors [15]. The TRE consists of two hexamer sequences, AGGTCA, with some sequence variation, arranged as direct repeats with a 4-bp gap. A class of nuclear receptors needs retinoid X receptor (RXR) as heterodimerization partner for their function. TR also forms a heterodimer complex with RXR, which binds to a TRE, stimulating or reducing gene transcription, whereas RXR generally binds the upstream hexamer and TR binds the downstream hexamer [14].

In this context, deiodinase enzymes deserve special attention because they play a significant function in adjusting circulating T3 as the intracellular action of TH is controlled by the quantity of local T3 accessible for receptor binding. The iodothyronine deiodinases include two activating enzymes, $5'$-deiodinase type 1 (D1) and $5'$-deiodinase type 2 (D2), and one inactivating enzyme, 5-deiodinase type 3 (D3). These enzymes are necessary for converting T4 to T3 (D1 and D2) and inactivating T3 and T4 to a nonbiological form (D3) and are differentially expressed developmentally and in adult tissues. The TH action is also regulated based on nutritional and iodine status [16,20,21]. Small variations in iodine intake are adequate to reset the thyroid system at different serum TSH levels in the negative feedback loop through modulating thyroid response to TSH [20]. Nutritional selenium deficiency is connected with the decreased activity of deiodinase as selenium is necessary for its catalytic activity [16,21], thus showing the importance of selenium in thyroid metabolism.

Regarding testis, the demonstration of thyroid transporters, thyroid receptors, and deiodinase enzymes suggest that mechanism of TH in testis is like any other tissues [22]. Expression of thyroid receptors and deiodinase enzymes have been shown in all three major testicular cell types such as Sertoli cells, germ cells, and Leydig cells [6]. Once TH is transported inside the testicular cells, deiodinase enzymes maintain its optimal levels for regulation of various testicular genes.

THYROID HORMONE AND TESTES

Role of Thyroid Hormone in Testicular Development

TH influences gametogenesis by regulating growth and differentiation of somatic cells in seminiferous epithelium [9,23]. During development, thyroid deficiency causes deleterious effects in testicular growth and maturation marked by a decrease in seminiferous tubule diameter, germ cell number per tubule, amplified degeneration, and arrested germ cell maturation [24–26] (Table 1). During fetal life, hypothyroidism was reported to have no effects on testicular development

TABLE 1 Regulation of Rat Testicular Oxidative Stress, Antioxidant Defense Parameters, and Testicular Physiology by Hyperthyroidism and Hypothyroidism and Effects of Antioxidant Treatments

Thyroid Disease	A. Hyperthyroidism
Changes in oxidative stress parameters	(1) Testicular oxidative stress is increased with elevated MDA [65,67,71] or TBARS levels, LOOH, H_2O_2, or PC contents [59,60,69,73,74] and NO concentration [65,71] during T3 or T4 induced hyperthyroidism.
	(2) Exposure to T3 or T4 decreases the percent of sperm head DNA showing induction of DNA damage in human sperm under high oxidative insult [76].
Deviations in the antioxidant defense system	Nonenzymatic antioxidants:
	(1) Short-term T4 administration to hypothyroid rats causes an increase in testicular GSH contents [65,70].
	(2) T3 treatment for 3 days to hypothyroid rats causes an elevation of GSSG and a decline in GSH contents resulting in a decreased GSH:GSSG ratio [69].
	(3) Testicular level of GSH is reduced by T4 [71] while T3 treatment decreases testicular total glutathione levels despite increasing GSH [74] and without changing GSSG levels [88]. The GSH:GSSG ratio remains higher during T4 or T3 induced hyperthyroidism [59,74].
	(4) Ascorbic acid content is also elevated in crude homogenate of hyperthyroid rat testis by T3 treatment [74].
	(5) Hyperthyroidism is associated with reduced level of β-carotene as compared with the normal group [115]; β-carotene provides an important antioxidant in keeping cells healthy and also in serving as a pool converted to vitamin A when needed [126].
	(6) Levels of vitamins A, E, and C concentration are decreased in hyperthyroid patients [115].

Continued

TABLE 1 Regulation of Rat Testicular Oxidative Stress, Antioxidant Defense Parameters, and Testicular Physiology by Hyperthyroidism and Hypothyroidism and Effects of Antioxidant Treatments—cont'd

Thyroid Disease	A. Hyperthyroidism
	Enzymatic antioxidants: (1) During acute hyperthyroid state, testis exhibits lower SOD activity and higher activities of CAT, GPx, GR, and G6PD enzymes [60,74]. In contrast, according to the study by Ourique et al., T3 treated hyperthyroid rat testis has lower CAT and GPx activities and higher GST activity [73]. (2) T4 induces a decrease in testicular SOD and CAT activities [71] while elevating GPx activity [59,65] with increase in both Se-D GPx and Se-I GPx activities [84]. Mitochondrial Se-I-GPx activity is also elevated due to T3 treatment [74]. In contrast, studies of El-Kashlan et al. [71] showed T4 treatment suppresses both GPx and GR activities. (3) According to Choudhury et al., hyperthyroidism induces CAT activity while it decreases GPx activity [69]. (4) Increased activity levels of most testicular antioxidant defense enzymes such as GPx, GR, GST, and CAT with decreased SOD activity have also been demonstrated in response to T3 induced hyperthyroidism [88].
Altered testicular physiology	(1) Transient juvenile hyperthyroidism causes an early termination of Sertoli cell proliferation and stimulates Sertoli cell maturation, resulting in premature canalization of seminiferous tubules, decreased testis size, and sperm production [6]. (2) Hyperthyroidism stimulates the differentiation of mesenchymal cells into progenitor Leydig cells [6]. (3) Hyperthyroidism is reported to lower genital sex organ weight; viable and total sperm count and motility; serum levels of LH, FSH, and T; testicular function markers and activities of testicular 3β-HSD and 17β-HSD; while inducing testicular DNA damage and dead and abnormal sperm counts [59,60,71,73,74]. (4) Testicular tissue of hyperthyroid rats shows histopathological changes characterized by degenerated, necrotic, shrunken, and disorganized seminiferous tubules with irregular basement membrane, incomplete spermatogenesis, increased interstitial space area, and wide lumens with few sperm [60,71]. (5) Immunohistochemical findings reveal that administration of T4 induces the expression of caspase-3 and Fas-L [71].
Effects of antioxidant treatments	(1) The coadministration of the DPP extract reduces the augmented level of MDA and NO and testicular DNA damage and apoptosis while it elevates CAT, SOD, GPx, and GR activities of hyperthyroid rat testis [71]. (2) The elevated testicular LPx and PC in response to T4 get reduced to the normal level by curcumin [59]. Treatment of curcumin to T4-treated rats results in elevation of testicular SOD and CAT activities [59]. Curcumin decreases the elevated testicular Se-D-GPx (GPx-1 and GPx-4) and Se-I-GPx of hyperthyroid rats to normal level [84]. The reduced oxidative stress condition is also due to the increased levels of GSH contents in testes of curcumin-fed hyperthyroid rats [59]. (3) Vitamin E decreases T4-induced testicular oxidative stress as marked by reduction in LPx and PC contents [59]. Treatment of vitamin E to T4-treated rats results in augmentation of testicular SOD and CAT activities. Vitamin E treatment also reduces the augmented testicular Se-D-GPx (GPx-1 and GPx-4) and Se-I-GPx of hyperthyroid rats to normal levels [84]. Vitamin E also increases GSH:GSSG ratio in T4-treated rats [59].

TABLE 1 Regulation of Rat Testicular Oxidative Stress, Antioxidant Defense Parameters, and Testicular Physiology by Hyperthyroidism and Hypothyroidism and Effects of Antioxidant Treatments—cont'd

Thyroid Disease	A. Hyperthyroidism
	(4) The RSV treatment decreases testicular LOOH and TBARS levels induced by T3 treatment while it increases CAT and GPx activities along with improving sperm motility in hyperthyroid rats [73].
	(5) The pinealectomy together with hyperthyroidism increase the MDA levels and reduce the levels of GSH. In hyperthyroidism induced by T4 after sham pinealectomy or pinealectomy, the testicular oxidative stress gets increased in hyperthyroid rats and the degree of damage is more marked with pinealectomy [67], demonstrating the important role of endogenous melatonin in reducing testicular oxidative damage during hyperthyroidism.
	(6) It has been found that while excess T3 and T4 induce DNA damage in human sperm, the addition of CAT and flavonoids Q and K inhibit such effects [76].
	(7) Normal testicular physiology is restored by vitamin E as noticed by elevation in total sperm and live sperm count in hyperthyroid rats treated with vitamin E [59].
	(8) Coadministration of DPP extract reverses the changes induced by hyperthyroidism in genital sex organs weight, sex hormones levels, 3β-HSD and 17β-HSD activities, and also normalizes both sperm count and motility with counteracting observed testicular DNA damage [71].
	(9) Testes from rats treated with DPP extract plus T4 exhibit less prominent histopathological changes when compared with those from the T4 induced hyperthyroid group with seminiferous tubules restored with their normal shape and diameter along with complete spermatogenic series [71].
	(10) Coadministration of DPP extract reduces the T4-induced overexpression of the proapoptotic markers (caspase-3 and Fas-L) to normal level [71].
Thyroid Disease	**B. Hypothyroidism**
Altered oxidative stress parameters	**(1)** While MDA level decreases [70], the levels of H_2O_2 and PC contents remain increased in the crude homogenate [69] of testis of hypothyroid rats. In addition, mitochondrial LPx and PC contents remain elevated in hypothyroid rat testis [63,69].
	(2) Increased PC level is also marked in hypothyroid immature rat testis [26].
	(3) The report by El-Kashlan et al. shows the augmentation of testicular MDA and NO by hypothyroidism [71]. However according to Zamoner et al., the oxygen consumption of testis in the newborn hypothyroid rats is significantly lower than the euthyroid controls without any difference in their LPx levels [68].
	(4) Increased prooxidant level and reduced antioxidant capacity render the hypothyroid mitochondria susceptible to oxidative injury [63] as marked by higher degree of oxidative damage imposed upon mitochondrial membrane lipids and proteins. While membrane proteins are shown to be more susceptible to carbonylation, thiol residue damage is evident in the mitochondrial matrix fraction due to hypothyroidism [63].
	(5) Transient hypothyroidism causes a decrease in testicular mitochondrial LPx while both the mitochondrial LPx and PC contents are elevated during persistent hypothyroidism [25].
	(6) The germ cells of transient hypothyroid rats exhibit higher LPx contents [72]. In contrast, STCs from rat testis show a decline in LPx, LOOH, H_2O_2, and protein oxidation in response to persistent and transient hypothyroidism [66].

Continued

TABLE 1 Regulation of Rat Testicular Oxidative Stress, Antioxidant Defense Parameters, and Testicular Physiology by Hyperthyroidism and Hypothyroidism and Effects of Antioxidant Treatments—cont'd

Thyroid Disease	B. Hypothyroidism
Deviations in the antioxidant defense system	**Nonenzymatic antioxidants** **(1)** In hypothyroid rats, testicular GSH level gets decreased compared to the control animals [25,69–71]. Besides, hypothyroid rat testis mitochondrial matrix also exhibits lower GSH and ascorbate contents [63] and higher GSSG contents leading to a decrease in the GSH:GSSG ratio [69]. Similar results of disturbed redox status is observed in immature rat testis by persistent hypothyroidism [26]. **(2)** In STCs of both persistent and transient neonatal hypothyroid rats, the OSI representing the ratio between GSSG and total GSH [79] remains elevated [66]. Germ cells of transient hypothyroid rats also exhibit lower GSH contents [72]. **(3)** Hypothyroid patients exhibit a decline in levels of vitamins A, E, and C concentration as compared to the control group [115].
	Enzymatic antioxidants **(1)** The activities of testicular SOD, GR, GPx, and CAT get significantly reduced in transient hypothyroid rats treated with PTU from birth to 30 days [25]. However, in adult rats, hypothyroidism induced after 90–120 days causes a decrease in both the testicular SOD and CAT activities [69,71] with an increase in GPX activity, hence reducing the ratio of SOD/CAT + GPX activities [69]. **(2)** Persistent hypothyroidism causes an elevation in SOD and CAT activities [25]. Persistent hypothyroidism reduces testicular GR and GPx activities including both Se-D-GPx and Se-I-GPx activities and mitochondrial GST levels [25,71,84]. **(3)** In hypothyroid immature rat testis, SOD, CAT, and GR activities are elevated while GPx and GST activities are reduced [26]. **(4)** The germ cells of transient hypothyroid rats exhibit lower CAT and SOD activities [72]. **(5)** In STCs of hypothyroid rats, SOD1 is upregulated transcriptionally and translationally as well as in activities while the SOD2 is decreased both translationally and in activities [66]. In STCs of persistent hypothyroid rat, both the transcription and the activity of CAT are induced [66]. Although transcript levels of GPx1 and GR did not change in STCs in response to hypothyroidism, their activities are elevated [66]. **(6)** Transient hypothyroidism is associated with reduced testicular SOD, CAT, GR, and GPx activities [25].
Changes in testicular physiology	**(1)** Neonatal transient hypothyroidism causes an increase in germ cell number resulting in enlargement of adult rat testis and an elevation of daily sperm production [25,30,31]. It prolongs the length of Sertoli cell proliferation by retarding their maturation and morphological differentiation, resulting in increased number of Sertoli cells in the adult testis [24,29–31]. It also causes an increase in the number of Leydig cells in adult rat testis [30,31,38] by arresting Leydig cell differentiation and promoting continuous proliferation of precursor mesenchymal cells.

TABLE 1 Regulation of Rat Testicular Oxidative Stress, Antioxidant Defense Parameters, and Testicular Physiology by Hyperthyroidism and Hypothyroidism and Effects of Antioxidant Treatments—cont'd

Thyroid Disease	B. Hypothyroidism
	(2) Continuous hypothyroidism from birth causes spermatogenic arrest at puberty resulting in a single layer of spermatogonia [27]. There have been also reports on the absence of round spermatids at 30 days in hypothyroid rat testis and the inability of the spermatogenic cells to complete meiosis [26,28]. Hypothyroidism induced from birth to adulthood is associated with delayed maturation of the testis, degeneration of germ cells, reduced seminiferous tubule diameter, and impaired spermatogenesis [6,24,25,28]. Persistent hypothyroidism in rats, from birth to 90 days, results in a significant decrease in germ cell (specifically primary spermatogonia and round spermatid) number, epididymal live sperm count, and GSI [25].
	(3) Decline in genital sex organ weight; sperm count and motility; serum levels of LH, FSH, and T; testicular function markers; and testicular 3β-HSD and 17β-HSD activities are observed in hypothyroidism with considerable testicular DNA damage [71].
	(4) Hypothyroid rat testicular tissue exhibits histopathological changes with degenerated, necrotic, shrunken, and disorganized seminiferous tubules with irregular basement membrane, incomplete spermatogenesis, increased interstitial space area, wide lumens, and few sperm [71].
	(5) Transient and persistent neonatal hypothyroidisms cause permanent upregulation of proapoptotic genes [43,71], hence increasing germ cell apoptosis [82].
Effects of antioxidant treatments	**(1)** The coadministration of the DPP extract reduces the augmented level of MDA and NO and testicular DNA damage and apoptosis while it elevates testicular CAT, SOD, GPx, and GR activities of hypothyroid rat testis [71].
	(2) Folic acid acts as an antioxidant and is also reported to reduce the MDA level in testes of hypothyroid rats and maintains the normal spermatogenesis by augmenting the level of testosterone, sperm count, and sperm motility [127].
	(3) Coadministration of DPP extract counteracted the observed changes in genital sex organ weight, sex hormone levels, 3β-HSD and 17β-HSD activities, sperm count and motility, and testicular DNA damage due to hypothyroidism [71].
	(4) Treatment with DPP extract to hypothyroid rats causes less noticeable testicular histopathological modifications with seminiferous tubules restoring their normal shape and diameter with complete spermatogenic series when compared with the hypothyroid animals [71].
	(5) Coadministration of DPP extract reduced the PTU-induced (hypothyroidism-induced) overexpression of caspase-3 and Fas-L proapoptotic markers to normal level [71].

References are shown in parentheses. *3β-HSD*, 3β-hydroxysteroid dehydrogenase; *17β-HSD*, 17β-hydroxysteroid dehydrogenase; *CAT*, catalase; *DPP*, date palm pollen; *FSH*, follicle stimulating hormone; *G6PD*, glucose-6-phosphate dehydrogenase; *GSH*, reduced glutathione; *GSH:GSSG*, reduced to oxidized glutathione ratio; *GPx*, glutathione peroxidase; *GR*, glutathione reductase; *GST*, glutathione S-transferase; *GSI*, gonadosomatic index; *GSSG*, oxidized glutathione; *H_2O_2*, hydrogen peroxide; *K*, kaempferol; *LOOH*, lipid hydroperoxide; *LPx*, lipid peroxide; *LH*, luteinizing hormone; *MDA*, malondialdehyde; *NO*, nitric oxide; *OSI*, oxidative stress index; *PC*, protein carbonyl; *Q*, quercetin; *PTU*, 6-n-propyl-2-thiouracil; *RSV*, resveratrol; *Se-I GPx*, Se-independent GPx; *Se-D GPx*, selenium dependent glutathione peroxidase; *SOD*, superoxide dismutase; *STCs*, seminiferous tubule cells; *T*, testosterone; *T3*, 3,3′,5-triiodo-L-thyronin; *T4*, L-thyroxine; *TBARS*, thiobarbituric acid-reactive substances.

[24]. However, hypothyroidism induced in newborn rats weakens testicular development affecting its growth, germ cell maturation, and seminiferous tubule formation at puberty [24–26]. Persistent hypothyroidism from birth also causes spermatogenic arrest at puberty marked by formation of only a single layer of spermatogonia [27], the lack of round spermatids as shown in 30 days hypothyroid rat testis [26,28]. Severe or prolonged neonatal hypothyroidism weakens the testicular development and function marked by reduced testicular weight and arrest of germ cell proliferation and differentiation, and increased degeneration of germ cells causing reduction in germ cell number with impaired spermatogenesis [6,9,24,27]. Testicular structural organization and physiology are also altered in response to different durations of hypothyroid condition. Both the testicular size and daily sperm production were elevated in adulthood when the hypothyroid animals allowed to recover to the euthyroid state [29]. The enlargement of adult rat testis and increase in daily sperm production are due to elevated germ cell number as demonstrated in juvenile hypothyroidism or neonatal transient hypothyroidism [25,30,31]. Temperature also plays an important role in regulating the neonatal hypothyroidism-induced changes in rat testicular size [32] as marked by lower testis mass; elevated germ cell degeneration; and decreased tubular size, germ cell numbers, and sperm density in the transient neonatal hypothyroid rats maintained at 34°C. The transient neonatal hypothyroid rats maintained under 21°C exhibited higher testis mass; lower body mass; and elevated tubular diameters, germ cell numbers, and sperm density [32].

Sertoli cells play a vital role in the initiation as well as maintenance of spermatogenesis and are source of many factors needed for germ cell survival within the seminiferous tubules [6]. The T3 receptors are highly expressed in proliferating Sertoli cells [33], indicating a major testicular target for TH. TH determines the duration of Sertoli cell division, delays their proliferation, stimulates differentiation, and is possibly involved in the maturational changes that reduce and abolish mitogenic responses to follicle stimulating hormone (FSH), as reported in many vertebrate species including rodents [6,9,34]. Transient neonatal/prepubertal hypothyroidism from birth up to day 30 postpartum prolongs the length of Sertoli cell proliferation by retarding their maturation and morphological differentiation, resulting in augmented number of Sertoli cells in the adult testis [24,30,31]. On the other hand, transient juvenile hyperthyroidism causes an early termination of Sertoli cell proliferation and stimulates Sertoli cell maturation, which subsequently results in premature canalization of seminiferous tubules, reduced testicular size, and reduced sperm production [6]. The T3 possibly regulates Sertoli cell proliferation by acting through particular cyclin-dependent kinase inhibitors (CDKIs), a family of proteins interacting directly with the cell cycle, and/or through a mechanism involving connexin43 (Cx43), a constitutive protein of gap junctions [6,35,36]. The TH also appears to affect the expression of many specific proteins associated with Sertoli cell differentiation through suppressing or upregulating them and also stimulates lactate production and protein synthesis in immature Sertoli cells and promotes amino acid accumulation [6,37].

Leydig cells are the principal source of testosterone (T) in males, and T is obligatory for the maintenance of reproductive function as well as appropriate functioning of many organ systems like muscle, bone, and skin. TH plays important roles in numerous features of Leydig cell development and function [38]. Through arresting Leydig cell differentiation and promoting continuous proliferation of precursor mesenchymal cells, juvenile hypothyroidism or neonatal transient hypothyroidism elevates the number of Leydig cells in adult rat testis [30,31,38]. On the contrary, hyperthyroidism promotes the differentiation of mesenchymal cells into progenitor Leydig cells [6]. Though THs also directly affect Leydig cell steroidogenesis, some TH-mediated alterations witnessed in Sertoli cells might indirectly influence Leydig cell differentiation as Sertoli cell–secreted proteins are known to have stimulatory effects on Leydig cells [6,31].

Impact of Altered Postnatal Thyroid Hormone Status on Adult Testes

Studies related to the role of TH on adult testis have inconsistent results. Though the previous studies demonstrated minor effects of induced hypothyroidism on testicular morphology, spermatogenesis, and serum T levels in adult rats [39,40], later studies established that hypothyroidism induced from birth to adulthood is linked with delayed maturation of the testis, degeneration of germ cells, decreased seminiferous tubule diameter, and impaired spermatogenesis [6,24,25,28] (Table 1). Persistent hypothyroidism induced by treating rats from birth to 90 days with 6-n-propyl-2-thiouracil (PTU) results in reduction in germ cell (specifically primary spermatogonia and round spermatid) number, epididymal live sperm count, and gonadosomatic index (GSI) [25] (Table 1). Sahoo et al. stated that the histoarchitectural disturbances in testes in persistent hypothyroidism lead to accumulation of germ cells and debris in the lumen and possibly cause a disruption in the normal sperm release from Sertoli cells and thereby decrease the sperm count in adults [25].

The effects of prolonged TH deficiency on testes from early neonatal life to the adult stage in rdw rats (having lower serum T4 levels because of a missense mutation in the thyroglobulin gene) showed the delayed structural development in the adult rdw rat testes. Soon after the full testicular maturation, normal morphology started to degenerate, and many germ cells underwent apoptosis, the germinal epithelium became thin, and finally resulted atrophic testes [6,41]. Comparable histological alterations were marked in adult rat testis exposed to chronic TH deficiency because of thyroidectomy performed early in life [6,42]. Transient and persistent neonatal hypothyroidisms cause permanent upregulation of proapoptotic genes in rat seminiferous tubule cells, which possibly could damage testicular physiological functions in adulthood [43]. Hypothyroidism arrests Leydig stem cell differentiation in the postnatal testis in rats but can be stimulated by supplementation with THs. In prolonged hypothyroid condition beyond the neonatal—prepubertal period, the fetal Leydig cells undergo cell atrophy and lose their T secretory capacity, which leads to the arrest in differentiation of adult population of Leydig cells [38]. On the other hand, in the neonatal—prepubertal animals, Sertoli cells in the seminiferous tubules continue to proliferate but fail to mature during the hypothyroid period. After withdrawal of hypothyroid status, the matured Sertoli cells number per testis is more like euthyroid testes as they went through a prolonged proliferative period due to hypothyroidism. This is one of the major reasons why transiently hypothyroid animals have larger testes at adulthood with increased sperm count with respect to the control animals [29]. Consistent hypothyroidism may decrease sperm count due to its influence on Sertoli cells. It has been reported that THs stimulate Sertoli cells to uptake glucose and in turn to secrete substances such as lactate, which is essential for the survival of germ cells and growth factors such as insulin-like growth factor-1 (IGF-1), which stimulate the synthesis of DNA in mitotic germ cells [44].

Observations in these studies point out that TH plays a vital role in the neonatal—prepubertal life in maintaining Sertoli and Leydig cell population in the adult testis and is critical to the general maintenance and reproductive functions in adulthood. Moreover, hypothyroidism in adult mice also elevates D2 expression significantly in testis [6]. While in the adult rat testes D2 expression is highly concentrated in elongated spermatids, other germ cells and Sertoli cells are virtually negative for this enzyme [45]. This suggests the possible role of TH, specifically on the spermiogenic phase in spermatogenesis in the adult rat testis [6].

Thyroid Receptors in Testicular Cells

TRs are widely dispersed in different testicular compartments. The presence of particular TH nuclear binding sites was first reported in Sertoli cell-enriched extracts [46] and in developing rat testis [47]. The TR expression is highest throughout the perinatal period and afterward gets dropped, but the T3 binding capacity is not totally absent in adult testis [44]. In human fetal and adult Sertoli cells only the TRα1 and TRα2 isoforms are expressed whereas TRβ isoform is absent [33]. While TRα2 is highly expressed at all stages, the TRα2/TRα1 ratio increases gradually from fetal to adult life. In rats, the TRα1 is the predominant isoform expressed both in immature proliferating Sertoli cells and mature adult Sertoli cells. The TRα1 expression was highest in late fetal and early neonatal life and confined to Sertoli cells, suggesting the chief target cells for T3 action in testis. The mRNAs of TRα2, TRα3, and TRβ1 were detected in Sertoli cells during development, but their corresponding proteins were found to be absent [48]. To establish the comparative functions of TRα1 and TRβ1 receptors in facilitating T3 effects on Sertoli cells and testicular development, Holsberger et al. [36] used TRα and TRβ knockout transgenic mice that lacked TRα or TRβ isoforms and observed that TRα! is the particular TR isoform that facilitates T3 effects in neonatal Sertoli cells.

Besides Sertoli cells, the active TR isoforms, including TRβ1, are present in Leydig cells, peritubular cells, and germ cells throughout neonatal development and also in the adult testis [6,44]. Rat mesenchymal stem cells, immature and adult Leydig cells, express the TRα isoform, their expression being maximal in the postnatal age, and decreases to almost negligible levels in adulthood. Studies also demonstrate that T3 binds specifically to nuclei of goat Leydig cells and consequently stimulates androgen production from these cells [49]. TRs are identified at different stages of developing rat germ cells such as gonocyte, spermatogonia, preleptotene, leptotene, pachytene, zygotene, and round and elongating spermatids. Both TRα and TRβ1 are expressed during different stages of germ cell development. TRβ1 first appears in intermediate-type spermatogonia while TRα first appear in type B spermatogonia [48]. The presence of TRs on germ cells implies a possible role of THs in supporting a different population of germ cells.

Expression of Thyroid Hormone Transporter and Manifestation of Iodothyronine Deiodinase

Specific TH membrane transporters were detected in testes [6]. The organic anion-transporting polypeptides (OATPs) form a family of influx transporters and are expressed in various tissues including testis in rodents and humans [6,50]. A specific OATP molecule named OATP1C1 [51], which transports T4 and reverse T3 (rT3) with high affinity, was identified in the human testis and was found to be expressed only in Leydig cells [52]. Three novel members of the OATPs family designated rat GsT-1 (gonad-specific transporter), rat GsT-2, and human GsT were identified in human and rat testis [6,53]. The rat GsT-1 and GsT-2 are highly expressed and transport T4 and T3 in Sertoli cells, spermatogonia, and Leydig cells as shown by functional studies. Furthermore, two novel splice variants of OATPs were found to be expressed in testicular cells such as OATP3A1-V1 in germ cells and OATP3A1-V2 in Sertoli cells but their physiological significance in regulating TH bioavailability to testicular cells is presently unknown [6].

Testicular 5'-deiodinase is an important factor in adjusting local bioavailability of active T3 and a key factor in testicular paracrine function. Testis expresses all three deiodinases (D1, D2, and D3) at different levels from weaning to adult life whereas D2 is the predominant activating enzyme in this organ [6,54]. D3 activity predominates in the developmental period but it decreases in adult life. D2 activity was increased in neonatal hypothyroid rat testis, signifying a D2 role in maintaining T3 concentration in testis when T4 levels are decreased in plasma [54].

THYROID DYSFUNCTION AND OXIDATIVE STRESS IN TESTES

Oxygen is indispensable for sustaining life as it is essential to maintain normal cell function. Mitochondria are the site where the incomplete reduction of oxygen takes place in its electron transport chain to produce reactive oxygen species (ROS). The ROS are the group of oxygen free radicals comprised of atoms, ions, or molecules with one or more unpaired electrons in their outer orbits. Such free radicals are superoxide (O_2^-), hydroxyl radical (HO•), hydrogen peroxide (H_2O_2), singlet oxygen ($^1O_2$), and so on, and these are extremely reactive until they bind to any atom or molecules to reach its octet state [55]. Oxidative stress (OS) was originally defined by Sies [56] as a disturbance in the prooxidant—antioxidant balance in favor of the former, leading to potential damage. Aerobic cells defend themselves from the OS generated due to the ROS by counteracting them by their highly evolved enzymatic and nonenzymatic antioxidant defenses [55] (Fig. 2). ROS, the by-products of tissue metabolism, are usually treated by physiological antioxidants. A decline in ROS formation is frequently due to an escalation in antioxidant capacity, while a decrease in the antioxidant capacity may be associated with increased ROS values. However, this is not always apparently so. Under physiological conditions, ROS can oxidize several biological molecules such as unsaturated fatty acids, sulphydryl proteins, and nucleic acids. Lipids are one of the preferential targets of ROS within the plasma membrane resulting in lipid peroxidation (LPx), which disrupts the bilayer

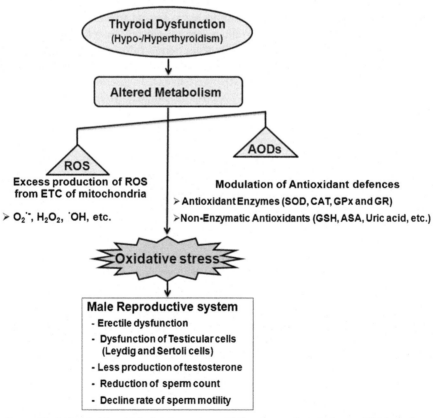

FIGURE 2 Schematic diagram illustrating that thyroid dysfunction causes oxidative stress and exerts abnormalities in male reproductive system. *CAT*, catalase; *ROS*, reactive oxygen species; *SOD*, superoxide dismutase; *GPx*, glutathione peroxidase; *GR*, glutathione reductase; *GSH*, reduced glutathione; *GST*; glutathione S-transferase; *ASA*, ascorbic acid; *AODs*, antioxidant defences.

structure, alters membrane attributes such as membrane fluidity, modifies the physiological functions of cell membranes, and contributes to cell membrane damage. THs are known to trigger OS in various tissues such as heart, blood, brain, muscle, kidney, liver, and testis [25,26,57−63]. Testis is associated with two highly energy-consuming physiological processes: spermatogenesis and steroidogenesis. Furthermore, testis is very rich in polyunsaturated fatty acids (PUFAs) (particularly 20:4 and 22:6), which are prone to peroxidation by prooxidant agents, and it has poor enzymatic and nonenzymatic antioxidant defense systems [64] (Fig. 2). OS has been recognized as one of the very significant factors that impact fertility status and has been studied extensively, including its role under influence of different thyroid states [25,26,59,60,63,65−70] (Table 1).

Hypothyroidism

Hypothyroidism is associated with a hypometabolic state and modifies both testicular oxidant generation and an antioxidant defense system. While in hypothyroid rat testes, OS parameters like malondialdehyde (MDA) level was reduced [70], and the levels of H_2O_2 and protein carbonyl (PC) contents were increased in the testicular crude homogenate [69]. In addition, testicular mitochondrial LPx and PC contents were augmented in hypothyroid rats [63,69] (Table 1). Distinct elevated testicular PC levels in hypothyroid immature rats also clearly signifies the prevalence of OS in hypothyroid condition [26]. El-Kashlan et al. also reported about the augmentation of testicular MDA and nitric oxide (NO) induced by hypothyroidism [71] (Table 1). Zamoner et al. reported significantly lower oxygen consumption of testis in the newborn hypothyroid rats than in the euthyroid controls; however, without any difference in their LPx levels [68]. Their observations also suggest that ROS levels do not increase, but reduced antioxidant activity could lead to OS in a hypothyroid state [68]. Elevated levels of prooxidants and decreased antioxidant capability rendered hypothyroid mitochondria vulnerable to oxidative damage [63], and it is reflected by augmented thiobarbituric acid-reactive substance (TBARS) levels and PC contents in mitochondrial membrane fractions, increased mitochondrial H_2O_2 contents, and thiol residue damage in mitochondrial matrix fraction [63]. Sahoo et al. also stated that although there was a decreased mitochondrial LPx in transient hypothyroidism, both the mitochondrial LPx and PC contents were increased in testis during persistent hypothyroidism [25].

Germ cells isolated from PTU-induced transient hypothyroid rats displayed higher LPx contents due to compromised antioxidant defense status [72]. In contrast, in another study on seminiferous tubule cells (STCs) from rat testis shows a decline in general OS indices like LPx, lipid hydroperoxide (LOOH), H_2O_2, and protein oxidation in response to persistent and transient hypothyroidism, while OS index was elevated in both the groups of hypothyroid rats [66].

Hyperthyroidism

For experimentally inducing hyperthyroidism, rats were either administered with T4 [59,65,67] or tri-iodothyronine (T3) [60,69,73,74], and their tissues were evaluated for oxidative damage. Mostly tissues display high susceptibility to oxidative damage [57,58] during hyperthyroidism, but the extent of OS also depends upon the tissue specificity and different TH isomers used to induce hyperthyroidism. Hypermetabolic state in hyperthyroidism stimulates free radical production [57] and inevitably induces LPx in different tissues depending on its severity [57,58,61−63,75]. OS is elevated in testis marked by increased MDA levels during T4-induced hyperthyroidism [65,67,71] or by augmented TBARS, LOOH, H_2O_2, or PC contents during T4 or tri-iodothyronine-induced hyperthyroidism [59,60,69,73,74] (Table 1). Testicular NO level was also elevated significantly following experimentally induced hyperthyroidism [65,71]. Dobrzyńska et al. studied the effects of the THs T4 and T3 on the induction of DNA damage in human sperm by comet assay, and DNA damage was quantified as a reduction in percent sperm head DNA compared to control [76]. According to the study, exposure to T3 or T4 decreased the percent of sperm head DNA. These results point towards a high oxidative insult of testis or sperm caused by the TH treatment.

THYROID DYSFUNCTION AND ANTIOXIDANT DEFENSES IN TESTES

Like other aerobic cells, testicular cells have antioxidant defense system comprising both small molecular weight antioxidants like ascorbic acid, vitamin E, reduced glutathione (GSH), uric acid, ubiquinone, and carotenoids; and antioxidant enzymes like superoxide dismutase (SOD), catalase (CAT), glutathione peroxidase (GPx), glutathione reductase (GR), and glutathione S-transferase (GST) for neutralizing generated ROS and also for inhibiting the oxidation of cellular macromolecules like lipids, proteins, and DNA by oxygen free radicals [75,77,78] (Fig. 2).

Hypothyroidism

The role of both persistent and transient hypothyroidism in modulating testicular antioxidant defense system was studied extensively including its impacts during testicular development and maturation [25,26,66,69–72] (Table 1). Testicular GSH level is decreased in hypothyroid rats compared to the control animals [25,69–71]. Along with GSH, ascorbate contents were also decreased in mitochondrial matrix of testis in hypothyroid rats [63]. In contrast, oxidized glutathione (GSSG) content was increased and because of which there is a decline in the ratio of reduced glutathione to oxidized glutathione (GSH:GSSG) during hypothyroidism, suggesting prevalence of OS in the testis [69]. A similar result of disturbed redox status was observed in immature rat testis by persistent hypothyroidism [26]. As a result, the OS index (OSI), represented as the ratio between GSSG and total GSH (OSI = $100 \times (2 \times GSSG)$/total GSH) [79] remained elevated in STCs of both persistent and transient neonatal hypothyroid rat testes [66]. The GSH contents were also found to be lower in testicular germ cells of transient hypothyroid rats [72]. High intracellular GSSG content might be responsible for triggering cell death [80] and decrease in intracellular GSH contents also accelerates germ cell apoptosis [81] as clearly evident from augmented germ cell apoptosis and elevated proapoptotic protein expression levels in testis in response to persistent and transient neonatal hypothyroidism [43,82].

Like nonenzymatic defenses, hypothyroidism also modulates testicular enzymatic defenses [25,26,66,68,69,71] (Table 1). The activities of testicular SOD, GR, GPx, and CAT were decreased significantly in transient hypothyroid rats treated from birth to 30 days [25]. However, in experimentally induced adult hypothyroid rats (induced after 90–120 days), both the testicular SOD and CAT activities were reduced [69,71] while GPx activity was elevated, resulting in a significant decline in the ratio of SOD/CAT + GPX [69]. Persistent hypothyroidism reduces the rat testicular mitochondrial GST levels and induces SOD and CAT activities [25] while it causes a reduction in GPx and GR activities [25,71]. These discrepancies have been attributed to alterations in the age of treated animals, period of treatment, and experimental methods for inducing hypothyroidism [25,26,31,38]. Moreover, testicular antioxidant defense parameters and OS status are known to be associated with aging [26,83].

Persistent hypothyroidism reduces both testicular selenium-dependent glutathione peroxidase (Se-D-GPx) and selenium-independent glutathione peroxidase (Se-I-GPx) activities [84]. Such decline in Se-D-GPx (which includes GPx-1 and GPx-4) and Se-I-GPx activities and increased SOD as well as CAT activities exhibit a key role of SOD and CAT antioxidant enzymes to combat OS than GPx in testes of rats during persistent hypothyroidism [25]. However, in hypothyroid immature rat testis, the activities of SOD, CAT, and GR were elevated while GPx and GST activities were reduced [26]. It is important to note that due to lack of CAT in testicular mitochondria, GPx plays an important role in neutralizing H_2O_2 in it. Lower GPx activity also influences T level as marked by decreased serum T level in hypothyroid rats [25,26]. It is noteworthy that T biosynthetic metabolic pathway needs protection against peroxidation [25,26]. Such altered antioxidant defense status in testis in rats before puberty affects testicular growth and development unfavorably by influencing spermatogenesis and steroidogenesis as marked by triggered germ cell apoptosis, decreased germ cell count [43,82,85], complete absence of round spermatids, reduced seminiferous tubule diameter, and declined T level [26]. Due to such type of adversely affected testicular physiology by hypothyroidism, fertility is hampered significantly in adulthood as evident from decreased viable germ cell number [72] and sperm counts [25].

Both the CAT and SOD antioxidant enzyme activities were decreased in testicular germ cells in transient hypothyroid rats [72]. Furthermore, a detailed study by Sahoo et al. revealed differential effects of PTU-induced neonatal hypothyroidism on the expression of two types of SOD (SOD1 and SOD2) at different levels (activity, translational, and transcriptional) in STCs [66]. While SOD1 gets upregulated transcriptionally, translationally as well as in activities, the SOD2 transcripts remain unchanged with fewer translated products and activities in STCs of hypothyroid rats than the control. Sahoo et al. stated that the unchanged mRNA level of SOD2 in hypothyroid rats could be due to the oxidation of transcription factors [66]. SOD2 expression is regulated not only at transcriptional level but also at the translational level through RNA binding proteins in mammalian cells [86]. The binding of proteins to RNA might have declined the SOD2 translated products and subsequently the activity [66]. On the contrary, there was an elevation of CAT transcripts and its activity in STCs of persistent hypothyroid rat in comparison to euthyroid and transient hypothyroid, but in case of translated products the condition was just reversed [66]. Such inconsistency between the level of transcription and translation of CAT might be because of decreased mRNA stability or reduced translational efficiency through binding of different transcription factors and RNA binding proteins [66]. In an earlier report, Van Remmen et al. opined that the CAT gene is under direct control of TH as evident from the presence of TRE (5′-AGGTCA-3′) as an inverted palindrome sequence (5′-TGACTCTCAGAGGTCA-3′) at −311 upstream of the ATG start codon within the CAT gene [87]. Although transcript levels of GPx1 and GR did not change in STCs in response to hypothyroidism, activities of both the enzymes were elevated [66]. Sahoo et al. stated that the elevation of GPx and GR in STCs could be a compensatory mechanism to maintain low levels of H_2O_2 and LPx at the cost of oxidation of GSH to GSSG and the increased GR activities in STCs might be to maintain the GSH pool to sustain the elevated GPx level [66]. These observations by Sahoo et al. demonstrate that neonatal transient or persistent hypothyroidism leads to permanent disruption of the antioxidant defense system of STCs in adulthood with altered redox status [66].

Hyperthyroidism

Hyperthyroidism-associated OS is caused by elevated production of ROS and compromised antioxidant defense status in several tissues. Rat testis is also affected by hyperthyroidism, exhibiting alterations in several enzymatic antioxidant defense parameters [59,60,65,69,70,73,74] (Table 1).

When hypothyroid rats were treated with T3 for 3 consecutive days, GSSG level was increased and GSH level was decreased, which resulted in a decline in the GSH:GSSG ratio [69]. Short-term T4 administration to hypothyroid or T4 treatment for 3 or 8 weeks to euthyroid rats results in an elevation in testicular GSH contents [65,70]. However, long-term T4 treatment resulted in a significant decline in testicular GSH contents in comparison with short-term treatments [65]. Also when euthyroid rats were treated with T3 for 5 consecutive days, it resulted in a significant increase in testicular GSH and ascorbic acid contents [74]. The GSH:GSSG ratio remains higher during T4- or T3-induced hyperthyroidism [59,74]. Interestingly, Zamoner et al. reported that hyperthyroidism decreases testicular total glutathione level despite increasing the GSH contents and without changing GSSG levels [88]. In contrast, the study by El-Kashlan et al. reported a decrease in testicular level of GSH due to hyperthyroidism [71].

Due to acute hyperthyroidism, SOD activity was declined while activities of most of the antioxidant enzymes like CAT, GPx, GR, and glucose-6-phosphate dehydrogenase (G6PD) were elevated in testis in response to the induced OS [60,74]. In contrast, studies conducted by Ourique et al. demonstrated decreased activities of CAT and GPx antioxidant enzymes and elevated GST activity in T3-treated hyperthyroid rat testis [73]. When rats were treated with T4 both testicular SOD and CAT activities declined [71] while GPx activity was augmented [59,65] with an increase in 20% and 30% in Se-D-GPx and Se-I-GPx activities, respectively [84]. Similar increase in Se-I-GPx activity was marked in testicular mitochondrial fraction (MF) after T3-induced hyperthyroidism [74]. Mitochondrial antioxidant defense profile might have a key role in controlling physiological functions like steroidogenesis and spermatogenesis in testis [59]. Such elevation in Se-D-GPx and Se-I-GPx activities in T4 treatment [84] and rise in Se-I-GPx activities in T3 treatment [74] may be an adaptive reaction to counteract toxic H_2O_2 produced as a result of impairment of normo-oxidant status of the organ. In contrast, El-Kashlan et al. [71] demonstrated that T4-induced hyperthyroidism suppresses the testicular activity of both GPx and GR. The study conducted by Choudhury et al. on rat testis after inducing hyperthyroidism showed an increase in CAT activity while there is a negative effect on level of testicular GPx [69]. Elevated activities of GPx, GR, GST, and CAT with decreased SOD activity have also been demonstrated in testis in response to T3-induced hyperthyroidism [88]. Such type of hyperthyroidism-induced OS and modulation in testicular antioxidant defenses may be a causative factor for impairment of fertility as evident from decreased total and viable sperm counts [59,60,74] and lower sperm motility [73].

THYROID DYSFUNCTION, MALE INFERTILITY, ANTIOXIDANT TREATMENT, AND TESTICULAR FUNCTION

Thyroid dysfunction is connected with abnormalities in testicular functions, erectile dysfunction, and loss of libido or impotence and infertility in men [6,89]. The contribution of T3 in regulation of Sertoli and Leydig cell proliferation, testicular maturation, and steroidogenesis is also well established. Clinical reports demonstrate that the patients with TH disorders are associated with some sexual dysfunction like decreased libido or erectile dysfunction, which gets reversed after achieving euthyroid condition [6,9,90]. It is well established that T3 receptors are expressed in Sertoli cells, which are one of the major cell types of testis that determine the size of the testis, germ cell numbers per testis, and sperm production rate in adulthood [91]. Thus testis is one of the target organs of TH and thyroid disorder can potentially affect testicular functions during early stages of development and maturation [9,25]. Hypothyroidism affects testicular size, weight, morphology, anatomy, growth and maturity, germ cell population, and serum T level based on the studies conducted in animal models [6,10,24,25,47,92,93]. Considering the clinical studies, hypothyroidism is very uncommon in males with an occurrence rate of only 0.1% in the general population [10,94]. Hypothyroid patients exhibited increased testicular size with less number of mature germ cells in seminiferous tubules [90,95] with adversely affected semen quality with compromised semen volume and progressive sperm motility and abnormal sperm morphology [89,96]. Like the studies based on hyperthyroidism in animal models, adverse effects on male reproductive organs and fertility were also reported in human subjects [10]. Hyperthyroidism delays Leydig cell development and causes reduction in testicular volume, sperm count, and motility with adverse effects on spermatogenesis as well as seminal parameters, and causes gynecomastia, decrease in libido, and abnormalities in metabolism of androgen and estrogen resulting in an elevated concentration of T, dihydrotestosterone, and estradiol [6,9,10,94,97—99].

Infertility is one of the major challenges in society. It has been reported that among infertile couples, it is estimated that 25% of cases are due to male factors [100]. The role of OS in male infertility has been extensively emphasized. Spermatozoa are like other aerobic cells, constantly exposed to the "oxygen paradox," and can be seriously attacked by the oxygen free radicals, resulting in defects with spermatogenesis. The beneficial or detrimental effects of ROS on sperm functions may depend on the nature, location, length of exposure, and concentration of ROS [101]. However, under normal physiological conditions, spermatozoa produce small amounts of ROS, particularly superoxide anion, which appears to play some crucial role needed for capacitation and acrosomal reaction [102]. Testicular cell and sperm plasma membranes contain higher amounts of PUFA, which are easily attacked by ROS; hence, they are comparatively more prone to OS. Therefore, it is necessary to maintain a balance between production of free radicals and its metabolism for appropriate function of testicular cells. Several reports have been revealed that under altered thyroid states (hypo- and hyperthyroidism) it exerts excess production of ROS and causes OS in testes [25,60,69].

A state of hypothyroidism is suggested as a complex hormonal dysfunction rather than a single hormonal defect [103]. While there are mixed reports on the luteinizing hormone (LH) and FSH levels in hypothyroid male rats [6], the study conducted by Wagner et al. showed that gonadotropin-releasing hormone (GnRH), LH, FSH, growth hormone (GH) and testicular T were decreased in rats during hypothyroid state, and by T4 treatment these alterations appeared to be ameliorated [6]. Hence, many of the testicular alterations detected in persistent hypothyroidism could be the outcome of some degree of reduced levels of the previously mentioned hormones. It has been demonstrated that the OS induced by hypothyroid condition is neither reversed by T3 administration [63] nor after the removal of reversible goitrogen PTU as studied in case of transient hypothyroidism [25]. During transient hypothyroidism, although the testicular mitochondrial LPx level was reduced, and testicular antioxidant defense capacity was severely affected as indicated by decreased activities of SOD, GR, and GPx in both MF along with postmitochondrial fractions (PMF) and CAT activity in PMF of rat testes [25,26]. The mitochondrial total GPx activity was also reduced during transient hypothyroidism and it was observed to be caused by the decreased activity of Se-D-GPx only [84]. Furthermore, the antioxidant capacity and OS status were also evaluated in the germ cells isolated from transient hypothyroid rat testis [72]. Prevalence of OS was observed in germ cells indicated by decreased GSH level, lower CAT and SOD activities, and higher LPx contents [72]. The elevated OS manifested by lower activities of overall antioxidant enzymes and higher LPx contents in germ cells [25,26,72] may be accountable for inducing apoptosis in germ cells [43,82,85], which results in reduction in sperm count in transient hypothyroid rats [25]. The cell fate of apoptosis is controlled by the ratio between pro- and antiapoptotic proteins and neonatal hypothyroidism imbalances this ratio in STCs of testis in adulthood as marked with unaltered expression of antiapoptotic protein Bcl-2 and elevated expression levels of Bax, Bad, caspase-3, and p53 proapoptotic proteins [43]. The elevated proapoptotic protein expression levels were not reversed to normal by withdrawing the PTU treatment in adult rats, suggesting permanent epigenetic modifications of the proapoptotic genes [43].

Administration of T3 hormone to PTU-induced hypothyroid rats increased CAT activity while it decreased GPx activity without changing SOD and GR activities in testicular PMFs [69]. The lower GSH and ascorbate content in mitochondrial matrix resulted from hypothyroidism is not nullified with the T3 treatment demonstrating the importance of mitochondrial thiol redox status for normal testicular physiology [63].

Antioxidants play an important role in neutralizing generated ROS and other free radicals in the body under altered physiological conditions, and those antioxidants encompass many phytochemicals, vitamins, organic molecules, and trace elements. Several antioxidants were studied to evaluate their beneficial effects on hypo- and hyperthyroid state triggered testicular OS and male fertility in general [59,67,71,73,76,77] (Table 1). Date palm pollen (DPP) extract has antioxidant effects and was used by the early Egyptians and ancient Chinese as a revitalizing agent, specifically as a therapy for male sterility, and is also used as dietary supplement worldwide [104—106]. In the studies conducted by El-Kashlan et al., the coadministration of the DPP extract lowered the augmented level of MDA and NO and testicular DNA damage and apoptosis while it elevated activities of CAT, SOD, GPx, and GR antioxidant enzymes in hypothyroid as well as hyperthyroid rat testis [71]. The potent radical nullifying activity of DPP extract is possibly because of its content of phenolic, flavonoid compounds, trace minerals, vitamins (A, E, and C), and certain amino acids [71,104]. The DPP extract was also known to diminish NO synthase activity [71]. Due to the high contents of gonadotropin-like substances and estrogenic materials such as estradiol, estriol, and estrone in Egyptian DPP, it improves male fertility and augments T and estradiol serum levels [71,105,106]. Moreover, DPP contains zinc required for T synthesis and also has a direct stimulatory effect on the pituitary gland, inducing LH release and on Leydig cells elevating 3β-hydroxysteroid dehydrogenase (3β-HSD) and 17β-hydroxysteroid dehydrogenase (17β-HSD) activities [71,104].

Curcumin is the most active constituent of turmeric having remarkable free radical scavenging ability as it inhibits generation of superoxide anion and hydroxyl radicals by preventing oxidation of Fe^{2+} to Fe^{3+} through Fenton reaction [107]. In their study, Sahoo et al. evaluated the protective properties of curcumin on hyperthyroid-induced testicular OS [59]. The elevated testicular LPx and PC due to T4 treatment was decreased to the normal level and testicular SOD and CAT activities were increased in curcumin-fed T4-treated rats [59]. However, curcumin treatment decreases the elevated testicular Se-D-GPx (GPx-1 and GPx-4) and Se-I-GPx activities of hyperthyroid rats to a normal level, which might be the result of decreased OS after curcumin administration [84]. Moreover, the reduced OS condition was evident from the elevated testicular GSH level in curcumin-administered hyperthyroid rats [59] and it might be the result of the triggered GSH biosynthesis by curcumin. Curcumin is known to induce transcription of the two Gcl genes, Gclc and Gclm, for glutamate cysteine ligase, the rate-limiting enzyme in glutathione synthesis, thus ultimately enhancing the cellular glutathione levels [108]. Reports claimed that N-acetyl L-cysteine, a precursor of GSH, reduces ROS-mediated DNA damage and improves sperm quality and motility [109].

Vitamin A is one of the potent antioxidants and acts as a scavenger of free radicals and also helps in maintaining the homeostasis of TH [110,111]. The interaction between the THs and vitamin A metabolism [111] and its deficiency has long been established. Vitamin A deficiency has multiple effects on thyroid function in animals [112]. Like vitamin A, vitamins E and C are also considered the most powerful chain-breaking antioxidants that scavenge superoxide, H_2O_2, and hydroxyl free radicals, led to prevent LPx and increase the sperm count [113,114]. Salwa and Abass reported significantly declined levels of vitamins A, E, and C concentration in both hypothyroidism and hyperthyroidism patients as compared to the control group [115]. Zamora et al. revealed that vitamin E quenches H_2O_2, which is required as an oxidizing agent for the oxidation of iodide, thus causing the declination of TH biosynthesis [116]. Several reports indicated that vitamin E deficiencies trigger testicular degeneration, resulting in reduction of sperm production in various animals like chickens, rats, hamsters, dogs, cats, pigs, boars, and monkeys [117]. Therefore, it has been suggested that dietary vitamin E improves the morphological integrity, motility, and overall quality of the semen [117–119]. Vitamin E was reported to reduce T4-induced testicular OS marked by decline in LPx and PC contents [59]. Moreover, vitamin E administration to T4-treated rats caused an augmentation in testicular SOD and CAT activities along with GSH:GSSG ratio [84]. However, vitamin treatment decreased the augmented Se-D-GPx (GPx-1 and GPx-4) and Se-I-GPx activities to normal levels in testes of T4-induced hyperthyroid rats possibly due to the declined OS after vitamin E administration [84]. The normal testicular physiology is restored by vitamin E as noticed by elevation in total sperm and live sperm count in hyperthyroid rats treated with vitamin E [59].

Resveratrol (RSV) is a natural polyphenol present mostly in grapes and wines [73,120]. It exhibits antioxidant properties by efficiently scavenging superoxide, hydroxyl, and metal-induced radicals; hence, it shows a protective effect against ROS-induced DNA damage and LPx in cell membranes [73,120]. The effect of RSV was explored on antioxidant status in the testes of T3-induced hyperthyroid rats [73]. The RSV treatment lowered testicular LOOH and TBARS levels and increased CAT and GPx activities along with improving sperm motility in hyperthyroid rats [73].

The pineal gland activates antioxidant systems via melatonin secretion. Melatonin reduces OS through its free radical scavenging and direct antioxidant effects [67,121]. Melatonin is reported to reduce LPx in the thyroid gland and gastric damage stimulated by indomethacin [67,122]. When hyperthyroidism was induced by T4 after sham pinealectomy or pinealectomy, the testicular OS was increased in hyperthyroid rats and the degree of damage became more noticeable with pinealectomy [67]. The pinealectomy together with hyperthyroidism increased the levels of MDA while reducing the levels of GSH. It is interesting to note that TH level gets amplified after pinealectomy and gets inhibited by melatonin [67,123]. Hence, the elevated OS is possibly due to the withdrawal of the inhibitor effect on THs because of pinealectomy [67]. Furthermore, according to the report [67], when endogenous melatonin is decreased by pinealectomy, the antioxidant activity gets withdrawn, resulting in an induced oxidative impairment in testis.

In human sperm and lymphocytes, flavonoids such as quercetin (Q) and kaempferol (K) have been detected, reducing the effects of food mutagens [124]. Dobrzyńska et al. investigated the impact of T4 and T3 hormones on extent of DNA damage and the protective effects of CAT, K, and Q in human sperm through comet assay [76]. While excess T3 and T4 induce DNA damage in human sperm, addition of CAT, Q, and K inhibited such effects [76]. Their studies confirmed the protective effects of flavonoids and CAT against ROS-induced DNA damage in human sperm because of their antioxidant activities. Carotenoids are the naturally occurring pigments that play a crucial role in protecting the cells by efficiently scavenging the free radicals [125]. According to the report by Russell, beta carotene acts as an antioxidant in protecting cells by neutralizing free radicals and also in serving as a pool converted to vitamin A as and when needed [126]. Studies revealed that hyperthyroidism is associated with reduced level of β-carotene compared to the normal group [115]. Folic acid acts as an antioxidant and is also reported to reduce the MDA level in testes of hypothyroid rats and maintains the normal spermatogenesis by augmenting the level of T, sperm count, and sperm motility [127]. Several studies also reported on different clinical trials validating the beneficial effects of antioxidants, their multiple combinations with different doses and durations in selected cases of male infertility including evidence supporting reduction in OS and improved sperm motility, particularly in asthenospermic patients after oral antioxidant therapy [128,129].

THYROID DYSFUNCTION AND ASSISTED REPRODUCTIVE TECHNOLOGY OUTCOME

Thyroid dysfunction is one of the major endocrine disorders in humans. THs influence sexual development and reproductive functions in both men and women. However, hypothyroidism is more prevalent than hyperthyroidism in both sexes; particularly hypothyroidism is more frequent in women of reproductive age (20−40 years) [130,131]. THs play a crucial role in normal reproductive physiology by directly affecting testes and ovaries and indirectly by interacting with sex hormone binding proteins. Thyroid dysfunction can lead to low production of T and sperm in case of men and menstrual irregularities and infertility in women [12]. Further, Santi et al. reported that hypothyroidism is associated with lipid oxidation and OS [132]. It has also been reported that the chances of spontaneous abortion during earlier pregnancy were greater in women with lower T4 levels than euthyroid pregnant women. Thus, thyroid dysfunction associated changes in physiopathological conditions and their mechanisms are yet to be understood properly. Among the proposed mechanisms, OS seems to be one of the major associations between them. Thyroid dysfunction causes autoimmune thyroid disease (AITD), and women having endometriosis and polycystic ovarian syndrome are more prone to AITD [133]. Under such conditions, treatment of T4 may be a helpful option to restore normal fertility, but its supplementation reduces the likelihood of an assisted reproductive technology (ART) procedure. The main reason may be due to the known phenomenon of TH-induced ROS production causing OS.

Assisted reproduction techniques including in vitro fertilization (IVF), intracytoplasmic sperm injection (ICSI), and in vitro maturation of oocytes are the options for both male and female infertility [134]. Exposure to ROS at physiological level and possessing natural antioxidant defenses are normal phenomena for both ovum and sperm. Optimal level of ROS in follicular fluid promotes a healthy development of oocytes [135]. However, an imbalance cellular redox status in the developing embryo results in suboptimal culture conditions and leads altered gene expression and impaired adenosine triphosphate generation [136], and subsequently possibly influencing impairment in placental and embryo growth [137]. Pasqualotto et al. reported that there is a correlation between OS biomarker, LPx level, and total antioxidant capacity (TAC) in the follicular fluid from women undergoing IVF treatment with pregnancy outcome [138]. This study indicated that the critical level of oxygen radicals is crucial for oocyte development and maturation. Further, a similar study by Das et al. conferred positive correlation between the biomarkers, LPx and TAC [138,139]. However, excessively high ROS generation around follicular fluid results in development of compromised embryos. Further, the study by Seino et al. reveals that a higher level of 8-hydroxy-2-deoxyguanosine (8-OHdG), a marker for DNA damage, affects the quality of oocytes and embryos in IVF and ICSI cycles and results in low fertilization rate and formation of poor quality embryos [140]. Spermatozoa are one of the sources of exogenous ROS, and under the influence of TH, the prevalence of ROS production is greater. Further, altered states of THs are associated with increased OS, which exerts a negative effect on testicular development, sperm motility, and overall quality of semen [141,142]. Under such conditions, after ART, the embryo or fetus is associated with a greater frequency of miscarriage.

CONCLUSION

Disruption of the normal euthyroid state disturbs the morphological and functional development of the testis as evident from the studies conducted not only in animal models but also from clinical reports. The testicular presence and expression of deiodinases, TH transporters, and TRs along with the significant role of TH on both Sertoli cell proliferation and maturation and Leydig cell differentiation and steroidogenic function clearly indicate a strong physiological association between TH and testicular function. Additionally, the key role of TH on modulating testicular OS and antioxidant defenses illustrates its strong association with testicular antioxidant defense status, thus subsequently its role on male fertility. Therefore, excess production of ROS under altered thyroid states might lead to infertility in males, and under such conditions, extraneous antioxidants could be a better option for the treatment against male infertility. In ART procedures, optimum combinations of antioxidant supplements in sperm preparation media might also be helpful in reducing the overloads of ROS.

LIST OF ABBREVIATIONS

17β-HSD 17β-hydroxysteroid dehydrogenase
3β-HSD 3β-hydroxysteroid dehydrogenase
AITD Autoimmune thyroid disease
ART Assisted reproductive technology
CAT Catalase
CDKI Cyclin-dependent kinase inhibitor
Cx43 Connexin43
D1 $5'$-deiodinase type 1
D2 $5'$-deiodinase type 2
D3 5-deiodinase type 3
DPP Date palm pollen
FSH Follicle stimulating hormone
G6PD Glucose-6-phosphate dehydrogenase
GH Growth hormone
GnRH Gonadotropin-releasing hormone
GPx Glutathione peroxidase
GR Glutathione reductase
GST Glutathione S-transferase
GsT Gonad-specific transporter
GSI Gonadosomatic index
GSH Reduced glutathione
GSH:GSSG Reduced to oxidized glutathione ratio
GSSG Oxidized glutathione
H_2O_2 Hydrogen peroxide
HO· Hydroxyl radical
ICSI Intracytoplasmic sperm injection
IGF-1 Insulin-like growth factor-1
IVF In vitro fertilization
IVM In vitro maturation of oocytes
K Kaempferol
LH Luteinizing hormone
LOOH Lipid hydroperoxide
LPx Lipid peroxide
MDA Malondialdehyde
NO Nitric oxide
OATPs Organic anion-transporting polypeptides
OSI Oxidative stress index
$^1O_2$ Singlet oxygen
$O_2{}^-$ Superoxide
PC Protein carbonyl
PCOS Polycystic ovarian syndrome
PUFA Polyunsaturated fatty acid
PTU 6-*n*-propyl-2-thiouracil
Q Quercetin
ROS Reactive oxygen species
RSV Resveratrol
RXR Retinoid X receptor
Se-I-GPx Selenium-independent glutathione peroxidase
Se-D-GPx Selenium-dependent glutathione peroxidase
SOD Superoxide dismutase
STC Seminiferous tubule cell
T3 3,3′,5-triiodo-L-thyronin
T4 L-thyroxine
T Testosterone
TAC Total antioxidant capacity
TBARS Thiobarbituric acid-reactive substance
TH Thyroid hormone

TH-TR Thyroid hormone and thyroid receptor complex
TR Thyroid hormone receptor
TRH Thyroid releasing hormone
TRE Thyroid response element
TSH Thyroid stimulating hormone

REFERENCES

[1] Martinez G, Daniels K, Chandra A. Fertility of men and women aged 15–44 years in the United States: National Survey of family growth. Natl Health Stat Rep April 2012;12:1–28.

[2] Agarwal A, Mulgund A, Hamada A, Chyatte MR. A unique view on male infertility around the globe. Reprod Biol Endocrinol April 26, 2015;13(1):37.

[3] Irvine DS. Epidemiology and aetiology of male infertility. Hum Reprod April 1, 1998;13(Suppl._1):33–44.

[4] Barker SB, Klitgaard HM. Metabolism of tissues excised from thyroxine-injected rats. Am J Physiol July 1, 1952;170(1):81–6.

[5] Oppenheimer JH, Schwartz HL, Surks MI. Tissue differences in the concentration of triiodothyronine nuclear binding sites in the rat: liver, kidney, pituitary, heart, brain, spleen and testis. Endocrinology September 1, 1974;95(3):897–903.

[6] Wagner MS, Wajner SM, Maia AL. The role of thyroid hormone in testicular development and function. J Endocrinol 2008;199(3):351–65.

[7] Rajender S, Monicaz MG, Walterz L, Agarw-all A. Thyroid, spermatogenesis, and male infertility. Front Biosci June 1, 2011;3:843–55.

[8] Panno ML, Salerno M, Lanzino M, De Luca G, Maggiolini M, Straface SV, Prati M, Palmero S, Bolla E, Fugassa E, Ando S. Follow-up study on the effects of thyroid hormone administration on androgen metabolism of peripubertal rat Sertoli cells. Eur J Endocrinol February 1, 1995;132(2):236–41.

[9] Jannini EA, Ulisse S, D'Armiento M. Thyroid hormone and male gonadal function. Endocr Rev 1995;16(4):443–59.

[10] Krajewska-Kulak E, Sengupta P. Thyroid function in male infertility. Front Endocrinol November 13, 2013;4:174.

[11] Sengupta P. Environmental and occupational exposure of metals and their role in male reproductive functions. Drug Chem Toxicol July 1, 2013;36(3):353–68.

[12] Krassas GE, Poppe K, Glinoer D. Thyroid function and human reproductive health. Endocr Rev 2010;31:702–5.

[13] Guerrero A, Pamplona R, Postero-Otin M, et al. Effect of thyroid status on lipid composition and peroxidation in the mouse liver. Free Radic Biol Med 1999;26(1–2):73–80.

[14] Brent GA. Mechanisms of thyroid hormone action. J Clin Invest September 4, 2012;122(9):3035.

[15] Cheng SY, Leonard JL, Davis PJ. Molecular aspects of thyroid hormone actions. Endocr Rev April 2010;31(2):139–70.

[16] Mullur R, Liu YY, Brent GA. Thyroid hormone regulation of metabolism. Physiol Rev April 1, 2014;94(2):355–82.

[17] Schweizer U, Weitzel JM, Schomburg L. Think globally: act locally: new insights into the local regulation of thyroid hormone availability challenge long accepted dogmas. Mol Cell Endocrinol July 16, 2008;289(1):1–9.

[18] Andersen S, Pedersen KM, Bruun NH, Laurberg P. Narrow individual variations in serum T4 and T3 in normal subjects: a clue to the understanding of subclinical thyroid disease. J Clin Endocrinol Metab March 1, 2002;87(3):1068–72.

[19] Ramadoss P, Abraham BJ, Tsai L, Zhou Y, Costa-e-Sousa RH, Ye F, Bilban M, Zhao K, Hollenberg AN. Novel mechanism of positive versus negative regulation by thyroid hormone receptor β1 (TRβ1) identified by genome-wide profiling of binding sites in mouse liver. J Biol Chem January 17, 2014;289(3):1313–28.

[20] Chung HR. Iodine and thyroid function. Ann Pediatr Endocrinol Metab March 1, 2014;19(1):8–12.

[21] Gereben B, Zavacki AM, Ribich S, Kim BW, Huang SA, Simonides WS, Zeöld A, Bianco AC. Cellular and molecular basis of deiodinase-regulated thyroid hormone signaling. Endocr Rev December 2008;29(7):898–938.

[22] Gao Y, Lee WM, Cheng CY. Thyroid hormone function in the rat testis. Front Endocrinol 2014;5.

[23] Palmero S, Prati M, Bolla F, Fugassa E. Tri-iodothyronine directly affects rat Sertoli cell proliferation and differentiation. J Endocrinol May 1, 1995;145(2):355–62.

[24] Francavilla S, Cordeschi G, Properzi G, Di Cicco L, Jannini EA, Palmero S, Fugassa E, Loras B, D'armiento M. Effect of thyroid hormone on the pre-and post-natal development of the rat testis. J Endocrinol April 1, 1991;129(1):35.

[25] Sahoo DK, Roy A, Bhanja S, Chainy GB. Hypothyroidism impairs antioxidant defence system and testicular physiology during development and maturation. Gen Comp Endocrinol March 1, 2008;156(1):63–70.

[26] Sahoo DK, Roy A. Compromised rat testicular antioxidant defence system by hypothyroidism before puberty. Int J Endocrinol January 16, 2012;2012.

[27] Maran RR, Sivakumar R, Arunakaran J, Ravisankar B, Ravichandran K, Sidharthan V, Jeyaraj DA, Aruldhas MM. Duration-dependent effect of transient neonatal hypothyroidism on Sertoli and germ cell number, and plasma and testicular interstitial fluid androgen binding protein concentration. Endocr Res January 1, 1999;25(3–4):323–40.

[28] Simorangkir DR, Wreford NG, De Kretser DM. Impaired germ cell development in the testes of immature rats with neonatal hypothyroidism. J Androl March 4, 1997;18(2):186–93.

[29] Cooke PS, Hess RA, Porcelli J, Meisami E. Increased sperm production in adult rats after transient neonatal hypothyroidism. Endocrinology 1991;129:244–8.

[30] Van Haaster LH, De Jong FH, Docter RO, De Rooij DG. The effect of hypothyroidism on Sertoli cell proliferation and differentiation and hormone levels during testicular development in the rat. Endocrinology September 1, 1992;131(3):1574–6.

[31] Maran RR. Thyroid hormones: their role in testicular steroidogenesis. Arch Androl January 1, 2003;49(5):375—88.

[32] Lagu SK, Bhavsar NG, Sharma RK, Ramachandran AV. Neonatal hypothyroidism-induced changes in rat testis size, dependence on temperature. Neuroendocrinol Lett December 2005;26(6):780—8.

[33] Jannini EA, Crescenzi A, Rucci N, Screponi E, Carosa E, De Matteis A, Macchia E, d'Amati G, D'Armiento M. Ontogenetic pattern of thyroid hormone receptor expression in the human testis. J Clin Endocrinol Metab September 1, 2000;85(9):3453—7.

[34] Holsberger DR, Cooke PS. Understanding the role of thyroid hormone in Sertoli cell development: a mechanistic hypothesis. Cell Tissue Res October 1, 2005;322(1):133—40.

[35] Gilleron J, Nebout M, Scarabelli L, Senegas-Balas F, Palmero S, Segretain D, Pointis G. A potential novel mechanism involving connexin 43 gap junction for control of Sertoli cell proliferation by thyroid hormones. J Cell Physiol October 1, 2006;209(1):153—61.

[36] Holsberger DR, Kiesewetter SE, Cooke PS. Regulation of neonatal Sertoli cell development by thyroid hormone receptor alpha1. Biol Reprod 2005;73(3):396—403.

[37] Palmero S, Bardi G, Bolla F, Fugassa E. Influence of thyroid hormone on Sertoli cell protein metabolism in the prepubertal pig. Boll Soc Ital Biol Sper 1996;72(5—6):163—70.

[38] Mendis-Handagama SM, Siril Ariyaratne HB. Leydig cells, thyroid hormones and steroidogenesis. Indian J Exp Biol 2005;43:939—62.

[39] Vilchez-Martinez JA. Study of the pituitary-testicular axis in hypothyroid adult male rats. J Reprod Fertil October 1, 1973;35(1):123—6.

[40] Weiss SR, Burns JM. The effect of acute treatment with two goitrogens on plasma thyroid hormones, testosterone and testicular morphology in adult male rats. Comp Biochem Physiol A January 1, 1988;90(3):449—52.

[41] Sakai Y, Yamashina S, Furudate SI. Developmental delay and unstable state of the testes in the rdw rat with congenital hypothyroidism. Dev Growth Differ August 1, 2004;46(4):327—34.

[42] Oncu M, Kavaklı D, Gokcımen A, Gulle K, Orhan H, Karaoz E. Investigation on the histopathological effects of thyroidectomy on the seminiferous tubules of immature and adult rats. Urol Int 2004;73(1):59—64.

[43] Sahoo SK, Dandapat J, Chainy GBN. Differential expression of apoptotic proteins in seminiferous tubule cells of adult rats by neonatal exposure to 6-n-propyl-2-thiouracil (PTU), a thyroid disrupting chemical. Indian J Exp Biol 2017;55:634—41.

[44] Canale D, Agostini M, Giorgilli G, Caglieresi C, Scartabelli G, Nardini V, et al. Thyroid hormone receptors in neonatal, prepubertal and adult rat testis. J Androl 2001;22:284—8.

[45] Wajner SM, dos Santos Wagner M, Melo RC, Parreira GG, Chiarini-Garcia H, Bianco AC, Fekete C, Sanchez E, Lechan RM, Maia AL. Type 2 iodothyronine deiodinase is highly expressed in germ cells of adult rat testis. J Endocrinol July 1, 2007;194(1):47—54.

[46] Palmero S, Maggiani S, Fugassa E. Nuclear triiodothyronine receptors in rat Sertoli cells. Mol Cell Endocrinol August 31, 1988;58(2):253—6.

[47] Jannini EA, Olivieri M, Francavilla S, Gulino A, Ziparo E, D'armiento MA. Ontogenesis of the nuclear 3,5,3'-triiodothyronine receptor in the rat testis. Endocrinology May 1, 1990;126(5):2521—6.

[48] Buzzard JJ, Morrison JR, O'Bryan MK, Song Q, Wreford NG. Developmental expression of thyroid hormone receptors in the rat testis. Biol Reprod 2000;62:664—9.

[49] Kumar A, Shekhar S, Dhole B. Thyroid and male reproduction. Indian J Endocrinol Metab January 2014;18(1):23.

[50] Westholm DE, Rumbley JN, Salo DR, Rich TP, Anderson GW. Organic anion-transporting polypeptides at the blood-brain and blood-cerebrospinal fluid barriers. Curr Top Dev Biol 2008;80:135.

[51] Kalliokoski A, Niemi M. Impact of OATP transporters on pharmacokinetics. Br J Pharmacol October 1, 2009;158(3):693—705.

[52] Pizzagalli F, Hagenbuch B, Stieger B, Klenk U, Folkers G, Meier PJ. Identification of a novel human organic anion transporting polypeptide as a high affinity thyroxine transporter. Mol Endocrinol October 1, 2002;16(10):2283—96.

[53] Suzuki T, Onogawa T, Asano N, Mizutamari H, Mikkaichi T, Tanemoto M, Abe M, Satoh F, Unno M, Nunoki K, Suzuki M. Identification and characterization of novel rat and human gonad-specific organic anion transporters. Mol Endocrinol July 1, 2003;17(7):1203—15.

[54] Bates JM, St Germain DL, Galton VA. Expression profiles of the three iodothyronine deiodinases, D1, D2, and D3, in the developing rat. Endocrinology February 1, 1999;140(2):844—51.

[55] Halliwell B, Gutteridge JMC. Free radicals in biology and medicine. 4th ed. Oxford, UK: Oxford University Press; 2007.

[56] Sies H. Hydroperoxides and thiol oxidants in the study of oxidative stress in intact cells and organs. In: Oxidative stress; 1985. p. 73—90.

[57] Venditti P, Balestrieri M, Di Meo S, De Leo T. Effect of thyroid state on lipid peroxidation, antioxidant defences, and susceptibility to oxidative stress in rat tissues. J Endocrinol October 1, 1997;155(1):151—7.

[58] Sahoo DK, Chainy GB. Tissue specific response of antioxidant defence systems of rat to experimentally-induced hyperthyroidism. Natl Acad Sci Lett 2007;30(7—8):247—50.

[59] Sahoo DK, Roy A, Chainy GBN. Protective effects of Vitamin E and curcumin on L-thyroxine-induced rat testicular oxidative stress. Chem Biol Interact 2008;176:121—8.

[60] Sahoo DK, Roy A, Bhanja S, Chainy GB. Experimental hyperthyroidism-induced oxidative stress and impairment of antioxidant defence system in rat testes. Indian J Exp Biol 2005;43:1058—67.

[61] Chattopadhyay S, Sahoo DK, Subudhi U, Chainy GB. Differential expression profiles of antioxidant enzymes and glutathione redox status in hyperthyroid rats: a temporal analysis. Comp Biochem Physiol C Toxicol Pharmacol September 30, 2007;146(3):383—91.

[62] Chattopadhyay S, Sahoo DK, Roy A, Samanta L, Chainy GB. Thiol redox status critically influences mitochondrial response to thyroid hormone-induced hepatic oxidative injury: a temporal analysis. Cell Biochem Funct March 1, 2010;28(2):126—34.

[63] Chattopadhyay S, Choudhury S, Roy A, Chainy GB, Samanta LT. 3 fails to restore mitochondrial thiol redox status altered by experimental hypothyroidism in rat testis. Gen Comp Endocrinol October 31, 2010;169(1):39—47.

[64] Peltola V, Huhtaniemi I, Ahotupa M. Antioxidant enzyme activity in the maturing rat testis. J Androl September 10, 1992;13(5):450—5.

[65] Asker ME, Hassan WA, El-Kashlan AM. Experimentally induced hyperthyroidism influences oxidant and antioxidant status and impairs male gonadal functions in adult rats. Andrologia August 1, 2015;47(6):644—54.

[66] Sahoo SK, Chainy GBN, Dandapat J. Neonatal hypothyroidism alters expression of antioxidant enzymes and redox status in adult rat seminiferous tubule cells. Curr Trends Biotechnol Pharm 2015;9:117.

[67] Mogulkoc R, Baltaci AK, Oztekin E, Aydin L, Tuncer I. Hyperthyroidism causes lipid peroxidation in kidney and testis tissues of rats: protective role of melatonin. Neuroendocrinol Lett December 1, 2005;26(6):806—10.

[68] Zamoner A, Barreto KP, Wilhelm Filho D, Sell F, Woehl VM, Guma FC, Pessoa-Pureur R, Silva FR. Propylthiouracil-induced congenital hypothyroidism upregulates vimentin phosphorylation and depletes antioxidant defenses in immature rat testis. J Mol Endocrinol March 1, 2008;40(3):125—35.

[69] Choudhury S, Chainy GBN, Mishro MM. Experimentally induced hypo- and hyper-thyroidism influence on the antioxidant defence system in adult rat testis. Andrologia 2003;35:131—40.

[70] Mogulkoc R, Baltaci AK, Oztekin E, Ozturk A, Sivrikaya A. Short-term thyroxine administration leads to lipid peroxidation in renal and testicular tissues of rats with hypothyroidism. Acta Biol Hung August 1, 2005;56(3—4):225—32.

[71] El-Kashlan AM, Nooh MM, Hassan WA, Rizk SM. Therapeutic potential of date palm pollen for testicular dysfunction induced by thyroid disorders in male rats. PLoS One October 1, 2015;10(10):e0139493.

[72] Sahoo DK, Roy A, Chainy GB. PTU-induced neonatal hypothyroidism modulates antioxidative status and population of rat testicular germ cells. Natl Acad Sci Lett 2006;29(3—4):133—5.

[73] Ourique GM, Finamor IA, Saccol EM, Riffel AP, Pes TS, Gutierrez K, Goncalves PB, Baldisserotto B, Pavanato MA, Barreto KP. Resveratrol improves sperm motility, prevents lipid peroxidation and enhances antioxidant defences in the testes of hyperthyroid rats. Reprod Toxicol 2013;37:31—9.

[74] Sahoo DK, Roy A, Chattopadhyay S, Chainy GBN. Effect of T3 treatment on glutathione redox pool and its metabolizing enzymes in mitochondrial and post-mitochondrial fractions of adult rat testes. Indian J Exp Biol 2007;45:338—46.

[75] Sahoo DK. Effects of thyroid hormone on testicular functions and antioxidant defence status. Biochemistry 2011;5(6).

[76] Dobrzyńska MM, Baumgartner A, Anderson D. Antioxidants modulate thyroid hormone-and noradrenaline-induced DNA damage in human sperm. Mutagenesis July 1, 2004;19(4):325—30.

[77] Sahoo DK. Testicular protection from thyroid hormone mediated oxidative stress. WebmedCentral Reprod 2013;4(5):WMC004252. https://doi.org/10.9754/journal.wmc.2013.004252.

[78] Dandekar SP, Nadkarni GD, Kulkarni VS, Punekar S. Lipid peroxidation and antioxidant enzymes in male infertility. J Postgrad Med July 1, 2002;48(3):186.

[79] Olsvik PA, Kristensen T, Waagbø R, Rosseland BO, Tollefsen KE, Baeverfjord G, Berntssen MH. mRNA expression of antioxidant enzymes (SOD, CAT and GSH-Px) and lipid peroxidative stress in liver of Atlantic salmon (*Salmo salar*) exposed to hyperoxic water during smoltification. Comp Biochem Physiol C Toxicol Pharmacol July 31, 2005;141(3):314—23.

[80] Park HA, Khanna S, Rink C, Gnyawali S, Roy S, Sen CK. Glutathione disulfide induces neural cell death via a 12-lipoxygenase pathway. Cell Death Differ 2009;16:1167.

[81] Ranawat P, Bansal MP. Decreased glutathione levels potentiate the apoptotic efficacy of selenium: possible involvement of p38 and JNK MAPKs—in vitro studies. Mol Cell Biochem 2008;309:21.

[82] Sahoo DK. Increased germ cell apoptosis during testicular development and maturation by experimentally induced transient and persistent hypothyroidism. WebmedCentral Apoptosis 2013;4(5):WMC004235. https://doi.org/10.9754/journal.wmc.2013.004235.

[83] Sahoo D, Roy A, Chainy G. Rat testicular mitochondrial antioxidant defence system and its modulation by aging. Acta Biol Hung December 1, 2008;59(4):413—24.

[84] Sahoo DK. Alterations of testicular selenium-dependent and independent glutathione peroxidase activities during experimentally L-thyroxine induced hyperthyroidism and n-propyl thiouracil induced hypothyroidism in adult rats. Res Rev Biosci 2012;6(3).

[85] Sarkar D, Singh SK. Neonatal hypothyroidism affects testicular glucose homeostasis through increased oxidative stress in prepubertal mice: effects on GLUT3, GLUT8 and Cx43. Andrology May 4, 2017;5.

[86] Abdelmohsen K, Kuwano Y, Kim HH, Gorospe M. Posttranscriptional gene regulation by RNA-binding proteins during oxidative stress: implications for cellular senescence. Biol Chem March 1, 2008;389(3):243—55.

[87] Van Remmen H, Williams MD, Yang H, Walter CA, Richardson A. Analysis of the transcriptional activity of the 5′-flanking region of the rat catalase gene in transiently transfected cells and in transgenic mice. J Cell Physiol January 1, 1998;174(1):18—26.

[88] Zamoner A, Barreto KP, Wilhelm Filho D, Sell F, Woehl VM, Guma FC, Silva FR, Pessoa-Pureur R. Hyperthyroidism in the developing rat testis is associated with oxidative stress and hyperphosphorylated vimentin accumulation. Mol Cell Endocrinol March 15, 2007;267(1):116—26.

[89] Krassas GE, Tziomalos K, Papadopoulou F, Pontikides N, Perros P. Erectile dysfunction in patients with hyper- and hypothyroidism: how common and should we treat? J Clin Endocrinol Metab 2008;93:1815—9.

[90] Krassas GE, Pontikides N. Male reproductive function in relation with thyroid alterations. Best Pract Res Clin Endocrinol Metabol 2004;18(2):183—95.

[91] Sharpe R, McKinnell C, Kivlin C, Fisher JS. Proliferation and functional maturation of Sertoli cells, and their relevance to disorders of testis function in adulthood. Reproduction 2003;125(6):769—84.

[92] Jiang JY, Umezu M, Sato E. Characteristics of infertility and the improvement of fertility by thyroxine treatment in adult male hypothyroid rdw rats. Biol Reprod December 1, 2000;63(6):1637—41.

[93] Cooke PS, Zhao YD, Bunick D. Triiodothyronine inhibits proliferation and stimulates differentiation of cultured neonatal Sertoli cells: possible mechanism for increased adult testis weight and sperm production induced by neonatal goitrogen treatment. Biol Reprod November 1, 1994;51(5):1000−5.

[94] Krassas GE, Perros P. Thyroid disease and male reproductive function. J Endocrinol Invest April 1, 2003;26(4):372−80.

[95] Wajner SM, Wagner MS, Maia AL. Clinical implications of altered thyroid status in male testicular function. Arq Bras Endocrinol Metab November 2009;53(8):976−82.

[96] Hernandez JC, Garcia JM, Garcia Diez LC. Primary hypothyroidism and human spermatogenesis. Arch Androl January 1, 1990;25(1):21−7.

[97] Clyde HR, Walsh PC, English RW. Elevated plasma testosterone and gonadotropin levels in infertile males with hyperthyroidism. Fertil Steril June 30, 1976;27(6):662−6.

[98] Rijntjes E, Wientjes AT, Swarts HJ, Rooij DG, Teerds KJ. Dietary-Induced hyperthyroidism marginally affects neonatal testicular development. J Androl November 12, 2008;29(6):643−53.

[99] Hudson RW, Edwards AL. Testicular function in hyperthyroidism. J Androl March 4, 1992;13(2):117−24.

[100] Sharlip ID, Jarow JP, Belker AM, Lipshultz LI, Sigman M, Thomas AJ, Schlegel PN, Howards SS, Nehra A, Damewood MD, Overstreet JW. Best practice policies for male infertility. Fertil Steril May 31, 2002;77(5):873−82.

[101] Agarwal A, Saleh RA. Role of oxidants in male infertility: rationale, significance, and treatment. Urol Clin N Am 2002;29:817−27.

[102] Agarwal A, Saleh RA, Bedaiwy MA. Role of reactive oxygen species in the pathophysiology of human reproduction. Fertil Steril 2003;79:829−43.

[103] Gomez Dumm CL, Cortizo AM, Gagliardino JJ. Morphological and functional changes in several endocrine glands induced by hypothyroidism in the rat. Cells Tissues Organs 1985;124(1−2):81−7.

[104] Hassan HM. Chemical composition and nutritional value of palm pollen grains. Glob J Biotechnol Biochem 2011;6(1):1−7.

[105] Abbas FA, Ateya AM. Estradiol, esteriol, estrone and novel flavonoids from date palm pollen. Aust J Basic Appl Sci 2011;5(8):606−14.

[106] El-Neweshy MS, El-Maddawy ZK, El-Sayed YS. Therapeutic effects of date palm (*Phoenix dactylifera* L.) pollen extract on cadmium-induced testicular toxicity. Andrologia December 1, 2013;45(6):369−78.

[107] Reddy ACP, Lokesh BR. Effect of curcumin and eugenol on iron-induced hepatic toxicity in rats. Toxicology 1996;107:39−45.

[108] Dickinson DA, Levonen AL, Moellering DR, Arnold EK, Zhang H, Darley-Usmar VM, Forman HJ. Human glutamate cysteine ligase gene regulation through the electrophile response element. Free Radic Biol Med October 15, 2004;37(8):1152−9.

[109] Lopes S, Jurisicova A, Sun JG, Casper RF. Reactive oxygen species: potential cause for DNA fragmentation in human spermatozoa. Hum Reprod 1998;13:896−900.

[110] Nockles CF, Ewing DL, Phetteplace H. Hypothyroidisms: an early signs of vitamin A deficiency in chickens. J Nutr 1984;114:1733−6.

[111] Morley JE, Damassa DA, Gordon J, Pekary AE, Hershman JM. 1978 Thyroid function and vitamin A deficiency. Life Sci 1978;22:1901−5.

[112] Arthur JR, Beckett M, Mitchell JH. Interactions between selenium and iodine deficiencies in man and animals. Nutr Res Rev 1999;12:55−73.

[113] Agarwal A, Nallella KP, Allamaneni SS, Said TM. Role of antioxidants in treatment of male infertility: an overview of the literature. Reprod Biomed Online 2004;8:616−27.

[114] Suleiman SA, Ali ME, Zaki ZM, el-Malik EM, Nasr MA. Lipid peroxidation and human sperm motility: protective role of vitamin E. J Androl 1996;17:530−7.

[115] Al-Rubae SHN, Al Musawi AK. An evaluation of antioxidants and oxidative stress in Iraqi patients with thyroid gland dysfunction. Afr J Biochem Res 2011;5:188−96.

[116] Zamora R, Hidalgo FJ, Tappel AL. Comparative antioxidant effectiveness of dietary carotene, Vitamin E, selenium and coenzyme Q10 in rat erythrocytes and plasma. J Nutr 1991;121:50−6.

[117] Marin-Guzman J, Mahan DC, Chung YK, Pate JL, Pope WF. Effects of dietary selenium and vitamin E on boar performance and tissue responses, semen quality, and subsequent fertilization rates in mature gilts. J Anim Sci 1997;75:2994−3003.

[118] Sonmez M, Yuce A, Turk G. The protective effects of melatonin and Vitamin E on antioxidant enzyme activities and epididymal sperm characteristics of homocysteine treated male rats. Reprod Toxicol 2007;23:226−31.

[119] Brzezinska-Slebodzinska E, Slebodzinski AB, Pietras B, Wieczorek G. Antioxidant effect of vitamin E and glutathione on lipid peroxidation in boar semen plasma. Biol Trace Elem Res 1995;47:69−74.

[120] Collodel G, Federico MG, Geminiani M, Martini S, Bonechi C, Rossi C, et al. Effect of trans-resveratrol on induced oxidative stress in human sperm and germinal cells. Reprod Toxicol 2011;31:239−46.

[121] Reiter RJ, Tan DX, Mayo JC, Sainz RM, Leon J, Czarnocki Z. Melatonin as an antioxidant: biochemical mechanisms and pathophysiological implications in humans. Acta Biochimica Pol January 1, 2003;50(4):1129−46.

[122] Karbownik M, Lewiński A. Melatonin reduces fenton reaction-induced lipid peroxidation in porcine thyroid tissue. J Cell Biochem November 1, 2003;90(4):806−11.

[123] Baltaci AK, Mogulkoc R, Kul A, Bediz CS, Ugur A. Opposite effects of zinc and melatonin on thyroid hormones in rats. Toxicology January 15, 2004;195(1):69−75.

[124] Anderson D, Dobryńska MM, Başaran N, Başaran A, Yu TW. Flavonoids modulate comet assay responses to food mutagens in human lymphocytes and sperm. Mutat Res Fund Mol Mech Mutagen June 18, 1998;402(1):269−77.

[125] Sies H, Stahl W. Vitamins E and C, beta-carotene, and other carotenoids as antioxidants. Am J Clin Nutr 1995;62:1315S−21S.

[126] Russell RM. The enigma of beta-carotene in carcinogenesis: what can be learned from animal studies. J Nutr 2004;134:262S−8S.

[127] Ibrahim W, Tousson E, Ali EMM, Mansour M. Folic acid alleviates oxidative stress and hyperhomocysteinemia involved in testicular dysfunction of hypothyroid rats. Gen Comp Endocrinol 2011;174:143−9.

[128] Gharagozloo P, Aitken RJ. The role of sperm oxidative stress in male infertility and the significance of oral antioxidant therapy. Hum Reprod May 5, 2011;26(7):1628—40.

[129] Cocuzza M, Agarwal A. Nonsurgical treatment of male infertility: specific and empiric therapy. Biologics September 2007;1(3):259.

[130] Wang C, Crapo LM. The epidemiology of thyroid disease and implications for screening. Endocrinol Metab Clin N Am 1997;1997:26189—218.

[131] Bjoro T, Holmen J, Kruger O, Midthjell K, Hunstad K, Schreiner T, et al. Prevalence of thyroid disease, thyroid dysfunction and thyroid peroxidase antibodies in a large, unselected population. The Health Study of NordTrondelag (HUNT). Eur J Endocrinol 2000;143:639—47.

[132] Santi A, Duarte MM, Moresco RN, Menezes C, Bagatini MD, Schetinger MR, Loro VL. Association between thyroid hormones, lipids and oxidative stress biomarkers in overt hypothyroidism. Clin Chem Lab Med 2010;48(11):1635—9.

[133] Petta CA, Arruda MS, Zantut-Wittmann DE, Benetti-Pinto CL. Thyroid autoimmunity and thyroid dysfunction in women with endometriosis. Hum Reprod 2007;22:2693—7.

[134] Gupta S, Malhotra N, Sharma D, Chandra A, Agarwal A. Oxidative stress and its role in female infertility and assisted reproduction: clinical implications. Int J Fertil Steril 2009;2:147—64.

[135] Attaran M, Pasqualotto E, Falcone T, Goldberg JM, Miller KF, Agarwal A, et al. The effect of follicular fluid reactive oxygen species on the outcome of in vitro fertilization. Int J Fertil Women's Med 2000;45:314—20.

[136] Hyslop PA, Hinshaw DB, Halsey Jr WA, Schraufstatter IU, Sauerheber RD, Spragg RG, et al. Mechanisms of oxidant-mediated cell injury. The glycolytic and mitochondrial pathways of ADP phosphorylation are major intracellular targets inactivated by hydrogen peroxide. J Biol Chem 1988;263:1665—75.

[137] Harvey AJ, Kind KL, Thompson JG. Redox regulation of early embryo development. Reproduction 2002;123:479—86.

[138] Pasqualotto EB, Agarwal A, Sharma RK, Izzo VM, Pinotti JA, et al. Effect of oxidative stress in follicular fluid on the outcome of assisted reproductive procedures. Fertil Steril 2004;81:973—6.

[139] Das S, Chattopadhyay R, Ghosh S, Ghosh S, Goswami SK, et al. Reactive oxygen species level in follicular fluid—embryo quality marker in IVF? Hum Reprod 2006;21:2403—7.

[140] Seino T, Saito H, Kaneko T, Takahashi T, Kawachiya S, Kurachi H. Eight-hydroxy-2′-deoxyguanosine in granulosa cells is correlated with the quality of oocytes and embryos in an in vitro fertilization-embryo transfer program. Fertil Steril 2002;77:1184—90.

[141] Resch U, Helsel G, Tatzber F, Sinzinger H. Antioxidant status in thyroid dysfunction. Clin Chem Lab Med 2002;40:1132—4.

[142] Trokoudes KM, Skordis N, Picolos MK. Infertility and thyroid disorders. Curr Opin Obstet Gyneocol 2006;18:446—51.

Chapter 2.8

Aging

Sezgin Gunes and Gülgez Neslihan Hekim Taşkurt

Ondokuz Mayis University, Samsun, Turkey

INTRODUCTION

Aging is a time-dependent progressive loss of physiologic integrity that leads to impairment of organ function and ultimately leads to death. Aging is a risk factor for many chronic and systemic diseases. Today, prolongation of average life expectancy along with a couple's desire to have children later in life due to socioeconomical reasons has caused aging to become a scientifically investigated issue, especially in terms of reproductive health.

In this chapter, we discuss the structural and functional changes in the male reproductive system in the course of aging. It proceeds with an overview of association of free radical theory of aging, sperm DNA fragmentation and repair, antioxidant capacity, apoptosis, and telomere length with aging of the male reproductive system. Moreover, this chapter highlights the oxidative stress and aging induced alterations in the male reproductive system.

MITOCHONDRIAL FREE RADICAL THEORY OF AGING

Many theories have been proposed to explain the aging process [1]. These theories basically suggest that aging is a programmed process or is the result of accumulation of damages in the organism [2]. In fact, it is not possible to justify aging with a single theory, since aging occurs as a consequence of various causes that damage the cells, tissues, and organs and reduce the repair capacity of this loss. One of the most important and investigated theories of aging have been the free radicals [3].

Harman proposed the "free radical theory of aging" for the first time [4]. According to his theory, "aging and the degenerative diseases associated with free radicals are attributed basically to the deleterious side attacks of free radicals on cell components and connective tissues." In 1972, Harman indicated that the free radicals are produced by the increase of oxygen consumption causing damage accumulation in the mitochondria, which ultimately result in death of mitochondria and proposed the "mitochondrial freerRadical theory of aging" (MFRTA) [5].

MFRTA can be summarized as damage by free radicals originating from electron transport chain (ETC) to macromolecules. Elevated reactive oxygen species (ROS) level results in impaired oxidative phosphorylation and decreased adenosine triphosphate (ATP) production in the cell. Eventually, MFRTA leads to activation of cell death pathways [6−10]. Mutations that encode proteins involved in mitochondrial function (either nuclear DNA or mitochondrial DNA [mtDNA]) often affect cells that use high energy, such as muscle and the cells of central nervous system. Therefore, loss of mitochondrial energy production is proposed to result in the development and progression of diseases associated with aging including atherosclerosis, myocardial hypertrophy, vascular dysfunction, and hypertension [10].

Mutations and deletions in mtDNA clonally expand with aging [11] as mentioned earlier, and there is a link between mtDNA mutations and aging phenotypes. Damage to ETC complex in these mice leads to decrease in ATP production and increase in apoptotic pathways. Knockin mice models also have shown early aging phenotypes characterized by fat loss, hair loss, kyphosis, osteoporosis, anemia, heart problems, and decline in fertility [12].

SPERM DNA DAMAGE/FRAGMENTATION, REACTIVE OXYGEN SPECIES, AND AGING

One of the most important causes of sperm DNA damage is oxidative stress induced by exogenous or endogenous factors or both [13]. The spermatozoa become highly vulnerable to ROS after spermiogenesis because most of their cytoplasm is removed and therefore they lack proper antioxidants [14]. Seminal ROS level and the number of sperm with DNA fragmentation are positively correlated with the number of seminal leukocytes [15]. However, not only ROS produced by leukocytes but also mitochondrial ROS is effective in eliciting sperm DNA damage The increased amount of ROS with both internal and external sources lead to damage of the sperm DNA [16]. Aging is also one of the factors that increase the production of ROS in the male reproductive system [17] (Fig. 1).

In the genome, ROS causes progressive damage that contributes to the aging process, including oxidized DNA bases and sugar, abasic regions, single-strand breaks (SSBs), and double-strand breaks (DSBs) [18,19]. Guanine has the lowest oxidation potential and therefore is the most easily oxidized base by the hydroxyl radical or the singlet oxygen [20]. Guanine-hydroxyl radical reaction results in C8-OH or Gua-N2-yl radicals. The main products of these radicals are 8-oxo-7,8-dihydroguanine (8oxoG), 2,6-diamino-4-hydroxy-5-formamidopyrimidine (Fapy-Gua), and oxazolone [21]. 8oxoG is considered an oxidative stress marker and its modified products are the most common DNA lesions. It is estimated that about 100,000 8oxoG lesions are formed every day in a cell. One to two of a million guanine in the nuclear genome and 1−3 of 100,000 G in mitochondrial DNA are 8oxoG [20]. Oxidized bases do not disrupt the double-helix structure of DNA and do not interfere with DNA replication [22]. However, 8oxoG may be paired with both cytosine and adenine and result in G:C → T:A transversion mutations [19,22]. 8oxoG accumulation is associated with many age-related pathological conditions [20] and leads to oxidative DNA lesions and mutations along with the increase in ROS production caused by the decreased enzyme activities in the base excision repair (BER) pathway [20,23].

The oxidative sperm DNA damage is repaired before the S-phase of first mitotic division of the zygote [24]. Oxidative damage in the sperm triggers arrest of the cell cycle at G2/M control point and phosphorylates cyclin-dependent kinases (CDKs) involved in this point in the mouse zygote [25]. At this stage, oxidative damage is repaired by the BER pathway. The repair of the oxidatively damaged DNA products, namely, 8-hydroxy-2′-deoxyguanosine, 8-oxo-7,8-dihydro-2′-deoxyguanosine, and 8-oxodG (8OHDG) lesions, is performed in male and female gametes [26]. 8-oxoguanine DNA glycosylase 1 (OGG1), the first enzyme of the BER pathway, has been identified in the spermatozoa. OGG1 creates abasic regions as the first step of repair in the paternal genome [26]. The downstream enzymes of the BER pathway are present in the oocyte [24]. Posttranslational modifications of these enzymes are initiated by fertilization and in the course of events 8OHDG excision occurs [17].

Studies have suggested a positive correlation between paternal aging and sperm DNA damage and fragmentation. The amount of ROS that increases with aging may be effective in increasing the sperm DNA damage. Studies have shown that the sperm DNA damage is most frequent in the eldest men. Alshahrani and colleagues have found that the sperm DNA damage in infertile men over 40 years was statistically higher than infertile males less than 30 years of age. The researchers found no association between different age groups and seminal ROS levels in these infertile men. On the other hand, all nonobstructive azoospermic infertile men were included in this study without any separation into subgroups. The effect of age on sperm DNA damage is important in the evaluation of males in fertility clinics, especially when they exceed the oocyte repair capacity [27]. The effect of aging on sperm DNA fragmentation in patients with oligoasthenoteratozoospermia (OAT) was investigated and the number of TUNEL positive spermatozoa increased significantly with age. This study showed that paternal aging in the infertile group was also associated with insufficient chromosome packing with protamines. However, DNA fragmentation and chromatin packing in the control group did not change with age [28]. Sperm DNA fragmentation in the male partner of couples with natural conception usually showed multiple repetitive miscarriages correlated with paternal age and miscarriage numbers [29]. Moreover, a study conducted among infertile males has demonstrated a significant correlation of the DNA fragmentation rate with the rate of numerical sperm

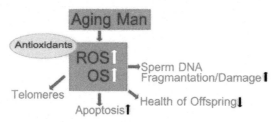

FIGURE 1 Aging of male reproductive system. *OS*, oxidative stress; *ROS*, reactive oxygen species.

chromosomal abnormalities. Although there was no significant difference between the paternal age of normal and abnormal karyotypes, DNA damage was more likely to be observed in sperm with chromosomal abnormality than in normal ones [30].

Sperm DNA fragmentation is higher in infertile males, but paternal age increases the rate of ROS and DNA fragmentation in both fertile and infertile males. A positive correlation between sperm DNA damage and paternal age was observed in a cohort over 4000 normozoospermic men [31]. In another study the ROS levels in fertile males 40 years of age and older were found to be significantly higher than the younger group [32]. A study conducted on healthy and nonsmoker men have found that increase of sperm DNA fragmentation correlates with aging. The predicted probability rate of sperm DNA fragmentation index was calculated as 95% for 80 years, while the index was 5% for 30-year-old men [33].

Although a metaanalysis indicated that male aging is associated with an increase in DNA fragmentation [34], some studies do not confirm these results. Furthermore, nonselected males who apply to the fertility clinic and normozoospermic males were divided into four groups according to their age. No correlation between age and sperm DNA fragmentation in either the control or the patient group was indicated. The same result was obtained when 35 years of age was settled as the cut-off value and arranged into only two groups: 35 years of age and younger [35]. Similarly, in a study conducted with infertile patients consulted in an assisted reproductive technique clinic demonstrated no significant increase in sperm DNA fragmentation in patients over 40 years of age [36]. On the other hand, sperm DNA fragmentation was evaluated by TUNEL in 140 infertile and 50 fertile men and the results showed that aging did not affect sperm DNA fragmentation but increased diploidy rate [37]. In these studies the lack of clarity of the patient group and the low number of patients included may have caused conflicting results.

Effects of Reactive Oxygen Species and Advanced Paternal Age on Health of Offspring

Mutant mouse experiments were performed to evaluate the effects of oxidative stress on male germ cells with increasing age. Senescence-accelerated mouse strains whose life spans are shorter than that of wild type rats are available for mutation accumulation naturally [38]. The P8 variant that is one of these mutant strains has lower OGG1 activity [39]. Studies conducted with the P8 variant showed that the percentage of sperm containing 8oxoG was statistically high in these mice [40].

Increased oxidative stress with aging leads to an increase in mutation rate due to decrease in efficiency of repair mechanisms and an increase in the cell death in the germ cell line [41,42]. Paternal aging is the one of the main sources of mutations in the next generation and the number of these mutations is correlated the age of the father [43]. The base substitutions are the most common paternally originated mutations [42]. This fact explains why children of older fathers are at higher risk to be born with single-gene disorders. These de novo diseases are the result of gain in function mutations in the genes of fibroblast growth factor receptor (*FGFR*), tyrosine kinase receptor, and RAS/mitogen activated protein kinase (MAPK) signaling [44]. As a result, impairment of RAS signaling pathway changes the growth and differentiation properties of spermatogonial stem cells [45]. These mutations, which occur during mitotic division of spermatogonial stem cells, are thought to give the advantage of selective growth to mutant cells. This selective-growth advantage is called selfish spermatogonial selection and exists in all males, leading to clonal expansion of mutant cells in the subsequent divisions [44]. Autosomal dominant diseases that have higher frequencies with advanced paternal age are Apert, Crouzon, Pfeiffer, Muenke Syndrome, achondroplasia, Costello and Noonan syndromes, and multiple endocrine neoplasia type 2A and type 2B, which result in point mutations at five genes (*FGFR2*, *FGFR3*, *HRAS*, *PTPN11*, *RET*) [44,45]. All of these disorders manifest congenital skeletal abnormalities, developmental deficiencies, cardiac disorders, skin hyperpigmentation, and cancer [33].

Advanced paternal age increases the risk of some multifactorial diseases in children as well as point mutations. Paternal aging is identified as a risk factor that increases the incidence of low birth weight, stillbirths, and premature births. Immediately after birth, the children whose fathers are over 45 years tend to have a lower health status [46]. In addition, the incidence of birth defects such as cleft palate, heart malformations, musculoskeletal-skin anomalies, and childhood cancers may increase in children of older fathers [47].

Furthermore, the increase of de novo mutations with paternal aging may cause some developmental and psychiatric disorders in the child. Retrospective and prospective studies and metaanalyses have shown that the incidence of some neuropsychiatric disorders in children of older fathers is higher. The risk of schizophrenia, autism, and bipolar disorder in children of men aged 50 years or over was found to be significantly higher than that of young fathers [48–54]. Probably the developmental delay, psychomotor impairment, or behavioral problems of children of older fathers have led to a high mortality rate due to accident or poisoning in these children [55].

Increased risk of neurodegenerative diseases in children of older fathers may be associated with epigenetic changes and higher rate of de novo mutations in the male germ cell line. An exon sequencing study reported that 39% of paternal de novo mutations were associated with autism-related genes [56]. In addition, sperm global 5-methylcytosine and 5-hydroxymethylcytosine levels were significantly correlated with paternal age [57] and some of these changes were in genes previously reported to be associated with schizophrenia and bipolar disorders [58].

ANTIOXIDANTS

Several antioxidant defense systems have been evolved to protect the organism against the destructive effects of increased levels of ROS in the cell during the evolutionary process. These antioxidants include many antioxidant enzymes and nonenzymatic compounds such as vitamins A, E, C, β-carotene, melatonin, and glutathione [59].

Oxidative stress develops when the level of ROS increases and this level cannot be compensated by antioxidant mechanisms. Aging elevates ROS level in cells, however the change in antioxidant defense varies with age. Studies have demonstrated either increased or decreased level of antioxidant with aging. On the contrary, growth hormone (GH) overexpressing mice showed almost half of the CAT activity. This data indicates that antioxidant protection is affected by hormonal regulation and the age-related changes in this mechanism shows variations among the species, strains, tissue, and sex [60].

Developmental profiles of the activity of the antioxidant enzymes including superoxide dismutase (SOD), catalase, glutathione peroxidase (GPx), glutathione transferase (GSH-Tr), and hexose monophosphate shunt were measured in the rat testis and liver. The results have shown the basal levels and developmental profiles of antioxidant enzymes in the testis differ greatly from those in the liver [61]. Age-related tissue oxidative stress alterations in rat testicular tissue demonstrated that the antioxidant defense system plays a crucial role in development and maturation of the rat testis. Elevations in the testicular lipid peroxidation levels and H_2O_2 along with reduction in levels of SOD, catalase, and ascorbic acid were shown in rat testicular tissue [62].

The membrane of spermatozoa is rich in unsaturated fatty acids and contains ROS-producing enzymes such as oxidases and is susceptible to oxidative stress [63]. This sensitivity is further increased because of the limited intrinsic antioxidant protection due to the fact that most of the cytoplasm is discarded during spermiogenesis. While germ cells continue to differentiate in the testes, Sertoli cells protect them from oxidative stress. After the removal of spermatozoa into the seminiferous tubule lumen, it is protected by epididymal and seminal plasma antioxidants [16].

Both the enzymatic and nonenzymatic antioxidant systems are present in the testis. All three forms of SOD are expressed in the testicular tissue. While GPxs are found in different forms in different cells of testicular tissue, catalase (CAT) has a single form [63]. Microarray analyzes indicated that Cat, Prdx3, and Prdx6 are highly expressed in pachytene spermatocytes, while Sod1 and Prdx4 show high expression in round spermatids [64]. Prdxs are antioxidants that regulate redox signaling and play a role in cell cycle, apoptosis, and aging process of spermatozoa. The enzyme constitutes the basic protection mechanism of spermatozoa and plays a role in capacitation reactions [59]. The testis also includes nonenzymatic factors for protection such as copper, vitamins C and E, melatonin, and resveratrol [63,65].

Antioxidant mechanisms are required for the maintenance of cellular functions. CAT overexpressing mice did not show germ cell or Sertoli cell loss due to aging. Additionally, ROS levels and 8oxoG lesions of germ cell decreased significantly in these mice [66]. Various animal experiments were conducted to elucidate the effect of testicular aging on antioxidant levels. Histological studies of testicular tissues of older Brown Norway rats have revealed site-specific changes in glutathione S transferase (GST) expression [67]. While age-related lipid peroxidation and H_2O_2 levels were increased in testis mitochondria of Wistar rats, decreased levels of glutathione, SOD, GPx, and glutathione reductase were observed [68]. GPx and SOD enzyme activities decreased in the epididymal spermatozoa of 21-month-old Brown Norway rats compared to 4 months of age and H_2O_2 and superoxide radical production increased in the spermatozoa of the old group [69]. In a recent study, researchers observed that prooxidant exposure reduced CAT expression in spermatids of both old and young rats [64]. Spermatids of young rats by downregulation of SOD1 reduce H_2O_2 production; therefore, the reduction in CAT level is compensated. In older spermatids, the level of SOD1 expression remained high, thus high SOD1 and low CAT levels result in an increase of H_2O_2 inducing the redox degradation [64].

Oxidative stress that cannot be eliminated by antioxidants with aging affects steroidogenesis. GSH deficiency, an antioxidant abundantly found in Leydig cells, resulted in approximately 40% reduction in testosterone production in isolated cells of old Brown Norway rats [70]. In vivo, GSH deprivation also reduced the testosterone production in both young and old rats. Researchers observed deterioration of the steroidogenic pathway in the Leydig cells with aging [70].

TRX 2 and 3 are two of the antioxidant enzymes that are specific to the male germline and found in mature spermatozoa. Deletion of the Trx gene leads to age-related alterations such as motility loss, increased DNA damage and ROS level, and impaired protamination in spermatozoa. Different antioxidants may be effective at different levels for the maintenance of germ cell quality with aging. In a study examining the effects of aging on germ cells of *Sod1*-null and *Cat*-null mice found that aging causes severe redox dysfunction in $Sod^{-/-}$ mice, but milder effects of oxidative stress in wild types and $Cat^{-/-}$ mice [71]. In young *Sod1*-null mice, the percentage of sperm containing 8oxoG was higher and the rate of 8oxoG increased with age. It is suggested that PRDX1, which is expressed in higher levels in wild types and $Cat^{-/-}$ mice, but found in low levels in young wild type and old $Sod^{-/-}$ mice is responsible for 8oxoG accumulation [71]. Animal models with functional deletions can help us understand the changes of specific antioxidant mechanisms with aging.

APOPTOSIS

The increase in mitochondrial ROS generation increases mtDNA damages and leads to impaired oxidative phosphorylation, mitochondrial degradation, and apoptosis. ROS is an important regulator in both extrinsic and intrinsic pathways of apoptosis. ROS has a direct function in the activation of death receptors in the extrinsic pathway and in the induction of apoptosis. Increased ROS level is involved in cellular signaling, which leads to the activation of death receptors involved in the extrinsic pathway [72].

The death ligand Fas activates nicotinamide adenine dinucleotide phosphate oxidase and enhances the production of H_2O_2 and superoxide radicals. These free radicals activate the proteosomal pathway of antiapoptotic proteins. Activation of Jun N-terminal protein kinase (JNK), an enzyme involved in the programmed cell death pathway activated by apoptosis signal regulatory kinase 1 (ASK1), is induced by ROS. Whether tumor necrosis factor α (TNF-α) and the ligand of TNF receptor (TNFR1) support cell death or survival depends on the level and duration ROS activation of JNK. While nonpersistent and low-level JNK activation induces antiapoptotic pathway, strong and long-term activation of JNK activates apoptosis via ASK1. The increased ROS level also causes an increase in the enzyme activity of ASK1 [73].

Apoptosis is observed at various stages of germ cell differentiation and is thought to balance proliferation rate between germ cells and Sertoli cells in the seminiferous epithelium [74] and plays an important role in physiological changes such as aging and causes alterations in testicles [75]. In testicular tissue, while cell proliferation decreases, apoptosis increases with aging [76]. Aging-accelerated transgenic mouse models showed increased levels of procaspase 3 and cleaved caspase 3 in the testis [76]. Apoptosis was investigated with TUNEL assay in the testis of elderly men and the relation of germ cell depletion with aging and apoptosis was studied [77]. The data have suggested that the increase in apoptosis among primary spermatocytes may result in germ cell loss in elderly men. Researchers found that the proportion of primary spermatocytes, round spermatids, and elongated spermatids to Sertoli cells decreased significantly in the testis in older men. Expression of Ki-67, a cell proliferation marker in spermatogonia, was lower in older men in comparison to control. Apoptosis rates of primary spermatocytes were higher and antiapoptotic Bcl-xl expression was lower in elderly men than young controls [77]. In agreement to this data, quantitatively assessed histological changes in aging testis demonstrated the ratio of round and elongated spermatids to Sertoli cells was lower in the elderly group than in the younger group [78]. Another study reported increased apoptosis index, significantly lower Sertoli cell number, and decreased proliferation index in men at 70 year or older. This study also showed a slight decrease in the spermatocytes number in the elder men compared to the young group. However, the spermatid number was significantly different between the two groups [78]. During the apoptosis, phosphatidylserine, which is normally localized on the cytoplasmic side of the membrane, migrates to the outer side of the membrane and is recognized by phagocytes on the cell surface. Outer membrane translocations of phosphatidylserine are considered to be an early apoptotic marker, and this marker has been shown to increase in sperm of men over 40 years of age [79].

Increased DNA fragmentation and apoptosis in testicular germ cells with aging may indicate that some DNA repair mechanisms lead to apoptosis [80]. The repair protein PARP 1 is activated by DNA strand breaks and can modify many molecules including histones, transcription factors, and a number of enzymes in the cell [81]. Therefore, it is suggested that this protein plays a role in many cellular processes including apoptosis. PARP1 activation leads to mitochondrial AIF release and thus activates caspase-independent cell death [82]. PARP1 is highly expressed in the testicular tissue and activated in the initial stages of apoptosis [80]. Apoptotic markers, PARP1 expression, active caspase 3 expression, and truncated PARP1 in the testis tissue of old men were found to be higher than in young men [80].

REACTIVE OXYGEN SPECIES, AGING, AND TELOMERE LENGTH

Human telomeres are approximately 5—12 kilobases DNA sequences consisting of tandem repeats of $(TTAGGG)_n$ at the ends of chromosomes. Telomeres are bound to a group of proteins called shelterins. These proteins confer a structure to telomeric DNA called the T-loop, which prevents DNA damage response proteins from mistakenly repairing telomeres.

Shelterin complex basically consists of six proteins, namely, TRF1, TRF2, POT1, RAP1, TIN2, and TPP1. Telomeric repeat binding factor 1 and 2 (TRF1 and 2) form the T-loop structure in the duplex telomeric repeats at the chromosome ends [83]. Loss of these proteins leads to telomeric 3′ end loss, p53 activation, and rearrangement at the chromosome ends [84]. TRF1, TRF2, and POT1 recognize hexameric telomere repeats. Then, TIN2, TPP1, and RAP1 bind to these three proteins [85].

Telomeres, along with their associated proteins, conserve the integrity of chromosomes and genetic information, protect the chromosomes from enzymatic degradation and recombination, and prevent the cell from entering senescence or apoptosis [86,87]. Telomeres also affect the nuclear localization of chromosomes and the movement of homologous chromosomes during cell division [86]. Due to the inability of the DNA polymerase to completely replicate the 5′ terminal sequence in replication, some of the terminal nucleotides are lost in each cell division, and ultimately the telomeres are shortened [88,89]. The loss of telomeric repeats disrupts the stability of the T-loop and the telomere-shelterin complex. This stability loss activates the DNA damage response and the cell enters a transient cycle arrest to allow time for the repair of DNA damage. However, if the damage cannot be repaired, this arrest becomes permanent [90]. When the length of telomeres reaches a critical level, the cell proliferation stops and senescence or apoptosis is induced [91,92].

Oxidative stress causes an increase in the loss of telomeric DNA [93,94]. The oxidative damage of telomeric DNA is less repaired than that of the other regions of the chromosomes. DNA damage signaling and DNA repair pathways are locally repressed in the telomeres, thus preventing the chromosomal rearrangement. In addition, guanine-rich repeats of the telomere are more prone to oxidation. Additionally, the BER pathway is not effective in the repair of oxidative damage that occurs in the single-stranded (ss) DNA of telomeres tails because OGG1 repairs only double-stranded (ds) DNA. Due to all these reasons, telomeres are more susceptible to oxidative stress than other regions of chromosomes [95]. Studies have also shown that oxidative damage in telomeric DNA also alters the binding activities of TRF1 and TRF2. While a single 8oxoG lesion in the telomere reduced the binding capacity of TRF1 and TRF2 at least 50%, the binding capacity is decreased by increase of 8oxoG [93]. The telomeric damage induced by oxidative stress leads to the shortening of the telomere, and the telomere loss causes an increase in chromosomal instability. Oxidative base damage together with telomeric dysfunction lead to abnormal nuclear morphologies such as micronucleus, nucleoplasmic bridges, and buds [96].

A recent study suggests that the effect of 8oxoG, the most common oxidative lesion on telomere length, may be bidirectional. The OGG1-deleted mice had longer telomeres in vivo but in the cultured cells of this animal there was an accelerated telomeric shortening due to the presence of oxidants [97]. As a result, the localization of oxidative base lesion may be effective on the telomere length. Oxidized bases may be found in both the structure of the DNA helix (8oxoG) and as free dNTPs (8oxoGTP) in the cells. Free dNTPs in the cell are more prone to oxidation than the nucleotides in the DNA strand. In light of this knowledge, the effect of free 8oxoGTP in the cell on telomere maintenance and integrity was investigated. Researchers have shown that when 8-oxoG is already present within the telomeric DNA sequence (either by insertion of oxidized nucleotides or by direct free radical−mediated oxidation), it promotes telomerase activity by destabilizing the G-quadruplex DNA structure. The inhibition and activation of telomerase depends on the mechanism by which 8-oxoG is inserted in telomeres and thereby mediates the biological outcome [98].

Telomeres are protected during male germ cell differentiation so that shortened telomeres do not pass on to the next generation and that telomere length is sufficient for the life of the child [99]. The telomere length of the offspring's chromosomes correlates with paternal telomere length. Spermatozoa telomeres play a role in guiding oocyte telomeres during preimplantation and development. This process occurs via an alternative prolongation named telomerase-independent telomere length maintenance [100]. In addition, due to high levels of telomerase expression in the testis, sperm chromosome telomeres extend with paternal aging. Knockin mouse models studies reported that the highest level of telomerase in the testis was measured in spermatogonia type A [101]. Although the telomeric sequences are longer among children of older fathers, the leukocyte telomere length shows individual differences due to telomerase and/or oxidative stress effects. In a study of the relative telomeric length of cells at different stages of spermatogenesis from testicular tissue samples of elderly and young men, it was observed that primary spermatocytes had the longest telomeres in both groups. Additionally, relative telomere length was found to be longer in primary spermatocytes than in spermatogonia and also shorter in spermatozoa than in spermatogonia. The telomere length of the elderly group was similar to that of the younger group, but the length differences between the stages were statistically significant. Researchers have suggested that the difference in telomere length does not arise from the end replication problem because there are only two cell divisions between primary spermatocytes and spermatozoa; indeed the oxidative stress may be effective in telomere length difference [99].

CONCLUSION

Aging causes tissue and organ damage in all aerobic organisms. The effect of free ROS on macromolecules in the cell is one of the most common explanations used to elucidate the aging process. ROS are produced continuously as a by-product of aerobic respiration and may cause oxidative damage to lipids, DNA, and proteins when not eliminated by antioxidants. In cells exogenous and endogenous sources of ROS increase with aging. Studies have shown that the increase in ROS level with aging is one of the causes of progressive changes in the male reproductive system. This situation draws attention to the potential consequences of becoming a father at older ages. Rigorous living conditions and a desire for a better life style cause postponing of parenthood until a later age. The effects of advanced age on disease risk of offspring remain unknown. The effects of aging on men's reproductive system and fertility potential are poorly understood. The effects of aging on the male reproductive system are multifactorial and influenced by both normal physiological processes and environmental causes. Further studies should investigate the onset of gonadal senesce and its regulation on aging men.

GLOSSARY

DNA damage Alterations of DNA that lead to a shift in the chemical structure of DNA.
DNA fragmentation Breaking of DNA strand(s) in pieces.
Free radical theory of aging Accumulation of deleterious side attacks of free radicals on cell components and connective tissues.
Mitochondrial free radical theory of aging The free radicals are produced by the increase of oxygen consumption, causing damage accumulation in the mitochondria that ultimately results in death of mitochondria.
Mitohormesis The response to mild mitochondrial stress that leads to adaptive reactions in animal models to leave the cell less susceptible to oxidative stress and extend the life span.
Oxygen poisoning The toxicity resulting from breathing oxygen with high partial pressure.
Telomerase A ribonucleoprotein that extends a species-dependent telomeric repeats to the 3' end of telomeres.
Telomere Terminal regions of chromosomes.

LIST OF ACRONYMS AND ABBREVIATIONS

8OHDG 8-oxodG
8oxoG 8-oxo-7,8-dihydroguanine
OGG1 8-oxoguanine DNA glycosylase 1
AIF Apoptosis inducing factor
ASK1 Apoptosis signal regulatory kinase 1
BER Base excision repair
CAT Catalase
CDK Cyclin-dependent kinase
DSB Double-strand break
ds Double-stranded
FGF Fibroblast growth factor
FGFR Fibroblast growth factor receptor
GSH Glutathione
GPx Glutathione peroxidase
GST Glutathione S transferase
GH Growth hormone
H_2O_2 Hydrogen peroxide
mtDNA Mitochondrial DNA
MAPK Mitogen activated protein kinase
OAT Oligoasthenoteratozoospermia
PRDX Peroxiredoxin
ROS Reactive oxygen species
SSB Single-strand break
ss Single-stranded
SOD Superoxide dismutase
TERT Telomerase reverse transcriptase
TRF Telomeric repeat binding factor
TRX Thioredoxin
TNFR1 Tumor necrosis factor
TNFα Tumor necrosis factor alpha

REFERENCES

[1] Park DC, Yeo SG. Aging. Korean J Audiol 2013;17(2):39–44.

[2] Jin K. Modern biological theories of aging. Aging Dis 2010;1(2):72–4.

[3] Liochev SI. Which is the most significant cause of aging? Antioxidants 2015;4(4):793–810.

[4] Harman D. Origin and evolution of the free radical theory of aging: a brief personal history, 1954-2009. Biogerontology 2009;10(6):773–81.

[5] Harman D. The biologic clock: the mitochondria? J Am Geriatr Soc 1972;20(4):145–7.

[6] Hekimi S, Lapointe J, Wen Y. Taking a "good" look at free radicals in the aging process. Trends Cell Biol 2011;21(10):569–76.

[7] Jang YC, Van Remmen H. The mitochondrial theory of aging: insight from transgenic and knockout mouse models. Exp Gerontol 2009;44(4):256–60.

[8] Lopez-Otin C, et al. The hallmarks of aging. Cell 2013;153(6):1194–217.

[9] Conley KE, Marcinek DJ, Villarin J. Mitochondrial dysfunction and age. Curr Opin Clin Nutr Metab Care 2007;10(6):688–92.

[10] Vajapey R, et al. The impact of age-related dysregulation of the angiotensin system on mitochondrial redox balance. Front Physiol 2014;5:439.

[11] Popadin K, et al. When man got his mtDNA deletions? Aging Cell 2014;13(4):579–82.

[12] Trifunovic A, et al. Premature ageing in mice expressing defective mitochondrial DNA polymerase. Nature 2004;429(6990):417–23.

[13] Gunes S, Al-Sadaan M, Agarwal A. Spermatogenesis, DNA damage and DNA repair mechanisms in male infertility. Reprod Biomed Online 2015;31(3):309–19.

[14] Agarwal A, Prabakaran SA, Said TM. Prevention of oxidative stress injury to sperm. J Androl 2005;26(6):654–60.

[15] Lobascio AM, et al. Involvement of seminal leukocytes, reactive oxygen species, and sperm mitochondrial membrane potential in the DNA damage of the human spermatozoa. Andrology 2015;3(2):265–70.

[16] Aitken RJ, Curry BJ. Redox regulation of human sperm function: from the physiological control of sperm capacitation to the etiology of infertility and DNA damage in the germ line. Antioxid Redox Signal 2011;14(3):367–81.

[17] Sabeti P, et al. Etiologies of sperm oxidative stress. Int J Reprod Biomed 2016;14(4):231–40.

[18] Mitra J, et al. New perspectives on oxidized genome damage and repair inhibition by pro-oxidant metals in neurological diseases. Biomolecules 2014;4(3):678–703.

[19] Pilger A, Rudiger HW. 8-Hydroxy-2'-deoxyguanosine as a marker of oxidative DNA damage related to occupational and environmental exposures. Int Arch Occup Environ Health 2006;80(1):1–15.

[20] Radak Z, Boldogh I. 8-Oxo-7,8-dihydroguanine: links to gene expression, aging, and defense against oxidative stress. Free Radic Biol Med 2010;49(4):587–96.

[21] Cadet J, Wagner JR. DNA base damage by reactive oxygen species, oxidizing agents, and UV radiation. Cold Spring Harb Perspect Biol 2013;5(2).

[22] Hegde ML, Izumi T, Mitra S. Oxidized base damage and single-strand break repair in mammalian genomes: role of disordered regions and posttranslational modifications in early enzymes. Prog Mol Biol Transl Sci 2012;110:123–53.

[23] Gorbunova V, et al. Changes in DNA repair during aging. Nucleic Acids Res 2007;35(22):7466–74.

[24] Lord T, Aitken RJ. Fertilization stimulates 8-hydroxy-2'-deoxyguanosine repair and antioxidant activity to prevent mutagenesis in the embryo. Dev Biol 2015;406(1):1–13.

[25] Zhang Y, et al. Oxidative stress-induced DNA damage of mouse zygotes triggers G2/M checkpoint and phosphorylates Cdc25 and Cdc2. Cell Stress Chaperones 2016;21(4):687–96.

[26] Smith TB, et al. The presence of a truncated base excision repair pathway in human spermatozoa that is mediated by OGG1. J Cell Sci 2013;126(Pt 6):1488–97.

[27] Alshahrani S, et al. Infertile men older than 40 years are at higher risk of sperm DNA damage. Reprod Biol Endocrinol 2014;12:103.

[28] Plastira K, et al. The effects of age on DNA fragmentation, chromatin packaging and conventional semen parameters in spermatozoa of oligoasthenoteratozoospermic patients. J Assist Reprod Genet 2007;24(10):437–43.

[29] Carlini T, et al. Sperm DNA fragmentation in Italian couples with recurrent pregnancy loss. Reprod Biomed Online 2017;34(1):58–65.

[30] Enciso M, Alfarawati S, Wells D. Increased numbers of DNA-damaged spermatozoa in samples presenting an elevated rate of numerical chromosome abnormalities. Hum Reprod 2013;28(6):1707–15.

[31] Belloc S, et al. Sperm deoxyribonucleic acid damage in normozoospermic men is related to age and sperm progressive motility. Fertil Steril 2014;101(6):1588–93.

[32] Cocuzza M, et al. Age-related increase of reactive oxygen species in neat semen in healthy fertile men. Urology 2008;71(3):490–4.

[33] Wyrobek AJ, et al. Advancing age has differential effects on DNA damage, chromatin integrity, gene mutations, and aneuploidies in sperm. Proc Natl Acad Sci U S A 2006;103(25):9601–6.

[34] Johnson SL, et al. Consistent age-dependent declines in human semen quality: a systematic review and meta-analysis. Ageing Res Rev 2015;19:22–33.

[35] Winkle T, et al. The correlation between male age, sperm quality and sperm DNA fragmentation in 320 men attending a fertility center. J Assist Reprod Genet 2009;26(1):41–6.

[36] Nijs M, et al. Correlation between male age, WHO sperm parameters, DNA fragmentation, chromatin packaging and outcome in assisted reproduction technology. Andrologia 2011;43(3):174–9.

[37] Brahem S, et al. The effects of male aging on semen quality, sperm DNA fragmentation and chromosomal abnormalities in an infertile population. J Assist Reprod Genet 2011;28(5):425–32.

[38] Takeda T, Hosokawa M, Higuchi K. Senescence-accelerated mouse (SAM): a novel murine model of senescence. Exp Gerontol 1997;32(1−2):105−9.

[39] Choi JY, et al. Thermolabile 8-hydroxyguanine DNA glycosylase with low activity in senescence-accelerated mice due to a single-base mutation. Free Radic Biol Med 1999;27(7−8):848−54.

[40] Smith TB, et al. The senescence-accelerated mouse prone 8 as a model for oxidative stress and impaired DNA repair in the male germ line. Reproduction 2013;146(3):253−62.

[41] Crow JF. The origins, patterns and implications of human spontaneous mutation. Nat Rev Genet 2000;1(1):40−7.

[42] Gregoire MC, et al. Male-driven de novo mutations in haploid germ cells. Mol Hum Reprod 2013;19(8):495−9.

[43] Kong A, et al. Rate of de novo mutations and the importance of father's age to disease risk. Nature 2012;488(7412):471−5.

[44] Maher GJ, Goriely A, Wilkie AO. Cellular evidence for selfish spermatogonial selection in aged human testes. Andrology 2014;2(3):304−14.

[45] Goriely A, Wilkie AO. Paternal age effect mutations and selfish spermatogonial selection: causes and consequences for human disease. Am J Hum Genet 2012;90(2):175−200.

[46] Sun Y, et al. Paternal age and Apgar scores of newborn infants. Epidemiology 2006;17(4):473−4.

[47] Green RF, et al. Association of paternal age and risk for major congenital anomalies from the National Birth Defects Prevention Study, 1997 to 2004. Ann Epidemiol 2010;20(3):241−9.

[48] Reichenberg A, et al. Advancing paternal age and autism. Arch Gen Psychiatry 2006;63(9):1026−32.

[49] Frans EM, et al. Advancing paternal age and bipolar disorder. Arch Gen Psychiatry 2008;65(9):1034−40.

[50] Brown AS, et al. Paternal age and risk of schizophrenia in adult offspring. Am J Psychiatry 2002;159(9):1528−33.

[51] Lopez-Castroman J, et al. Differences in maternal and paternal age between schizophrenia and other psychiatric disorders. Schizophr Res 2010;116(2−3):184−90.

[52] Sorensen HJ, et al. Effects of paternal age and offspring cognitive ability in early adulthood on the risk of schizophrenia and related disorders. Schizophr Res 2014;160(1−3):131−5.

[53] Miller B, et al. Meta-analysis of paternal age and schizophrenia risk in male versus female offspring. Schizophr Bull 2011;37(5):1039−47.

[54] Tsuchiya KJ, et al. Paternal age at birth and high-functioning autistic-spectrum disorder in offspring. Br J Psychiatry 2008;193(4):316−21.

[55] Zhu JL, et al. Paternal age and mortality in children. Eur J Epidemiol 2008;23(7):443−7.

[56] O'Roak BJ, et al. Sporadic autism exomes reveal a highly interconnected protein network of de novo mutations. Nature 2012;485(7397):246−50.

[57] Jenkins TG, et al. Paternal aging and associated intraindividual alterations of global sperm 5-methylcytosine and 5-hydroxymethylcytosine levels. Fertil Steril 2013;100(4):945−51.

[58] Jenkins TG, et al. Age-associated sperm DNA methylation alterations: possible implications in offspring disease susceptibility. PLoS Genet 2014;10(7):e1004458.

[59] O'Flaherty C. Peroxiredoxins: hidden players in the antioxidant defence of human spermatozoa. Basic Clin Androl 2014;24:4.

[60] Brown-Borg HM, Rakoczy SG. Catalase expression in delayed and premature aging mouse models. Exp Gerontol 2000;35(2):199−212.

[61] Peltola V, Huhtaniemi I, Ahotupa M. Antioxidant enzyme activity in the maturing rat testis. J Androl 1992;13(5):450−5.

[62] Samanta L, Roy A, Chainy GB. Changes in rat testicular antioxidant defence profile as a function of age and its impairment by hexachlorocyclohexane during critical stages of maturation. Andrologia 1999;31(2):83−90.

[63] Aitken RJ, Roman SD. Antioxidant systems and oxidative stress in the testes. Oxid Med Cell Longev 2008;1(1):15−24.

[64] Selvaratnam J, Paul C, Robaire B. Male rat germ cells display age-dependent and cell-specific susceptibility in response to oxidative stress challenges. Biol Reprod 2015;93(3):72.

[65] Turner TT, Lysiak JJ. Oxidative stress: a common factor in testicular dysfunction. J Androl 2008;29(5):488−98.

[66] Selvaratnam J, Robaire B. Overexpression of catalase in mice reduces age-related oxidative stress and maintains sperm production. Exp Gerontol 2016;84:12−20.

[67] Mueller A, Hermo L, Robaire B. The effects of aging on the expression of glutathione S-transferases in the testis and epididymis of the Brown Norway rat. J Androl 1998;19(4):450−65.

[68] Sahoo DK, Roy A, Chainy GB. Rat testicular mitochondrial antioxidant defence system and its modulation by aging. Acta Biol Hung 2008;59(4):413−24.

[69] Weir CP, Robaire B. Spermatozoa have decreased antioxidant enzymatic capacity and increased reactive oxygen species production during aging in the Brown Norway rat. J Androl 2007;28(2):229−40.

[70] Chen H, et al. Effect of glutathione depletion on Leydig cell steroidogenesis in young and old brown Norway rats. Endocrinology 2008;149(5):2612−9.

[71] Selvaratnam JS, Robaire B. Effects of aging and oxidative stress on spermatozoa of superoxide-dismutase 1- and catalase-null mice. Biol Reprod 2016;95(3):60.

[72] Li X, Becker KA, Zhang Y. Ceramide in redox signaling and cardiovascular diseases. Cell Physiol Biochem 2010;26(1):41−8.

[73] Circu ML, Aw TY. Reactive oxygen species, cellular redox systems, and apoptosis. Free Radic Biol Med 2010;48(6):749−62.

[74] Gomez-Lopez N, et al. The apoptotic pathway in fertile and subfertile men: a case-control and prospective study to examine the impact of merocyanine 540 bodies on ejaculated spermatozoa. Fertil Steril 2013;99(5):1242−8.

[75] Gunes S, et al. Effects of aging on the male reproductive system. J Assist Reprod Genet 2016;33(4):441−54.

[76] Pastor LM, et al. Proliferation and apoptosis in aged and photoregressed mammalian seminiferous epithelium, with particular attention to rodents and humans. Reprod Domest Anim 2011;46(1):155−64.

[77] Kimura M, et al. Balance of apoptosis and proliferation of germ cells related to spermatogenesis in aged men. J Androl 2003;24(2):185—91.

[78] Jiang H, et al. Quantitative histological analysis and ultrastructure of the aging human testis. Int Urol Nephrol 2014;46(5):879—85.

[79] Colin A, et al. The effect of age on the expression of apoptosis biomarkers in human spermatozoa. Fertil Steril 2010;94(7):2609—14.

[80] El-Domyati MM, et al. Deoxyribonucleic acid repair and apoptosis in testicular germ cells of aging fertile men: the role of the poly(adenosine diphosphate-ribosyl)ation pathway. Fertil Steril 2009;91(5 Suppl):2221—9.

[81] Maymon BB, et al. Role of poly(ADP-ribosyl)ation during human spermatogenesis. Fertil Steril 2006;86(5):1402—7.

[82] Feng X, et al. Silencing of Apoptosis-Inducing factor and poly(ADP-ribose) glycohydrolase reveals novel roles in breast cancer cell death after chemotherapy. Mol Cancer 2012;11:48.

[83] Broccoli D, et al. Human telomeres contain two distinct Myb-related proteins, TRF1 and TRF2. Nat Genet 1997;17(2):231—5.

[84] Griffith JD, et al. Mammalian telomeres end in a large duplex loop. Cell 1999;97(4):503—14.

[85] de Lange T. Shelterin: the protein complex that shapes and safeguards human telomeres. Genes Dev 2005;19(18):2100—10.

[86] Gancarcikova M, et al. The role of telomeres and telomerase complex in haematological neoplasia: the length of telomeres as a marker of carcinogenesis and prognosis of disease. Prague Med Rep 2010;111(2):91—105.

[87] Nussey DH, et al. Measuring telomere length and telomere dynamics in evolutionary biology and ecology. Methods Ecol Evol 2014;5(4):299—310.

[88] Eisenberg DT. An evolutionary review of human telomere biology: the thrifty telomere hypothesis and notes on potential adaptive paternal effects. Am J Hum Biol 2011;23(2):149—67.

[89] Oeseburg H, et al. Telomere biology in healthy aging and disease. Pflugers Arch 2010;459(2):259—68.

[90] Correia-Melo C, Hewitt G, Passos JF. Telomeres, oxidative stress and inflammatory factors: partners in cellular senescence? Longev Healthspan 2014;3(1):1.

[91] Else T. Telomeres and telomerase in adrenocortical tissue maintenance, carcinogenesis, and aging. J Mol Endocrinol 2009;43(4):131—41.

[92] Lobetti-Bodoni C, et al. Telomeres and telomerase in normal and malignant B-cells. Hematol Oncol 2010;28(4):157—67.

[93] Opresko PL, et al. Oxidative damage in telomeric DNA disrupts recognition by TRF1 and TRF2. Nucleic Acids Res 2005;33(4):1230—9.

[94] von Zglinicki T. Oxidative stress shortens telomeres. Trends Biochem Sci 2002;27(7):339—44.

[95] Aeby E, et al. Peroxiredoxin 1 protects telomeres from oxidative damage and preserves telomeric DNA for extension by telomerase. Cell Rep 2016;17(12):3107—14.

[96] Coluzzi E, et al. Oxidative stress induces persistent telomeric DNA damage responsible for nuclear morphology change in mammalian cells. PLoS One 2014;9(10):e110963.

[97] Wang Z, et al. Characterization of oxidative guanine damage and repair in mammalian telomeres. PLoS Genet 2010;6(5):e1000951.

[98] Fouquerel E, et al. Oxidative guanine base damage regulates human telomerase activity. Nat Struct Mol Biol 2016;23(12):1092—100.

[99] Jorgensen PB, et al. Age-dependence of relative telomere length profiles during spermatogenesis in man. Maturitas 2013;75(4):380—5.

[100] de Frutos C, et al. Spermatozoa telomeres determine telomere length in early embryos and offspring. Reproduction 2016;151(1):1—7.

[101] Pech MF, et al. High telomerase is a hallmark of undifferentiated spermatogonia and is required for maintenance of male germline stem cells. Genes Dev 2015;29(23):2420—34.

Part III

Clinical Methods to Determine and Treat Oxidative Stress

Chapter 3.1

Reactive Oxygen Species Methodology Using Chemiluminescence Assay

Rakesh Sharma, Manesh Kumar Panner Selvam and Ashok Agarwal

American Center for Reproductive Medicine, Cleveland Clinic, Cleveland, OH, United States

INTRODUCTION

The excessive production of reactive oxygen species (ROS) is associated with pathology of male infertility. ROS is produced by both intrinsic and extrinsic sources and affects sperm quality. Main contributors include leukocytes, especially granulocytes and immature and morphologically abnormal spermatozoa [1,2]. ROS are associated with the cellular damage and have a major impact on spermatogenesis by attacking the sperm lipids, proteins, and DNA, and affect sperm function [3,4]. Increased ROS levels in infertile men induces sperm DNA fragmentation by attacking the nuclear and mitochondrial DNA. Increased levels of ROS are associated with increased miscarriage or pregnancy loss [5–7]. Pathophysiological state in the spermatozoa is created due to the increased levels of ROS. The inability of the available antioxidants present in the seminal fluid to neutralize this makes them susceptible to oxidative stress (OS). OS causes damage to the sperm membrane and alters its permeability and fluidity, and disturbs the normal sperm functions. It also affects both natural and assisted reproduction. Low pregnancy rates have been reported in men with high ROS levels [8–11]. Therefore measuring the accurate levels of ROS is important, as this test can be offered as a diagnostic test or screening test for differentiating fertile population from infertile or men with unexplained/idiopathic infertility [12].

ROS are highly reactive and have a short half-life [13]. Robust and sensitive assays are required for the measurement of ROS. Measurement of ROS provides a better understanding of sperm metabolism in the spermatozoa-related male infertility condition. In this chapter, the various methods for measurement of ROS are described. The measurement of ROS by chemiluminescence method is more common and is described in detail in this chapter.

METHODS FOR MEASURING REACTIVE OXYGEN SPECIES

Different assays are available for measurement of ROS. They are mainly categorized into direct and indirect methods. Direct assay measures the net ROS levels in the semen sample, but the indirect assay provides the negative effect of ROS on spermatozoa. Each technique has its own merits and demerits. Some of the important techniques are presented in Table 1.

MEASUREMENT OF REACTIVE OXYGEN SPECIES BY CHEMILUMINESCENCE

Measurement of ROS by chemiluminescence assay is used in advanced research clinical laboratories for the assessment of ROS in fresh semen sample. It is a direct method for measurement of ROS and a useful tool in the clinical andrology laboratory to identify infertile men with unexplained infertility and OS. Luminol (5 amino-2,3-dihydro-1,4-phthalazinedione) and lucigenin (10,10′-dimethyl-9,9′-biacridinium nitrate) are the two common probes used to measure ROS. Luminol measures global ROS (i.e., both the intra- and extracellular ROS [O_2^-, H_2O_2 and OH^-]) as they are not

TABLE 1 Direct and Indirect Techniques for Measurement of Reactive Oxygen Species in Semen

Technique	Principle/Probe	Instrument	Type of Sample
Direct			
Chemiluminescence	Luminol	Luminometer	Extracellular and intracellular
	Lucigenin		Extracellular
Nitro blue tetrazolium (NBT)	NBT reduced to formazan by superoxide ions	Spectrophotometer	Extracellular
Cytochrome C reduction test	Ferricytochrome C	Spectrophotometer	Extracellular
Fluorescein probe	2'-7'-Dichlorodihydrofluorescein diacetate (DCFH-DA)	Flow cytometer	Spermatozoa
Oxidation-induced fluorochrome probe	Dihydroethidium (DHE)	Confocal microscope	Spermatozoa
Electron spin resonance	Paramagnetic species	Electron spin resonance spectroscopy	Extracellular and intracellular
Indirect			
Myeloperoxidase or Endtz test	Peroxidase activity	Colorimeter	Spermatozoa
Lipid peroxidation levels	Thiobarbituric acid-reactive substances	Colorimeter	Oxidized components in seminal plasma
Chemokines	Specific antibodies ELISA	ELISA reader	Seminal plasma
Antioxidant, micronutrients, vitamins	Column chromatography	HPLC	Seminal plasma
Ascorbate	Column chromatography	HPLC	Seminal plasma
Antioxidants—total antioxidant capacity	2,2'-Azinodi-[3-ethylbenzthiazolinesulfonate] (ABTS)	Luminometer	Seminal plasma
DNA damage	TUNEL	Flow cytometer	Spermatozoa

HPLC, high-performance liquid chromatography; *ROS*, reactive oxygen species; *ELISA*, enzyme linked immunosorbent assay; *TUNEL*, terminal deoxynucleotidyl transferase dUTP nick end labeling.

charged and permeable through the membrane, whereas lucigenin is positively charged and impermeable and can measure only extracellular ROS (O_2^- and OH^- free radicals) [14,15]. Chemiluminescence is the most sensitive detection method currently available [16].

Principle

Chemiluminescence is the light emitted by a chemical reaction. The active component used is either luminol or lucigenin, which reacts with various types of ROS at neutral pH. Luminol is first oxidized in a one-electron step, which leads to the formation of a free radical. It reacts in its univalently oxidized form with ROS to generate an unstable endoperoxide that decomposes to an electronically excited product. This product releases a photon as it falls to the ground state. In the case of lucigenin it is first reduced to a cation radical. Then it reacts in its univalently reduced form with ROS to produce dioxetane, which breaks down to generate photons. These probes cannot measure the individual free radicals but measure global ROS levels in the sample. Luminescence signals are expressed in relative light units (RLU), a direct measure of free radicals produced.

$$\text{Luminol (free radical)} + \text{ROS} \rightarrow \text{Endoperoxide (unstable)} \rightarrow \text{Photons}$$

$$\text{Lucigen (cation)} + \text{ROS} \rightarrow \text{Dioxetane} \rightarrow \text{Photons}$$

TYPES OF LUMINOMETERS

Chemiluminescence signals are measured using luminometers. All luminometers contain photodiodes or photo-multiplier tubes to detect the chemiluminescence signals. These detectors are either placed below or to the side of the sample tubes to capture the signals. Basically they are designed to measure the signals as photons or electric current when the photons strike the photomultiplier tube. The results are expressed as or millivolts/sec, counted photons/min (cpm), or RLUs [17].

Single or Double Tube Luminometer

Single or double tube luminometers can measure the chemiluminescence of one or two samples at a time. This type of luminometer is considered economical when compared with multitube or microplate luminometers [18,19]. Single tube luminometers can be used to analyze up to 40 samples per day and are ideal for small research laboratories [20].

Examples: TD 20/20 (Turner Biosystems Inc., Sunnyvale, CA, USA), FB-12 (Zylux Corporation, Oak Ridge, TN, USA), Traithler (Bioscan, Washington, DC, USA), Zylux FB 15 (Bio-World, Dublin, OH, USA).

Multitube Luminometer

Multiple samples can be analyzed simultaneously using multitube luminometers. They are expensive, hence used widely in commercial laboratories. Certain luminometers (Berthold LB9505 and LB953) are integrated with a kinetic mode and temperature maintenance unit, which allows the measurement of chemiluminescence at different temperatures [21]. They also are equipped with automated injectors to dispense the reagents. Real-time production of the signals can be monitored and visualized on the monitor.

Examples: Autolumat LB 953 (Berthold Technologies, Oak Ridge, TN, USA), Optocomp-2 (MGM Instruments, Inc., Hamden, CT, USA).

Microplate Luminometer

Multiple samples can be analyzed by loading them into a single 96-well plate. Reading of all the samples is done simultaneously using microplate luminometer. These luminometers are used in commercial scale and research laboratories handling multiple samples at a single time.

Examples: Luminoskan (GMI, Inc., Albertville, MN, USA), GloMax-96 Microplate Luminometer, Centro Luminescence Microplate Reader LB 960 (Berthold Technologies, Oak Ridge, TN, USA), MicroLumi (Harta Instruments, Gaithersburg, MD).

Measurement of Reactive Oxygen Species in Semen by AutoLumat Luminometer

The AutoLumat luminometer can measure the ROS in liquefied seminal ejaculate (unprocessed semen), processed semen (spermatozoa free from seminal plasma), and are obtained by a swim-up technique or by density gradient—separated sperm [1].

INSTRUMENT AND CONSUMABLES

1. Disposable polystyrene tubes with caps (15 mL)
2. Pipettes (5 and 10 μL)
3. Serological pipettes (1, 2, and 10 mL)
4. Centrifuge
5. Disposable sperm counting chamber
6. Dimethyl sulfoxide (DMSO)
7. Luminol (5-amino-2,3-dihydro-1,4-phthalazinedione)
8. Hydrogen peroxide (H_2O_2)
9. Polystyrene round-bottom tubes (6 mL)
10. Luminometer (Model: AutoLumat plus LB 953, Oakridge, TN)
11. Dulbecco's phosphate-buffered saline solution $1 \times$ (PBS)

Reagents

Luminol stock solution (100 mM): Add 177.09 mg of luminol to 10 mL of DMSO solution in a polystyrene tube and mix well. The tube must be wrapped with aluminum foil to avoid light exposure to luminol. Stock solution can be stored at room temperature until expiration date.

Working luminol solution (5 mM): Always prepare the working solution (5 mM) freshly before the start of experiment. Dilute 20 μL of stock solution with 380 μL DMSO in polystyrene tube wrapped with foil (Fig. 1A). Working luminol solution must be protected from the light and used within 24 h from the time of preparation.

DMSO solution: Commercially available ready-to-use solution. Store in an amber-colored bottle at room temperature until expiration date (Fig. 1B).

Hydrogen peroxide: 30% commercially available solution is used and stored at 4°C.

Semen Analysis

Following an abstinence of 2−3 days, sample is collected in a sterile wide-mouth collection cup and placed in an incubator at 37°C for 20 min to undergo complete liquefaction. Hyperviscous samples are treated with 5 mg α-chymotrypsin (viscosity treatment system; Vitrolife; CA) to break the viscosity of the sample. Examine the initial physical semen characteristics including semen volume, pH, and color. Load 6 μL of well-mixed semen sample onto a sperm counting chamber to manually assess the concentration and percent motility. Also count the round cells and perform Endtz test if the concentration is $\geq 1 \times 10^6$/mL required.

Sample Preparation for Reactive Oxygen Species

Prepare blank (3 tubes), negative control (3 tubes), test sample (2 tubes), and positive control (3 tubes). Number the tubes (12 × 75 mm) from 1 to 11, and add reagents as follows (Fig. 2).

1. Blank (tube 1−3): Add 400 μL of PBS.
2. Negative control (tube 4−6): Add 400 μL of PBS + 10 μL working solution of luminol.
3. Test sample (tube 7−8): Add 400 μL of well-mixed semen sample + 10 μL working solution of luminol.
4. Positive control (tube 9−11): Add 400 μL of PBS + 50 μL of H_2O_2 + 10 μL working solution of luminol.

The reaction is carried out in darkn or under subdued light. Carefully add the reagent/sample to the bottom of the tube. Mix the luminol uniformly with the sample by vortexing and ensure that the sample is free from bubbles. Place all labeled tubes in the luminometer in the following order: blank (tubes labeled 1−3), negative control (tubes labeled 4−6), test sample (tubes labeled 7−8) and positive control (tubes labeled 9−11) (Figs. 3 and 4) [12,22]. It is important to check that the sample tube holder chain does not contain any other tubes from a previous run.

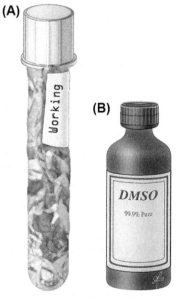

(A)

(B)

FIGURE 1 (A) Working luminol solution; wrapped in aluminum foil due to light sensitivity. (B) Bottle of dimethyl sulfoxide (DMSO).

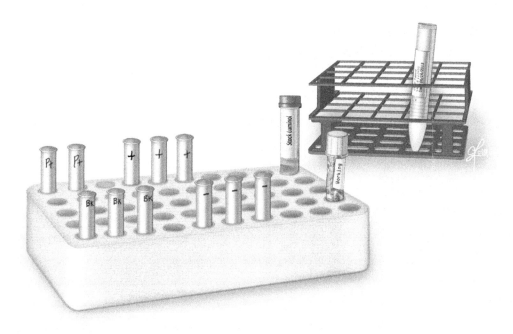

FIGURE 2 Setup for reactive oxygen species (ROS): three blank controls, three negative controls, two patient sample tubes, and three positive controls.

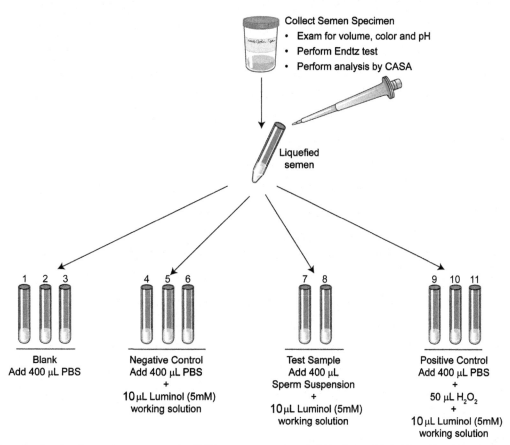

FIGURE 3 Preparing the tubes for reactive oxygen species (ROS) measurement. A total of 11 tubes are labeled from S1 to S11: blank, negative control, test sample, and positive control. Luminol is added to all tubes except the blank. Hydrogen peroxide is added only to the positive control. *PBS*, phosphate-buffered saline.

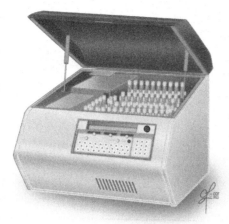
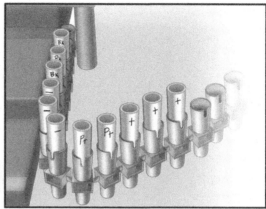

FIGURE 4 Placing of tubes into luminometer.

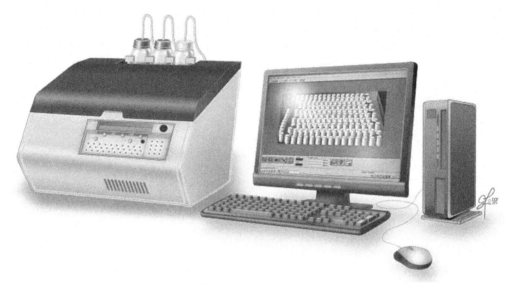

FIGURE 5 The luminometer connected with a computer and monitor.

Instrument Setup

1. Check that the luminometer and computer is connected (Fig. 5).
2. Turn on the luminometer and click the Berthold tube master icon on the desktop to initiate the program/software.
3. Navigate to the Setup menu and select Measurement Definition; continue with New Measurement. Next perform the following operations:
   a. Measurement Name (initials, date, measurement, and patient initials; e.g., RK3-13-13ROSXX). Copy the information and click OK. It will then show Measurement Definition on the toolbar (initials, date, analyte and measurement, patient initials; e.g., RK 3-13-13 ROS XX).
   b. Click the Luminometer Measurement protocol and select Rep. assay from the drop-down menu. Set and save the following parameters:
      i. Read time: 1 s
      ii. Background read time: 0 s
      iii. Total time: 900 s, Cycle time 30 s
      iv. Delay Inj M read (s): 0 s
      v. Injector M (μL): 0 s
      vi. Temperature (°C): 37°C
      vii. Temperature control (0 = OFF): 1 = ON

4. Go to the Setup menu, select Assay Definition, and click New Assay. Enter the assay details (initials, date, analyte and measurement, patient initials) and click OK or paste the information and click OK to confirm. In the drop-down menu under Measurement Method, select the measurement option and enter the file name (initials, date, analyte and measurement, patient initials) to verify the provided information is correct. Finally, navigate to Column Menu and hide everything except the following: sample ID, status, RLU mean, read date and read time.

5. In the Sample Type menu select Normal and click OK. Go to the option file, select New, click Workload, and click OK. Save the work load (initials, date, analyte and measurement, patient initials) in the Work Load file. The file name will be displayed in the Title Bar after saving it. The specimens are now ready for ROS measurement.

Measurement of Reactive Oxygen Species

1. Once the tubes are placed in the instrument, click Start to scan the tubes. The total number of tubes detected by the luminometer is displayed on the monitor.

2. Click Next, select the Assay type, and subsequently choose Next and then click Finish. Immediately, Excel worksheet is displayed on the monitor screen.

3. The instrument starts reading the tubes; during this period do not disturb the computer and also make sure that everything is working properly.

4. After the completion of the readings save the Excel worksheet and also save the measurement, Measurement Files (*.txr) with the same name (e.g., RK 3-13-13 ROS XX) for future reference.

5. Before closing the files, print:
   a. Excel worksheet along with chart 1
   b. Berthold sheet (Fig. 6)
   c. Work Load sheet (Fig. 7)

Calculation and Result Interpretation

Calculate the average RLU for Negative control, Test samples, and Positive control. Sample ROS is calculated by subtracting its average from negative control average. Finally Normalized or Corrected ROS is calculated by dividing Sample ROS with Sperm concentration/mL (Fig. 8).

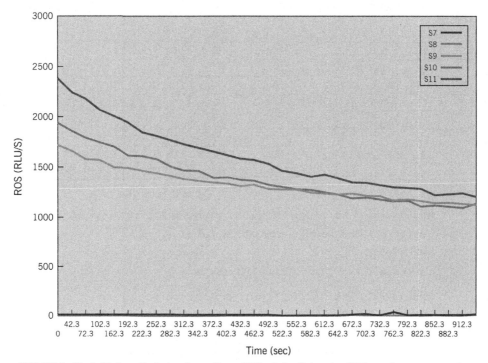

FIGURE 6 Berthold sheet displaying the readings. *RLU*, relative light units; *ROS*, reactive oxygen species.

Time	S1	S2	S3	S4	S5	S6	S7	S8	S9	S10	S11
0	6	4	9	10	13	10	19	12	1943	1719	2386
42.3	6	7	7	6	12	10	19	12	1857	1657	2248
72.3	9	7	7	10	7	12	18	9	1786	1576	2179
102.3	6	9	4	9	10	10	19	12	1742	1565	2068
132.3	9	9	7	10	7	10	16	12	1701	1493	2003
162.3	6	6	6	10	12	10	19	15	1614	1486	1943
192.3	6	7	4	9	7	15	21	13	1611	1462	1845
222.3	6	9	7	10	6	7	16	13	1582	1442	1812
252.3	7	9	10	9	10	12	16	9	1506	1408	1770
282.3	6	6	6	10	9	9	18	12	1462	1377	1729
312.3	7	9	6	12	10	12	16	12	1462	1358	1691
342.3	7	7	6	10	10	10	13	12	1391	1344	1657
372.3	4	7	7	7	9	9	18	10	1393	1330	1623
402.3	7	6	4	12	9	9	12	10	1372	1307	1583
432.3	7	10	7	9	9	15	13	10	1361	1319	1567
462.3	7	7	6	7	9	12	12	9	1319	1276	1534
492.3	6	9	7	12	9	12	9	7	1300	1275	1462
522.3	6	7	7	9	7	12	12	9	1278	1269	1437
552.3	6	12	6	10	6	13	13	10	1266	1238	1402
582.3	7	6	6	9	6	10	10	15	1244	1225	1424
612.3	10	7	6	9	9	10	10	9	1223	1216	1384
642.3	9	6	4	9	10	9	10	18	1182	1231	1344
672.3	6	9	9	7	9	13	9	27	1191	1207	1338
702.3	7	7	12	10	7	10	15	9	1169	1207	1310
732.3	9	7	7	9	7	10	12	38	1151	1157	1294
762.3	6	4	7	9	13	9	12	12	1163	1169	1287
792.3	12	7	9	7	7	9	10	7	1100	1156	1282
822.3	6	4	6	10	7	15	13	10	1114	1132	1212
852.3	3	9	10	9	9	9	15	10	1097	1142	1219
882.3	7	6	4	10	10	12	12	12	1085	1125	1234
812.3	7	9	9	9	13	18	13	10	1135	1117	1195

FIGURE 7 Work load sheet.

Sample	Sample ID	Status	RLU Mean	Read Date	Read Time
1		Done	6269	11/17/2010	1:35:54 PM
2	Blank	Done	6713	11/17/2010	1:35:56 PM
3		Done	6189	11/17/2010	1:35:57 PM
4		Done	8454	11/17/2010	1:35:59 PM
5	Negative Control	Done	8104	11/17/2010	1:36:00 PM
6		Done	9993	11/17/2010	1:36:02 PM
7	Test Sample	Done	12954	11/17/2010	1:36:03 PM
8		Done	11368	11/17/2010	1:36:05 PM
9		Done	1261225	11/17/2010	1:36:06 PM
10	Positive Control	Done	1207794	11/17/2010	1:36:08 PM
11		Done	1458674	11/17/2010	1:36:10 PM

Example

Patient average (P_{av}) = 12161 RLU / sec   Sperm count = 12.6×10^6 /mL

Negative Control average (NC_{av}) = 8850.3 RLU / sec

Corrected value = $P_{av} - NC_{av}$

12161 - 8850.3 RLU / sec = 3310.7 RLU / sec

Corrected ROS = $\dfrac{3310.7}{12.6}$ = 262.7   RLU / sec / $\times 10^6$ sperms

Result = ROS positive

FIGURE 8 Berthold sheet showing a typical ROS calculation. *RLU*, relative light units; *ROS*, reactive oxygen species.

Reference Values of Reactive Oxygen Species

Laboratory reference values can be established by analyzing a large cohort of samples from healthy and infertile subjects. In our laboratory, we have established the reference values as follows: Normal range: <93 RLU/s/10^6 sperm/mL and Critical value: ≥ 93 RLU/s/10^6 sperm/mL [12].

ASSAY QUALITY CONTROL

1. Always keep the interior of the instrument clean with antistatic spray, especially the chain belt.
2. To reduce static and maintain the humidity inside the machine, place a container filled with distilled water inside the machine.
3. Background noise check: Monitor the instrument background reading from the rate meter regularly. It should not be ≥ 20 RLU.
4. Check the reagents for contamination. First, check the PBS buffer. Next, check the luminol solution; always prepare the luminol solution in DMSO.

ADVANTAGES AND DISADVANTAGES OF MEASURING REACTIVE OXYGEN SPECIES BY CHEMILUMINESCENCE

Advantages

1. Chemiluminescence is a robust technique with high sensitivity and specificity.
2. Luminol measures global ROS levels; that is, both extracellular and intracellular (superoxide anion, hydrogen peroxide, hydroxyl radical).
3. Software for measuring ROS is simple and user friendly.

Disadvantages

1. It is a time-consuming technique.
2. The equipment is expensive.
3. Variables such as semen age, volume, repeated centrifugation, temperature control, pH of luminol, and background luminescence may interfere with measurement.

LIMITATIONS OF ASSAY

1. Assay cannot be performed in patient samples with low volume. A total of 800 μL of sample is required to run the samples in duplicate.
2. Test is not suitable for azoospermic samples (absence of spermatozoa). Corrected ROS cannot be determined in such samples as ROS has to be normalized with sperm concentration.
3. Hyperviscous samples with delayed and poor liquefaction interfere with chemiluminescent signals.
4. ROS cannot be measured in frozen semen samples.
5. Presence of leukocytes (leukocytospermia) affects the ROS levels.

FACTORS AFFECTING CHEMILUMINESCENT SIGNALS

1. Instrumental factor: Calibration, determination of sensitivity, dynamic range, and units used to determine the ROS affects the measurement and also the sensitivity and type of probe used affects the ROS readings.
2. Semen age: Generally chemiluminescent activity tends to decline with time taken for analyzing the sample [23]. The experiment must be conducted within 1 h from the time the sample was received [24].
3. Centrifugation: During centrifugation shearing force is generated, leading to artificial increase in chemiluminescent signal. Avoid repeated centrifugation of the samples.
4. Luminol pH: Chemiluminescent luminol is highly sensitive to change in pH [25].
5. Chemical artifacts: Even in the absence of spermatozoa, biomolecules such as nicotinamide adenine dinucleotide phosphate, cysteine, ascorbate acid, or uric acid can generate chemiluminescent signals interfering with the actual readings.

These nonspecific signals generated by the artifacts can be avoided by including negative controls (without sperm) in the assay.

6. Light exposure: Chemiluminescence signal is affected by extraneous light. Exposure of the glass or polypropylene tubes to the room light results in phosphorescence activity, which may interfere with the assay [20].

NEWER TECHNIQUE TO MEASURE OXIDATIVE STRESS

Quantification of ROS in the sample does not provide the complete picture of OS. It does not provide any information on the antioxidant status of the sample. A new novel technique was introduced to determine the OS in the sample at real time by measuring the oxidation reduction potential (ORP) of the semen sample using the MiOXSYS System [26]. This technique requires less volume of semen sample (30 µL) and measurement can be carried out on the frozen semen samples. ORP is the estimate of both the oxidants and antioxidants present in the semen; that is, it measures the redox potential. Higher ORP values are indicative of OS.

CONCLUSION

In addition to the routine semen analysis, ROS measurement helps in diagnosis and management of infertility in men. Among the different assays developed, luminometers are widely used for quantification of ROS in the semen samples. The chemiluminescence assay provides andrology laboratories with a reliable, validated diagnostic method for detecting ROS levels in patient semen samples with clearly established reference values. A good quality control check of the technique will produce reliable results.

REFERENCES

[1] Agarwal A, Tvrda E, Sharma R. Relationship amongst teratozoospermia, seminal oxidative stress and male infertility. Reprod Biol Endocrinol 2014;12(1):45.

[2] Aitken R. The role of free oxygen radicals and sperm function. Int J Androl 1989;12(2):95−7.

[3] Agarwal A, Cocuzza M, Abdelrazik H, Sharma RK. Oxidative stress measurement in patients with male or female factor infertility. In: Handbook of chemiluminescent methods in oxidative stress assessment. India: Transworld Research Network; 2008. p. 195−218.

[4] Agarwal A, Virk G, Ong C, du Plessis SS. Effect of oxidative stress on male reproduction. World J Men's Health 2014;32(1):1−17.

[5] Zini A, San Gabriel M, Libman J. Lycopene supplementation in vitro can protect human sperm deoxyribonucleic acid from oxidative damage. Fertil Steril 2010;94(3):1033−6.

[6] Agarwal A, Hamada A, Esteves SC. Insight into oxidative stress in varicocele-associated male infertility: part 1. Nat Rev Urol 2012;9(12):678−90.

[7] Cho C-L, Esteves SC, Agarwal A. Novel insights into the pathophysiology of varicocele and its association with reactive oxygen species and sperm DNA fragmentation. Asian J Androl 2016;18(2):186−93.

[8] Zorn B, Vidmar G, Meden-Vrtovec H. Seminal reactive oxygen species as predictors of fertilization, embryo quality and pregnancy rates after conventional in vitro fertilization and intracytoplasmic sperm injection. Int J Androl 2003;26(5):279−85.

[9] Hammadeh M, Radwan M, Al-Hasani S, Micu R, Rosenbaum P, Lorenz M, et al. Comparison of reactive oxygen species concentration in seminal plasma and semen parameters in partners of pregnant and non-pregnant patients after IVF/ICSI. Reprod Biomed Online 2006;13(5):696−706.

[10] Kothari S, Thompson A, Agarwal A, du Plessis SS. Free radicals: their beneficial and detrimental effects on sperm function. Indian J Exp Biol 2010;48:425−35.

[11] Gosalvez J, Tvrda E, Agarwal A. Free radical and superoxide reactivity detection in semen quality assessment: past, present, and future. J Assist Reprod Genet 2017;34:1−11.

[12] Agarwal A, Gupta S, Sharma R. Reactive oxygen species (ROS) measurement. In: Andrological evaluation of male infertility. Springer; 2016. p. 155−63.

[13] Rani V, Asthana S, Vadhera M, Yadav UCS, Atale N. Tools and techniques to measure oxidative stress. In: Free radicals in human health and disease. Springer; 2015. p. 43−56.

[14] Agarwal A, Deepinder F. Determination of seminal oxidants (reactive oxygen species). In: Infertility in the male. Cambridge University Press; 2009. p. 618−32.

[15] Aitken RJ, De Iuliis GN, Baker MA. Direct methods for the detection of reactive oxygen species in human semen samples. In: Studies on Men's health and fertility. Humana Press; 2012. p. 275−99.

[16] Khan P, Idrees D, Moxley MA, Corbett JA, Ahmad F, von Figura G, et al. Luminol-based chemiluminescent signals: clinical and non-clinical application and future uses. Appl Biochem Biotechnol 2014;173(2):333−55.

[17] Kashou AH, Sharma R, Agarwal A. Assessment of oxidative stress in sperm and semen. In: Spermatogenesis. Methods in Molecular Biology (Methods and Protocols). Humana Press; 2013;927:351−61.

[18] Fingerova H, Oborna I, Novotny J, Svobodova M, Brezinova J, Radova L. The measurement of reactive oxygen species in human neat semen and in suspended spermatozoa: a comparison. Reprod Biol Endocrinol 2009;7(1):118.

[19] Homa ST, Vessey W, Perez-Miranda A, Riyait T, Agarwal A. Reactive Oxygen Species (ROS) in human semen: determination of a reference range. J Assist Reprod Genet 2015;32(5):757–64.

[20] Vessey W, Perez-Miranda A, Macfarquhar R, Agarwal A, Homa S. Reactive oxygen species in human semen: validation and qualification of a chemiluminescence assay. Fertil Steril 2014;102(6):1576–83.

[21] Zhu H, Jia Z, Trush MA, Li YRA. Highly sensitive chemiluminometric assay for real-time detection of biological hydrogen peroxide formation. React Oxygen Species 2016;1(3):216–27.

[22] Sharma RK, Agarwal A. Role of reactive oxygen species in male infertility. Urology 1996;48(6):835–50.

[23] Aitken RJ, Clarkson JS. Cellular basis of defective sperm function and its association with the genesis of reactive oxygen species by human spermatozoa. J Reprod Fertil 1987;81(2):459–69.

[24] Kobayashi H, Gil-Guzman E, Mahran AM, Sharma RK, Nelson DR, Thomas AJ, et al. Quality control of reactive oxygen species measurement by luminol-dependent chemiluminescence assay. J Androl 2001;22(4):568–74.

[25] Aitken RJ, Baker MA, O'Bryan M. Andrology lab corner: shedding light on chemiluminescence: the application of chemiluminescence in diagnostic andrology. J Androl 2004;25(4):455–65.

[26] Agarwal A, Roychoudhury S, Bjugstad KB, Cho C-L. Oxidation-reduction potential of semen: what is its role in the treatment of male infertility? Therap Adv Urol 2016;8(5):302–18.

Chapter 3.2

NBT Test

Eva Tvrda

Slovak University of Agriculture in Nitra, Nitra, Slovak Republic

INTRODUCTION: FREE RADICALS: TWO-EDGED MOLECULES IN MALE REPRODUCTION

All aerobic cells, including spermatozoa, are continuously confronted by the alleged "oxygen paradox" [1]: oxygen that is a crucial element supporting aerobic metabolism, which poses a threat to cell survival. Cellular respiration is closely accompanied by the creation of by-products called free radicals or reactive oxygen species (ROS) [2,3], which, in small amounts, are required for normal cell behavior [4]. However, if their levels become too high, oxidative stress (OS) develops, with unpredictable consequences on the cell's survival [5].

Low ROS levels play important roles in the promotion of molecular pathways involved in sperm production, maturation, acrosomal reaction, and fusion with the ovum [6–9]. Inversely, ROS overproduction can cause alterations to the sperm structural integrity and functional activity resulting in decreased motility, premature capacitation and acrosome reaction, abnormalities in phosphatidylserine translocation, morphological aberrations, and compromised sperm–oocyte interactions [6,10,11]. At the same time, oxidative insults may result in lipid peroxidation, protein deterioration, aberrations to cell, and molecular signaling, leading to cell death. Furthermore, seminal OS has been associated with sperm DNA fragmentation, which may in turn lead to poor embryo development and increased risk of miscarriage [12–15].

The genesis and etiologies of seminal OS in subjects presenting with sub- or infertility have only recently been unraveled, providing a number of strategies to enhance the diagnostic and management tools for OS-associated male reproductive dysfunction. As such, new laboratory methodologies quantifying ROS production by male gametes are crucial to comprehend both physiological and pathological roles of ROS on the sperm behavior. Furthermore, there is a definitive urgency for practical andrology to be able to determine and/or measure seminal OS [10,13,16–18].

Superoxide: The Backbone of Cellular Oxidative Balance

The discovery that cells have the ability to generate considerable amounts of superoxide ($O_2^{\cdot-}$) through their normal metabolism [19] and that diverse scavenging enzymes, most notably, superoxide dismutase (SOD), detoxify aerobic cellular systems against the potentially harmful effects of this ROS [20,21], have triggered significant scientific attention in diverse areas of physiology and pathology. As such it is not a surprise that free radical–associated biology was originally thought to be superoxide-centric, primarily due to the fact that superoxide is mostly the predominant ROS generated by cellular systems [22].

Superoxide is considered to be the primary ROS produced by aerobic cells, including spermatozoa [8]. This radical is a regular by-product of oxidative phosphorylation [23], created between complexes I and III of the electron transport chain [24] as a result of a monovalent reduction of oxygen and the incorporation of one electron [25].

In the male gamete, $O_2^{\cdot-}$ is predominantly generated through two reduced forms of β-nicotinamide adenine dinucleotide phosphate (NADPH) oxidases that are comparable to those localized in phagocytes [26]: the nicotinamide adenine dinucleotide (NADH)-dependent oxidoreductase found in the inner mitochondrial membrane [27], and the NADPH-oxidase located in the cytoplasmic membrane [28]. The hypothesis that these enzymes are primarily responsible for low-level generation of $O_2^{\cdot-}$ important in cell signaling events in spermatozoa is based essentially on two events. First,

Oxidants, Antioxidants, and Impact of the Oxidative Status in Male Reproduction. https://doi.org/10.1016/B978-0-12-812501-4.00018-3

adding physiological NADPH doses to purified spermatozoa has led to an increase in $O_2^{\cdot-}$ production, subsequently resulting in a decline of the sperm function [29,30]. Second, such increased $O_2^{\cdot-}$ production was counteracted by SOD, which protects male reproductive cells against potentially harmful effects of NADPH [29,31]. Additionally, glucose-6-phosphate dehydrogenase, an enzyme found in the cytoplasm, regulates the rate of glucose circulation and the intracellular amounts of NADPH available through the hexose monophosphate shunt, which in turn provides electrons to fuel $O_2^{\cdot-}$ production through NADPH oxidase [29,32]. Last, another relevant source of $O_2^{\cdot-}$ in spermatozoa is electron leakage from the mitochondrial electron transport chain [33].

Surprisingly, $O_2^{\cdot-}$ acts as a reductant in addition to its mild oxidation properties. In the majority of dismutations, one superoxide behaves as an oxidant while the other exhibits reducing activities [20,21].

Although $O_2^{\cdot-}$ is rather unreactive [25], in the presence of H^+ the radical enters into a spontaneous or SOD-catalyzed dismutation, leading to the generation of hydrogen peroxide (H_2O_2), a membrane permeable molecule [33], which is considered to be primarily responsible for peroxidative damage of the sperm plasma membrane [6,34]. Hydrogen peroxide may be directly scavenged either by the components of the glutathione cycle or catalase, catalyzing its breakdown into water and oxygen.

Moreover, $O_2^{\cdot-}$ as well as H_2O_2 may be transformed into the highly reactive hydroxyl radical ($OH^\bullet$) via the Fenton and Haber-Weiss reaction, comprising a reduction of ferric ion (Fe^{3+}) to its ferrous form (Fe^{2+}) in the presence of $O_2^{\cdot-}$, followed by a subsequent H_2O_2 conversion to $OH^\bullet$. Furthermore, $O_2^{\cdot-}$ may interact with nitric oxide (NO) to generate peroxynitrite ($ONOO^-$), which has been associated with an increased rate of apoptosis or necrosis [35,36].

CURRENT METHODS FOR SUPEROXIDE DETECTION IN SEMEN

As high ROS levels have been repeatedly affiliated with male reproductive dysfunction, quantification of their seminal levels may significantly contribute to the initial assessment as well as follow-ups of sub- or infertile patients [37–39]. Currently, over 30 different assays are available to evaluate and study seminal OS.

The charged superoxide anion is a short-lived molecule with poor membrane permeability. The radical is quickly transformed to H_2O_2 by SOD, which is why tests for $O_2^{\cdot-}$ detection in semen must compete for superoxide as a substrate [40]. Diverse probes have been suggested for low-level $O_2^{\cdot-}$ identification in spermatozoa. Compounds such as lucigenin [41,42] or 2-methyl-6-(p-methoxyphenyl)-3,7-dihydroimidazo([1,2]-a) pyrazin-3-one (MCLA) [40] are used in chemiluminescence-based techniques. Other techniques are ferricytochrome c reduction [43], electron spin resonance and trapping [44], and dihydroethidium (DHE), a fluorescence-based method [45]. All these methods have been suggested to reliably detect superoxide. Another popular albeit indirect option to evaluate the $O_2^{\cdot-}$ amount is to assess the SOD activity using commercial kits and following the methodical instructions supplied by the manufacturer [46].

Nevertheless, all of these methods have limitations. Luminometric techniques often lack the necessary sensitivity for the identification of intracellular $O_2^{\cdot-}$ in male gametes. At the same time, artificial $O_2^{\cdot-}$ generation has frequently been observed in the presence of lucigenin as this probe has detected superoxide even in the absence of any $O_2^{\cdot-}$ promoting substances [47]. Data obtained from chemiluminiscence assays must be interpreted cautiously as a variety of factors may affect the resulting signal, such as incubation time, pH, seminal plasma contamination, or leukocytospermia [48]. Ferricytochrome c reduction lacks sensitivity because of its high molecular mass and significant background signal [30]. Furthermore, it may become difficult to use ferricytochrome c in the presence of intact cells [40]. In the meantime, MCLA only measures extracellular superoxide as this fluorescent probe is membrane impermeable [49].

Although DHE fluorescence has been used to detect $O_2^{\cdot-}$ in numerous mammalian cells or tissues with success [45,50,51], the probe seems to provide only qualitative data on $O_2^{\cdot-}$ production due to its ability to catalyze $O_2^{\cdot-}$ dismutation. As such, the assay does not quantify the target radical, but it simply indicates the percentage of highly active cells without providing information on the concentration or cellular content of ROS under evaluation [18,50].

Despite a significant progress in the development of novel techniques to evaluate seminal OS, simpler and cheaper methods with well-defined and clinically important detection ranges still have to be designed. These methods should be based on the physiological or pathological effects of ROS on sperm functions and should be quantitative in nature for ROS to become a reliable marker of semen quality in clinical andrology.

THE NITROBLUE TETRAZOLIUM TEST: A COLORIMETRIC MARKER OF SUPEROXIDE IN SEMEN

The distinctive biochemical features of tetrazolium salts that have led to their extensive use in histochemistry and cytology are closely related to the positively charged quaternary tetrazole ring core comprising four nitrogens. Furthermore, three aromatic groups that usually involve phenyl moieties surround this structural core. Following a slight reduction, tetrazolium salts change from colorless or mildly colored compounds into bright formazan crystals because of the disruption of the tetrazole ring. Ditetrazolium salts including nitroblue tetrazolium (NBT), neotetrazolium, and tetranitroblue tetrazolium are primarily used in histological applications, which has been primarily attributed to significant binding properties of their formazan products to tissue proteins, hence minimizing diffusion products [52].

The NBT test has emerged as a straightforward yet efficient laboratory technique to provide data on the intracellular oxidative balance and neutrophil behavior [53]. This assay is based on the use of NBT, a yellow, water-soluble, nitro-substituted aromatic tetrazolium salt (2,2′-bis(4-nitrophenyl)-5,5′-diphenyl-3,3′-(3,3′-dimethoxy-4,4′-diphenylene) ditetrazolium chloride), with the ability to interact with intracellular superoxide to create formazan, which may be subsequently observed spectrophotometrically or microscopically [26,54]. The sperm cytoplasm comprises glucose-6-phosphate dehydrogenase employing glucose to generate NADPH through the hexose monophosphate shunt. NADPH subsequently provides electrons for $O_2^{\cdot-}$ production via the NADPH oxidase localized in male gametes, which in turn catalyzes the conversion of NBT to formazan. Moreover, oxidases found in the cytoplasm enable the shift of electrons from NADPH to formazan [18,53]. Hence, the NBT assay uncovers the intracellular ROS-generating ability and as such may help identify the cellular origin of ROS in heterogeneous samples, including semen [18,54].

The principle of the NBT assay is straightforward: target cells are incubated in the presence of the tetrazolium salt and subsequently take up NBT into their cytoplasm where it is transformed by superoxide radicals to purple-blue and water insoluble formazan crystals [53]. While formazan is trapped intracellularly, it may be observed within the cells using an optical microscope. As an alternative, formazan may be released from the cells with the help of a solubilization agent and subsequently quantified by measuring the absorbance of the resulting purple-blue mixture [55,56].

The NBT salt is usually provided as powder, dissolved in phosphate buffered saline (PBS) at a concentration ranging from 0.01% to 0.1% and stirred at 37°C for 1 h before use. The NBT protocol may be used for whole ejaculates, washed spermatozoa, or isolated leukocytes. After the addition of NBT to the cell suspension, the mixtures are generally incubated at 37°C for 30−60 min [18,54].

Following incubation, two approaches may be used:

1. Samples are washed with PBS and centrifuged to remove the residual tetrazolium, leaving only the cell pellet comprising formazan. To quantify the final product, the cells are solubilized using 2 M potassium hydroxide (KOH), and the resulting color reaction is assessed using either a spectrophotometer or a microplate reader. Most NBT protocols use wavelengths ranging from 530 [57] to 630 nm [55,56] to determine the formazan production. ROS production is expressed as μg of formazan per 10^7 cells, which may be obtained from a standard curve of absorbance values relevant for known concentrations of the formazan substrate ([18]; Fig. 1).

2. An alternative approach is based on a microscopic evaluation of the color reaction rather than cell solubilization. In this case, following incubation, the cell suspensions are centrifuged, smears are prepared from the pellet and air-dried. The resulting smears are stained with the Wright stain, and a total of 100 cells are scored under 100× magnification. Spermatozoa are usually classified either as cells with formazan occupying more than 50% of the cytoplasm and 50% or less of the cytoplasm ([54]; Fig. 2).

The Oxisperm kit, a commercially available assay, has emerged as a simplified alternative to the traditional NBT protocol. In this case, the NBT salt is provided in the form of a reactive gel and can be used to evaluate the color intensity following the reaction either directly in the ejaculate, in the spermatozoa separated from the seminal plasma, or in the seminal plasma. The mixture of the reactive gel with the sample to be assessed is gelified at 4°C for 5 min and subsequently incubated for 45 min at 37°C. The resulting color of the mixture is compared with a color scheme provided to estimate the corresponding OS level. Alternatively, a colorimeter or imaging analysis system can be used to measure the absorbance at wavelengths ranging from 530 to 630 nm [58,59]. The reactive gel does not allow the formazan crystals to precipitate; therefore, the color intensity can be homogeneously assessed following the reaction.

Freshly obtained leukocytes stimulated with phorbol myristate acetate (Fig. 3A) [60] usually serve as a positive control of the reaction. This assay can be useful, particularly in leukocytospermic patients, by assessing the level of activity registered in the leukocytes (Fig. 3B). Oxisperm can also be used to evaluate the combined color response in each ejaculate fraction (seminal plasma [SP] or sperm [S]) as well as in a neat semen sample (NS). Using this approach, four different patterns of combined color can be distinguished (Fig. 4). Pattern type-1 represents individuals presenting with a negative response to the NBT assay in NS, SP, or spermatozoa (Fig. 4 (1)). Pattern type-2 represents individuals presenting with a positive response in all three types of sample (Fig. 4 (2)). Pattern type-3 represents individuals exhibiting a positive reaction in a neat ejaculate and the SP as well as a negative response in spermatozoa (Fig. 4 (3)). Finally, pattern type-4 represents individuals presenting with a positive response to NBT in a neat specimen and sperm fraction as well as a negative reaction in the SP (Fig. 4 (4)).

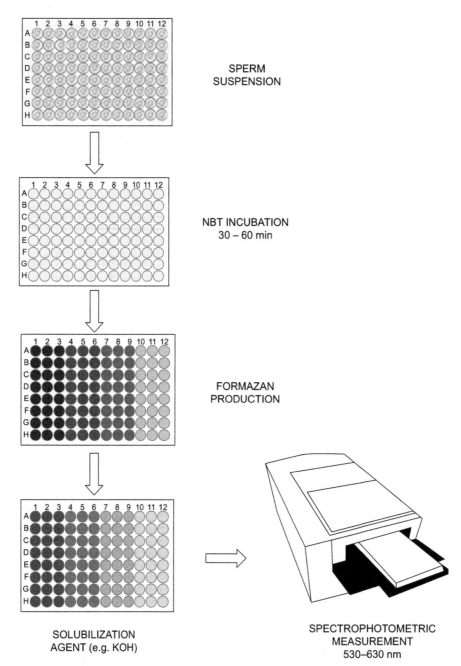

FIGURE 1 Nitroblue tetrazolium protocol using a spectrophotometric approach.

Bright field microscopy can also be used to assess the distribution of the affected spermatozoa (Fig. 5). In this case, spermatozoa can be free of any visible signal of the formazan salt (Fig. 5A), and these cells are considered unaffected. In other cases, formazan can be concentrated in the midpiece to a different extent (Fig. 5A–D), or can be seen in the sperm head (Fig. 5E–G). The associations between the proportion of affected spermatozoa in the ejaculate/pattern type in different individuals (Fig. 5) and the final reproductive outcome have not been investigated.

CLINICAL AND EXPERIMENTAL DATA: PRINCIPLES AND INTERPRETATIONS

Generally, most clinical laboratories do not test men with reproductive dysfunction for the presence of OS as currently available tests are expensive, difficult to perform, or require complex and costly equipment when compared to a routine semen analysis. In addition, cut-off values, positive and negative predictive values, as well as sensitivity and specificity

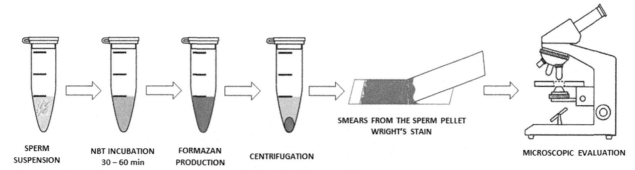

SPERM
SUSPENSION

NBT INCUBATION
30 – 60 min

FORMAZAN
PRODUCTION

CENTRIFUGATION

SMEARS FROM THE SPERM PELLET
WRIGHT'S STAIN

MICROSCOPIC EVALUATION

FIGURE 2 Nitroblue tetrazolium protocol using a microscopic approach.

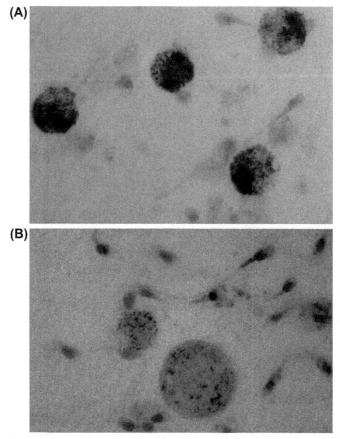

FIGURE 3 (A) Freshly obtained leukocytes stimulated with phorbol myristate acetate. (B) Subject affected with leukocytospermia exhibiting leukocytes with equivalent labeling to those showed in (A). Some of the spermatozoa were also positively labeled after Oxisperm reaction.

have yet to be fully and independently evaluated for these tests. Since an effective OS management plan and/or treatment may improve male subfertility, there is an urgency to perform assays to identify seminal OS so that the results can be placed into context with other semen parameters, including sperm motility, morphology, and DNA integrity [18]. In addition, an overdose of antioxidants may lead to unwanted results due to so-called reductive stress [61,62], which is as dangerous for the male germ cell and its functionality as OS [61,63].

As the NBT reaction may provide essential information on the oxidative balance in a simple, fast, and cost-effective manner, several studies have focused on the development and/or standardization of the NBT staining technique in whole ejaculates as well as individual cells such as spermatozoa and leukocytes.

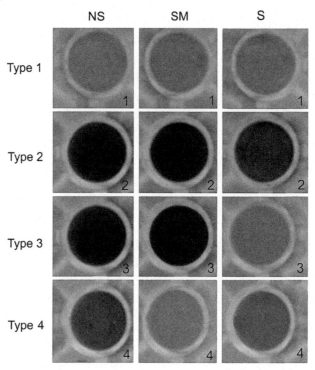

FIGURE 4 Different types (1)—(4) of individual response to nitroblue tetrazolium reaction after assessing the presence of formazan in a recently ejaculated neat sample (NS), in the seminal plasma (SP), or in isolated spermatozoa (S).

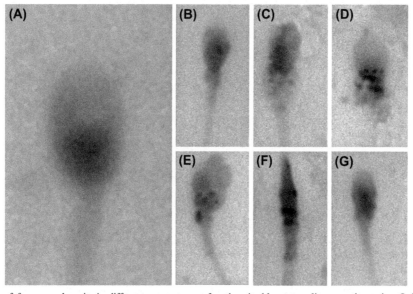

FIGURE 5 Localization of formazan deposits in different spermatozoa after the nitroblue tetrazolium reaction using Oxisperm. Enlarged selected spermatozoa show no traces of formazan deposits (A). Formazan deposits are preferably localized in the midpiece (B)—(D) and/or sperm head (E)—(G).

The first studies to report on spermatozoa capacity to reduce NBT and the usefulness of the NBT test to assess human sperm metabolic capacity were published by Mercado-Pichardo et al. [57,64]. Both reports assessed whether washed spermatozoa from fertile, healthy donors or patients with fertility issues were capable of NBT reduction in a manner similar to that of leukocytes. Formazan blue formation obtained in both cases suggested that NADH oxidoreductase is present and active in the mitochondria of spermatozoa collected from healthy as well as subfertile subjects and that the NBT test could be considered a promising tool to evaluate semen quality in clinical settings.

In order to distinguish superoxide-generating activity in the most prominent cells present in semen (spermatozoa and leukocytes) based on their morphological properties obtained by the deposition of formazan, Esfandiari et al. [54] used the histochemical version of the NBT test in whole ejaculates, leukocytes, and abnormal spermatozoa collected from 9 healthy males as well as 21 infertile subjects. At the same time, the study assessed possible relationships between the nitroblue tetrazolium staining and the ROS-total antioxidant capacity (TAC) score, which is an index to measure and express the extent of seminal OS using chemiluminescence [65]. The proportion of NBT-positive cells was significantly higher in semen samples contaminated with leukocytes in comparison with those collected from nonleukocytospermic subjects and fertile sperm donors. A significant positive correlation was found between seminal ROS levels and the nitroblue tetrazolium-positive reaction in leukocytes and semen fractions contaminated with leukocytes obtained by a density gradient separation. Moreover, ROS levels were positively correlated with the occurrence of cytoplasmic droplets in spermatozoa from whole ejaculates as well as morphologically defective spermatozoa. At the same time, the ROS-TAC score was inversely correlated with the nitroblue tetrazolium reaction in leukocytes and spermatozoa with cytoplasmic droplets. Based on the data obtained, Esfandiari et al. [54] emphasized that the NBT test may be used to study the presence of seminal leukocytes and their contribution to the seminal oxidative profile as a suitable alternative to myeloperoxidase staining or other relevant cytochemical techniques. Finally, the report hypothesizes that the NBT test is equally efficient in studying the ROS-generating activity of abnormal or immature male gametes.

Electing to improve a more traditional photometric approach, Tunc et al. [18] performed the NBT test on ejaculates collected from 21 fertile donors and 36 patients presenting with an etiology of male infertility and correlated these results with standard markers of sperm function including spermatozoa motility, DNA integrity, and apoptosis. Seminal levels of ROS were, on average, fourfold higher in the infertile men. ROS production by spermatozoa was positively correlated with sperm DNA damage as well as apoptotic changes and was negatively correlated with the sperm motion behavior. The results presented in this report confirmed that spermatozoa can reduce NBT to formazan and also provided more evidence on the mechanics involved in ROS-derived oxidative insults to the sperm plasma membranes, mitochondria, and DNA.

Similarly, Amarasekara et al. [66] used the NBT assay as a diagnostic tool to evaluate seminal OS as a marker of male factor infertility in a cohort study including 102 subfertile and 30 healthy and fertile Sri Lankan males. ROS production was significantly higher in men presenting with asthenozoospermia and unexplained infertility than in the case of fertile or other subfertile groups included in the study. Moreover, highly significant associations were found between formazan generation, sperm concentration, motility, and morphology exclusively in the infertile group.

Iommiello et al. [59] evaluated possible relationships between the oxidative imbalance caused by $O_2^{\cdot-}$ in human semen samples with the DNA fragmentation index and occurrence of round cells. The authors evaluated 56 ejaculates obtained from infertile males following the World Health Organization (WHO) 2010 guidelines, while the OS assessment was performed using the Oxisperm kit. Sperm DNA damage and chromatin integrity were evaluated with the sperm chromatin structure assay. Samples exhibiting a high degree of superoxide production were positively correlated with DNA damage and round cells. The study strongly emphasized the need to evaluate the relationship between OS and sperm DNA damage in order to develop novel therapeutic procedures and to enhance the outcomes of assisted reproduction.

EXISTING ISSUES

Although the NBT assay represents a convenient and inexpensive diagnostic tool to evaluate seminal OS, some discrepancies must still be addressed before the full potential of this relatively simple laboratory method can be realized in clinical routine.

Chemistry of the Nitroblue Tetrazolium Reduction

The primary issue to be taken into consideration is the exact involvement of specific enzymes present in semen in the chemistry of the NBT test. Armstrong et al. [26] examined the activity of NADPH-oxidase and hence the ability of spermatozoa to generate formazan similarly to leukocytes. In order to monitor sperm ROS production, spermatozoa from 18 healthy donors were isolated using Percoll gradient and subjected to electron paramagnetic resonance (EPR), chemiluminescence, and NBT to monitor ROS production. At the same time, phorbol 12-myristate 13-acetate (PMA) was used to activate the NADPH-oxidase. Unlike leukocytes, spermatozoa did not produce EPR spectra, did not increase their chemiluminescent signals, and most importantly, did not reduce NBT with or without PMA stimulation. It is unclear why this discrepancy exists, as NADPH-oxidase has been repeatedly emphasized to contribute to seminal OS [67−69]. Armstrong et al. [26] hypothesized that NADPH-oxidase previously localized in mitochondria present in the sperm midpiece and responsible for an overproduction of ROS might not be identical to the NADPH oxidase typical for neutrophils [70]. An alternative explanation might be found in the existence of different sperm populations with different ROS-producing abilities. At the same time, ROS production depends upon the degree of sperm maturation, with immature spermatozoa being the primary source of ROS alongside leukocytes [71]. Because the report used the Percoll-gradient method to select mature and functionally active spermatozoa, it could be probable that no significant ROS source was present in the sample at the time of analysis [26].

Moreover, as recently pointed out by Aitken [72], superoxide anion will give up an electron to reduce NBT. However, in reality, any enzyme capable of effecting NBT reduction as an electron donor may have the ability to generate a response similar to a ROS signal. As such, while $O_2^{\cdot-}$ may be capable of reducing NBT, the same response could be generated by a number of oxidoreductases using alternative electron donors, including cytochrome P450 and cytochrome b5-reductases. Based on this contradictory knowledge, the interpretation of the results and the validity of the conclusions drawn from clinical studies have to be based on the understanding of the fundamental chemistry and properties of NBT.

Leukocytospermia

Leukocyte contamination of semen may be another cause of concern for the NBT interpretation. It is widely acknowledged that seminal leukocytes contain NADPH oxidase and therefore may also contribute to some of the formazan occurrence within ejaculates [26,70]. Nevertheless, a swim-up or Precoll gradient generating pure sperm fractions may provide reliable results, indicating the ability of spermatozoa to produce formazan even when contaminating leukocytes are absent [54,57,64]. Furthermore, while the spermatozoa of infertile men generate less than half the amount of formazan in comparison to leukocytes on a per cell basis, as observed by Tunc et al. [18], ROS production by spermatozoa seems to be the principal indicator of net ROS production in semen because of their extensive numerical dominance over leukocytes.

Concentration of Spermatozoa

Spermatozoa concentration may also be an important factor determining the success of the NBT assay. Keshtgar et al. [73] evaluated the effectiveness of the NBT test in ROS assessment and compared the NBT test with the chemiluminescent method in semen samples collected from healthy donors. In this study, no significant differences were found between the stained slides from the control and test groups, and no significant formazan sedimentation was seen in the cells. Furthermore, no significant differences were observed between the control and trolox groups in terms of optical absorption of formazan granules in the NBT reaction with oxygen free radicals. As such, ROS evaluation with the NBT test was not as precise as originally expected, at least in a medium containing less than 20×10^6 sperm/mL. Based on these results, the authors did not recommend this method for accurate evaluation of seminal OS in samples with a low sperm concentration. Nevertheless, the NBT assay could be effective in samples containing higher concentrations of spermatozoa or in oligozoospermic samples following gradient centrifugation.

Lack of Clinical Data

Even though the NBT assay is quite straightforward and inexpensive to perform, its practical use in clinical andrology is hampered by a relative absence of reported physiological or pathological cut-off values. Although previous studies have, to a certain extent, established specific value ranges for the amount of formazan to assess the reproductive condition of individual subjects with a high sensitivity and specificity, these studies comprise a relatively small number of participants and need to be confirmed by larger multicenter trials. As such, the lack of demonstrated correlations with clinical outcomes represents one of the major pitfalls of the NBT test.

CONCLUSION: CLINICAL IMPACT AND FUTURE STATUS OF THE NITROBLUE TETRAZOLIUM TEST

The NBT test may be used to study seminal OS, to assess the individual contribution of cellular components of semen to ROS generation, to identify spermatozoa damaged by oxidative insults, as well as the state of activation of leukocytes present in semen. Such a precise, affordable, and easy-to-perform assay shows promise to become a part of the routine clinical andrology workup for the identification and assessment of seminal OS without any costly technical equipment such as a luminometer or flow cytometer [23,60]. Considering that the majority of the studies emphasizing the benefits associated with the NBT assay in clinical settings have been performed on a relatively small number of fertile or subfertile subjects, we can assume that the NBT assay may be clinically useful once large-scale, multicenter clinical trials have been performed. Finally, the data collected from the NBT test should be matched up with other available techniques used for the evaluation of sperm structural integrity, functional activity, oxidative balance, and DNA integrity.

ACKNOWLEDGMENTS

The author is grateful to Prof. Dr. Jaime Gosálvez from the Universidad Autónoma de Madrid, Spain for his kind assistance with gathering information concerning the Oxisperm kit and provision of photographs. This research was supported by the Slovak Research and Development Agency grant no. APVV-15-0544.

REFERENCES

[1] Sies H. Strategies of antioxidant defense. Eur J Biochem 1993;215:213–9.

[2] Boveris A, Chance B. The mitochondrial generation of hydrogen peroxide. General properties and effect of hyperbaric oxygen. Biochem J 1973;134:707–16.

[3] Chance B, Sies H, Boveris H. Hydroperoxide metabolism in mammalian organs. Physiol Rev 1979;59:527–605.

[4] Makker K, Agarwal A, Sharma R. Oxidative stress & male infertility. Indian J Med Res 2009;129:357–67.

[5] Sies H. Oxidative stress: oxidants and antioxidants. Exp Physiol 1997;82:291–5.

[6] Aitken RJ, Irvine DS, Wu FC. Prospective analysis of sperm-oocyte fusion and reactive oxygen species generation as criteria for the diagnosis of infertility. Am J Obstet Gynecol 1991;164:542–51.

[7] de Lamirande E, Gagnon C. Human sperm hyperactivation and capacitation as parts of an oxidative process. Free Radic Biol Med 1993;14:157–66.

[8] de Lamirande E, Jiang H, Zini A, Kodama H, Gagnon C. Reactive oxygen species and sperm physiology. Rev Reprod 1997;2:48–54.

[9] Sanchez R, Sepulveda C, Risopatron J. Human sperm chemotaxis depends on critical levels of reactive oxygen species. Fertil Steril 2010;93:150–3.

[10] Aitken RJ, Clarkson JS, Fishel S. Generation of reactive oxygen species, lipid peroxidation, and human sperm function. Biol Reprod 1989;41:183–97.

[11] Whittington K, Ford WCL. The effect of incubation periods under 95% oxygen on the stimulated acrosome reaction and motility of human spermatozoa. Mol Hum Reprod 1998;4:1053–7.

[12] Aitken RJ, Gordon E, Harkiss D, Twigg JP, Milne P, Jennings Z, et al. Relative impact of oxidative stress on the functional competence and genomic integrity of human spermatozoa. Biol Reprod 1998;59:1037–46.

[13] Henkel R, Hajimohammad M, Stalf T, Hoogendijk C, Mehnert C, Menkveld R, et al. Influence of deoxyribonucleic acid damage on fertilization and pregnancy. Fertil Steril 2004;81:965–72.

[14] Zorn B, Vidmar G, Meden-Vrtovec H. Seminal reactive oxygen species as predictors of fertilization, embryo quality and pregnancy rates after conventional in vitro fertilization and intracytoplasmic sperm injection. Int J Androl 2003;26:279–85.

[15] Ozmen B, Koutlaki N, Youssry M, Diedrich K, Al-Hasani S. DNA damage of human spermatozoa in assisted reproduction: origins, diagnosis, impacts and safety. Reprod Biomed Online 2007;14:384–95.

[16] Tvrdá E, Kňažická Z, Bárdos L, Massányi P, Lukáč N. Impact of oxidative stress on male fertility - a review. Acta Vet Hung 2011;59:465–84.

[17] Henkel R, Hoogendijk CF, Bouic PJ, Kruger TF. TUNEL assay and SCSA determine different aspects of sperm DNA damage. Andrologia 2010;42:305–13.

[18] Tunc O, Thompson J, Tremellen K. Development of the NBT assay as a marker of sperm oxidative stress. Int J Androl 2010;33:13–21.

[19] McCord JM, Fridovich I. The reduction of cytochrome c by milk xanthine oxidase. J Biol Chem 1968;243:5753–60.

[20] McCord JM, Keele Jr BB, Fridovich I. Superoxide dismutase: an enzymic function for erythrocuprein (hemocuprein). J Biol Chem 1969;244:6049–55.

[21] McCord JM, Keele Jr BB, Fridovich I. An enzyme-based theory of obligate anaerobiosis: the physiological function of superoxide dismutase. Proc Natl Acad Sci U S A 1971;68:1024–7.

[22] Hybertson BM, Gao B, Bose SK, McCord JM. Oxidative stress in health and disease: the therapeutic potential of Nrf2 activation. Mol Aspect Med 2011;32:234–46.

[23] Turrens JF, Boveris A. Generation of superoxide anion by the NADH dehydrogenase of bovine heart mitochondria. Biochem J 1980;191:421–7.

[24] Koppers AJ, De Iuliis GN, Finnie JM. Significance of mitochondrial reactive oxygen species in the generation of oxidative stress in spermatozoa. J Clin Endocrinol Metab 2008;93:3199–207.

[25] Griveau JF, Le Lannou D. Reactive oxygen species and human spermatozoa: physiology and pathology. Int J Androl 1997;20:61–9.

[26] Armstrong JS, Bivalacqua TJ, Chamulitrat W, Sikka S, Hellstrom WJ. A comparison of the NADPH oxidase in human sperm and white blood cells. Int J Androl 2002;25:223–9.

[27] Caldwell K, Blake ET, Sensabaugh GF. Sperm diaphorase: genetic polymorphism and a sperm-specific enzyme in man. Science 1976;191:1185–7.

[28] Gavella M, Lipovac V. NADH-dependent oxidoreductase (diaphorase) activity and isozyme pattern of sperm in infertile men. Arch Androl 1992;28:135–41.

[29] Aitken R, Fisher H, Fulton N, Gomez E, Knox W, Lewis B, et al. Reactive oxygen species generation by human spermatozoa is induced by exogenous NADPH and inhibited by the flavoprotein inhibitors diphenylene iodonium and quinacrine. Mol Reprod Dev 1997;47:468–82.

[30] Richer S, Ford W. A critical investigation of NADPH oxidase activity in human spermatozoa. Mol Hum Reprod 2001;7:237–44.

[31] Griveau J, Le Lannou D. Influence of oxygen tension on reactive oxygen species production and human sperm function. Int J Androl 1997;20:195–200.

[32] Said TM, Agarwal A, Sharma RK, Mascha E, Sikka SC, Thomas Jr AJ. Human sperm superoxide anion generation and correlation with semen quality in patients with male infertility. Fertil Steril 2004;82(4):871−7.

[33] Halliwell B. Free radicals and other reactive species in disease. Encyclopedia Life Sci 2005. https://doi.org/10.1038/npg.els.0003913.

[34] Aitken RJ. Molecular mechanisms regulating human sperm function. Mol Hum Reprod 1997;3:169−73.

[35] Cantoni O, Palomba L, Guidarelli A. Cell signaling and cytotoxicity by peroxynitrite. Environ Health Perspect 2002;110:823−5.

[36] Du Plessis SS, Agarwal A, Halabi J, Tvrda E. Contemporary evidence on the physiological role of reactive oxygen species in human sperm function. J Assist Reprod Genet 2015;32:509−20.

[37] Agarwal A, Mulgund A, Sharma R, Sabanegh E. Mechanisms of oligozoospermia: an oxidative stress perspective. Syst Biol Reprod Med 2014;60:206−16.

[38] Agarwal A, Tvrda E, Sharma R. Relationship amongst teratozoospermia, seminal oxidative stress and male infertility. Reprod Biol Endocrinol 2014;12:45.

[39] Ko EY, Sabanegh Jr ES, Agarwal A. Male infertility testing: reactive oxygen species and antioxidant capacity. Fertil Steril 2014;102:1518−27.

[40] Burnaugh L, Sabeur K, Ball BA. Generation of superoxide anion by equine spermatozoa as detected by dihydroethidium. Theriogenology 2007;67(3):580−9.

[41] Athayde KS, Cocuzza M, Agarwal A, Krajcir N, Lucon AM, Srougi M, et al. Development of normal reference values for seminal reactive oxygen species and their correlation with leukocytes and semen parameters in a fertile population. J Androl 2007;28:613−20.

[42] Kashou AH, Sharma R, Agarwal A. Assessment of oxidative stress in sperm and semen. Meth Mol Biol 2013;927:351−61.

[43] Gavella M, Lipovac V, Vucic M, Sverko V. In vitro inhibition of superoxide anion production and superoxide dismutase activity by zinc in human spermatozoa. Int J Androl 1999;22:266−74.

[44] Chatterjee S, Gagnon C. Production of reactive oxygen species by spermatozoa undergoing cooling, freezing, and thawing. Mol Reprod Dev 2001;59:451−8.

[45] De Iuliis GN, Wingate JK, Koppers AJ, McLaughlin EA, Aitken RJ. Definitive evidence for the nonmitochondrial production of superoxide anion by human spermatozoa. J Clin Endocrinol Metab 2006;91:1968−75.

[46] Wheeler CR, Salzman JA, Elsayed NM. Automated assays for superoxide dismutase, catalase, glutathione peroxidase, and glutathione reductase activity. Anal Biochem 1990;184:193−9.

[47] Liochev SI, Fridovich I. Lucigenin as mediator of superoxide production: revisited. Free Radic Biol Med 1998;25:926−8.

[48] Kobayashi H, Gil-Guzman E, Mahran AM. Quality control of reactive oxygen species measurement by luminol-dependent chemiluminescence assay. J Androl 2001;22:568−74.

[49] Saez F, Motta C, Boucher D, Grizard G. Prostasomes inhibit the NADPH oxidase activity of human neutrophils. Mol Hum Reprod 2000;6:883−91.

[50] Myhre O, Andersen JM, Aarnes H, Fonnum F. Evaluation of the probes 2′,7′-dichlorofluorescin diacetate, luminol, and lucigenin as indicators of reactive species formation. Biochem Pharmacol 2003;65:1575−82.

[51] Rothe G, Valet G. Flow cytometric analysis of respiratory burst activity in phagocytes with hydroethidine and 2′,7′-dichloroflourescein. J Leukoc Biol 1990;47:440−8.

[52] Berridge MV, Herst PM, Tan AS. Tetrazolium dyes as tools in cell biology: new insights into their cellular reduction. Biotechnol Annu Rev 2005;11:127−52.

[53] Baehner RL, Boxer LA, Davis J. The biochemical basis of nitroblue tetrazolium reduction in normal human and chronic granulomatous disease polymorphonuclear leukocytes. Blood 1976;48:309−13.

[54] Esfandiari N, Sharma RK, Saleh RA, Thomas Jr AJ, Agarwal A. Utility of the nitroblue tetrazolium reduction test for assessment of reactive oxygen species production by seminal leukocytes and spermatozoa. J Androl 2003;24:862−70.

[55] Rook GA, Steele J, Umar S, Dockrell HM. A simple method for the solubilisation of reduced NBT, and its use as a colorimetric assay for activation of human macrophages by gamma-interferon. J Immunol Meth 1985;82:161−7.

[56] Choi HS, Kim JW, Cha YN, Kim C. A quantitative nitroblue tetrazolium assay for determining intracellular superoxide anion production in phagocytic cells. J Immunoassay Immunochem 2006;27:31−4.

[57] Mercado-Pichardo E, Vilar-Rojas C, Wens-Flores MD. Reduction capacity on nitroblue tetrazolium (NBT) of the normal human spermatozoa. Arch Invest Med 1981;12:107−14.

[58] de la Casa M, Canadas MC, Jonhston SD, Gosálvez J. Semi-quantitative assessment of superoxide anions in neat semen using OxiSperm (R): a survey to compare visual, spectrophotometric and image analysis results. In: Paper presented at the 31st annual meeting of the European Society of Human Reproduction and Embryology (ESHRE), Lisbon Portugal; 14−17 June 2015.

[59] Iommiello VM, Albani E, Di Rosa A, Marras A, Menduni F, Morreale G, et al. Ejaculate oxidative stress is related with sperm DNA fragmentation and round cells. Int J Endocrinol 2015. https://doi.org/10.1155/2015/321901.

[60] Hassan NF, Campbell DE, Douglas SD. O-phenylenediamine oxidation by phorbol myristate acetate-stimulated human polymorphonuclear leukocytes: characterization of two distinct oxidative mechanisms. Clin Immunol Immunopathol 1987;42:274−80.

[61] Henkel R. Leukocytes and oxidative stress: dilemma for sperm function and male fertility. Asian J Androl 2011;13:43−52.

[62] Chen SJ, Allam JP, Duan YG, Haidl G. Influence of reactive oxygen species on human sperm functions and fertilizing capacity including therapeutical approaches. Arch Gynecol Obstet 2013;288:191−9.

[63] Brewer A, Banerjee Mustafi S, Murray TV, Rajasekaran NS, Benjamin IJ. Reductive stress linked to small HSPs, G6PD and NRF2 pathways in heart disease. Antioxidants Redox Signal 2013;18:1114−27.

[64] Mercado-Pichardo E, Luna del Villar J, Wens-Flores MA. Reduction capacity of nitroblue tetrazolium (NBT) of sperms from patients with fertility problems. Arch Invest Med 1981;12:499−503.

[65] Sharma RK, Pasqualotto FF, Nelson DR, Thomas Jr AJ, Agarwal A. The reactive oxygen species—total antioxidant capacity score is a new measure of oxidative stress to predict male infertility. Hum Reprod 1999;14:2801−7.

[66] Amarasekara DS, Wijerathna S, Fernando C, Udagama PV. Cost-effective diagnosis of male oxidative stress using the nitroblue tetrazolium test: useful application for the developing world. Andrologia 2014;46:73−9.

[67] Marchetti C, Obert G, Deffosez A, Formstecher P, Marchetti P. Study of mitochondrial membrane potential, reactive oxygen species, DNA fragmentation and cell viability by flow cytometry in human sperm. Hum Reprod 2002;17:1257−65.

[68] Sabeti P, Pourmasumi S, Rahiminia T, Akyash F, Talebi AR. Etiologies of sperm oxidative stress. Int J Reprod Biomed 2016;14:231−40.

[69] Gosalvez J, Coppola L, Fernandez JL, Lopez-Fernandez C, Gongora A, Faundez R, Kim J, Sayme N, de la Casa M, Santiso R, Harrison K, Agarwal A, Johnston S, Esteves SC. Multi-centre assessment of nitroblue tetrazolium reactivity in human semen as a potential marker of oxidative stress. Reprod Biomed Online 2017. https://doi.org/10.1016/j.rbmo.2017.01.014.

[70] de Lamirande E, Harakat A, Gagnon C. Human sperm capacitation induced by biological fluids and progesterone, but not by NADH or NADPH, is associated with the production of superoxide anion. J Androl 1998;19:215−25.

[71] Huszar G, Vigue L. Correlation between the rate of lipid peroxidation and cellular maturity as measured by creatine kinase activity in human spermatozoa. J Androl 1994;15:71−7.

[72] Aitken J. Nitroblue tetrazolium (NBT) assay. Reprod Biomed Online 2017. https://doi.org/10.1016/j.rbmo.2017.09.005.

[73] Keshtgar S, Forootan JF, Ghani E, Iravanpoor F. Effectiveness of NBT test in evaluation of ROS generation by human sperm. In: Paper presented at the 1st International congress on reproductive ethics and 3rd National congress on ethics and modern methods of infertility treatment, Jahrom Iran; 18−20 December 2013.

Chapter 3.3

Total Antioxidant Capacity Measurement by Colorimetric Assay

Sajal Gupta, Meaghanne Caraballo and Ashok Agarwal

American Center for Reproductive Medicine, Cleveland Clinic, Cleveland, OH, United States

INTRODUCTION

Reactive oxygen species (ROS) have been implicated as causative factors for many diseases including male infertility [1–3]. Elevated levels of ROS in semen samples are generated from immature spermatozoa and leukocytes present in the semen [2]. On the other hand, seminal fluid is rich in antioxidants that are able to neutralize these ROS. There are several published literature reports that have observed a correlation between low antioxidant capacity and male infertility [3,4]. Assessment of total antioxidant capacity (TAC) is a diagnostic tool in male infertility evaluation. However, the antioxidant capacity has to be assessed in combination with the amount of ROS produced in the semen and the sperm DNA damage to provide a complete picture of the impact of oxidative stress on semen quality and sperm function. Therefore, TAC determination is a crucial component of the assessment of redox status in semen samples of infertile male patients [5].

METHODS FOR MEASURING ANTIOXIDANTS

Assessment of antioxidants in biological fluid can be performed for individual antioxidants or as aggregate of all antioxidants, which is also referred to as TAC. Antioxidants present in the semen offer formidable protection against excessive oxidative stress. The assays are based on principles of enhanced chemiluminescence (ECL), spectrophotometry-based ferric reducing of antioxidant power (FRAP) assay, principle of formation of 2,2′,-azinobis-3-ethylbenzothiazoline-6-sulphonate (ABTS+) radical and electrochemical methodology—based voltametry.

TYPES OF ASSAYS FOR TOTAL ANTIOXIDANT MEASUREMENT

Chemiluminescence Assays (ECL Assays)

The enhanced chemiluminecsence assay detects nonenzymatic antioxidants in seminal plasma using very stringent conditions. Therefore, the assay is very cumbersome with limitations of preparing fresh reagents each time. Luminol plus para-iodophenol are the chemical inducers of luminescence utilized in the assay. The chemical inductors are then mixed with immunoglobulin linked to horseradish to produce the ROS. In the next step hydrogen peroxide is added to the mixture. Trolox is a water-soluble tocopherol analog and is used as the reference standard in this assay. To evaluate the results, a comparison is made between the ability of the seminal plasma versus Trolox to inhibit the induced chemiluminescence [6].

Spectrophotometric Assay: Ferric Reducing of Antioxidant Power Assay

TAC is also measured by utilizing the FRAP assay, and the measurement is conducted with the help of a spectrophotometer. In this assay, the colorless oxidized Fe^{3+} form of iron is converted to a blue-colored Fe^{2+} tri-pyridyl triazine

(TPTZ)-reduced form, which is due to the action of the electron donation from antioxidants [7]. The assay measures a change in the absorbance at a wavelength of 593 nm. The reagent for the FRAP assay is constituted with mixing of TPTZ, HCl, and $FeCl_3$ [7].

Assay-based on Formation of ABTS Radical: ELISA Assay

The TAC assessment technique based on colorimetry was described by Miller et al. in 1993 [8]. The compound 2,2′-azinobis-(3-ethyl-benzothiazoline-6-sulphonic acid) (ABTS) is incubated with met-myoglobin, which is a peroxidase, and with hydrogen peroxide [9]. This coincubation results in the production of a stable product, ABTS+, which produces a stable green color and is measured at a wavelength of 600 nm. The antioxidants in the seminal plasma will suppress the green color in an intensity proportional to its concentration [10].

MEASUREMENT OF ANTIOXIDANT CAPACITY BY COLORIMETRIC ASSAY

ROS are natural products of cellular metabolism in physiological amounts and are essential to trigger capacitation and induce acrosome reaction leading to successful fertilization. Free radicals are unstable due to the presence of one unpaired electron in their outer orbit causing high chemical reactivity. Therefore, such molecules react very easily with cellular components and damage lipids, proteins, and DNA. The sperm plasma membrane contains an extraordinarily high amount of polyunsaturated fatty acids, and in addition to that, have only very limited antioxidant defense mechanisms, including low concentrations of ROS-scavenging enzymes due to absence of cytoplasm [11,12]. Living organisms have developed complex antioxidant systems to counteract the effects of ROS and reduce damage. Antioxidants can help protect the spermatozoa and cells by using three mechanisms: prevention, interception, and repair [13]. The antioxidant system includes enzymes such as superoxide dismutase, catalase, and glutathione peroxidase; macromolecules such as albumin, ceruloplasmin, and ferritin; and an array of small molecules, including ascorbic acid, α-tocopherol, β-carotene, reduced glutathione, uric acid, and bilirubin [14]. A step-by-step protocol for the TAC assessment by ELISA assay is provided next. This is an in-house protocol developed in the Andrology Lab [15].

Instrument and Consumables

1. Antioxidant Assay Kit (Cat # 709001; Cayman Chemical, Ann Arbor, Michigan) (Fig. 1)
2. Epoch Biotek Gen 5 Absorbance Microplate Reader (BioTek Instruments, Inc., Winooski, Vermont) (Fig. 2)
3. 96-well plate (seen in Fig. 2)
4. Horizontal plate shaker (Eppendorf MixMate) (Fig. 3)
5. Pipettes (20, 200 and 100 μL)
6. Pipette tips (20, 200 and 100 μL)
7. Multichannel pipettes (8 channel, 30–300 μL) (Fig. 9)
8. Ultrapure water (Cat # 400000; Cayman Chemicals, Ann Arbor, Michigan) (Fig. 5)
9. Polystyrene centrifuge tubes (50 and 15 mL) (Fig. 7)
10. Eppendorf Safe Lock tubes (12 x 75 mm) (Figs. 4–8)
11. Plastic boats for reagents (Cat # P5078-23, Vistalab Technologies) (Fig. 9)
12. Microfuge (Fig. 6)

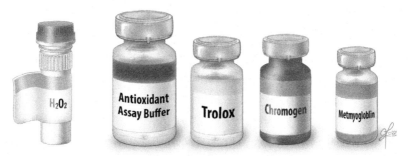

FIGURE 1 Antioxidant assay kit.

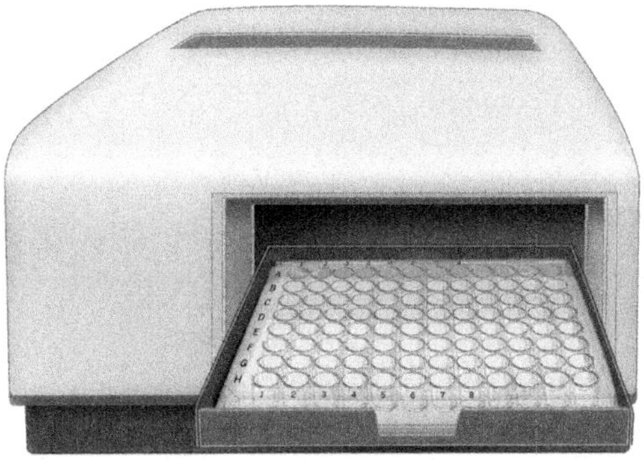

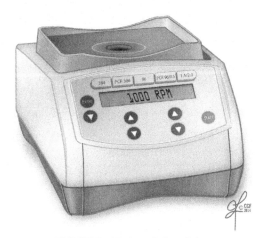

FIGURE 2   Epoch Biotek Gen 5 absorbance microplate reader.

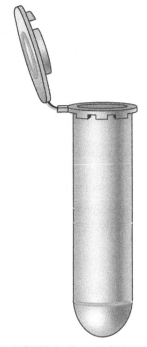

FIGURE 3   Horizontal plate shaker.

FIGURE 4   Eppendorf tubes.

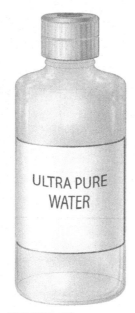

FIGURE 5   Ultrapure water.

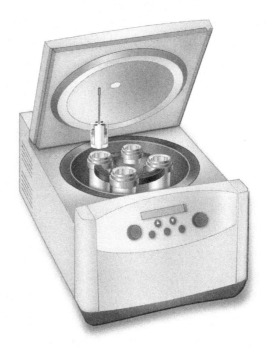

FIGURE 6   Microfuge, for centrifugation of thawed seminal plasma.

Assay Reagents

1. Antioxidant assay buffer (10×)
2. Lyophilized met-myoglobin
3. Trolox standard (6-hydroxy-2, 5, 7, 8-tetramethylchroman-2-carboxylic acid)
4. Hydrogen peroxide (441 µM)
5. Chromogen (containing ABTS)

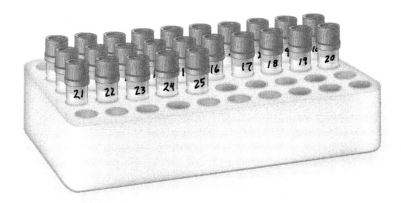

FIGURE 7   Seminal plasma samples ordered and numbered for identification.

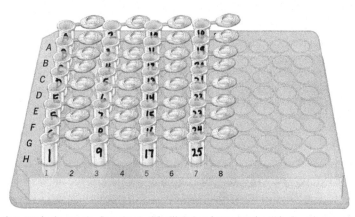

FIGURE 8   Samples A–G: Trolox standard controls. Samples 1–25: diluted patients samples (10 µL patient seminal plasma +90 µL assay buffer).

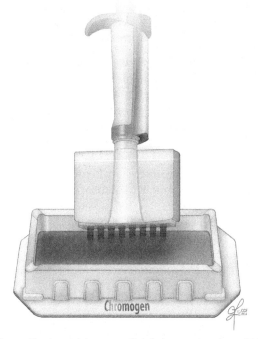

FIGURE 9   Reagent boat containing reconstituted chromogen and a multichannel pipette.

Methodology

Specimen Collection

A semen sample should be collected by masturbation and ejaculation into a clean wide-mouthed plastic specimen cup between 48 and 72 h of sexual abstinence. The sample should be collected in the privacy of a room near the laboratory. If not, it should be delivered to the laboratory within 1 h of collection. Lubrication should not be used to facilitate the semen collection, except for those provided by the laboratory. The sample should be protected from extreme temperatures (not less than 20°C and not more than 40°C) when transporting to the laboratory if collected outside the facility grounds. After complete liquefaction (37°C for 20 min), the sample has to be centrifuged at 300g for 10 min at room temperature. Finally, the clear seminal plasma has to be aliquoted into cryogenic vials and frozen at −80°C until the time of the TAC assay.

Instrument Setup

1. Open the Gen 5 software, 2.09 in One Micro Manipulator Reader software.
2. Power on the Epoch Biotek Gen 5 absorbance microplate reader.
3. Choose the Experiments icon from the Task Manager tab.
4. Choose the proper Protocol per laboratory requirements.
5. Select the green Read New tab, enter the Assay Kit Lot Number, and select OK.
6. In the data box for the plate reader, select 750.
7. The Load Plate icon will appear; select OK to run a test on the software and the reader connection.
8. Test Run Setup: Select the green Read New Button, enter the Assay Kit lot number, and select OK. Verify that the data box for the plate reader is selected at 750 nm.

Principle of the Assay

Seminal plasma TAC measurement is done using the Antioxidant Assay Kit supplied by Cayman Chemical, Ann Arbor, Michigan Cat # 709001 (Fig. 1). TAC assay is dependent on the capability of the antioxidants in the seminal plasma to inhibit the oxidation of ABTS (2,2′-azino-di-[3-ethylbenzthiazoline sulphonate]) to ABTS·+ by met-myoglobin [1] [14]. As a result of the induced reaction the antioxidants suppress the absorbance at 750 nm to a level that is equivalent to their concentration. The capacity of the antioxidants present in the sample to prevent ABTS oxidation was compared to standard Trolox (6-hydroxy-2,5,7,8 etramethylchroman-2-carboxylic acid); Trolox is a water-soluble tocopherol analog. Results are reported as micromoles of Trolox equivalent.

Assay steps are given next.

Reagent Preparation for Total Antioxidant Capacity

1. Antioxidant assay buffer is used diluted using a ratio 1:9, 1 mL of assay buffer concentrate to 9 mL of ultrapure water in a 15 mL conical tube. The reconstituted vial is stable for 6 months when stored at 4°C.
2. Lyophilized met-myoglobin is reconstituted with 600 μL of assay buffer (prepared in the previous step). Once reconstituted, it is sufficient for 60 wells. The reconstituted reagent is stable for 1 month when stored at −20°C.
3. The Trolox standard (6-hydroxy-2, 5, 7, 8-tetramethylchroman-2-carboxylic acid) is used to prepare the standard curve. One milliliter of ultrapure water is added to the lyophilized Trolox; the reconstituted vial is stable for 24 h at 4°C.
4. Hydrogen peroxide 441 μM working solution is prepared from 8.82 M solution of hydrogen peroxide. Dilute 10 μL of hydrogen peroxide reagent with 990 μL of ultrapure water. Further dilute by removing 20 μL and diluting with 3.98 mL of ultrapure water to give a 441 μM working solution. The working solution is stable for 4 h at room temperature.
5. Chromogen (containing ABTS) is reconstituted with 6 mL of ultrapure water. It is sufficient for 40 wells. The reconstituted vial is stable for 24 h at 4°C. Chromogen is light sensitive and must be prepared in indirect light.

Sample Preparation for Total Antioxidant Capacity

1. Bring all reagents and samples to room temperature for 30 min prior to starting the assay. All reagents are prepared per the manufacturer's instructions.
2. The frozen seminal plasma is brought to room temperature and centrifuged in a microfuge at 300g for 7 min. Remove the clear seminal plasma and dilute each sample 1:9 (10 μL sample + 90 μL assay buffer) in a microfuge tube.

3. Prepare Eppendorf Safe Lock tubes for the Trolox standards (seven tubes), internal controls (previously ran patients), and current patient samples. Label the Trolox standard tubes A—G and the patient tubes numerically (e.g., 1, 2, 3, etc.).
  a. Trolox standard (tubes A—G): Add the required amount of reconstituted Trolox and assay buffer to each tube as shown in Table 1.
  b. Patient sample (numerical tubes): Remove the clear seminal plasma and dilute each sample of seminal plasma, 1:9 (10 μL sample + 90 μL assay buffer) in a microfuge tube.

TABLE 1 Preparation of Trolox standards for TAC assay

Tube	Reconstituted Trolox (μL)	Assay Buffer (μL)	Final Concentration (mM Trolox)
A	0	1000	0
B	30	970	0.044
C	60	940	0.088
D	90	910	0.135
E	120	880	0.18
F	150	850	0.225
G	220	780	0.330

4. Trolox standards and patient samples are added in duplicate to each well in the 96-well plate. Each sample is recorded in a plate template form (Appendix A).
5. Add 10 μL of Trolox standard and samples in duplicate and 10 μL of met-myoglobin per well.
6. In the dark add 150 μL of chromogen per well. A multichannel pipette should be used to pipette the chromogen. Chromogen can be pipetted from a flat container or reagent boat.
7. With the lights still turned off, initiate the reaction by adding 40 μL of hydrogen peroxide working solution using a multichannel pipette from a reagent boat. Complete this step as quickly as possible ($\sim$45 s). Set the timer for 5 min, 5 s.
8. Cover the plate with a plate cover and incubate on a shaker at room temperature. Remove the plate from the shaker with $\sim$30 s left on the timer and remove the plate cover.
9. Place the plate onto the plate holder on the Epoch Biotek Gen 5 Absorbance Microplate Reader. At the end of the incubation time select OK and read the absorbance at 750 nm.

Calculating Assay Results

Calculating the average absorbance of each Trolox standard and sample determines the reaction rate. The standard curve records the average absorbance of the standards as a function of the final Trolox concentration. The total antioxidant concentration of each sample is calculated using the equation obtained from the linear regression of the standard curve by substituting the average absorbance values for each sample into the equation:

$$\text{Antioxidant (μM)} = [(\text{Unknown average absorbance} - \text{Y intercept})/\text{slope}] \times \text{dilution} \times 1000(14).$$

Reference Values and Ranges

The normal value for TAC is greater than or equal to ($\geq$) 1950 μM Trolox [14].

Assay Quality Control

The standard reading of the Trolox standards (vials A—G) should be within the expected range. Standard A ranges are equal to 0.35 to 0.45 and standard G ranges are equal to 0.100 to 0.150. If the readings are significantly different (higher or lower), the samples must be rerun. Internal controls or previously run samples should be within 500 ± μM of the previous results.

Tips for Troubleshooting

Tips are provided for resolving common issues with the assay, including in sample preparation, reagent preparation, sample incubation, and reagent addition for the assay [14].

1. Samples should be completely thawed for 20 min and centrifuged at $300g$ for 7 min to pellet the debris and spermatozoa.
2. All reagents should be at room temperature for 30 min prior to starting the assay.
3. The water used to prepare the reagents should be ultrapure water and used before the expiration date (6 months).
4. To avoid great fluctuation in the readings, both chromogen and met-myoglobin should be from the same lot.
5. It is important that the incubation time after the addition of hydrogen peroxide is exactly 5 min and 5 s. The reaction starts as soon as hydrogen peroxide is added to each well, and there is a reaction termination step. The absorbance will keep changing with time.
6. Thirty seconds before the completion of the 5 min and 5 s, place the plate on the plate reader.
7. If you make any errors when adding the reagent(s) or sample to each well, note this fact in the template and final results.
8. The Trolox standard reading (A and G) well should be within the expected range (i.e., 0.35 to 0.45 for well A and 0.100 to 0.150 for well G). If the readings are significantly different (higher or lower), the samples must be rerun.

CONCLUSIONS

The colorimetric assay is a relatively inexpensive, simple, and reliable assay for assessment of total antioxidant capacity, which is less time consuming. It was also reported to have a strong correlation with other established assays such as the enhanced chemiluminescence method. The TAC estimation is an important marker associated with male infertility and impaired sperm function.

REFERENCES

[1] (a) Gangel EK. AUA and ASRM produce recommendations for male infertility. American Urological Association, Inc and American Society for Reproductive Medicine. Am Fam Physician 2002;65:2589–90.
(b) Tremellen K. Oxidative stress and male infertility—a clinical perspective. Hum Reprod Update 2008;14:243–58.
[2] Aitken RJ. A free radical theory of male infertility. Reprod Fertil Dev 1994;6:19–23 [discussion 23–24].
[3] Lewis SE, Boyle PM, McKinney KA, Young IS, Thompson W. Total antioxidant capacity of seminal plasma is different in fertile and infertile men. Fertil Steril 1995;64:868–70.
[4] Lewis SE, Sterling ES, Young IS, Thompson W. Comparison of individual antioxidants of sperm and seminal plasma in fertile and infertile men. Fertil Steril 1997;67:142–7.
[5] Smith R, Vantman D, Ponce J, Escobar J, Lissi E. Total antioxidant capacity of human seminal plasma. Hum Reprod 1996;11:1655–60.
[6] Said TM, Kattal N, Sharma RK, Sikka SC, Thomas Jr AJ, Mascha E, et al. Enhanced chemiluminescence assay vs colorimetric assay for measurement of the total antioxidant capacity of human seminal plasma. J Androl 2003;24:676–80.
[7] Pahune PP, Choudhari AR, Muley PA. The total antioxidant power of semen and its correlation with the fertility potential of human male subjects. J Clin Diagn Res 2013;7:991–5.
[8] Miller NJ, Rice-Evans C, Davies MJ, Gopinathan V, Milner A. A novel method for measuring antioxidant capacity and its application to monitoring the antioxidant status in premature neonates. Clin Sci (Lond) 1993;84:407–12.
[9] Sharma RK, Pasqualotto FF, Nelson DR, Thomas Jr AJ, Agarwal A. The reactive oxygen species-total antioxidant capacity score is a new measure of oxidative stress to predict male infertility. Hum Reprod 1999;14:2801–7.
[10] Roychoudhury S, Sharma R, Sikka S, Agarwal A. Diagnostic application of total antioxidant capacity in seminal plasma to assess oxidative stress in male factor infertility. J Assist Reprod Genet 2016;33:627–35.
[11] Agarwal A, Durairajanayagam D, du Plessis SS. Utility of antioxidants during assisted reproductive techniques: an evidence based review. Reprod Biol Endocrinol 2014;12:112.
[12] Parks JE, Lynch DV. Lipid composition and thermotropic phase behavior of boar, bull, stallion, and rooster sperm membranes. Cryobiology 1992;29:255–66.
[13] Sies H. Strategies of antioxidant defense. Eur J Biochem 1993;215:213–9.
[14] Makker K, Agarwal A, Sharma R. Oxidative stress & male infertility. Indian J Med Res 2009;129:357–67.
[15] Agarwal A, Gupta S, Sharma R. Andrological evaluation of male infertility. 2016.

APPENDIX A

PLATE TEMPLATE

	1	2	3	4	5	6	7	8	9	10	11	12
A												
B												
C												
D												
E												
F												
G												
H												

Chapter 3.4

Oxidation-Reduction Potential Methodology Using the MiOXSYS System

Ashok Agarwal and Albert D. Bui

American Center for Reproductive Medicine, Cleveland Clinic, Cleveland, OH, United States

INTRODUCTION

Infertility affects approximately 48.5 million couples worldwide [1]. While about 50% of all cases are attributable to both female and male causes, 20%—30% of the infertility cases are solely due to male factors [2]. Approximately 7% of men worldwide are infertile [3].

The basic semen analysis is the conventional method to evaluate a male's ability to conceive [4,5]. However, the test contains high intraindividual variability and high interobserver variability [4]. The test as per World Health Organization guidelines is also inconsistently performed among laboratories in the United States and the United Kingdom [6,7]. Thus there is a need for more advanced tests that can accurately assess sperm quality and determine the etiology of male infertility.

Oxidative stress (OS) is one of the main causes of male infertility and describes an imbalanced redox state between oxidants and reductants, which can result from either increased production of reactive oxygen species (ROS) or a deficiency of antioxidants [8—11]. ROS are oxygen-derived free radicals that are required at low levels for sperm capacitation, hyperactivation, acrosome reaction, and oocyte fusion [12]. However, excess ROS are lethal to spermatozoa as these oxidants compromise their semipermeable plasma membrane, DNA, and apoptotic mechanisms [13—16]. Ultimately, the accumulated damage to sperm leads to unsuccessful fertilization, pregnancy loss, and poor assisted reproductive technology (ART) outcomes [17,18]. Commonly used assays to measure OS only evaluate single biomarkers. Examples of such assays include chemiluminescence for ROS, total antioxidant capacity (TAC) for antioxidants, and the determination of malondialdehyde (MDA) for post-hoc damage due to lipid peroxidation. However, these tests are laborious, time-consuming, expensive, and require sophisticated instruments and large sample volumes [19]. Therefore the ideal test should be simple and can simultaneously measure all oxidants and antioxidants that contribute to OS in a semen sample.

Oxidation-reduction potential (ORP) provides a snapshot of the current redox balance in semen samples as it explains the relationship between oxidants and antioxidants. Measuring ORP in semen samples is a novel method to measure OS in the field of andrology. It has shown promise in predicting abnormal semen parameters and differentiating fertile from infertile semen samples [20—24]. In this chapter, the methods measuring ORP by the MiOXSYS system in semen samples are described in detail.

CLINICAL SIGNIFICANCE OF OXIDATION-REDUCTION POTENTIAL

Studies conducted by the Cleveland Clinic American Center for Reproductive Medicine and collaborators worldwide have advanced our understanding of the MiOXSYS system and its application in male infertility. The initial study sought to establish MiOXSYS as a tool to measure OS in both semen and seminal plasma [20]. With a small cohort of 26 controls and 33 infertile men, the investigators observed a negative correlation between ORP values with concentration and total sperm count in both groups. Surprisingly, these correlations persisted even after 120 min of sperm liquefaction. From this information, measuring ORP in semen and seminal plasma was complementary to a basic semen analysis in observing semen with possible OS. Subsequent studies enrolled more patients with the intent of assigning a reference value that not only best predicts abnormal semen parameters but also differentiates fertile from infertile men [21,22]. A normalized ORP cutoff of $1.36 \text{ mV}/10^6/\text{mL}$ was adequate to provide the optimal information with a sensitivity of 69.6%, specificity of 83.1%, positive predictive value of 85.3%, and a negative predictive value of 65.9%. Additionally, an ORP of $>1.57 \text{ mV}/10^6/\text{mL}$ could predict at least one abnormal semen parameter. Oligozoospermia is best predicted with an ORP measurement greater than $2.59 \text{ mV}/10^6/\text{mL}$. These values were crucial in demonstrating that ORP measurement is a robust test that can identify infertile patients with dysfunctional sperm. The latest studies confirmed that ORP is related to abnormal semen parameters and is consistently elevated in infertile patients compared to that of controls both nationally and internationally [23,24]. Overall, measuring ORP is reproducible and reliable in clinically diagnosing male infertility.

METHODS FOR MEASURING OXIDATIVE STRESS

OS can be measured with many different assays, both directly and indirectly. Direct assays measure total ROS in the semen sample while the indirect assays either provide total antioxidant levels or measure markers of lipid peroxidation. There are distinct advantages and disadvantages with every technique. Table 1 compares the more commonly utilized techniques to measuring OS.

TABLE 1 Comparison of Various Techniques to Measure Oxidative Stress in the Seminal Plasma

Technique	Instrument	Advantages	Disadvantages
Direct			
ORP	• MiOXSYS	• Provides a snapshot of the redox balance in real time • Levels of all oxidants and reductants are measured • Less time consuming • Inexpensive materials • Simple methodology • Both fresh and frozen semen and seminal plasma can be measured	• Semen age, high viscosity, and repeated centrifugation may alter results of measurements
ROS by chemiluminescence	• Luminometer	• Robust chemiluminescence • High sensitivity and specificity • Intracellular and extracellular ROS are detected	• 15–30 min to yield test results • Cost and size of equipment • Semen age, volume, repeated centrifugation, temperature, and background luminescence may alter results of measurements
Indirect			
TAC	• Colorimeter • Luminometer	• Reliable and predictive of antioxidant capacity • Total antioxidants in seminal plasma measured	• Cannot differentiate the amounts of enzymatic and nonenzymatic antioxidants independently • Long duration of inhibition time • Cost of microplate readers
ROS-TAC	• Statistical analyses	• Superior to ROS or TAC alone	• Calculated through statistical analyses • Does not directly measure ROS or TAC
MDA	• Colorimeter and fluorometer for MDA-TBA adduct • HPLC	• Assesses lipid peroxidation	• Rigorous controls required • Nonspecific test • Only detects post-hoc damage

HPLC, high performance liquid chromatography; *MDA*, malondialdehyde; *ROS*, reactive oxygen species; *TAC*, total antioxidant capacity; *TBA*, thiobarbituric acid.
Table adapted from Agarwal et al. Ther Adv Urol. 2016;8 (5):302-318.

OXIDATION-REDUCTION POTENTIAL MEASUREMENT: REVIEW OF THE CURRENT TECHNOLOGY

There are many available probes and analyzers on the market designed to detect ORP. However, these devices are used mainly to assess water quality, metal finishing, and ozone treatment [25−29]. To our knowledge, the MiOXSYS system is the only device that has been used to measure ORP in human semen samples. After a thorough comparison of technical specifications and user manuals, the MiOXSYS system appears to offer distinct advantages over many of the current technologies. Its measuring capacity ranges from 0.1 to 400 mV while only requiring a very small sample volume (30 μL).

MEASUREMENT OF OXIDATION-REDUCTION POTENTIAL BY THE MIOXSYS SYSTEM

Measuring ORP in biological samples has been successful in major trauma and strenuous exercise [30−33]. Examples of such fluids that can be analyzed include whole blood, cerebrospinal fluid, sweat, saliva, and urine [34]. Advanced andrology laboratories quickly adapted the ORP assessment technique for detecting OS in semen samples. Using the MiOXSYS system, andrology laboratories can directly obtain a composite measurement of known and unknown oxidants and antioxidants that play a role in OS and male infertility. This technology consists of a galvanostat-based analyzer and disposable sensor tests with a built-in three-electrode system [35]. The electrochemical circuit is completed once the sample fills the reference cell while the sensor is inserted into the analyzer. A sample with a significantly higher ORP value than that of the control sample confirms the presence of OS as the redox balance is shifted toward a prooxidant state [36].

Principle

Technically, the MiOXSYS system measures the transfer of electrons from a reductant (antioxidants) to an oxidant (ROS). ORP, also known as the redox potential (E), can be calculated with the Nernst equation [34]:

$$E(ORP) = E^\circ - RT/nF \ \ln([Red]/[Ox])$$

E° standard reduction potential; R, universal gas constant; T, absolute temperature; n, number of moles of exchanged electrons; F, Faraday's constant; [Red], concentration of reduced species; [Ox], concentration of oxidized species.

The analyzer contains an ultrahigh impedance electrometer and the sensor contains three electrodes (platinum working and counterelectrodes and a 3 M KCl, Ag/AgCl reference electrode). Once the sample is loaded onto the sample application port, it will eventually hydrate the hydrophilic KCl gel above the reference cell. Hydrating the KCl helps maintain a constant potential. The sample will be evaluated for 2 min where an ORP will be calculated from an average of the last 10 s of the run [35]. ORP is expressed in millivolts, which is proportional to the degree of OS.

INSTRUMENTS AND CONSUMABLES

1. Phase contrast microscope
2. Disposable Pasteur pipette
3. Serological pipettes
4. Graduated centrifuge tube
5. Glass slides and cover slips
6. Disposable sperm counting chamber and/or Makler chamber
7. Pipettes (5, 25, and 50 μL)
8. Dilution cups (2 mL)
9. Phosphate buffered saline (PBS, 1×)
10. pH paper (range 6.0−8.0)
11. MiOXSYS analyzer
12. MiOXSYS sensor
13. MiOXSYS analyzer calibration key

Semen Collection and Preparation

Semen samples should be collected in a sterile wide-mouth collection cup after 48−72 h of sexual abstinence. The sample is allowed to liquefy by placing it in an incubator for 20 min at 37°C. Within 30 min of ejaculation, the samples have to be inspected for initial physical characteristics such as semen volume, viscosity, pH, and color. When the sample is liquefied, a basic semen analysis is performed. Denote the time at which motility was read if the sample is more than 1 h old.

Instrument Setup

Press the power button on the MiOXSYS analyzer. If a green LED appears on the power button, the unit is on. If using AC power, the display screen will be backlit. "Insert sensor" will appear on the display screen once the MiOXSYS analyzer is ready.

Analyzing the Sample

1. Sample insertion:
   a. Unwrap an individual MiOXSYS sensor and insert it face-up while holding it at the front-side edges.
   b. The sensor electrodes must face the MiOXSYS analyzer with the socket insertion end aligned with the sensor socket. The sensor must be fully inserted to begin sample analysis (Figs. 1 and 2).
   c. "Waiting for sample" will appear on the display screen once the MiOXSYS sensor is correctly inserted.
   d. The MiOXSYS analyzer will analyze the sample for 2 min after it is loaded. A timer countdown will appear on the display screen.

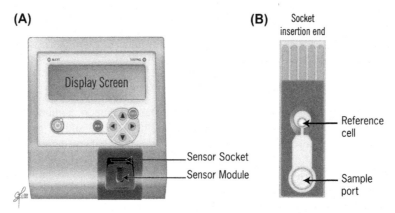

FIGURE 1 Setup of the (A) MiOXSYS analyzer and (B) sensor.

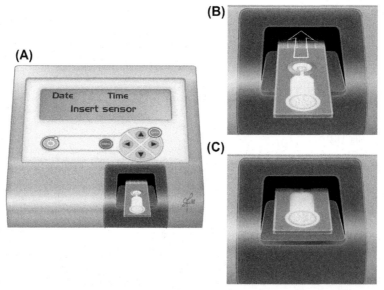

FIGURE 2 Sample run on the MiOXSYS analyzer. Fully insert sensor into the analyzer for appropriate sample analysis (A-C).

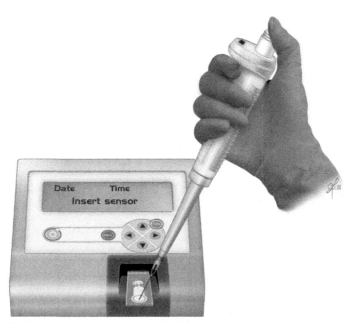

FIGURE 3 View of the sensor showing the application port for loading of the sample.

2. Sample application:
   a. Fresh or frozen semen or seminal plasma samples can be used for ORP analysis.
   b. 30 μL of the sample should be applied with a pipette.
   c. Sample volume should be consistent for each test during a study.
   d. Apply the sample to the sample application port on the inserted sensor. The entire port should be covered (Fig. 3).
3. Sample run:
   a. The testing will automatically begin once the sample reaches the reference cell of the sensor. Blinking of a blue testing LED indicates proper execution of the test.
   b. "Processing sample" and the time remaining will appear on the display screen once the test is initiated.
   c. While the test is in progress, do not press any buttons or remove the sensor.
   d. An error code will appear on the display screen if an error occurs during testing. A red alert LED will also illuminate. It is important to file the error reading for personal records. To clear the error, follow the instructions on the screen.
4. Test results:
   a. Once the test is complete, audible beeps will be emitted.
   b. Record all data for proper record keeping before removing the sensor. The following test results will appear on the display screen (Fig. 4):
      i. Date
      ii. Time
      iii. ORP (in millivolts or mV)
   c. After recording the data, immediately remove the MiOXSYS sensor from the sensor socket. Discard the sensor per the guidelines of disposing biological fluids.
   d. "Insert sensor" will appear on the display screen once the used MiOXSYS sensor is removed. To perform additional tests, repeat the steps starting from "Sample Insertion."
   e. Once all measurements have been completed, press and hold the power button to turn off the analyzer. If the MiOXSYS analyzer is on but inactive, it will automatically turn off. The display screen will show a 15 s timeout warning. A warning beep will also be heard with every second of the countdown. Reset the timeout clock by pressing any button.

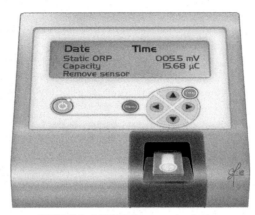

FIGURE 4   MiOXSYS test results display.

Calculation and Result Interpretation

1. Calculate the average ORP for the sample. Furthermore, the normalized ORP is calculated by dividing the average ORP by sperm concentration/mL. The final ORP should be expressed as $mV/10^6$ sperm/mL. An example calculation of ORP is provided in Table 2.

Reference Values of Oxidation-Reduction Potential

Through multiple studies exploring the ability of ORP to differentiate fertile from infertile men, we report the following reference values: Normal range: $<1.36 \, mV/10^6$ sperm/mL and critical value: $>1.36 \, mV/10^6$ sperm/mL.

ASSAY QUALITY CONTROL

1. Since the external control solution kits are supplied separately by the vendor, every new received batch of MiOXSYS sensors should be verified upon arrival and before use.
2. Follow the appropriate federal, state, and local guidelines in testing the external controls.

ADVANTAGES AND DISADVANTAGES OF OXIDATION-REDUCTION POTENTIAL MEASUREMENT BY MIOXSYS

Advantages:

1. Expenses are primarily due to the cost of the sensor strip ($35–$50).
2. The analyzer is easy to use as it does not require extensive technical training or elaborate software.
3. The analyzer is portable and requires a very small sample volume (30 μL).
4. A short amount of time is needed to conduct a test (5 min).
5. ORP measurements are stable up to 120 min after collection.
6. Fresh and frozen semen and seminal plasma can be analyzed.
7. Samples do not require additional processing, purification, or isolation before analysis.

TABLE 2 Example Calculation of Oxidation-Reduction Potential (ORP)

Sample#	Patient Identification	Date	Time	ORP (mV)
1	Patient A	08/02/17	11:16 a.m.	78.1
2	Patient A	08/02/17	11:27 a.m.	78.4

Sperm concentration = 52.3×10^6/mL.
Patient average ORP = (78.1 + 78.4)/2 = 78.25.
Normalized ORP = 78.25/52.3 = 1.50 $mV/10^6$ sperm/mL.

8. Low intraobserver and interobserver variability among ORP values.
9. It predicts poor sperm quality, particularly oligozoospermia with 88% sensitivity and 91.2% specificity.
10. It provides high sensitivity, specificity, and accuracy, which warrant its use as a potential diagnostic tool.

Disadvantages:

1. Normalized ORP cannot be calculated in azoospermic samples.
2. Further studies need to be repeated to standardize the reference values between different laboratories among different ethnic populations.
3. The role of ORP in monitoring antioxidant therapies for reproductive diseases and predicting pregnancy or ART outcomes is unknown.

FACTORS AFFECTING MEASUREMENT

1. Advanced semen age (span of time from collection to analysis) may affect the accuracy of ORP measurement.
2. Poor liquefaction leading to high viscosity will not allow the sample to adequately flow from the sample port to the reference cell.
3. Repeated centrifugation will generate shear forces to spermatozoa which can be responsible for increases in ORP.

MANAGEMENT OF ABNORMAL OXIDATION-REDUCTION POTENTIAL

Many factors, both intrinsic and extrinsic, exacerbate OS, which may be reflected through an abnormal ORP value. These factors include alcohol consumption, cigarette smoking, varicocele, obesity, diabetes, strenuous exercise, psychological stress, aging, environmental pollutants, ionizing radiation, and infections [37,38]. To minimize OS, it is important to treat the underlying cause. Varicocelectomy and antioxidant supplementation has shown to be beneficial in combating OS-induced sperm damage [39,40]. Lastly, lifestyle modifications may help improve quality of life and perhaps halt the progression of OS [41,42]. However, more studies are necessary in evaluating specific ORP response to OS treatment.

CONCLUSION

Measurement of ORP is clinically useful in assessing male infertility. It provides a complete picture of an individual's OS status, describing the relative proportions of oxidants and reductants in the seminal plasma. Overall, the MiOXSYS system consistently predicts ORP values that are well correlated with poor semen parameters and male infertility. As future studies are conducted, ORP's ability to monitor the effect of antioxidant treatments and to predict ART outcomes will be better understood.

REFERENCES

[1] Mascarenhas M, Flaxman S, Boerma T, Vanderpoel S, Stevens G. National, regional, and global trends in infertility prevalence since 1990: a systematic analyses of 277 health surveys. PLoS Med 2012;9:e1001356.
[2] Agarwal A, Mulgund A, Hamada A, Chyatte M. A unique view on male infertility around the globe. Reprod Biol Endocrinol 2015;13:37.
[3] Nieschlag E, Behre H, Nieschlag S. Andrology. Male reproductive health and dysfunction. 3rd ed. Heidelberg, Dordrecht, London, New York: Springer; 2010.
[4] Esteves S. Clinical relevance of routine semen analysis and controversies surrounding the 2010 World Health Organization criteria for semen examination. Int Braz J Urol 2014;40(4):443−53.
[5] Esteves S, Hamada A, Kondray V, Pitchika A, Agarwal A. What every gynecologist should know about male infertility: an update. Arch Gynecol Obstet 2012;286(1):217−29.
[6] Keel B, Stembridge T, Pineda G, Serafy Sr N. Lack of standardization in performance of the semen analysis among laboratories in the United States. Fertil Steril 2002;78(3):603−8.
[7] Riddell D, Pacey Whittington K. Lack of compliance by the UK andrology laboratories with World Health Organization recommendations for sperm morphology assessment. Hum Reprod 2005;20(12):3441−5.
[8] Aitken R, Clarkson J, Hargreave T, Irvine D, Wu F. Analysis of the relationship between defective sperm function and the generation of reactive oxygen species in cases of oligozoospermia. J Androl 1989;10(3):214−20.
[9] Sharma R, Agarwal A. Role of reactive oxygen species in male infertility. Urology 1996;48(6):835−50.
[10] Agarwal A, Sharma R, Nallella K, Thomas A, Alvarez J, Sikka S. Reactive oxygen species as an independent marker of male factor infertility. Fertil Steril 2006;86(4):878−85.

[11] Smith R, Vantman D, Ponce J, Escobar J, Lissi E. Total antioxidant capacity of human seminal plasma. Hum Reprod 1996;11(8):1655−60.

[12] de Lamirande E, Jiang H, Zini A, Kodama H, Gagnon C. Reactive oxygen species and sperm physiology. Rev Reprod 1997;2(1):48−54.

[13] Agarwal A, Saleh R, Bedaiwy M. Role of reactive oxygen species in the pathophysiology of human reproduction. Fertil Steril 2003;79(4):829−43.

[14] Dorostghoal M, Kazeminejad S, Shahbazian N, Pourmehdi M, Jabbari A. Oxidative stress status and sperm DNA fragmentation in fertile and infertile men. Andrologia 2017. https://doi.org/10.1111/and.12762.

[15] Wang X, Sharma R, Sikka S, Thomas A, Falcone T, Agarwal A. Oxidative stress is associated with increased apoptosis leading to spermatozoa DNA damage in patients with male factor infertility. Fertil Steril 2003;80(3):531−5.

[16] Sakkas D, Mariethoz E, St John J. Abnormal sperm parameters in humans are indicative of an abortive apoptotic mechanism linked to the Fas-mediated pathway. Exp Cell Res 1999;251(2):350−5.

[17] Du Plessis S, Makker K, Desai N, Agarwal A. Impact of oxidative stress on IVF. Exp Rev Obstet Gynecol 2008;3(4):539−54.

[18] Esteves S, Rogue M, Agarwal A. Outcome of assisted reproductive technology in men with treated and untreated varicocele: systematic review and meta-analysis. Asian J Androl 2016;18(2):254−8.

[19] Agarwal A, Roychoudhury S, Bjugstad K, Cho C. Oxidation-reduction potential of semen: what is its role in the treatment of male infertility? Ther Adv Urol 2016;8(5):302−18.

[20] Agarwal A, Sharma R, Roychoudhury S, Du Plessis S, Sabanegh E. MiOXSYS: a novel method of measuring oxidation reduction potential in semen and seminal plasma. Fertil Steril 2016;106(3):566−73. e10.

[21] Agarwal A, Roychoudhury S, Sharma R, Gupta S, Majzoub A, Sabanegh E. Diagnostic application of oxidation-reduction potential assay for measurement of oxidative stress: clinical utility in male factor infertility. Reprod Biomed Online 2017;34(1):48−57.

[22] Agarwal A, Wang S. Clinical relevance of oxidation-reduction potential in the evaluation of male infertility. Urology 2017;104:84−9.

[23] Agarwal A, Arafa M, Chandrakumar R, Majzoub A, AlSaid S, Elbardisi H. A multicenter study to evaluate oxidative stress by oxidation-reduction potential, a reliable and reproducible method. Andrology 2017. https://doi.org/10.1111/andr.12395.

[24] Arafa M, Agarwal A, AlSaid S, Majzoub A, Sharma R, Bjugstad K, AlRumaihi K, Elbardisi H. Semen quality and infertility status can be identified through measures of oxidation-reduction potential. Andrologia 2017. https://doi.org/10.1111/and.12881. e12881.

[25] Ye Z, Wang S, Chen T, Gao W, Zhu S, He J, Han Z. Inactivation mechanism of *Escherichia coli* induced by slightly acidic electrolyzed water. Sci Rep 2017;7(1):6279.

[26] Bergendahl J, Stevens L. Oxidation reduction potential as a measure of disinfection effectiveness for chlorination of wastewater. Environ Prog Sustain Energy 2005;24(2):214−22.

[27] Victorin K, Hellstrom K, Rylander R. Redox potential measurements for determining the disinfecting power of chlorinated water. J Hyg 1972;70(2):313−23.

[28] McFarland M, Glarborg C, Ross M. Chemical treatment of chelated metal finishing wastes. Water Environ Res 2012;84(12):2086−9.

[29] Hjorth M, Pedersen C, Feilberg A. Redox potential as a means to control the treatment of slurry to lower H$_2$S emissions. Sensors (Basel, Switzerland) 2012;12(5):5349−62.

[30] Shapiro H. Redox balance in the body: an approach to quantitation. J Surg Res 1972;13(3):138−52.

[31] Rael L, Bar-OR R, Aumann R, Slone D, Mains C, Bar-Or D. Oxidation-reduction potential and paraoxonase-arylesterase activity in trauma patients. Biochem Biophys Res Commun 2007;361(2):561−5.

[32] Rael L, Bar-Or R, Mains C, Slone D, Levy A, Bar-Or D. Plasma oxidation-reduction potential and protein oxidation in traumatic brain injury. J Neurotrauma 2009;26(8):1203−11.

[33] Stagos D, Goutzourelas N, Bar-Or D, Ntontou A, Bella E, Becker A, Statiri A, Kafantaris I, Kouretas D. Application of a new oxidation-reduction potential assessment method in strenuous exercise-induced oxidative stress. Redox Rep 2015;20(4):154−62.

[34] Bar-Or R, Bar-Or D, Rael L, inventors. Method and apparatus for measuring oxidation-reduction potential. Aytu Bioscience, Inc, assignee; United States patent US 9,528,959; Dec 27 2016.

[35] Rael L, Bar-Or R, Kelly M, Carrick M, Bar-Or D. Assessment of oxidative stress in patients with isolated traumatic brain injury using disposable electrochemical test strips. Electroanalysis 2015;27:2567−73.

[36] Kohen R, Nyska A. Oxidation of biological systems: oxidative stress phenomena, antioxidants, redox reactions, and methods for their quantification. Toxicol Pathol 2002;30(6):620−50.

[37] Sabeti P, Pourmasumi S, Rahiminia T, Akyash F, Talebi A. Etiologies of sperm oxidative stress. Int J Reprod Biomed (Yazd, Iran) 2016;14(4):231−40.

[38] Bisht S, Dada R. Oxidative stress: major executioner in disease pathology, role in sperm DNA damage and preventative strategies. Front Biosci (Scholar Edition) 2017;9:420−47.

[39] Jensen C, Ostergren P, Dupree J, Ohl D, Sonksen J, Fode M. Varicocele and male infertility. Nat Rev Urol 2017. https://doi.org/10.1038/nrurol.2017.98.

[40] Majzoub A, Agarwal A. Antioxidant therapy in idiopathic oligoasthenoteratozoospermia. Indian J Urol 2017;33(3):207−14.

[41] Dada R, Kumar S, Chawla B, Bisht S, Khan S. Oxidative stress induced damage to Paternal genome and impact of meditation and yoga − Can it reduce incidence of childhood cancer? Asian Pac J Cancer Prev 2016;17(9):4517−25.

[42] Wright C, Milne S, Leeson H. Sperm DNA damage caused by oxidative stress: modifiable clinical, lifestyle and nutritional factors in male infertility. Reprod Biomed Online 2014;28(6):684−703.

Chapter 3.5

Treatment of Sperm Oxidative Stress: A Collaborative Approach Between Clinician and Embryologist

Kelton Tremellen

Flinders University, Bedford Park, SA, Australia

INTRODUCTION

Oxidative damage to sperm and resulting impaired fertility potential occurs when there is an imbalance between the production of potentially harmful reactive oxygen species (ROS) and their neutralization by protective antioxidants contained within seminal plasma, male reproductive tract secretions, and the sperm [1,2]. Oxidative stress (OS) is a very common problem, reported to affect up to 70% of men seeking fertility treatment, and is commonly present even in normozoospermic men in infertile relationships [1]. An excess of ROS, commonly referred to as free radicals, damages the sperm lipid membrane, which then limits motility and fertilization capacity due to altered acrosomal membrane function [1,2]. Furthermore, even if fertilization does occur, oxidative damage to the paternal DNA has the potential to impair embryo quality, thereby limiting conception but also increasing the risk of miscarriage [1–3]. Finally, there is some evidence that oxidative damage to sperm may lead to gene mutations or epigenetic modifications of the paternal genome, which have serious health consequences for the resulting child such as an increased risk of cancer [3–5]. For all of these reasons, it is imperative that both clinicians and scientists involved in the treatment of infertile couples are mindful of the potential harm that sperm OS can cause.

Despite OS being a common pathology, it is alarming that the majority of assisted reproductive treatment (ART) clinics make no attempt to analyze their patient's sperm for oxidative damage, nor do they provide any empirical antioxidant treatment [1]. As such, sperm OS can be thought of as a reproductive iceberg; a large potential threat to reproductive outcomes, but generally ignored due to its low profile of importance in the minds of the majority of in vitro fertilization (IVF) physicians and scientists.

In order to best protect men's sperm from oxidative attack the treating physician and reproductive scientist must understand what processes initiate OS so that they can best nullify these damaging processes. Therefore this chapter will outline the underlying clinical and laboratory causes for OS, plus how best to minimize this potential damaging process from both a clinical and laboratory perspective.

CLINICAL CAUSES OF OXIDATIVE STRESS AND THEIR TREATMENT

The first step in the clinical management of potential sperm OS is to recognize its presence. The major reversible causes of sperm OS, plus their treatment, are covered by the helpful mnemonic **TESTICULAR**, as outlined in Table 1, but will be discussed in more detail as follows.

Toxins

Exposure to environmental toxins is a common factor aggravating sperm OS. These toxins may be present within the local environment (air or water), or as a result of occupational exposure. Large epidemiological studies have linked high levels

TABLE 1 Clinical Causes of Sperm Oxidative Stress and Their Management: The TESTICULAR Approach

Cause of Oxidative Stress	Specific Management Options
1. **T**oxins (air pollution, pesticides, metal fumes)	Minimize time outdoors on high pollution days, use indoor air filters; safety equipment (respirators, protective clothing); good ventilation around exposure to toxins.
2. **E**jaculatory frequency (long periods of abstinence)	Optimal sperm DNA integrity is achieved following 1−2 days of abstinence.
3. **S**tress (psychological)	Minimization of stress through yoga and meditation reduces sperm oxidative stress, plus improves general well-being.
4. **T**emperature (occupational heat exposure, baths and saunas, electric blankets)	Appropriate heat shields and air conditioning to minimize occupational exposure to heat; avoid long hot baths and saunas plus sleeping with electric blanket on; wear loose fitting clothing in hot weather.
5. **I**nfection/inflammation (STIs, accessory gland and systemic infections)	Treat infections with antibiotics; minimize residual ROS production by activated leukocytes using NSAIDs.
6. **C**ancer (and its treatment)	Surgical removal of cancer to resolve proinflammatory/oxidant state. Store sperm before starting cancer therapy.
7. **U**nhealthy lifestyle (poor diet, lack of exercise, obesity)	Diet low in red and processed meats but high in fresh fruit/vegetables/nuts/legumes and oily fish; maintain normal BMI and frequent moderate exercise; avoid prolonged cycling.
8. **A**natomical (varicocele)	Surgical ligation of clinically apparent varicoceles that are associated with impaired semen quality.
9. **R**adiation (mobile phones, Wi-Fi, ionizing radiation)	Use land line over mobile phone when possible; avoid storage of mobile phone in trouser pocket; keep laptop computer off the lap.

BMI, body mass index; *NSAID*, nonsteroidal antiinflammatory drug; *ROS*, reactive oxygen species; *STI*, sexually transmitted infections.

of exposure to air pollution, with reductions in sperm motility and morphology, plus alterations in chromatin, making the sperm more susceptible to DNA damage [6,7]. Polycyclic aromatic hydrocarbons (PAHs), common environmental toxins formed during incomplete combustion of organic materials (oil-based fuels, wood, coal, and tobacco), and their associated particulate matter are believed to be responsible [7,8], with inhalation of these pollution particles being associated with both systemic inflammation and OS [9]. Clinical management of this harmful exposure is difficult, but minimizing time spent outdoors on days of high pollution, wearing face masks, and the use of air purifiers within the home are some practical options.

Pesticides such as lindane, methoxychlor, and dioxin-TCDD are all linked with impaired sperm quality, with OS being one of the major underlying mechanisms [10]. Exposure to these environmental contaminants can be minimized by consuming organically produced food, extensive washing of fruit and vegetables before eating, and preferentially drinking and cooking only with filtered water. Farmers' occupational exposure to pesticides can be minimized through appropriate protective clothing, respirators, and washing after contact with toxins, reducing their risk of impaired sperm quality to that of the general population [10].

Another common occupational toxin linked with sperm OS and male subfertility is inhalation of metal fumes produced during welding, soldering, and the construction of lead-acid batteries [11,12]. Again, appropriate personal protection equipment and ventilation are the keys to minimization of these toxins' negative impact on sperm health.

Ejaculatory Frequency

Studies have now linked infrequent ejaculation with a reduction in sperm quality [13], possibly because prolonged storage in the epididymis exposes sperm to increased risk of OS damage [1]. Infrequent ejaculation can be the result of sexual difficulties exacerbated by the stress of infertility, but is also a relatively common side effect of the selective serotonin reuptake inhibitor class of antidepressants, which impair ejaculation and have been linked with increased sperm DNA fragmentation [14]. As short periods of sexual abstinence (1−2 days) are reported to result in optimal sperm DNA quality, infertile men should be advised to avoid long periods of abstinence prior to providing a semen sample for assisted reproduction or attempting natural conception. This point should be made very clear to all patients undergoing infertility treatment as it is a common misconception that a prolonged period of abstinence may assist ART or natural conception because it maximizes the number of available sperm.

Stress

Psychological stress has been implicated in sperm OS and male subfertility [15], with the removal of this type of stress (completion of university examinations) being reported to result in a reduction in sperm oxidative damage [16]. Furthermore, the adoption of meditation and yoga practices to reduce stress has recently been reported to result in a reduction in sperm oxidative damage and improvements in DNA integrity [17]. While this report was not a randomized control study, it would appear sensible to suggest these types of interventions to reduce psychological distress in those men severely emotionally impacted by their infertility status, especially as yoga and meditation may also improve these men's general well-being.

Temperature

The testicles are contained within the scrotum because spermatogenesis optimally occurs at a temperature at least 2 degrees below core body temperature [18]. However, when the testicles are exposed to excessive heat through high environmental temperatures (e.g., working in a smelter or hot kitchen, prolonged use of a laptop computer on the lap [18,19], or frequent use of saunas and baths), there is a decline in sperm quality mediated by OS [18,20]. Management of heat stress obviously involves avoidance of heat related recreational activity (baths, saunas, and exercise in extreme heat), wearing loose-fitting clothing, and avoiding prolonged direct contact between the testicles and heat sources (laptop computers, electric blankets). Interestingly, some researchers even advocate the use of nocturnal scrotal cooling using air streams [21] or underwear containing cooling gel inserts (Snowballs; https://www.snowballsunderwear.com/pages/design) as an effective treatment of heat-related male infertility.

Infection/Inflammatory

Infection of the male reproductive tract (male accessory gland infection or sexually transmitted infections [STIs]) [22,23], or chronic viral (hepatitis B, HIV), bacterial (tuberculosis), and parasitic infections (Schistosomiasis) have all been linked to sperm OS [24,25]. Furthermore, noninfective inflammatory conditions such as inflammatory bowel disease and many rheumatic autoimmune diseases have also been associated with a decline in sperm quality and impaired testosterone production [26,27].

The proposed common mechanistic link is that both infective and noninfective (autoimmune) conditions trigger the release of proinflammatory cytokines, many of which reach the male reproductive tract where they are capable of upregulating local leukocyte production of ROS, while also depleting antioxidant reserves [25]. The net end result of this process is of course an increased risk of OS damage to sperm [22]. Any man suspected of having a genitourinary infection based on symptoms, sexual history, examination (tender or thickened epididymis or vas, tender prostate), or abnormal semen analysis (altered semen viscosity or color, increased pH, or the presence of leukocytospermia) should be screened for STIs and have a semen culture, plus relevant ultrasound assessment of the scrotal contents and male accessory glands in order to localize the potential infective source [25]. Any identified infection should then be treated with antibiotics, often requiring multiple and prolonged courses of treatment in the case of male accessory gland infection, as this approach has been shown to produce superior bacteriological cure rates and a reduction in OS-related sperm damage, plus boost natural conception rates [28]. Furthermore, as inflammation and its associated increase in ROS production may continue beyond eradication of bacterial infection, some authors have suggested using nonsteroidal antiinflammatory agents to further reduce sperm oxidative attack [29]. Similarly, antiinflammatory agents such as monoclonal antibodies toward the proinflammatory cytokine TNFα have been suggested as useful therapies to reverse inflammatory OS and improve sperm quality (vitality, motility, and normal forms) in men with autoimmune disease [30].

Cancer

Cancers of the testis, Hodgkin lymphoma, and leukemia, the most common cancers affecting men of reproductive age, have all been linked with impaired sperm quality [31]. While it is possible that a mass effect may explain the link between testicular cancer and impaired spermatogenesis, this is not likely to be the case with nontesticular cancers. Furthermore, given that the majority of testicular tumors involve only one testicle, other systemic processes must also be responsible for the observed impairment in spermatogenesis. Importantly, cancer is known to be associated with inflammation and a resulting OS state throughout the body [32], and therefore it is logical that sperm production and quality would be impaired in untreated cancer. The resolution of this fighting immune response against cancer following orchiectomy may help explain why semen parameters often rapidly improve postsurgery, despite the presence of only one residual testicle [31].

Both chemotherapy and radiotherapy have been associated with inducing OS, both directly and indirectly via tumor cell necrosis and associated inflammation [33,34]. Obviously this cannot be modified, but it is important to consider sperm cryopreservation for cancer patients of reproductive age before they commence potentially damaging cancer therapy.

Unhealthy Lifestyle

An unhealthy diet is an increasing problem in the developed world because of increased consumption of packaged food high in sugar and fat content, but low in beneficial micronutrients such as antioxidants. Large epidemiological studies have linked frequent consumption of red and processed meat, known triggers for OS, with a decline in sperm quality [35]. Furthermore, a high consumption of fruit and vegetables, especially those containing β-carotene, lutein, and lycopene antioxidants [36], has been linked with improved sperm quality [37]. Overall optimal sperm quality is best supported by eating a minimum amount of red and processed meats (salami and the like), plus plenty of fruit, vegetables, legumes, whole grains, and nuts [35]. Furthermore, one randomized controlled trial (RCT) has linked consumption of omega-3 fatty acid supplements containing docosahexaenoic acid (DHA) and eicosapentaenoic acid, both abundant in oily fish such as salmon and sardines, with improvements in seminal antioxidant capacity plus sperm motility, concentration, and morphology [38]. Furthermore, another similar study found that the use of DHA supplements had the ability to reduce sperm DNA damage and improve seminal antioxidant status [39]. Therefore men are advised to increase their intake of oily fish to boost sperm quality.

Heavy alcohol intake, generally considered as the consumption of at least six standard drinks per day (60 g total), has been associated with a systemic prooxidant state and a reduction in semen quality [40]. While this reduction in semen quality is multifactorial (impaired leutinizing hormone and follicle stimulating hormone pituitary drive, direct alcohol toxicity to Leydig cells), the association between heavy alcohol consumption and the presence of increased number of seminal leukocytes does suggest a male reproductive tract inflammatory response, with the potential for ROS production and resulting oxidative damage to sperm [40]. Similarly, cigarette smoking has been associated with an increase in seminal OS and impaired spermatogenesis, plus an increase in sperm DNA damage, which has been linked with serious health consequences for the next generation [41]. Interestingly, the combination of high acute consumption of alcohol and cigarettes was associated with sperm oxidative damage and a decline in semen quality in a recent report examining semen quality before and after University examination celebrations [42]. As such, alcohol intake should be kept to a minimum, preferably below two standard drinks per day, and smoking totally avoided.

Obesity is associated with a decline in sperm quality and an increase in sperm oxidative damage, possibly related to an increase in macrophage activation state within semen [43]. The underlying cause for this obesity-related proinflammatory state is multifactorial, but recently studies have linked obesity with a breakdown in the barrier function of the intestinal mucosa, allowing bacteria to pass from the gut lumen into the circulation, where they initiate an inflammatory response that is likely to result in an increase in ROS production and impaired spermatogenesis [44,45]. Weight loss through diet, exercise, or bariatric surgery, however, is known to improve sperm quality [44,46]. A recent RCT of moderate exercise (treadmill walking or jogging for 30–45 min 3–6 days week) in 419 infertile men has reported that exercise did result in a reduction in seminal inflammation, sperm OS, and improvements in sperm quality, plus a significant increase in conception rates [47]. However, as a cautionary note, bicycle riding as a form of exercise has been linked with a reduction in sperm quality [48], possibly mediated by the heating of the testicles by tight-fitting bike clothes or contact with the bike seat, and therefore this type of exercise is probably not ideal for infertile men with evidence of sperm OS.

Anatomical

The presence of a palpable varicocele, seen in up to 40% of infertile men, has been conclusively linked with an increase in sperm OS and a subsequent decline in sperm quality [49]. However, the association between subclinical (nonpalpable), ultrasound-defined varicoceles with sperm OS and infertility is less uncertain. Multiple studies have now reported a reduction in sperm OS with surgical varicocele repair, and significant improvements in both semen quality and chances of natural conception, provided surgical repair is performed only on those men with clinically apparent varicoceles and semen abnormalities (reviewed in [49]). Therefore, we would advocate for consideration of surgical repair of varicocele in this subgroup, but not for those men with varicoceles that are only identified on ultrasound or who have normal sperm parameters.

Radiation

While exposure to ionizing radiation will result in sperm damage, both directly and indirectly via generation of ROS [50], this is a relatively uncommon occurrence due to appropriate occupational health precautions. However, exposure to the radiofrequency electromagnetic radiation (RFER) is extremely common with the widespread use of mobile phones and Wi-Fi networks. A metaanalysis of 10 studies examining the impact of mobile phone use on sperm quality reported that exposure to mobile phones was associated with significant reduction in sperm motility and viability, but no clear impact on sperm concentration [51]. Another review reported that all seven studies measuring ROS after RFER exposure observed an increase in ROS production, and 4 out of 5 of these reports also found an alarming resulting increase in sperm DNA damage [52]. Similarly, people using Wi-Fi connected devices may be exposed to electromagnetic energy, which may be especially problematic for reproductive potential when that device is in close physical proximity to the testicles, such as a laptop computer placed in a man's lap. An interesting ex vivo study reported that exposure of donor quality sperm to 4 h of radiation from a wireless Internet-connected laptop produced a reduction in sperm motility and increase in sperm DNA damage through a nonthermal mechanism [53]. As such, we would advise all men that it is safest to avoid the use of laptop computers on their lap, plus minimize their exposure to mobile phone RFER by keeping their phones in a coat pocket rather than trouser pocket and using traditional land-line phone connections rather than their mobile phone whenever possible.

ANTIOXIDANT SUPPLEMENTS TO AUGMENT SPERM QUALITY

After the production of ROS has been reversed or minimized by improvements in behavior, surgery, and other associated therapies, it makes obvious good sense to augment the infertile man's antioxidant defenses in order to provide optimal protection of sperm from any residual ROS. Over the last three decades multiple different supplements, each with differing doses and types of antioxidants, have been studied in both controlled and noncontrolled settings. A full discussion of the merits and weaknesses of these studies is beyond the scope of this chapter, but is well covered in recent reviews [54−56]. However, some general comments in relation to antioxidant supplements to optimize sperm health are still warranted.

First, the majority of antioxidant supplements in clinical use rely on more than one active ingredient, primarily as different antioxidants work at different sites or through different mechanisms, thereby improving the ROS scavenging capacity of the supplement. For example, an antioxidant such as vitamin C has been shown to spare and/or recycle vitamin E, thereby making sense that both of these antioxidants should be included in an ideal synergistic preparation [54]. Table 2 outlines the ingredients and strengths used in some of the most commonly used antioxidant supplements designed specifically for augmenting male fertility. From this table it is apparent that vitamin C, vitamin E, lycopene, glutathione, N-acetyl cysteine, acetyl L-carnitine, coenzyme Q10, zinc, and selenium are commonly used antioxidants. Antiinflammatory agents such as omega-3 fatty acids and garlic oil are also used in some supplements to reduce

TABLE 2 Typical Contents of Antioxidant Preparations Used to Treat Sperm Oxidative Stress

Active Antioxidant Ingredient	Typical Daily Dose
1. Vitamin C	200−1000 mg
2. Vitamin E	200−600 mg
3. Selenium	100−200 mcg
4. Zinc	15−40 mg
5. L-carnitine	1−3 g
6. *N*-Acetyl cysteine (NAC)	600 mg
7. Co enzyme Q10 (CoQ10)	60−300 mg
8. Lycopene	4−6 mg
9. Glutathione	500 mg
10. Omega-3 fish oil (DHA/EPA)	1.5−2 g

DHA, docosahexaenoic acid; *EPA*, eicosapentaenoic acid.

inflammatory ROS production. Finally, micronutrients such as zinc and selenium assist in protamine packaging of sperm, making the paternal DNA less susceptible to oxidative attack [54].

Second, it is impossible to make scientifically robust general statements concerning the ability of antioxidants to improve semen quality because of the huge variation in ingredients and doses used in the various studies, the relative small size of these studies, and their failure to test for the presence of oxidative damage before enrolment. However, overall the prevailing consensus is that antioxidant supplements do have the capacity to improve sperm motility and concentration, although they probably do not improve morphology [54–56]. Furthermore, many studies have shown antioxidants can reduce oxidative damage to sperm (markers of sperm membrane lipid peroxidation and DNA oxidative damage), with some also reporting improvements in natural conception [54–56]. Furthermore, a Cochrane review has concluded that pretreatment of men with antioxidants prior to IVF or intrauterine insemination therapy improves their partners' chances of successful conception and live birth [57]. Therefore, as there is considerable evidence that antioxidant supplements may improve sperm health while being inexpensive and relatively free of significant side effects, it appears sensible to suggest their use in all men experiencing male subfertility or couples experiencing infertility of unknown cause where sperm OS is often the underlying cryptic pathology [58]. Finally, since sperm production takes on average 70 days, it is likely that maximal benefit will not be seen for up to 2–3 months after initiation of antioxidant therapy.

As a final word of caution, some authors have suggested that the use of oral antioxidants in the setting of male infertility may have the potential for harm [59]. The use of an oral antioxidant preparation containing vitamins C and E, β-carotene, zinc, and selenium for a period of 3 months was reported to result in a reduction in sperm DNA fragmentation, but also an increase in sperm DNA condensation. As high degrees of sperm DNA decondensation may be linked with asynchronous chromosome condensation and poor embryo development, it has been suggested that antioxidant treatment should not be recommended to men whose semen sample show a high degree of decondensation over a threshold of 20% on sperm chromatin structure assay (SCSA) assessment [59]. However, as the Cochrane review does show an overall benefit in pregnancy rates from treating the male with antioxidants prior to ART treatment [57], it is currently debatable if this decondensation issue is a significant clinical concern.

LABORATORY PROCEDURES TO MINIMIZE OXIDATIVE DAMAGE TO SPERM DURING ASSISTED REPRODUCTIVE TECHNIQUE TREATMENT

The handling of sperm in the clinical laboratory in preparation for assisted reproduction poses significant risk of oxidative damage for a number of reasons [2,60].

First, sperm are normally contained postejaculation within seminal plasma, a physiological medium that contains many antioxidants that help protect sperm from oxidative attack. During sperm processing for ART, seminal plasma is removed, placing sperm at increased risk of oxidative attack [61]. Second, the physical separation of sperm by centrifugation has the potential for increasing oxidative damage, as centrifugal forces are known to increase ROS production by sperm [62]. Furthermore, some density gradients used in the separation of sperm from seminal plasma have been identified as containing transitional metals such as iron, which are known to stimulate ROS production by the Fenton reaction [63]. Centrifugation may also bring sperm in close proximity with leukocytes in the cellular pellet, with production of ROS by leukocytes being 1000 times greater than sperm themselves, thereby creating very significant potential for sperm damage [2,60]. Finally, cryopreservation, a commonly used laboratory tool for sperm storage, is known to induce ROS mediated damage to sperm [64]. Taken together, there is certainly the potential for a coordinated oxidative assault on sperm in the laboratory if appropriate precautions are not taken.

In order to minimize iatrogenic oxidative damage to sperm, the following laboratory approaches have been suggested (Table 3).

1. Minimize centrifuge-related OS by using short duration low g-force processing to separate the sperm from the seminal plasma if possible, as hard and prolonged centrifugation increases sperm oxidative damage [65]. Other sperm recovery processes such as electrophoretic separation [66], annexin V magnetic activated cell separation of apoptotic sperm [67], and the use of zeta-potential [68] have also been described as superior methods for isolating viable sperm with less oxidative damage compared to traditional techniques such as density-gradient centrifugation, although none of these later techniques are in common clinical use.

2. Addition of antioxidants (catalase, glutathione, N-acetyl cysteine, vitamins C and E) plus chelating agents like ethylenediaminetetraacetic acid that remove prooxidant transition metals (iron, copper) from sperm processing and culture media have all been reported to have the potential to reduce sperm oxidative damage (reviewed in 56 and 60). The

TABLE 3 Steps to Reduce Sperm Oxidative Stress in the In Vitro Fertilization Laboratory

Nine steps to minimizing sperm oxidative stress in the IVF laboratory

1. If a prior semen analysis has suggested the possibility of OS (leukocytospermia or other sentinel signs of OS), please report this to the treating clinician so that an appropriate treatment plan can be initiated before the ART cycle.
2. Ask patients to abstain for only 1–2 days prior to producing a semen sample for IVF/IUI treatment.
3. When processing sperm use the minimum amount of centrifugation possible to obtain the required number of sperm (lowest g-force, shortest possible spin times).
4. Prepare sperm with the least possible delay between sample production and utilization for fertilization (ideally less than 2–4 h).
5. Use sperm wash/preparation media that contains protective antioxidants.
6. Avoid exposing sperm to potential OS stressors such as bright lights, pH fluctuations, and temperature changes.
7. Consider requesting a surgically collected sperm sample with likely superior DNA integrity if the ejaculate sample has known or probable poor DNA quality, or there has been a poor blastocyst formation rate in the past using ejaculate sperm.
8. Use cryopreservation media containing antioxidants and avoid repeat freeze-thawing of sperm. Ideally use fresh sperm over frozen if clinically possible.
9. Allow for natural selection in IVF by using routine insemination rather than ICSI, unless ICSI is mandated by very low semen quality or past poor fertilization rates. Oxidative damaged sperm are unlikely to participate in fertilization, reducing the chances of producing an embryo containing damaged paternal DNA.

ART, assisted reproductive technology; *ICSI*, intracytoplasmic sperm injection; *IUI*, intrauterine insemination; *IVF*, in vitro fertilization; *OS*, oxidative stress.

addition of antioxidants such as vitamins C and E, catalase, and glutathione to cryopreservation media has also been reported to be of some benefit in terms of improving sperm postthaw motility and DNA integrity [69].

3. Exposure to bright environmental light sources, plus fluctuations in pH or temperature, all have the potential for creating OS [60]. Therefore sperm should ideally be processed in labs with indirect lighting (light reflected off walls), with appropriate culture buffer systems and temperature control [60].

4. Men should be instructed to only abstain for 1–2 days before producing a semen sample for use in ART as this improves sperm DNA integrity [13]. Furthermore, those men with a history of high semen viscosity should be asked to produce their sample into culture media, which often allows for easier and more rapid recovery of high-quality sperm.

5. Minimization of the time between production of a semen sample, its processing, and ultimate use for fertilization to less than 2 h, as this has been shown to minimize culture-related ROS damage [70].

6. The technique used for achieving fertilization may also have some impact on reproductive outcomes in the setting of IVF. While intracytoplasmic sperm injection (ICSI) has the advantage of achieving fertilization more rapidly than routine insemination, thereby minimizing the time that sperm is exposed to in vitro OS [60], ICSI does pose a significant potential for harm as an oxidatively damaged sperm with poor DNA integrity may be chosen for ICSI and can still create an embryo. However, this embryo has reduced live-birth potential and may possibly produce significant health issues later in life [4]. Conversely, sperm with oxidative-damaged DNA and acrosomal membrane are unlikely to achieve natural fertilization as they have been reported to not bind to the oocyte zona pellucida [71], thereby providing an important protective biological filter. As such, we advocate routine insemination as the favored approach in IVF, unless very poor semen quality mandates ICSI.

7. The use of surgically extracted testicular sperm has some advantages over ejaculate-derived sperm in the setting of high degrees of DNA damage [72,73]. It is believed that most oxidative damage to sperm occurs after the sperm has left the protective environment of the Sertoli cells and are being stored in the epididymis [74]. As such, studies have confirmed improved sperm DNA integrity and resulting embryo quality/pregnancy rates when using surgically extracted sperm compared to those from an ejaculate sample [72,73]. However, many men with sperm present in their ejaculate are resistant to the concept of surgical testicular sperm extraction to improve sperm DNA quality. A brief description, colloquially explained as taking sperm straight from the factory production line (testis) before it has a chance to be scratched (DNA damaged) in the car lot (epididymis and ejaculate), is often a useful explanation for enlisting cooperation from the male partner!

CONCLUDING REMARKS

OS is a very common pathology affecting many men in infertile relationships, even normozoospermic individuals. Since most clinical laboratories do not test for the presence of OS, it is vital that the treating clinician be aware of the sentinel signs and clinical causes of oxidative attack, so that they have the opportunity to suggest changes to lifestyle and treat any underlying pathology, plus instigate antioxidant supplement therapy. This approach will not only maximize a couple's chances of natural conception, but also increase the efficiency of any ART treatment required. Similarly, careful handling of sperm in the IVF laboratory is important for optimizing sperm health and reproductive outcomes. Failure to address sperm OS may result in DNA damage, with associated poor embryo development, increased miscarriage risk, plus possible health implications for next generation. A collaborative approach between patient, clinician, and embryologist will give each couple the best chances of becoming parents to a healthy child.

LIST OF ACRONYMS AND ABBREVIATIONS

ART Assisted reproductive technology
DHA Docosahexaenoic acid
EDTA Ethylenediaminetetraacetic acid
EPA Eicosapentaenoic acid
FSH Follicle stimulating hormone
IUI Intrauterine insemination
IVF In vitro fertilization
LH Leutinizing hormone
MAGI Male accessory gland infection
NSAID Nonsteroidal antiinflammatory drug
OS Oxidative stress
PAH Polycyclic aromatic hydrocarbons
RCT Randomized controlled trial
RFER Radio-frequency electromagnetic radiation
ROS Reactive oxygen species
SSRI Selective serotonin reuptake inhibitors
TNFα Tumor necrosis factor alpha

REFERENCES

[1] Tremellen K. Oxidative stress and male infertility—a clinical perspective. Hum Reprod Update 2008 May—June;14(3):243—58. https://doi.org/10.1093/humupd/dmn004.

[2] Opuwari CS, Henkel RR. An update on oxidative damage to spermatozoa and oocytes. BioMed Res Int 2016;2016:9540142. https://doi.org/10.1155/2016/9540142.

[3] De Iuliis GN, Thomson LK, Mitchell LA, Finnie JM, Koppers AJ, Hedges A, et al. DNA damage in human spermatozoa is highly correlated with the efficiency of chromatin remodeling and the formation of 8-hydroxy-2′-deoxyguanosine, a marker of oxidative stress. Biol Reprod September 2009;81(3):517—24. https://doi.org/10.1095/biolreprod.109.076836.

[4] Aitken RJ, De Iuliis GN, McLachlan RI. Biological and clinical significance of DNA damage in the male germ line. Int J Androl February 2009;32(1):46—56. https://doi.org/10.1111/j.1365-2605.2008.00943.x.

[5] Tunc O, Tremellen K. Oxidative DNA damage impairs global sperm DNA methylation in infertile men. J Assist Reprod Genet 2009 September—October;26(9—10):537—44. https://doi.org/10.1007/s10815-009-9346-2.

[6] Selevan SG, Borkovec L, Slott VL, Zudová Z, Rubes J, Evenson DP, et al. Semen quality and reproductive health of young Czech men exposed to seasonal air pollution. Environ Health Perspect September 2000;108(9):887—94.

[7] Wu L, Jin L, Shi T, Zhang B, Zhou Y, Zhou T, et al. Association between ambient particulate matter exposure and semen quality in Wuhan, China. Environ Int January 2017;98:219—28. https://doi.org/10.1016/j.envint.2016.11.013.

[8] Jeng HA, Pan CH, Chao MR, Lin WY. Sperm DNA oxidative damage and DNA adducts. Mutat Res Genet Toxicol Environ Mutagen December 2015;794:75—82. https://doi.org/10.1016/j.mrgentox.2015.09.002.

[9] Risom L, Møller P, Loft S. Oxidative stress-induced DNA damage by particulate air pollution. Mutat Res December 30, 2005;592(1—2):119—37.

[10] Mehrpour O, Karrari P, Zamani N, Tsatsakis AM, Abdollahi M. Occupational exposure to pesticides and consequences on male semen and fertility: a review. Toxicol Lett October 15, 2014;230(2):146—56. https://doi.org/10.1016/j.toxlet.2014.01.029.

[11] Bonde JP. The risk of male subfecundity attributable to welding of metals. Studies of semen quality, infertility, fertility, adverse pregnancy outcome and childhood malignancy. Int J Androl August 1993;16(Suppl 1):1—29.

[12] Naha N, Chowdhury AR. Inorganic lead exposure in battery and paint factory: effect on human sperm structure and functional activity. J UOEH June 1, 2006;28(2):157—71.

[13] Agarwal A, Gupta S, Du Plessis S, Sharma R, Esteves SC, Cirenza C, et al. Abstinence time and its impact on basic and advanced semen parameters. Urology August 2016;94:102—10. https://doi.org/10.1016/j.urology.2016.03.059.

[14] Tanrikut C, Feldman AS, Altemus M, Paduch DA, Schlegel PN. Adverse effect of paroxetine on sperm. Fertil Steril August 2010;94(3):1021—6. https://doi.org/10.1016/j.fertnstert.2009.04.039.

[15] Nordkap L, Jensen TK, Hansen ÅM, Lassen TH, Bang AK, Joensen UN, et al. Psychological stress and testicular function: a cross-sectional study of 1,215 Danish men. Fertil Steril January 2016;105(1):174—87. https://doi.org/10.1016/j.fertnstert.2015.09.016. e1-2.

[16] Eskiocak S, Gozen AS, Kilic AS, Molla S. Association between mental stress & some antioxidant enzymes of seminal plasma. Indian J Med Res December 2005;122(6):491—6.

[17] Rima D, Shiv BK, Bhavna C, Shilpa B, Saima K. Oxidative stress induced damage to paternal genome and impact of meditation and yoga - can it reduce incidence of childhood cancer? Asian Pac J Cancer Prev January 9, 2016;17(9):4517—25.

[18] Jung A, Schuppe HC. Influence of genital heat stress on semen quality in humans. Andrologia December 2007;39(6):203—15.

[19] Sheynkin Y, Jung M, Yoo P, Schulsinger D, Komaroff E. Increase in scrotal temperature in laptop computer users. Hum Reprod February 2005;20(2):452—5.

[20] Ahmad G, Agarwal A, Esteves SC, Sharma R, Almasry M, Al-Gonaim A, et al. Ascorbic acid reduces redox potential in human spermatozoa subjected to heat-induced oxidative stress. Andrologia March 1, 2017. https://doi.org/10.1111/and.12773 [Epub ahead of print].

[21] Jung A, Eberl M, Schill WB. Improvement of semen quality by nocturnal scrotal cooling and moderate behavioural change to reduce genital heat stress in men with oligoasthenoteratozoospermia. Reproduction April 2001;121(4):595—603.

[22] Ochsendorf FR. Infections in the male genital tract and reactive oxygen species. Hum Reprod Update 1999 September—October;5(5):399—420.

[23] Potts JM, Pasqualotto FF. Seminal oxidative stress in patients with chronic prostatitis. Andrologia October 2003;35(5):304—8.

[24] McKenna G, Schousboe M, Paltridge G. Subjective change in ejaculate as symptom of infection with Schistosoma haematobium in travellers. BMJ October 18, 1997;315(7114):1000—1.

[25] La Vignera S, Vicari E, Condorelli RA, D'Agata R, Calogero AE. Male accessory gland infection and sperm parameters (review). Int J Androl October 2011;34(5 Pt 2):e330—47. https://doi.org/10.1111/j.1365-2605.2011.01200.x.

[26] Tiseo BC, Cocuzza M, Bonfa E, Srougi M, Silva CA. Male fertility potential alteration in rheumatic diseases: a systematic review. Int Braz J Urol 2016 January—February;42(1):11—21. https://doi.org/10.1590/S1677-5538.IBJU.2014.0595.

[27] Valer P, Algaba A, Santos D, Fuentes ME, Nieto E, Gisbert JP, et al. Evaluation of the quality of semen and sexual function in men with inflammatory bowel disease. Inflamm Bowel Dis July 2017;23(7):1144—53. https://doi.org/10.1097/MIB.0000000000001081.

[28] Vicari E. Effectiveness and limits of antimicrobial treatment on seminal leukocyte concentration and related reactive oxygen species production in patients with male accessory gland infection. Hum Reprod December 2000;15(12):2536—44.

[29] Vicari E, La Vignera S, Calogero AE. Antioxidant treatment with carnitines is effective in infertile patients with prostatovesiculoepididymitis and elevated seminal leukocyte concentrations after treatment with nonsteroidal anti-inflammatory compounds. Fertil Steril December 2002;78(6):1203—8.

[30] Villiger PM, Caliezi G, Cottin V, Förger F, Senn A, Østensen M. Effects of TNF antagonists on sperm characteristics in patients with spondyloarthritis. Ann Rheum Dis October 2010;69(10):1842—4. https://doi.org/10.1136/ard.2009.127423.

[31] Agarwal A, Desai NR, Ruffoli R, Carpi A. Lifestyle and testicular dysfunction: a brief update. Biomed Pharmacother October 2008;62(8):550—3. https://doi.org/10.1016/j.biopha.2008.07.052.

[32] Kundu JK, Surh YJ. Emerging avenues linking inflammation and cancer. Free Radic Biol Med May 1, 2012;52(9):2013—37. https://doi.org/10.1016/j.freeradbiomed.2012.02.035.

[33] Chen Y, Jungsuwadee P, Vore M, Butterfield DA, St Clair DK. Collateral damage in cancer chemotherapy: oxidative stress in nontargeted tissues. Mol Interv June 2007;7(3):147—56.

[34] Zhao W, Robbins ME. Inflammation and chronic oxidative stress in radiation-induced late normal tissue injury: therapeutic implications. Curr Med Chem 2009;16(2):130—43.

[35] Gaskins AJ, Colaci DS, Mendiola J, Swan SH, Chavarro JE. Dietary patterns and semen quality in young men. Hum Reprod October 2012;27(10):2899—907. https://doi.org/10.1093/humrep/des298.

[36] Zareba P, Colaci DS, Afeiche M, Gaskins AJ, Jørgensen N, Mendiola J, et al. Semen quality in relation to antioxidant intake in a healthy male population. Fertil Steril December 2013;100(6):1572—9. https://doi.org/10.1016/j.fertnstert.2013.08.032.

[37] Chiu YH, Gaskins AJ, Williams PL, Mendiola J, Jørgensen N, Levine H, et al. Intake of fruits and vegetables with low-to-moderate pesticide residues is positively associated with semen-quality parameters among young healthy men. J Nutr May 2016;146(5):1084—92. https://doi.org/10.3945/jn.115.226563.

[38] Safarinejad MR. Effect of omega-3 polyunsaturated fatty acid supplementation on semen profile and enzymatic anti-oxidant capacity of seminal plasma in infertile men with idiopathic oligoasthenoteratospermia: a double-blind, placebo-controlled, randomised study. Andrologia February 2011;43(1):38—47. https://doi.org/10.1111/j.1439-0272.2009.01013.x.

[39] Martínez-Soto JC, Domingo JC, Cordobilla B, Nicolás M, Fernández L, Albero P, et al. Dietary supplementation with docosahexaenoic acid (DHA) improves seminal antioxidant status and decreases sperm DNA fragmentation. Syst Biol Reprod Med December 2016;62(6):387—95.

[40] La Vignera S, Condorelli RA, Balercia G, Vicari E, Calogero AE. Does alcohol have any effect on male reproductive function? A review of literature. Asian J Androl March 2013;15(2):221—5. https://doi.org/10.1038/aja.2012.118.

[41] Esakky P, Moley KH. Paternal smoking and germ cell death: a mechanistic link to the effects of cigarette smoke on spermatogenesis and possible long-term sequelae in offspring. Mol Cell Endocrinol November 5, 2016;435:85—93. https://doi.org/10.1016/j.mce.2016.07.015.

[42] Silva JV, Cruz D, Gomes M, Correia BR, Freitas MJ, Sousa L, et al. Study on the short-term effects of increased alcohol and cigarette consumption in healthy young men's seminal quality. Sci Rep April 3, 2017;7:45457. https://doi.org/10.1038/srep45457.

[43] Tunc O, Bakos HW, Tremellen K. Impact of body mass index on seminal oxidative stress. Andrologia April 2011;43(2):121—8. https://doi.org/10.1111/j.1439-0272.2009.01032.x.

[44] Tremellen K. Gut Endotoxin Leading to a Decline IN Gonadal function (GELDING) - a novel theory for the development of late onset hypogonadism in obese men. Basic Clin Androl June 22, 2016;26:7. https://doi.org/10.1186/s12610-016-0034-7.

[45] Tremellen K, McPhee N, Pearce K. Metabolic endotoxaemia related inflammation is associated with hypogonadism in overweight men. Basic Clin Androl March 8, 2017;27:5. https://doi.org/10.1186/s12610-017-0049-8.

[46] Oliveira PF, Sousa M, Silva BM, Monteiro MP, Alves MG. Obesity, energy balance and spermatogenesis. Reproduction June 2017;153(6):R173–85. https://doi.org/10.1530/REP-17-0018.

[47] Hajizadeh Maleki B, Tartibian B. Moderate aerobic exercise training for improving reproductive function in infertile patients: a randomized controlled trial. Cytokine April 2017;92:55–67. https://doi.org/10.1016/j.cyto.2017.01.007.

[48] Gaskins AJ, Afeiche MC, Hauser R, Williams PL, Gillman MW, Tanrikut C, et al. Paternal physical and sedentary activities in relation to semen quality and reproductive outcomes among couples from a fertility center. Hum Reprod November 2014;29(11):2575–82. https://doi.org/10.1093/humrep/deu212.

[49] Tiseo BC, Esteves SC, Cocuzza MS. Summary evidence on the effects of varicocele treatment to improve natural fertility in subfertile men. Asian J Androl 2016 March–April;18(2):239–45. https://doi.org/10.4103/1008-682X.172639.

[50] Einor D, Bonisoli-Alquati A, Costantini D, Mousseau TA, Møller AP. Ionizing radiation, antioxidant response and oxidative damage: a meta-analysis. Sci Total Environ April 1, 2016;548–549:463–71. https://doi.org/10.1016/j.scitotenv.2016.01.027.

[51] Adams JA, Galloway TS, Mondal D, Esteves SC, Mathews F. Effect of mobile telephones on sperm quality: a systematic review and meta-analysis. Environ Int September 2014;70:106–12. https://doi.org/10.1016/j.envint.2014.04.015.

[52] Houston BJ, Nixon B, King BV, De Iuliis GN, Aitken RJ. The effects of radiofrequency electromagnetic radiation on sperm function. Reproduction December 2016;152(6):R263–76.

[53] Avendaño C, Mata A, Sanchez Sarmiento CA, Doncel GF. Use of laptop computers connected to internet through Wi-Fi decreases human sperm motility and increases sperm DNA fragmentation. Fertil Steril January 2012;97(1):39–45. https://doi.org/10.1016/j.fertnstert.2011.10.012. e2.

[54] Tremellen K. Antioxidant therapy for the enhancement of male reproductive health: a critical review of the literature. In: Parekattil SJ, Agarwal A, editors. Male Infertility. Contemporary clinical approaches, andrology, ART and antioxidants. Springer; 2012. p. 389–400.

[55] Lanzafame FM, La Vignera S, Vicari E, Calogero AE. Oxidative stress and medical antioxidant treatment in male infertility. Reprod Biomed Online November 2009;19(5):638–59.

[56] Zini A, Al-Hathal N. Antioxidant therapy in male infertility: fact or fiction? Asian J Androl May 2011;13(3):374–81. https://doi.org/10.1038/aja.2010.182.

[57] Showell MG, Mackenzie-Proctor R, Brown J, Yazdani A, Stankiewicz MT, Hart RJ. Antioxidants for male subfertility. Cochrane Database Syst Rev 2014;12:CD007411. https://doi.org/10.1002/14651858.CD007411.pub3.

[58] Aktan G, Doğru-Abbasoğlu S, Küçükgergin C, Kadıoğlu A, Ozdemirler-Erata G, Koçak-Toker N. Mystery of idiopathic male infertility: is oxidative stress an actual risk? Fertil Steril April 2013;99(5):1211–5. https://doi.org/10.1016/j.fertnstert.2012.11.045.

[59] Ménézo YJ, Hazout A, Panteix G, Robert F, Rollet J, Cohen-Bacrie P, Chapuis F, Clément P, Benkhalifa M. Antioxidants to reduce sperm DNA fragmentation: an unexpected adverse effect. Reprod Biomed Online April 2007;14(4):418–21.

[60] Agarwal A, Durairajanayagam D, du Plessis SS. Utility of antioxidants during assisted reproductive techniques: an evidence based review. Reprod Biol Endocrinol November 24, 2014;12:112. https://doi.org/10.1186/1477-7827-12-112.

[61] Twigg J, Irvine DS, Houston P, Fulton N, Michael L, Aitken RJ. Iatrogenic DNA damage induced in human spermatozoa during sperm preparation: protective significance of seminal plasma. Mol Hum Reprod May 1998;4(5):439–45.

[62] Aitken RJ, Clarkson JS. Significance of reactive oxygen species and antioxidants in defining the efficacy of sperm preparation techniques. J Androl 1988 November–December;9(6):367–76.

[63] Aitken RJ, Finnie JM, Muscio L, Whiting S, Connaughton HS, Kuczera L, et al. Potential importance of transition metals in the induction of DNA damage by sperm preparation media. Hum Reprod October 10, 2014;29(10):2136–47. https://doi.org/10.1093/humrep/deu204.

[64] Thomson LK, Fleming SD, Aitken RJ, De Iuliis GN, Zieschang JA, Clark AM. Cryopreservation-induced human sperm DNA damage is predominantly mediated by oxidative stress rather than apoptosis. Hum Reprod September 2009;24(9):2061–70. https://doi.org/10.1093/humrep/dep214.

[65] Shekarriz M, DeWire DM, Thomas Jr AJ, Agarwal A. A method of human semen centrifugation to minimize the iatrogenic sperm injuries caused by reactive oxygen species. Eur Urol 1995;28(1):31–5.

[66] Aitken RJ, Hanson AR, Kuczera L. Electrophoretic sperm isolation: optimization of electrophoresis conditions and impact on oxidative stress. Hum Reprod August 2011;26(8):1955–64. https://doi.org/10.1093/humrep/der162.

[67] Said TM, Agarwal A, Zborowski M, Grunewald S, Glander HJ, Paasch U. Utility of magnetic cell separation as a molecular sperm preparation technique. J Androl 2008 March–April;29(2):134–42.

[68] Nasr Esfahani MH, Deemeh MR, Tavalaee M, Sekhavati MH, Gourabi H. Zeta sperm selection improves pregnancy rate and alters sex ratio in male factor infertility patients: a double-blind, Randomized Clinical Trial. Int J Fertil Steril 2016 July–September;10(2):253–60.

[69] Amidi F, Pazhohan A, Shabani Nashtaei M, Khodarahmian M, Nekoonam S. The role of antioxidants in sperm freezing: a review. Cell Tissue Bank December 2016;17(4):745–56.

[70] Toro E, Fernández S, Colomar A, Casanovas A, Alvarez JG, López-Teijón M, et al. Processing of semen can result in increased sperm DNA fragmentation. Fertil Steril December 2009;92(6):2109–12. https://doi.org/10.1016/j.fertnstert.2009.05.059.

[71] Liu DY, Baker HW. Human sperm bound to the zona pellucida have normal nuclear chromatin as assessed by acridine orange fluorescence. Hum Reprod June 2007;22(6):1597–602.

[72] Esteves SC, Sánchez-Martín F, Sánchez-Martín P, Schneider DT, Gosálvez J. Comparison of reproductive outcome in oligozoospermic men with high sperm DNA fragmentation undergoing intracytoplasmic sperm injection with ejaculated and testicular sperm. Fertil Steril December 2015;104(6):1398−405. https://doi.org/10.1016/j.fertnstert.2015.08.028.

[73] Mehta A, Bolyakov A, Schlegel PN, Paduch DA. Higher pregnancy rates using testicular sperm in men with severe oligospermia. Fertil Steril December 2015;104(6):1382−7. https://doi.org/10.1016/j.fertnstert.2015.08.008.

[74] Vernet P, Aitken RJ, Drevet JR. Antioxidant strategies in the epididymis. Mol Cell Endocrinol March 15, 2004;216(1−2):31−9.

Part IV

Current Approaches: The OMICS

Chapter 4.1

Genomics and Epigenetics

Biren V. Patel and James M. Hotaling
University of Utah, Salt Lake City, UT, United States

INTRODUCTION

Deoxyribonucleic acid (DNA) is the blueprint for life on earth. Over the last 50 years, substantial advances have been made in the study of DNA (genomics) and there appears to be a long runway of discoveries that lay ahead.

The word genomics is derived from Greek, with *gen* meaning "create, become, birth or creation." In simplest terms, DNA is composed of four chemical units called nucleotide bases, and their sequence order determines the instructions of the information. The four bases are adenine (A), thymine (T), cytosine (C), and guanine (G). C always pairs with G and T always pairs with A. These bases are attached to a backbone of sugar (deoxyribose) and phosphate [1]. By convention, we read the DNA sequence from the $5'$ end of the sugar chain to the $3'$ end.

The complete set of DNA for an organism is its genome, and the human genome contains approximately three billion DNA base pairs. A specific segment of DNA that encodes the instructions for a protein formation (or a set of protein formation) is termed a gene and the human genome contains 25,000 discovered genes (and counting) [1]. These genes are read by multiple proteins that synthesize a complementary strand called a messenger RNA (mRNA), which then serves as a guide to assemble novel proteins from nucleic acids.

The genome is grouped in 23 pairs of chromosomes with 22 autologous and 1 pair of sex chromosomes. Every offspring inherits one copy of each chromosome from each parent. Mutations can occur in many ways, including spontaneously or during recombination (a process in meiosis where homologous chromosomes pair in dividing germ cells).

EPIGENETICS

Epigenetics can have profound effects on male reproduction. It is a relatively new field and is literally defined as "in addition to changes in genetic sequence." Epigenetics represents all the discovered mechanisms of *heritable* modification for gene expression [2]. The most commonly cited include methylation, acetylation, phosphorylation, and ubiquitylation (sumoylation). In a relatively short timeframe, many diet and environmental agents have been discovered that drive these epigenetic mechanisms. Examples include heavy metals, tobacco smoke, hydrocarbons, hormones, bacteria, viruses, radiation, and pesticides [3].

Deoxyribonucleic Acid Methylation

Methylation is perhaps the simplest mechanism to understand and is defined as the addition of a methyl group ($-CH_3$) to a DNA molecule by DNA-methyltransferases (Dnmt), almost always in mammals to the carbon-5 (C5) position of cytosine to form 5-methyl cytosine (Fig. 1) [3].

DNA methylation was first discovered around the same time that DNA was identified in the 1940s [4]. It was not until the 1980s, however, that scientists began to appreciate DNA methylation's role in gene expression and cell differentiation [5].

The family of methyltransferases that transfer the methyl group from S-adenyl methionine to cytosine are numerous and complex in their function. They transfer mostly to CpG sites, which are regions of DNA with a cytosine followed by a guanine when read from the $5'$ end.

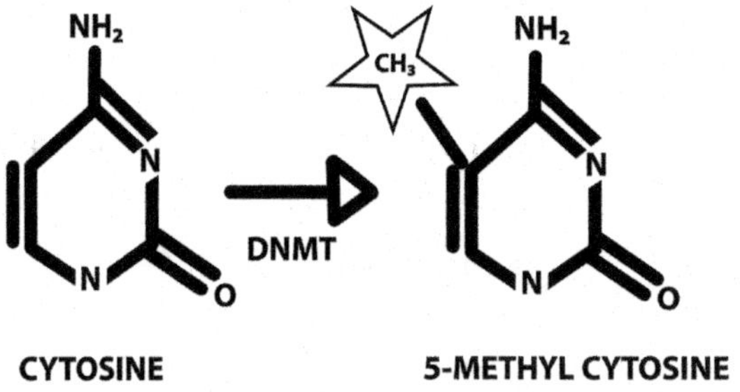

FIGURE 1 **DNA methylation.** The methylation of cytosine by Dnmts is a crucial epigenetic mechanism. *Dnmt*, DNA-methyltransferase.

The cytosine nucleotides on both strands are methylated. The proteins that take part in methylation can be broken up into three categories: writers, erasers, and readers [4]. Writers are the methyltransferases that add the methyl group. Erasers are proteins that modify and remove methylation. Readers are proteins that bind to the methyl group to make transcription less likely (usually).

The erasers perform their job via either a passive or an active mechanism. The passive mechanism simply entails inhibiting or removing Dnmt-1, the main DNA methyltransferase, which is constantly active. Stopping this protein allows newly synthesized DNA to have unmethylated cytosine nucleotides. The active mechanism has not been fully elucidated but consists of a series of hypothesized enzymatic pathways that degrade the 5-methyl cytosine to thymine, or similarly derived nucleotide residue, creating a DNA mismatch. This residue is then replaced by a newly synthesized, unmethylated cytosine by the cell's DNA repair system.

Many of these CpG sites are located upstream from genes so methylation of DNA correlates inversely to gene expression. DNA methylation reduces gene expression by inhibiting proper binding of transcription factors via conformational changes. The cascade of proteins drawn to the methyl groups may also actively create a silenced state by modifying transcription factors directly. This mechanism is still largely undiscovered and being explored [6].

Histones

Outside of DNA, the major players in epigenetics are histones. They are highly alkaline proteins from four major families (H2A, H2B, H3, and H4) that combine as dimers to create a core structure around which DNA wraps. This is called a nucleosome. Nucleosomes are linked by another histone family protein (H1) and further packaged into tighter and denser storage units. Histones are highly conserved. They have a positively charged N-terminus tail with many lysine and arginine residues. These tails actually protrude from the nucleosome structure and are the location of most histone-related epigenetic modifications. The result is the amazing condensation of DNA from 4 m in total length during the G_2 phase to 120 μm during mitosis [7].

Non-DNA Methylation

Like DNA, methylation also occurs in histones. The addition of methyl groups is performed by a histone methyltransferase but unlike DNA methylation, which inactivates a region of the genome, methylation of histones can either activate or repress transcription. This is determined by the particular histone protein (e.g., H3 or H4) and the specific amino acid (e.g., lysine 9 or lysine 20) that undergoes methylation and the precise location of the modification within the broader genome. The N-terminus tail with its rich concentration of lysine and arginine is the primary site of methylation. A single lysine residue can have several methyl additions forming methyl-lysine, dimethyl-lysine, and trimethyl-lysine (Fig. 2).

Similarly, a single arginine residue can have multiple sites of methylation.

Acetylation of Histones

Histone acetylation is the process of adding an acetyl group ($-CH_3CO$) to lysine residues of histones (Fig. 3).

The acetylation process was first described in 1961 and was one of the earliest discovered histone modifications [8]. The process is carried out by histone acetyltransferases (HATs), and the addition of an acetyl group to histones generally increases gene expression.

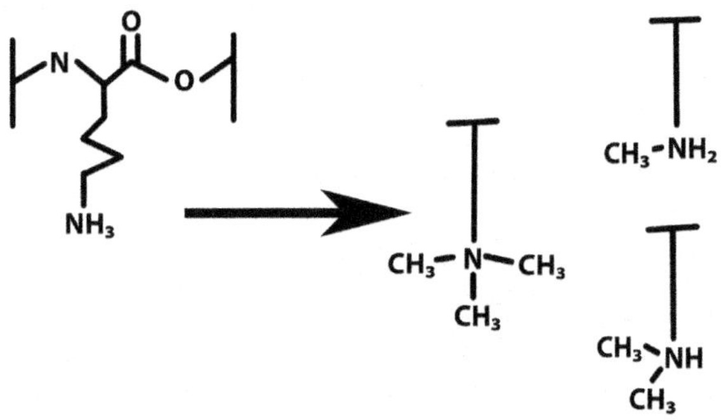

FIGURE 2 Histone methylation. Lysine can be methylated once, twice, or three times to form methyl-lysine, dimethyl-lysine, and trimethyl-lysine, respectively.

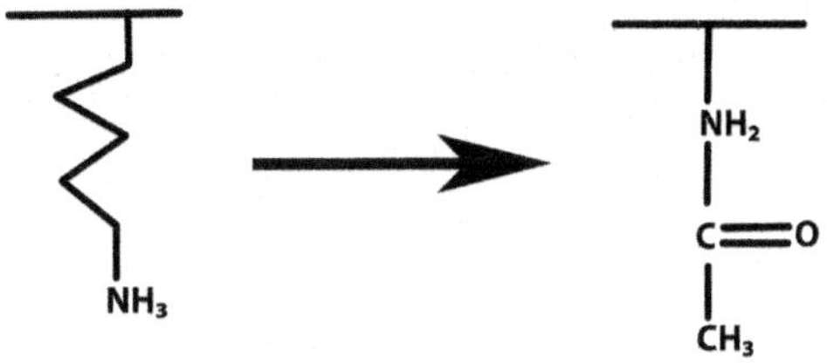

FIGURE 3 Histone acetylation. The addition of an acetyl group to the lysine residue on a histone tail.

Acetylation was thought to confer a negative charge to the histone proteins, which would theoretically disturb nucleosome formation and allow relaxation of the compacted DNA-histone complex. This in turn would allow the transcription machinery access to the DNA. More recent studies, however, suggest that lysine acetylation also creates bindings sites for transcription initiation [8,9]. These binding sites can be occupied by bromodomains, an extensive family of evolutionary conserved regions on proteins that have been shown to regulate transcription [10].

Acetylation is, in fact, a very dynamic process (HATs have half-lives measured in minutes) that allows rapid mobilization for gene transcription in response to any environmental stimuli. The swift speed of HATs allows acetylation to also have nonepigenetic functions. Areas of DNA damage are known to induce histone acetylation, presumably to allow access for DNA repair proteins.

Phosphorylation

Phosphorylation is a commonly seen mechanism in many aspects of cellular biology. In the field of epigenetics, phosphorylation refers to the addition of a phosphoryl group $(PO_3)^-$ to histones via a pathway involving a kinase protein. Nucleosome tails can be phosphorylated by various kinases. This phosphorylation occurs in serine, threonine, and tyrosine amino acids. Many of the early discovered gene expressions induced by phosphorylation are related to oncogenes, such as epidermal growth factor, c-fos, and c-myc [11].

Because of the broad set of functions served by phosphorylation within a cell, it can be difficult to determine when epigenetic changes are taking place. Histone phosphorylation has been shown to regulate chromosome condensation ahead of cell cycle events such as replication or apoptosis [12,13]. Even the linker histone, H1, has also been shown to undergo phosphorylation to coordinate ribosome genesis and cell growth [14].

Ubiquitylation and Sumoylation

Ubiquitylation (or ubiquitination) is the process of adding ubiquitin (an 8.5 kDa, 76-amino acid regulatory protein) to a substrate. This process was first discovered as part of a pathway for protein degradation [15]. Ubiquitin is joined to lysine residues by peptide bonds that can be cleaved by deubiquitinases. Like phosphorylation, ubiquitylation is used in a variety of processes such as signaling, DNA repair, and cell cycle control. The discovery of its role in epigenetics is more recent. The reversible ubiquitylation of histone H2B has been shown to lead to either transcription activation or repression, depending on cell conditions and the specific residue receiving the ubiquitin [16,17].

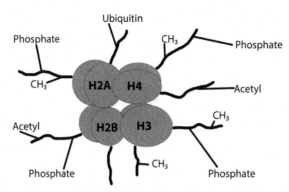

FIGURE 4 **Modifications of histone tails.** The histone tails undergo epigenetic modification. DNA (not shown) is wrapped twice around the nucleosome core.

Sumoylation is a somewhat related term describing a similar process to ubiquitylation. The acronym SUMO refers to small ubiquitin-like modifier. These modifiers are small proteins with a variety of potential functions including stabilization, localization, and regulation of other proteins. It is still mostly unknown so it can be considered a catch-all category by some. dDsk2, a ubiquitin-like protein previously known to help target proteins for degradation, has also been shown to serve as regulatory molecules for DNA transcription [18]. Another SUMO, a specialized version of the transcription factor Sp3, was found in *Drosophila* to recruit proteins to repress transcription [19]. With these epigenetic mechanisms, it is important to remember that there is significant cross-talk between pathways. Histone modification has been shown to affect DNA methylation and vice versa (Fig. 4 and Table 1).

EPIGENETICS IN MALE REPRODUCTION

Considerable research has been done on epigenetics related to the male reproductive tract. The testes are a fundamentally different organ from nonreproductive tissue. In fact, they contain eight times more hypomethylated (transcriptionally active) loci than somatic tissue [20,21]. The testes can also have different molecular analogues from somatic tissue. An important protein to consider is BORIS, an acronym for the uniquely named Brother of Regulator of Imprinting Sites [22]. This protein is closely related to the highly conserved and much studied CTCF, a DNA binding protein with roles in transcription regulation, imprinting genes, X-chromosome inactivation, and cell proliferation control. While CTCF is expressed throughout most cells in the body, BORIS expression is restricted to germ line cells where it plays a key role in setting early methylation patterns. CTCF knockouts in mice result in early embryonic death, but BORIS knockouts result in subfertility with defective spermatogenesis [23]. Expression of BORIS in normally BORIS-negative cells (i.e., somatic tissue) promotes aberrant epigenetic dysregulation, leading to cell growth and malignancy [22].

It is comforting to know, however, that biology has provided potential checks and balances to the power of epigenetics. Reprogramming is a mechanism that can stop erroneous methylation patterns from being transmitted through the germline. For example, in primordial mice germ cells, the entire genome—which previously had patterns of methylation inherited from parents—undergoes rapid removal of DNA methylation. This demethylation is selective for single-copy genes and occurs after the primordial germ cells have migrated to the genital ridge. The timing and specificity of the reprogramming suggests that cells have considerable control in epigenetic regulation of potentially aberrant methylation patterns [24].

Many studies have looked at the rates of methylation in infertile or subfertile men and found abnormalities. Several hypermethylated loci (NTF3, MT1A, PAX8, and PLAGL1) were found to be associated with poorer sperm concentration, motility, and morphology in one study looking at 69 men at an infertility center [25]. Another study showed that the hypermethylation of the promoter gene for methylenetetrahydrofolate reductase (MTHFR), a critical enzyme for methylation steps, was observed in testicular biopsies of 53% of men with nonobstructive azoospermia versus 0% of men with obstructive azoospermia. DNA from peripheral blood showed no difference in the methylation profile of the promoter region when compared to fertile controls. This suggests that these aberrant methylation changes were solely in the testis [26]. The association between MTHFR promoter hypermethylation, infertility, and other adverse health outcomes such as recurrent pregnancy loss has been seen in many other studies [27,28].

Another area of epigenetic control unique to spermatozoa and male reproduction is the set of basic nuclear proteins called protamines. Male germ cells pack their chromatin into volumes smaller than virtually any other cell in the body. This feat requires a pathway where the majority of histones are first replaced with proteins called protamines [29]. Though these

TABLE 1 Examples of Epigenetics in DNA and Histones

Name/References	Epigenetic Change	Effect	Example
DNA methylation [4]	Addition of methyl group to cytosine in DNA strand and usually in CpG sites	Usually transcriptional repression	Dnmt1 = maintains DNA methylation pattern through replication; most abundant methyltransferase in mammalian cell; most studied epigenetic mechanism
Histone methylation[a]	Addition of 1, 2, or 3 methyl groups to either lysine or arginine residues	Transcription activation or repression	Trimethylation of histone H3 at lysine 4 (H3L4) is associated with transcriptional activation while dimethylation of histone H3 at lysine 9 (H3L9) is associated with transcriptional repression
Histone acetylation [10]	Addition of acetyl groups to lysine residues	Usually transcriptional activation; acetylated lysine residues are usually recognized by bromodomain (a highly conserved protein sequence)	Lysine 3 or 36 on histone 3 or lysine 20 on histone 4 (H3L3, H3L36, H4L20) can be acetylated and are recognized by the bromodomain region of transcriptional activators CREB-binding protein and P300/CBP-associated factor
Histone phosphorylation [14]	Addition of phosphate groups to serine, threonine, and tyrosine	Transcription activation or repression; important in cross-talk with other epigenetic factors	Phosphorylation of many residues on histone H1 upregulates the transcription of RNA polymerase in interphase and helps control the cell cycle
Histone ubiquitylation (ubiquitination) [16]	Addition of ubiquitin	Transcription activation or repression; important in cross-talk with other epigenetic factors	Histone H2B ubiquitylation is seen in the fruit fly, yeast, the plant species Arabidopsis, and mice spermatogenesis. It was seen to both upregulate and downregulate transcription depending on the scenario and gene while playing a role in cell cycle control, development, gametogenesis, and cell signaling.
Histone sumoylation [18]	Addition of small ubiquitin-sized protein	Transcription activation or repression; important in cross-talk with other epigenetic factors	dDsk2 is a conserved ubiquitin receptor that plays a role in helping target ubiquitinated proteins for destruction but also plays a critical role to help transcribe developmental genes in the fruit fly.

DNA, deoxyribonucleic acid.
[a]*Gupta, S., Kim, S.Y., Artis, S., Molfese, D.L., Schumacher, A., Sweatt, J.D. et al. Histone methylation regulates memory formation. J Neurosci 2010; 30(10):3589–99.*

protamines are rapidly cleared after successful fertilization, there is evidence that they themselves undergo unique epigenetic modifications [30]. This histone-to-protamine transition is a tightly controlled process that allows the cell to determine which genes are available for early transcription.

Drugs

Numerous drugs have been shown to exert epigenetic control across generations. When administered in early gestation to pregnant mice, the antiandrogen drug Vinclozolin produced altered DNA methylation patterns in both maternally and paternally imprinted domains in the offspring [31]. The male mice offspring, in particular, also had reduced sperm concentration compared to controls. In another study, both Vinclozolin and Methoxychlor, an estrogenic compound, disrupted sperm methylation patterns for up to four generations after exposure to gestating maternal rats [32].

Diet

Diet can alter normal epigenetic profiles [33,34]. The amount of zinc, folate, methionine, betaine, and alcohol intake can alter the availability for methyl groups for DNA and histone modification [35,36]. The longevity of second generation mice has been shown to be positively associated with either preconception or pregnant maternal dietary methyl supplementation [37]. Even low levels of vitamin D have been associated with altered DNA methylation patterns at multiple loci in mice for two generations downstream from the exposed group [38]. Several Swedish studies have tried to examine the effect of diet on health outcomes using historical records. They found that grandchildren had longer survival and decreased risk of diabetes if their paternal grandfather experienced at least one poor harvest; that is, overeating and obesity in the paternal grandfathers could have potential epigenetic effects down to their grandchildren [39,40].

Environment

Pesticides, jet propellant, and bisphenol-A were studied in mice and found to alter epigenetic patterns for three generations after the initial exposure [34,41]. Environmental studies in humans have suggested similar outcomes. High levels of 2,3,7,8-tetrachlorodibenzodioxin, from a chemical plant accident in Italy, were associated with poorer sperm concentration and motility in individuals who had been exposed to the accident in infancy [42]. Individuals exposed to the accident during adulthood, however, showed no sperm parameter changes. This suggests the existence of a critical window in development where insults are more likely to cause damage to germ lines.

OXIDATIVE STRESS

Oxidative stress, the imbalance of removal of reactive oxidative species (ROS), and its effect on male fertility is an area of intense interest in the research community because oxidative stress has the potential for large epigenetic ramifications. The majority of the ROS originate from leukocytes (from infection or inflammation) and immature spermatozoa. The protective system employed by the body involves both enzymatic and nonenzymatic components [43]. The enzymatic system includes superoxidase dismutase, catalase, and glutathione peroxidase. The nonenzymatic system includes vitamins A, C, E, and B. Glutathione, pantothenic acid, coenzyme Q10, zinc, copper, and selenium are also included [43].

ROS are particularly damaging to spermatozoa because cell membranes contain a high concentration of unsaturated fatty acids. These fatty acids are highly susceptible to oxidation, and spermatozoa, given their small size, generally lack the protective enzymatic system found in other cells [44]. The loss of membrane function can have deleterious effects on fertilization rates, embryo development, and miscarriage rates [44–46]. Reactive species can also directly damage DNA via strand breaks and nicks. ROS are capable of increasing the mutation rate by altering nucleotides to their derivatives, for example, 8-hydroxy-2-deoxyguanosine (8-OHdG) or O^6-methylguanine. These derivatives are not recognized as accurately by the cell and their addition results in increased proofreading and replication errors. If the bases are substantially altered or suboptimally repaired, Dnmts are also unable to properly methylate DNA [47].

REACTIVE OXIDATIVE SPECIES AND EPIGENETICS

Epigenetic changes from ROS are observed in many disease processes in both males and females. ROS have been shown to not just play a direct role through cellular damage in the pathogenesis of cardiovascular disease but also to alter the DNA methylation and histone modification patterns [48]. In women, retrograde menstruation, with its deposits of hemoglobin and iron, causes local oxidative stress, and this has been linked with decreased DNA methylation potentially modifying susceptible genes. This could explain the predisposition of some patients to endometriosis [49].

Numerous studies have associated excessive ROS and male infertility. Smoking, drinking, radiation, toxins, inflammation, and infection have all been shown to elevate ROS [47,50]. The levels of testicular cytokines, small regulatory proteins that regulate development of germ cells and epigenetic programming, are altered by ROS. The levels of cytokines IL-6, IL-8, and TNF-α, in particular, increase sharply with oxidative stress [50].

Protamine Transition

The critical histone-to-protamine transition is a pivotal step in the stability of DNA transmission. ROS change the dynamics of this process directly through toxicity and indirectly through cytokine-mediated inflammation. The proper functions of protamines include stabilization of DNA modifications and prevention of sperm gene expression. An abnormal ratio of histone-to-protamine transition results in epigenetic instability. In one large Chinese study looking at 118 men with high levels of seminal ROS compared to 106 controls, Jiang and et al. found abnormal sperm histone-to-protamine ratios and alteration of 93 different cytokines in the experimental group [50]. Many of these cytokines (CXCL5, CXCL16, and TNF-α) are correlated with altered protamine expression.

Cigarette smoke contains a high concentration of free radicals that induce ROS in virtually all tissue, including the testis [51]. The normal ratio in fertile men of histone-to-protamine exchange is about 85%, and the ratio of two different types of protamines (SP1 and SP2) is about 1:1. The histone-to-protamine ratio and mRNA expression of SP1 and SP2 were assessed in 147 heavy smokers and 175 controls receiving fertility treatment by Yu et al. [52]. Their study showed that heavy smoking was associated with abnormalities in the histone-to-protamine transition with increased SP1-to-SP2 ratio. Another study in European smokers found similar results [53]. Heavy smokers were found to have elevated testicular ROS as measured by seminal markers of oxidative stress (malondialdehyde, 8-hydroguanosine, and cotinine) and found to have elevated SP1/SP2 ratios. Both studies suggested a strong association between oxidative stress and aberrant SP2 expression.

DNA Fragmentation

ROS can directly cause sperm DNA fragmentation, which is a measure of the level of DNA damage. There is growing evidence that it correlates directly to abnormal epigenetic programming. Damaged DNA generally leads to increased DNA methylation and decreased histone acetylation [54]. Many mechanisms have been proposed. Altered base pairs prevent DNA from serving as a proper substrate for enzymes (e.g., Dnmts, HATs, etc.). DNA damage may also alter proper chromatin packing, causing abnormal histone binding access for epigenetic machinery.

A small Turkish study compared fertile and infertile males and found a correlation between the level of seminal oxidative stress and sperm DNA fragmentation [55]. The researchers identified elevation in several oxidative stress markers (protein carbonyl groups, nitrotyrosine, and malondialdehyde), as assayed by the terminal deoxynucleotide transferase-mediated dUTP nick-end labeling (TUNEL) test, which correlated with abnormally high DNA fragmentation rates. Similar results were also seen in another study conducted at an exercise laboratory [56]. Levels of seminal ROS (malondialdehyde and 8-isoprostane) and sperm DNA fragmentation (TUNEL test) correlated and were higher in the experimental group. This study was unique in that it looked at 56 elite, extreme-training athletes and compared them to a control of 52 active, nonathlete men. Their results suggest that excessive and strenuous exercise may tip the balance in favor of oxidative stress. The protective system, measured by the ROS fighting enzymes superoxidase dismutase and catalase in the seminal fluid, was also seen to be lower in the elite athlete group, suggesting that it may have been overwhelmed.

The research done by Tunc and et al. corroborates these studies [57]. Oxidative stress, as measured by the modified colorimetric nitro blue tetrazolium test, was shown to increase sperm DNA fragmentation (TUNEL) and impede the process of sperm DNA methylation. The interesting part of this study was the trial arm of 50 male factor infertile patients. They received 3 months of antioxidant therapy (a capsule of folate, vitamin C, vitamin E, lycopene, zinc, selenium, and garlic oil) and then were retested. After 3 months there were significant decreases in seminal ROS levels and sperm DNA fragmentation. Global sperm DNA methylation was shown to be increased. While the results are promising, great care should be taken before extrapolating this study. There was no control arm and the modest improvements in the semen analyses parameters after 3 months could have happened by chance alone. What should be taken from all of these studies is that ROS can be harmful to spermatogenesis both directly and epigenetically and more robust research needs to be performed.

Other Mechanisms

Since the bulk of the research on epigenetics is done with DNA methylation, it can be easy to forget the other epigenetic mechanisms. ROS have been shown to induce global changes in histone modifications such as phosphorylation, acetylation, and ubquitylation [58–60]. Many of these mechanisms are the consequences of DNA damage, which alter the ability of intracellular signaling to recruit repair machinery and salvage DNA. Phosphorylation, in particular, has been studied extensively in protamines (Table 2) [60].

FINAL THOUGHTS

Epigenetics has fundamentally changed how we understand the impact of the environment on gene expression. Although we are just beginning to unravel exactly how these changes impact the germline, the impact of diet and lifestyle on ROS and their associated epigenetic changes has broad implications for reproductive medicine and future generations.

TABLE 2 Summary of Selected Reactive Oxygen Species–Induced Epigenetic Studies

Effect	Example
Altered protamine transition and cytokines [50]	118 men with high levels of seminal ROS were compared with 106 controls. Semen parameters, histone-to-protamine ratios, and over 400 cytokines were evaluated. ROS was correlated with poorer sperm parameters including concentration, volume, vitality, and progressive motility. ROS levels were also positively correlated with both abnormal histone-to-protamine ratios and abnormal histone transition. High levels of ROS were associated with elevations in 93 different cytokines including CXCL5, CXCL8, IL-16, CCL8, CCL22, CCL20, CXCL16, IL-1B, IL-6, IL-7, IL-10, CSF3, CCL3, CCL4, and TNF-α.
DNA methylation and histone acetylation [54]	Sperm samples were obtained from 25 infertile men. Damaged DNA was assessed by the level of DNA fragmentation and those with more than 30% fragmentation rate had much higher levels of DNA methylation. Histone acetylation (histone 4, lysine 12) showed negative correlation as the level of DNA damage increased.
Histone acetylation and phosphorylation [58]	ROS caused DNA single-strand breaks leading to phosphorylation of histone 3. This phosphorylation cross-talked with other mechanisms to cause hyperacetylation of histone 3 (lysine 9, 14, 18, and 23) and histone 4 (lysine 5, 8, 12, and 16). These changes are suspected to be an attempt of the cell to recruit DNA repair machinery to the sites of damage.
Histone phosphorylation [60]	Diazinon, an organophosphorus pesticide widely used in agriculture and pest control and potent generator of ROS, was found to have deleterious effects in mice. After treatment with diazinon, the quality of the sperm and promatine structure were evaluated. Viable sperm and motility were decreased. There was also poorer morphology. There was also a 50% hyperphosphorylation of protamines, which may be a direct result of damage to their structures.

DNA, deoxyribonucleic acid; *ROS*, reactive oxidative species.

As the cost of biological research continues to decrease, the future of ROS and epigenetics looks bright. However, the complexities are significant and careful work will be necessary to untangle the exact impact of ROS and epigenetics on fertility. It is difficult to extrapolate what animal studies mean for humans and what, if any, clinical correlations epigenetic changes have. Humans have unique genomes and environmental exposures that make it difficult to control variables when trying to predict outcomes. A clear, simple picture of epigenetic cause and effect is not possible just yet. But research is progressing rapidly.

REFERENCES

[1] National Human Genome Research Institute. A brief guide to genomics. August 27, 2015. Retrieved from: https://www.genome.gov/18016863/a-brief-guide-to-genomics/.

[2] Weinhold B. Epigenetics: the science of change. Environ Health Perspect 2006;114(3):A160–7.

[3] Zemach A, McDaniel I, Silva P, Zilberman D. Genome-wide evolutionary analysis of eukaryotic DNA methylation. Science 2010;328(5980):916–9.

[4] Moore LD, Le T, Fan G. DNA methylation and its basic function. Neuropsychopharmacol Rev 2013;38(1):23–38.

[5] Compere SJ, Palmiter RD. DNA methylation controls the inducibility of the mouse metallothionein-I gene lymphoid cells. Cell 1981;25(1):233–40.

[6] Xie W, Barr CL, Kim A, Yue F, Lee AY, Eubanks J, et al. Base-resolution analyses of sequence and parent-of-origin dependent DNA methylation in mouse genome. Cell 2012;148(1):816–31.

[7] Redon C, Pilch D, Rogakou E, Sedelnikova O, Newrock K, Bonner W. Histone H2A variants H2AX and H2AZ. Curr Opin Genet Dev 2002;1(12):162–9.

[8] Zentner GE, Henikoff S. Regulation of nucleosome dynamics by histone modifications. Nat Struct Mol Biol 2013;20(3):259–66.

[9] Allfrey VG, Faulkner R, Mirsky AE. Acetylation and methylation of histones and their possible role in regulation of RNA synthesis. Proc Natl Acad Sci USA 1964;51(5):786–94.

[10] Ren C, Zeng L, Zhou MM. Preparation, biochemical analysis, and structure determination of the bromodomain, an acetyl-lysine binding domain. Methods Enzymol 2016;573(1):321–43.

[11] Rossetto D, Avvakumov N, Côté J. Histone phosphorylation: a chromatin modification involved in diverse nuclear events. Epigenetics 2012;7(10):1098–108.

[12] Sauve DM, Anderson HJ, Ray JM, James WM, Roberge M. Phosphorylation-induced rearrangement of the histone H3 NH2-terminal domain during mitotic chromosome condensation. J Cell Biol 1999;145(2):225–35.

[13] Ajiro K. Histone H2B phosphorylation in mammalian apoptotic cells: an association with DNA fragmentation. J Biol Chem 2010;275(1):439–43.

[14] Zheng Y, John S, Pesavento JJ, Schultz-Norton JR, Schiltz RL, Baek S, et al. Histone H1 phosphorylation is associated with transcription by RNA polymerases I and II. J Cell Biol 2010;189(3):407–15.

[15] Wilkinson KD. The discovery of ubiquitin-dependent proteolysis. Proc Natl Acad Sci USA 2005;102(43):15280−2.

[16] Wright DE, Wang CY, Kao CF. Flickin' the ubiquitin switch: the role of H2B ubiquitylation in development. Epigenetics 2011;6(10):1165−75.

[17] Chandrasekharan MB, Huang F, Sun ZW. Histone H2B ubiquitination and beyond. Epigenetics 2010;5(6):460−8.

[18] Kessler R, Tisserand J, Font-Burgada J, Reina O, Coch L, Attolini CS, et al. dDsk2 regulates HsBub1 and RNA polymerase II pausing at dHP1c complex target genes. Nat Commun 2015;6(7049). https://doi.org/10.1038/ncomms8049.

[19] Stielow B, Sapetschnig A, Kruger I, Kunert N, Brehm A, Boutros M, et al. Identification of SUMO-dependent chromatin-associated transcriptional repression components by a genome-wide RNAi screen. Mol Cell 2008;29(6):742−54.

[20] Rajender S, Avery K, Agarwal A. Epigenetics, spermatogenesis and male infertility. Mutat Res 2011;727(3):62−71.

[21] Oakes CC, La Salle S, Smiraglia DJ, Robaire B, Trasler JM. A unique configuration of genome-wide DNA methylation patterns in the testis. Proc Natl Acad Sci USA 2007;104(1):228−33.

[22] Klenova EM, Morse HC, Ohlsson R, Lobanenkov VV. The novel BORIS + CRCF gene family is uniquely involved in the epigenetics of normal biopsy and cancer. Semin Cancer Biol 2002;12(5):399−414.

[23] Pugacheva E, Rivero-Hinojosa S, Espinoza C, Mendez-Catala C, Kang S, Suzuki T, et al. Comparative analyses of CTCF and BORIS occupancies uncover two distinct classes of CTCF binding genomic regions. Genome Biol August 14, 2015. https://doi.org/10.1186/s13059-015-0736-8.

[24] Hajkova P, Erhardt S, Lane N, Haaf T, El-maarri O, Reik W, et al. Epigenetic reprogramming in mouse primordial germ cells. Mech Dev 2002;117(1−2):15−23.

[25] Houshdaran S, Cortessis VK, Siegmund K, Yang A, Laird PW, Sokol RZ. Widespread epigenetic abnormalities suggest broad DNA methylation erasure defect in abnormal human sperm. PLoS One 2007;2(12):e1289.

[26] Khazamipour N, Noruzinia M, Fatehmanesh P, Keyhanee M, Puhol P. MTHFR promoter hypermethylation in testicular biopsies of patients with non-obstructive azoospermia: the role of epigenetics in male infertility. Hum Reprod 2009;24(9):2361−4.

[27] Wu W, Shen O, Qin Y, Niu X, Lu C, Xia Y, et al. Idiopathic male infertility is strongly associated with aberrant promoter methylation of methylenetetrahydrofolate reductase (MTHFR). PLoS One 2010;5(11):e13884.

[28] Rotonod JC, Bosi S, Bazzan E, Di Domenico M, De Mattei M, Selvatici R, et al. Methylenetetrahydrofolate reductase gene promoter hyper-methylation in semen samples of infertile couples correlates with recurrent spontaneous abortion. Hum Reprod 2010;27(12):2632−8.

[29] Dada R, Kumar M, Jesudasan R, Fernandez JL, Gosalvez J, Agarwal A. Epigenetics and its role in male infertility. J Assist Reprod Genet 2011;29(3):213−23.

[30] Marushige Y, Marushige K. Transformation of sperm histone during formation and maturation of rat spermatozoa. J Biol Chem 1975;250(1):39−45.

[31] Stouder C, Paoloni-Giacobino A. Transgenerational effects of the endocrine disruptor vinclozolin on the methylation pattern of imprinted genes in the mouse sperm. Reproduction 2010;139(2):373−9.

[32] Anway MD, Kupp AS, Uzumcu M, Skinner MK. Epigenetic transgenerational actions of endocrine disruptors and male fertility. Science 2005;308(5727):1466−9.

[33] Schagdarsurengin U, Steger K. Epigenetics in male reproduction: effect of paternal diet on sperm quality and offspring health. Nat Rev Urol 2016;13(10):584−95.

[34] Haotian W, Hauser R, Krawetz SA, Pilsner JR. Environmental susceptibility of the sperm epigenome during windows of male germ cell development. Curr Environ Health Rep 2015;2(4):356−66.

[35] McGowan PO, Meaney MJ, Szyf M. Diet and the epigenetic (re)programming of phenotypic differences in behavior. Brain Res July 29, 2008. https://doi.org/10.1016/j.brainres.2008.07.074.

[36] Cooney CA. Are somatic cells inherently deficient in methylation metabolism? A proposed mechanism for DNA methylation loss, senescence and aging. Growth Dev Aging 1993;57(4):261−73.

[37] Cooney CA, Dave AA, Wolff GL. Maternal methyl supplementation in mice affect epigenetic variation and DNA methylation of offspring. J Nutr 2002;132(8 Suppl.):2393S−400S.

[38] Xue J, Schoenrock SA, Valdar W, Tarantino LM, Ideraabdullah FY. Maternal vitamin D depletion alters DNA methylation at imprinted loci in multiple generations. Clin Epigenet October 12, 2016. https://doi.org/10.1186/s13148-016-0276-4.

[39] Bygren LO, Kaati G, Edvinsson S. Longevity determined by paternal ancestors' nutrition during their slow growth period. Acta Biotheor 2001;49(1):53−9.

[40] Kaati G, Bygren LO, Edvinnson S. Cardiovascular and diabetes mortality determined by nutrition during parents' and grandparents' slow growth period. Eur J Hum Genet 2002;10(11):682−8.

[41] Manikkam M, Tracey R, Guerrero-Bosagna C, Skinner MK. Plastics derived endocrine disruptors (BPA, DEHP and DBP) induce epigenetic transgenerational inheritance of obesity, reproductive disease and sperm epimutations. PLoS One 2013;8(1):e55387.

[42] Mocarelli P, Gerthoux PM, Patterson DG, Milani S, Limonta G, Bertona M, et al. Dioxin exposure, from infancy through puberty, produces endocrine disruption and affects human semen quality. Environ Health Perspect 2008;116(1):70−7.

[43] Walczak-Jedrzejowska R, Wolski JK, Slowikowska-Hilczer J. The role of oxidative stress and antioxidants in male fertility. Cent Eur J Urol 2012;66(1):60−7.

[44] Zini A, San Gabriel M, Baazeem A. Antioxidants and sperm DNA damage: a clinical perspective. J Assist Reprod Genet 2009;26(8):427−32.

[45] Aitkin RJ, De Iuliis GN, Finnie JM, Hedges A, McLachlan RI. Analysis of the relationship between oxidative stress, DNA damage and sperm vitality in a patient population: development of diagnostic criteria. Hum Reprod 2010;25(10):2415−26.

[46] Tremellen K. Oxidative stress and male infertility − a clinical perspective. Hum Reprod Update 2008;14(3):243−58.

[47] Franco R, Schoneveld O, Georgakilas AG, Panayiotidis MI. Oxidative stress, DNA methylation and carcinogenesis. Cancer Lett 2008;266(1):6−11.

[48] Kietzmann T, Petry A, Shvetsova A, Gerhold JM, Gorlach A. The epigenetic landscape related to reactive oxygen species formation in the cardiovascular system. Br J Pharmacol March 23, 2017. https://doi.org/10.1111/bph.13792.

[49] Ito F, Yamada Y, Shigemitsu A, Akinishi M, Kaniwa H, Miyake R, et al. Role of oxidative stress in epigenetic modification in endometriosis. Reprod Sci January 1, 2017. https://doi.org/10.1177/1933719117704909.

[50] Jiang L, Zheng T, Huang J, Mo J, Zhou H, Liu M, et al. Association of semen cytokines with reactive oxygen species and histone transition abnormalities. J Assist Reprod Genet 2016;33(9):1239−46.

[51] Isik B, Ceylan A, Isik R. Oxidative stress in smokers and non-smokers. Inhal Toxicol 2007;19(9):767−9.

[52] Yu B, Qi Y, Liu D, Gao X, Chen H, Bai C, et al. Cigarette smoking is associated with abnormal histone-to-protamine transition in human sperm. Fertil Steril 2014;101(1):51−7.

[53] Hammadeh M, Hamad M, Montenarh M, Fischer-Hammadeh C. Protamine contents and P1/P2 ratio in human spermatozoa from smokers and non-smokers. Hum Reprod 2010;25(1):2708−20.

[54] Rajabi H, Mohseni-Kouchesfehani H, Eslami-Arshaghi T, Salehi M. Sperm DNA fragmentation affects epigenetic feature in human male pronucleus. Andrologia March 6, 2017. https://doi.org/10.1111/and.12800.

[55] Aktan G, Dogru-Abbasoglu S, Kucukgergin C, Kadioglu A, Ozdemirler-Erata G, Kocak-Toker N. Mystery of idiopathic male infertility: is oxidative stress an actual risk? Fertil Steril 2013;99(5):1211−5.

[56] Tartibian B, Maleki B. Correlation between seminal oxidative stress biomarkers and antioxidants with sperm DNA damage in elite athletes and recreationally active men. Clin J Sports Med 2012;22(2):132−9.

[57] Tunc O, Tremellen K. Oxidative DNA damage impairs global sperm DNA methylation in infertile men. J Assist Reprod Genet 2009;26(9−10):537−44.

[58] Monks T, Xie R, Tikoo K, Lau S. ROS-induced histone modifications and their role in cell survival and cell death. Drug Metab Rev 2006;38(4):755−67.

[59] Faure AK, Pivot-Pajot C, Kerjean A, Hazzouri M, Pelletier R, Peoc'h M, et al. Misregulation of histone acetylation in sertoli-cell only syndrome and testicular cancer. Mol Hum Reprod 2003;9(12):757−63.

[60] Pina-Guzman B, Solis-Heredia MJ, Quintanilla-Vega B. Diazinon alters sperm chromatin structure in mice by phosphorylating nuclear protamines. Toxicol Appl Pharmacol 2005;202(2):189−98.

Chapter 4.2

Transcriptomics and Oxidative Stress in Male Infertility

Sezgin Gunes and Asli M. Mahmutoglu

Ondokuz Mayis University, Samsun, Turkey

INTRODUCTION

Infertility is the inability to conceive a baby despite regular and unprotected intercourse for a year and affects 8%–12% of couples all around the world [1,2]. Male factor infertility represents nearly half of this reproductive problem [3] and originates from different reasons including congenital abnormalities, sexual dysfunction, genetic causes, testicular damage, hypogonadism, oncological diseases, and reproductive tract obstruction [4]. However, the known reasons are inadequate to clarify the underlying mechanisms of idiopathic infertility that comprises 30%–40% of male factor infertility [5]. Oxidative stress (OS) has been proposed to be responsible for idiopathic male infertility [6,7]. OS is a condition that arises when the antioxidant scavenging system of the cell does not overwhelm the high level of reactive oxygen species (ROS) [8]. Low levels of ROS are indispensable for certain physiological processes; some of these processes are stimulated by ezrin protein and nuclear factor kappa B (NF-κB) transcription factor induced by ROS [8,9]. However, overproduction of ROS gives rise to lipid peroxidation and DNA damage in spermatozoa [10]. Although, OS is one of the pathological mechanisms of male infertility [11] and even in idiopathic infertility, the underlying molecular mechanism of the pathology due to OS is not clear [6]. Conventional semen analysis includes the analysis of physical characteristics of semen [12] and substantial diagnostic methods (e.g., invasive methods) of male factor infertility are frequently insufficient to characterize of male reproductive potential. Recent advancements in reproductive sciences based on the omic technologies, namely, transcriptomics, proteomics, and metabolomics, are projected as better evaluators of both diagnosis and treatment of male infertility [13].

Transcriptomic analysis allows the characterization of testis tissue, epididymis, and sperm transcriptome profiles of fertile, infertile, and/or fertile versus infertile men in a variety of model and nonmodel animals [14–21]. Sperm transcriptome provides novel markers for the regulation of spermatogenesis, which comprises expression of multiple genes sequentially and regularly [22,23]. OS-induced gene expression changes have also been revealed by transcriptomic approaches [24,25]. Despite the presence of relatively advanced molecular techniques and knowledge about the role of OS in idiopathic male infertility, a limited number of studies investigating the association between gene expression changes and OS related with male infertility has been published thus far [26–28].

In this chapter, the main focus is on differential gene expression profiles of testis, spermatozoa, and epididymides in infertile men studied via transcriptomic approaches. It proceeds with an overview of the methods, especially the most preferred ones, used in the transcriptomic analysis. Moreover, this chapter highlights the OS-induced transcriptomic alterations in testis, spermatozoa, and epididymis in male infertility.

METHODS USED IN TRANSCRIPTOMIC ANALYSES

The transcriptome encompasses the gene expression at RNA level [29]. To date, transcript quantification has been performed by various techniques such as Northern blot, reverse transcription polymerase chain reaction (RT-PCR), reverse transcription quantitative real-time PCR (RT-qPCR), serial analysis of gene expression (SAGE), microarray, and RNA-Seq

[30,31]. Throughput levels of Northern blot, RT-PCR, and RT-qPCR techniques are lower than microarray and RNA-Seq techniques as they allow measurement of a limited number of transcripts at a time [32]. Since high throughput techniques are the preferred ones, we document the microarray and RNA-Seq methods in detail.

Microarray Technique

Microarray analysis is based on the molecular hybridization between probe and target that is a nucleotide sequence (e.g., cDNA, cRNA) on a solid substrate [33–35]. Microarray technique enables detection of the expression levels of numerous genes simultaneously [36], under certain biological processes, physiological conditions, and/or disease states [12]. This method also gives an opportunity to discover new tools for diagnosis of male infertility [37].

Microarray technique includes several steps. The first step is RNA extraction, which is an essential step for all transcriptomic analysis [30]. The quality of RNA obtained from isolation process is one of the key factors for successful microarray profiling [18]. Following the RNA isolation, if RNA quantity is not enough for the study or researchers want to decrease the cost, mRNA pooling can be done or the quantity of DNA may be increased by PCR amplification [38]. The second step is synthesis and labeling of cDNA. Extracted RNA is reverse-transcribed into cDNA, and then cDNA is labeled with fluorescent dyes [39]. In the hybridization step, probes attached to a glass slide are hybridized to the targets that are labeled fluorescently [35]. Washing process allows the removal of unhybridized molecules from the slide, and transcripts are scanned with a laser [39], and specific software interprets the intensity of the fluorescence signal based on the hybridization level of probe and target [35]. Ultimately, microarray analysis gives expression changes of multiple genes and these are interpreted via bioinformatics tools [12]. The expression of certain genes is mostly validated by RT-qPCR [34].

Microarray technique has several limitations as well as advantages including requirement of a reference transcript for probe construction and limited sequence resolution [30]. Researchers have started to choose the RNA-Seq method due to certain advantages over microarray technique [31].

RNA Sequencing

The importance of whole transcriptome analysis in the understanding of the structure and function of the genome, the identification of biomarkers of diseases, and the clarifying of genetic regulatory networks related to various cellular, biological, and physiological processes cannot be ignored [40]. RNA-Seq technique (also known as cDNA sequencing and RNA deep sequencing) makes possible whole-transcriptome analysis by using next-generation sequencing [41,42]. This method enables the quantification of gene expression levels; precisely, the identification of 5′ and 3′ ends, exon/intron boundaries, transcription start sites, splicing variants of genes, the identification of single nucleotide polymorphisms, and other populations of RNA such as tRNA, rRNA, and miRNA. In addition to these, the analysis provides data about the transcriptional structure, which has an impact on cellular localization, splicing, and RNA's translation and turnover [43–45].

The standard RNA-Seq method involves several steps including RNA isolation, cDNA synthesis, library construction, sequencing, and data analysis; however, some of the steps can differ according to sequencing platforms (e.g., Roche 454, PacBio, SOLiD, Illumina, Ion Torrent, Helicos, and Complete genomics) [46]. RNA extraction is the first step in RNA-Seq experiments [47]. Following RNA extraction, rRNAs constituting approximately 9 out of 10 of the total RNA in the cell are removed by one of two methods, poly(A) selection or rRNA depletion methods [48]. Poly(A)+ RNA selection can be performed by capturing either cellulose membranes/columns or magnetic beads that are coated with oligo-dT molecules. This can be also done by the oligo-dT priming method, but it introduces 3′ bias [46,47]. rRNA can be depleted by different approaches including using sequence-specific probes and specific (namely Ovation RNA-Seq), probe-directed degradation and C_0T-hybridization methods. In eukaryotic cells, the most preferred technique is oligo-dT bead-based purification of poly(A)+ RNA being cost-effective and user-friendly [47]. The next step after RNA depletion or poly(A) selection is fragmentation that can be also performed after cDNA synthesis. The large part of the sequencing platforms has size limitations; therefore, RNAs need to be fragmented. Fragmentation can be achieved by enzymes, divalent cations, and alkali solutions [31,44,47]. Depending on the sequencing platforms instead of RNAs, double-stranded cDNAs can also be fragmented by enzymes called DNases [44,47]. Fragmented or nonfragmented RNAs are reverse-transcribed into cDNA with oligo-dT or random hexamer primers. cDNAs are then ligated to adapters for amplification (8–12 cycles) and sequencing [44,46,47]. Sequencing can be done in single-end (one direction) or paired-end (both direction) when transcripts are ready. One-direction sequencing for transcripts quantification is fast and cheap, while both-direction sequencing provides stable products (alignment and/or assemblies) and is suitable for discovering transcript isoforms and gene annotation [30].

RNA-Seq analysis generates a wide range of raw sequence reads comprising fluorescence signals. These signals need to be transformed into base sequences, and each base in the sequence needs to be controlled for quality via calculation of a quality score [49]. Quality control, which is an essential step in data analysis of RNA-Seq [50], is performed by analysis of guanine-cytosine content, high duplication read reflecting sequencing errors, over representation of k-mers (sequence is relatively shorter than length of reads), and the existence of adaptors [48,51]. Analysis of transcript sequences can be done onto either a reference genome or a de novo assembly of RNA-Seq, which is an applicable option in the absence of reference genome [30,51]. RNA-Seq presents various options to researchers; however, it has certain challenges such as methodological challenges including transcriptome composition, length, and fragmentation bias [40].

Several RNA-Seq methods are available for transcriptomic analysis [47]. In one study, RNA-Seq methods have been compared in sperm. Generally, human spermatozoal RNAs are known to have partial or high fragmentation and low quantity, causing difficulty in RNA-Seq but this feature makes sperm a good candidate to compare the sequencing methods. Sixteen libraries were prepared by using RNA that is extracted from human spermatozoa with different commercial RNA-Seq library amplification protocols. No differences in RNA profiling have been reported relating to the quantity of input RNA and the RNA purification step option in the study [52].

TRANSCRIPTOMICS AND MALE INFERTILITY

In mammals, the mature spermatozoa include a heterogeneous population of RNAs that are suggested to be components of the nuclear matrix, and located in the various parts of the head and the tail region. The abundance of spermatozoal RNAs varies from species to species, and their quantity in human spermatozoa is about 10−400 fg [53−55]. It is well known that spermatozoa take part in fertilization and embryo development via transmitting a unique suite of paternal RNAs (mRNA, miRNA, etc.) to the oocyte [43]. The identification of different types and functions of spermatozoal RNAs has been revealed in humans and various animals using advanced genomic approaches such as transcriptomic analysis [56,57].

The transcriptome is defined as the full set of coding and noncoding RNAs, which are transcribed at a specific developmental stage and/or are present at various physiological conditions within a cell type or tissue. Transcriptomics involves the study of all transcripts and provides information about gene structure and function for clarifying molecular mechanism of a biological process [29] and/or disease [37]. Transcriptomic analysis of testis, epididymis, and spermatozoa in humans, mice, bovines, chickens, cattle, yaks, and stallions in relation to male fertility and/or infertility have been reported [26,57−63]. Transcriptomic studies of male factor infertility in humans are summarized in Table 1. The mRNA contents of human spermatozoa have been reported to be a genetic fingerprint for a specific individual's ejaculate [64]. In proven fertile men, mRNA profiles of spermatozoa have been found to be concordant with those of testis, suggesting that fertile men had an mRNA fingerprint in their spermatozoa that represents a historical record of gene expression during spermatogenesis. Gene ontology (GO) analysis of these mRNAs has verified the functions of spermatozoal RNAs in early embryo development [65]. Over the last decade, studies investigating the associations between transcriptomics and male factor infertility have increased in parallel with advances in transcriptomic approaches [14,66−68].

A prospective study was performed to discover new downregulated genes in the testicular tissue of infertile men with Sertoli cell−only syndrome (SCOS) or maturation arrest (MA) and normal spermatogenesis by using microarray technique. They have reported downregulation in the expression of 300 genes, and of these genes, 10 were found to be related to infertility [69]. Differences in the mRNA expression profiles of spermatozoa between idiopathic infertile and proven fertile men have been notified and 136 genes related to infertility were reported to be underexpressed [70]. Teratozoospermic individuals have demonstrated the near-absence of proteosomal RNAs involved in the major cellular system, ubiquitin proteasome pathway, resulting in failure in spermatogenesis. Remarkably, Platts and colleagues showed that the proteasomal transcripts were underrepresented; however, the ubiquitin transcripts' fingerprints were disrupted in the teratozoospermic group compared to fertile controls. RNA transcripts corresponding to the proteasomal proteins mapped in Kyoto Encyclopedia of Genes and Genomes (KEGG) were found to be disrupted more than fivefold and as high as 21-fold in teratozoospermia. In the same study, alterations in the ratio of constitutive and inducible proteasomal core subunits of inducible PSMB1, PSMB5, and PSMB7 relative to PSMB8, PSMB9, and PSMB10 were investigated. The ratios of the normozoospermic and teratozoospermic groups were 2:1 and 3:1, respectively. The authors have also argued that the reduction of proteasomal mRNA transcripts may prevent morphogenesis of spermatozoa by inhibiting the positioning of the acrosomal cap, nuclear condensation of spermatozoa, and maturation of sperm tail and midpiece [71].

RNA contents of sperm cells from four asthenozoospermic infertile men were compared with those from four normozoospermic fertile controls [72]. In the asthenozoospermic group, alterations in the abundance of RNA transcripts were detected, and five of them (*OAZ3*, *ANXA2*, *BRD2*, *mtND2*, and *mtNB3*) were employed for validation of expression profile by real-time PCR. The expression of *OAZ3*, *ANXA2*, and *BRD2* genes has been proposed to be significantly associated with

TABLE 1 Transcriptomic Studies on Male Fertility and/or Infertility in Humans

Study Participants	Source(s)	Method	Result(s)	References
• Normozoospermic • Azoospermic men	Spermatozoa	RT-PCR	Sperm transcript was a fingerprint for specific individual's ejaculate.	[64]
• Fertile men	Spermatozoa Testis	Microarray	Fertile men had unique mRNA contents in their spermatozoa.	[65]
• Fertile • Infertile men	Spermatozoa	SAGE	Infertile men presented approximately 3000 unique tags.	[96]
• Patients with normal spermatogenesis • Patients with MA and SCOS	Testis	Microarray	300 genes were differentially expressed in infertile men with SCOS or MA represented. Ten novel genes were found to be infertility related.	[69]
• Fertile men • Teratozoospermic patients	Spermatozoa	Microarray	Transcriptional alterations were found in infertile men.	[71]
• Patients with cryptorchidism controls	Spermatozoa	Microarray	Thirty-eight genes were downregulated in men with cryptorchidism compared to controls.	[19]
• Proven fertile men • Infertile patients	Spermatozoa	Microarray	Expression of hundreds of genes was different from that of fertile men.	[70]
• Patients with nonobstructive azoospermia • Normal controls	Testis	Microarray	miRNAs involved in the regulation of spermatogenesis.	[97]
• Oligozoospermic patients with AZFc deletion • Idiopathic infertile men	Testis	Microarray	The absence of DAZ gene expression might induce certain cellular mechanisms.	[98]
• Patients who achieved a pregnancy by IUI • Patients who did not achieve a pregnancy by IUI	Spermatozoa	Microarray	The expression of 741 exclusive transcripts (ESTs) was only detected in spermatozoa of patients with achieved pregnancy.	[99]
• Patients who achieved a pregnancy with fresh or frozen spermatozoa • Patients who did not achieve a pregnancy with fresh or frozen spermatozoa	Spermatozoa	Microarray	A wide range of mRNA transcripts were differentially expressed in men with achieved pregnancy.	[75]
• Fertile men • Asthenozoospermic men	Spermatozoa	Microarray	Asthenozoospermic men showed differences in gene expression compared to fertile men.	[72]
• Fertile men • Oligozoospermic patients	Spermatozoa	Microarray	Transcriptome profile of spermatozoa was not similar to that of fertile men.	[73]

Patients/Groups	Sample	Technique	Finding	Ref.
Healthy men Infertile men	Semen	Microarray	Fifty-two miRNAs expression was found to be specific to abnormal semen of infertile males.	[100]
Proven fertile men Asthenozoospermic men Idiopathic infertile men	Spermatozoa	Microarray	Over 2000 transcripts were different between three groups.	[14]
Azoospermic men with nonmosaic KS Controls	Testis	Microarray	KS patients showed 903 differentially expressed transcripts expressed by somatic cells of testis.	[74]
Patients with obstructive azoospermia	Testis	RNA-Seq	Gene ontology analysis has revealed differentially expressed genes involved in the regulation of spermatogenesis.	[101]
Men with globozoospermia Men with obstructive azoospermia	Testis	RT-PCR	Downregulation of KIFC1 gene was found in the testis of globozoospermia.	[102]
Patients with hypospermatogenesis Patients with hypospermatogenesis and AZFc deletion Patients with SCOS Patients with MA Men with normal spermatogenesis	Testis	Microarray	Deregulation of specific miRNAs was detected in all groups except patients with hypospermatogenesis group.	[68]
Azoospermic patients with KS Controls	Testis	Microarray	Patient with KS represented 1050 differentially expressed transcripts.	[66]
Patients with spermatogonial arrest Patients with normal spermatogenesis	Spermatogonia	RNA-Seq (single-cell expression analysis)	Heterogeneity was revealed among the cells by single-cell expression analysis.	[67]

IUI, intrauterine insemination; KS, Klinefelter syndrome; MA, maturation arrest; RT-PCR, reverse transcription polymerase chain reaction; SAGE, serial analysis of gene expression; SCOS, Sertoli cell-only syndrome.

progressive motility [72]. The expression of genes involved in motility and spermatogenesis has decreased almost 33-fold in oligozoospermic men compared with their normozoospermic controls. OS regulation (e.g., *PARK7*) and DNA repair genes (e.g., *NIPBL*) were indicated to be some of them. In the same study, Montjean and colleagues demonstrated up to 42.96-fold decrease in the expression of genes associated with spermatogenesis, motility, and antiapoptotic process of germ cells (CREM, MEA-1, PRM2, SPATA-4, SPZ-1). Additionally, a striking drop (up to 29-fold) in histone modification genes expression (DDX3X, JMJD1A) was observed. DNA methylation and noncoding RNAs are important regulators of transcription, therefore these regulators may alter the gene expression in developing spermatozoa leading to decline in sperm count [73]. Microarray analysis of spermatozoal RNAs from normozoospermic infertile (n = 20), asthenozoospermic (n = 20) and fertile men (n = 20) have revealed differences in gene expression. Of the total of 2081 differentially expressed transcripts, some are suggested to be specific to asthenozoospermic patients (e.g., *RPS16, GDI2, PARK7 RPS24*), while others are specific to normozoospermic males (e.g., *CAPNS1, RPL19, SMNDC1*) [14]. A transcriptomic approach has identified a molecular mechanism leading to testis degeneration in Klinefelter syndrome (KS), and the data found that 903 transcripts demonstrated significantly altered expression profiles in testis of nonmosaic KS patients versus controls. While 247 of these transcripts were downregulated, 656 were upregulated, and many of them were expressed by somatic cells of the testis [74].

The majority of upregulated genes were involved in the apoptosis of testicular cells; however, downregulated transcripts were associated with failure of spermiogenesis and morphological abnormalities The majority of upregulated genes were involved in the apoptosis of testicular cells; however, downregulated transcripts were associated with failure of spermiogenesis and morphological abnormalities [66]. Garcia-Herrero and colleagues compared the mRNA profile of spermatozoa that achieved pregnancy by intracytoplasmic sperm injection (ICSI) with those that failed to do so and reported a large number of differentially expressed transcripts [75]. In the most recent study, transcriptomic profiling of preimplantation bovine embryos was suggested to be affected by male infertility status. Although the exact mechanism causing this situation is not known yet, it is thought that DNA methylation might be responsible for it [60].

TRANSCRIPTOMIC STUDIES ON MALE INFERTILITY AND OXIDATIVE STRESS

Significant variation in whole cell/tissue transcriptome is reported in different model systems from yeast to mammals. Transcriptome analysis of taf25-3 mutant strain of *Saccharomyces cerevisiae* has revealed differential gene expression levels in the existence of OS as compared to the pZHW4 control strain by using RNA-Seq analysis [25]. Taf25-3 mutant strain generated by the global transcription machinery engineering approach has increased tolerance of H_2O_2-induced OS [76]. OS has caused changes in a total 1006 transcript expressions, of which 336 were downregulated and 670 upregulated, while an absence of OS differential expression of 1023 genes in taf25-3 strain was reported. According to GO and KEGG pathway enrichment analysis of 10 million clean reads in the study, the most enriched signaling or metabolic pathways were reported to be carbohydrate metabolism; fatty acid degradation; glycolysis/gluconeogenesis; and glutamate, alanine, and aspartate metabolism [25]. Glutathione (GSH) is synthesized from glycine, cysteine, and glutamate amino acids catalyzed by gamma-glutamylcysteine (GCS) and GSH synthetase enzymes and is involved in the cell proliferation and OS defense.

Cell proliferation and the expression of genes involved in OS defense have been regulated by AP1, a transcription factor consisting of c-fos and c-jun proteins. Tertiary-butyl hydroperoxide (THBP)-induced OS has been reported to cause upregulation of c-jun and c-fos transcripts in testis [77]. In mouse testis, OS has also given rise to expression changes in certain miRNAs, miR122, miR-34a, and miR181b taking part in the spermatogenesis arrest, antioxidant responses, and inflammation pathway [78]. Syed and Hecht conducted a research to identify the molecular mechanism of testicular lesions in meiotic prophase cells. Degeneration of pachytene spermatocytes is characteristic of a testicular lesion. In the study, pachytene spermatocytes were cultured with 2-methoxyethanol or methoxyacetic acid to induce testicular lesions. Exposure to these chemicals resulted in overregulation of genes induced by OS in Sertoli cells as compared to controls [79]. Although a large number of reports document OS-induced alteration of transcriptome in cells and tissue of various organisms, there is paucity of information on direct effects of OS of human sperm transcriptome.

Antioxidant protection is essential for eliminating the negative effects of ROS-induced OS during the embryo implantation, in testis and epididymis, since spermatozoa are highly vulnerable to ROS by virtue of the high levels of polyunsaturated fatty acids in their plasma membrane. Spermatozoon, testis, and epididymis have a variety of enzymatic and nonenzymatic antioxidants including superoxide dismutase (SOD), extracellular SOD (EC-SOD), phospholipid hydroperoxide GPx (PHGPx), catalase (CAT), alpha-tocopherol, thiols, glutathione peroxidase (GPX), and GSH reductase [80,81]. The presence of antioxidant enzymes in rat epididymis was revealed by using Northern blot analysis. Expression of SOD, GPX, CAT, and PHGPX mRNAs were detected in all regions of the epididymis; however, EC-SOD and EC-GPx were detected only in certain regions of the epididymis, in corpus and caput, respectively [82]. The intracellular level of GPX depends on the activation of gamma-glutamyl transpeptidase (GGT) enzyme taking part in the synthesis of GSH.

Xanthine oxidase (ROS-generating agent) has been suggested to induce OS resulting in GGT mRNA expression level in the initial segment of rat epididymis [83]. The expression of genes encoding antioxidant enzymes has showed variations among epididymal and testicular tissues in bison. For instance, CAT transcripts were abundantly found in the caput and cauda epididymis, whereas PHGPx transcripts were mostly represented in bison testis [84]. p53-target genes play a role in OS responses in different cells and tissues. Microarray analysis of gene expression has demonstrated that long-term OS induced by diquat gave rise to a significant increase in the expression profile of thiol antioxidant genes such as *Gclc*, *Mt1*, *Txnrd*, and *Srxn1* in Sod1$^{-/-}$ mice. The ablation of *Sod1* and *Gpx1* gene in the Sod1$^{-/-}$ and Gpx1$^{-/-}$ mice resulted in sensitivity to OS. Induction of p53-target genes (e.g., *Gadd45a*, *Trp53inp1*, *Plk3*, *Ndrg1*) has been proposed to lead a common response to endo- and exogenous (ablation of Sod1 and Gpx1 gene, and diquat treatment, respectively) OS. Activation of these genes as a response to OS is known to be protected among different cells, organs, and species [24]. In testicular tissues of rats with varicocele, ROS resulted from long-term hypoxia have induced upregulation of p53 protein, and this caused testicular hypofunction, ultimately resulting in male infertility [85].

Monticone and colleagues have implied that the highest level of mitochondrial fission regulator (Mtfr1) transcripts was found in testis of wild type mouse. *Mtfr1* gene encodes a mitochondrial protein. Researchers have conducted their studies by using Mtfr1-deficient mice to comprehend the function of the *Mtfr1* gene. Decreases in the expression levels of ROS scavenging genes due to failure in the *Mtfr1* gene expression have been reported by using DNA array analysis. *Mtfr1* has been suggested to be involved in the regulation of ROS scavenging genes in the male gonad [86].

Oligozoospermic infertile men displayed unique transcriptomic profiles in their spermatozoa as compared to fertile controls, and a substantial reduction was reported in the expression of genes involved in OS regulation such as *PARK7* (*DJ1*) [73]. A high level of ROS has also been detected in infertile men with oligozoospermia [87]. In this case, high levels of ROS can be one of the plausible reasons for transcriptomic changes in oligozoospermic infertile men.

Microarray analysis of testis transcriptome in a model organism, zebrafish, has demonstrated that 2,3,7,8-tetrachlorodibenzodioxin (TCDD) caused alterations in the transcript expressions that took part in steroidogenesis, cell morphology, hormone metabolism, molecular transport, testis development, lipid metabolism, and xenobiotic response. TCDD is a toxic endocrine-disrupting chemical and is associated with decreased reproductive capacity and induction of OS in testis. *ca2*, *apobb*, and *abcc2* genes have been reported to be involved in tissue defense and xenobiotic-response pathways, and relatively high expression levels of *abcc2* (<60-fold) and *apobb* (<35-fold) genes were found in testis. Decreased expression level of the *nudt15* xenobiotic-responsive gene has been suggested to be a factor in TCDD-induced pathology. *nudt15* plays a role in the protection against oxygen radicals and translational errors. In the same organism, increased expression of *ugt5g* and *ugta1* genes, involved in cellular fate, cell cycle, and OS pathways and response were observed [88].

Heat stress may induce ROS production from different structures and organelles including cytoplasm, peroxisomes, and mitochondrial membranes resulting in OS [89]. Heat stress has been reported to cause a significant increase in the expression of mRNAs of GPX1 and GST antioxidant genes [90]. Heat shock proteins play a vital role in spermatogenesis and the defenses against heat, chemicals, and radiation. DNA microarray analysis (pooling mRNA) demonstrated that of 2208 differentially expressed genes, 151 genes were underexpressed and 27 genes were overexpressed in response to heat shock [91]. GO analysis has revealed that 7 of these 27 genes with high expression profiles were regulators and effectors of stress response, namely, Hsp25, Hsp40, and Hsp60, while the constitutive high expression of testicular Hsp86 was underexpressed in response to hyperthermia. Furthermore, genes involved in apoptosis (*CDC25a*, *Bak1*, *Bax*, procaspase 2), DNA repair (*RAD23*, *ERRCC5*), and OS metabolism (*SOD2*, *SOD3*, glutathione reductase 1) were up- or down-regulated at the mRNA level in response to heat shock [91]. Hsp72 is one of the heat-shock proteins that are involved in the protection against apoptosis and OS. In bovine Sertoli cells, puerarin (Chinese herbal medicine with an impact on the reducing oxidative damage) treatment suppressed the increase in Hsp72 expression and ROS production via attenuation of apoptosis as well as oxidative damage resulting from heat stress [92].

OS plays a fundamental role in the pathophysiology of varicocele-associated male infertility [93]. OS has been proposed to cause testicular damage in varicocele via ROS generation resulting from toxic adrenal and renal metabolites, hypoxia, and heat. Exposure to stressful cellular factors including OS, heat, and hypoxia might cause apoptosis [94]. The association of seminal miRNAs with OS and apoptotic markers in a cohort consisting of fertile and infertile men (n = 220) was investigated in four groups. The groups consisted of fertile men (n = 52), fertile men with varicocele (n = 43), oligoasthenoteratozoospermic (OAT) men without varicocele (n = 62), and OAT men with varicocele (n = 63). The level of OS markers (malondialdehyde [MDA] and GPX) and protein expression level of seminal apoptotic markers (BAX and BCL2) were evaluated. Expression of seminal miRNAs, miRNA-34c5, miRNA-122, and miRNA-181a were analyzed by qRT-PCR. The lowest level of miRNA-34c5, miRNA-122, and miRNA-181a were detected in OAT men with varicocele as compared to three other groups—varicocele, grade, and bilaterality. A positive correlation between seminal miRNAs and sperm concentration, motility, and morphology was found. However, seminal MDA and protein expression of BAX were found to be negatively associated with BCL2 level [28].

Elevations in the generation of ROS can be stimulated by the absence of prohibitin (PHB) proteins in somatic cells. PHB is an evolutionarily conserved protein in the mitochondrial membrane of sperm and consists of PHB1 and PHB2 homologous subunits. Expression of PHB proteins was suggested to cause an increase in the ROS level and an alteration in the mitochondrial membrane potential in infertile men, therefore it might promote sperm motility [95]. A study was performed to characterize the location and expression of PHB proteins in male reproductive systems of rat and human. In addition, the role of these proteins during OS response has also been investigated. PHB1 and PHB2 expression were detected in different human tissues including heart, liver, muscle, lung, spleen, testis, and epididymis using semi-quantitative RT-PCR. However, the highest expression levels of PHB1 and PHB2 were found in epididymis and limited expression levels were reported in testis. Immunohistochemical analysis revealed that PHB1 and PHB2 localized in the cytoplasm of all cell types in human testis and epididymis, and that PHB1 localized on the entire tail region of spermatozoa whereas PHB2 localized on the equatorial region of spermatozoa. Interestingly, doxorubicin-stimulated (3 mg/kg) OS caused a decrease in mRNA and protein expression levels in testis and no change was reported in the epididymis of rat [27].

CONCLUSIONS

In this chapter, we summarized the studies investigating the associations between OS and/or male infertility by using transcriptomic analysis. All of these studies have clearly indicated that both OS and male factor infertility have caused transcriptomic changes. However, more studies are needed to clarify the association between OS-induced transcriptomic alterations in spermatozoa of infertile men. The combination of transcriptomic, proteomic, and metabolomic approaches can also be useful to identify this correlation.

GLOSSARY

Gene expression The process by which information from a gene is used in the synthesis of a functional gene product.
Gene ontology (GO) Structured, controlled vocabularies and classifications of gene function across species and research areas.
Microarray A multiplex array of oligonucleotides used for high-throughput screening of transcript abundance.
Noncoding RNA Functional RNA molecule that is transcribed, but not translated into a protein.
Transcript An RNA molecule copied (transcribed) from a DNA template.
Transcriptome Complete set of all RNA molecules transcribed from a DNA template.

LIST OF ACRONYMS AND ABBREVIATIONS

CAT Catalase
EC-SOD Extracellular SOD
GCS Gamma-glutamylcysteine
GO Gene ontology
GPX Glutathione peroxidase
GR Glutathione reductase
GSH Glutathione
H₂O₂ Hydrogen peroxide
HOCL Hypochlorous acid
ICSI Intracytoplasmic sperm injection
IUI Intrauterine insemination
KEGG Kyoto Encyclopedia of Genes and Genomes
KS Klinefelter syndrome
LOO Lipid peroxyl
LOOH Lipid peroxide
MA Maturation arrest
Mtfr1 Mitochondrial fission regulator
NF-κB Nuclear factor kappa B
NO Nitric oxide

NSP Not-so-random primers

O$_2^-$ Superoxide ion

O$_3$ Ozone

OAT Oligoasthenoteratozoospermic

OH$^-$ Hydroxyl ion

PHB Prohibitin

PHGPx Phospholipid hydroperoxide glutathione peroxidase

ROS Reactive oxygen species

RT-PCR Reverse transcription polymerase chain reaction

RT-qPCR Quantitative real-time PCR

SAGE Serial analysis of gene expression

SCOS Sertoli cell-only syndrome

SOD Superoxide dismutase

TCDD 2,3,7,8-tetrachlorodibenzodioxin

THBP Tertiary-butyl hydroperoxide

REFERENCES

[1] Inhorn MC, Patrizio P. Infertility around the globe: new thinking on gender, reproductive technologies and global movements in the 21st century. Hum Reprod Update 2015;21(4):411−26.

[2] Sharlip ID, Jarow JP, Belker AM, Lipshultz LI, Sigman M, Thomas AJ, et al. Best practice policies for male infertility. Fertil Steril 2002;77(5):873−82.

[3] Neto FT, Bach PV, Najari BB, Li PS, Goldstein M. Genetics of male infertility. Curr Urol Rep 2016;17(10):70.

[4] Punab M, Poolamets O, Paju P, Vihljajev V, Pomm K, Ladva R, et al. Causes of male infertility: a 9-year prospective monocentre study on 1737 patients with reduced total sperm counts. Hum Reprod 2017;32(1):18−31.

[5] Turchi P. Prevalence, definition, and classification of infertility. In: Clinical management of male infertility. Springer; 2015. p. 5−11.

[6] Aktan G, Dogru-Abbasoglu S, Kucukgergin C, Kadioglu A, Ozdemirler-Erata G, Kocak-Toker N. Mystery of idiopathic male infertility: is oxidative stress an actual risk? Fertil Steril 2013;99(5):1211−5.

[7] Mayorga-Torres BJM, Camargo M, Cadavid AP, du Plessis SS, Cardona Maya WD. Are oxidative stress markers associated with unexplained male infertility? Andrologia 2017;49(5).

[8] Agarwal A, Virk G, Ong C, du Plessis SS. Effect of oxidative stress on male reproduction. World J Mens Health 2014;32(1):1−17.

[9] Bisht S, Faiq M, Tolahunase M, Dada R. Oxidative stress and male infertility. Nat Rev Urol 2017;14.

[10] Gharagozloo P, Aitken RJ. The role of sperm oxidative stress in male infertility and the significance of oral antioxidant therapy. Hum Reprod 2011;26(7):1628−40.

[11] Aitken RJ, Smith TB, Jobling MS, Baker MA, De Iuliis GN. Oxidative stress and male reproductive health. Asian J Androl 2014;16(1):31−8.

[12] Garrido N, Garcia-Herrero S, Meseguer M. Assessment of sperm using mRNA microarray technology. Fertil Steril 2013;99(4):1008−22.

[13] Kovac JR, Pastuszak AW, Lamb DJ. The use of genomics, proteomics, and metabolomics in identifying biomarkers of male infertility. Fertil Steril 2013;99(4):998−1007.

[14] Bansal SK, Gupta N, Sankhwar SN, Rajender S. Differential genes expression between fertile and infertile spermatozoa revealed by transcriptome analysis. PLoS One 2015;10(5):e0127007.

[15] Bissonnette N, Levesque-Sergerie JP, Thibault C, Boissonneault G. Spermatozoal transcriptome profiling for bull sperm motility: a potential tool to evaluate semen quality. Reproduction 2009;138(1):65−80.

[16] Chan WY, Lee TL, Wu SM, Ruszczyk L, Alba D, Baxendale V, et al. Transcriptome analyses of male germ cells with serial analysis of gene expression (SAGE). Mol Cell Endocrinol 2006;250(1−2):8−19.

[17] Das PJ, McCarthy F, Vishnoi M, Paria N, Gresham C, Li G, et al. Stallion sperm transcriptome comprises functionally coherent coding and regulatory RNAs as revealed by microarray analysis and RNA-seq. PLoS One 2013;8(2):e56535.

[18] El Fekih S, Nguyen MH, Perrin A, Beauvillard D, Morel F, Saad A, et al. Sperm RNA preparation for transcriptomic analysis: review of the techniques and personal experience. Andrologia 2017;49.

[19] Nguyen MT, Delaney DP, Kolon TF. Gene expression alterations in cryptorchid males using spermatozoal microarray analysis. Fertil Steril 2009;92(1):182−7.

[20] Sonenshine DE, Bissinger BW, Egekwu N, Donohue KV, Khalil SM, Roe RM. First transcriptome of the testis-vas deferens-male accessory gland and proteome of the spermatophore from *Dermacentor variabilis* (Acari: Ixodidae). PLoS One 2011;6(9):e24711.

[21] Xie S, Zhu Y, Ma L, Lu Y, Zhou J, Gui Y, et al. Genome-wide profiling of gene expression in the epididymis of alpha-chlorohydrin-induced infertile rats using an oligonucleotide microarray. Reprod Biol Endocrinol 2010;8:37.

[22] Carrell DT, Aston KI, Oliva R, Emery BR, De Jonge CJ. The "omics" of human male infertility: integrating big data in a systems biology approach. Cell Tissue Res 2016;363(1):295−312.

[23] Chalmel F, Rolland AD. Linking transcriptomics and proteomics in spermatogenesis. Reproduction 2015;150(5):R149−57.

[24] Han ES, Muller FL, Perez VI, Qi W, Liang H, Xi L, et al. The in vivo gene expression signature of oxidative stress. Physiol Genomics 2008;34(1):112−26.

[25] Zhao H, Chen J, Liu J, Han B. Transcriptome analysis reveals the oxidative stress response in *Saccharomyces cerevisiae*. RSC Adv 2015;5(29):22923—34.

[26] Lalancette C, Platts AE, Johnson GD, Emery BR, Carrell DT, Krawetz SA. Identification of human sperm transcripts as candidate markers of male fertility. J Mol Med (Berl) 2009;87(7):735—48.

[27] Li Y, Wang HY, Liu J, Li N, Wang YW, Wang WT, et al. Characterization of prohibitins in male reproductive system and their expression under oxidative stress. J Urol 2016;195(4 Pt 1):1160—7.

[28] Mostafa T, Rashed LA, Nabil NI, Osman I, Mostafa R, Farag M. Seminal miRNA relationship with apoptotic markers and oxidative stress in infertile men with varicocele. Biomed Res Int 2016;2016:4302754.

[29] Dong Z, Chen Y. Transcriptomics: advances and approaches. Sci China Life Sci 2013;56(10):960—7.

[30] Lowe R, Shirley N, Bleackley M, Dolan S, Shafee T. Transcriptomics technologies. PLoS Comput Biol 2017;13(5):e1005457.

[31] Malone JH, Oliver B. Microarrays, deep sequencing and the true measure of the transcriptome. BMC Biol 2011;9(1):34.

[32] Nonis A, De Nardi B, Nonis A. Choosing between RT-qPCR and RNA-seq: a back-of-the-envelope estimate towards the definition of the break-even-point. Anal Bioanal Chem 2014;406(15):3533—6.

[33] Bumgarner R. Overview of DNA microarrays: types, applications, and their future. Curr Protoc Mol Biol 2013;101. Chapter 22:Unit 22 1.

[34] Jaluria P, Konstantopoulos K, Betenbaugh M, Shiloach J. A perspective on microarrays: current applications, pitfalls, and potential uses. Microb Cell Fact 2007;6:4.

[35] Miura S, Himaki T, Takahashi J, Iwahashi H. The role of transcriptomics: physiological equivalence based on gene expression profiles. Rev Agric Sci 2017;5:21—35.

[36] Zhang W, Carriquiry A, Nettleton D, Dekkers JC. Pooling mRNA in microarray experiments and its effect on power. Bioinformatics 2007;23(10):1217—24.

[37] He Z, Chan W-Y, Dym M. Microarray technology offers a novel tool for the diagnosis and identification of therapeutic targets for male infertility. Reproduction 2006;132(1):11—9.

[38] Shih JH, Michalowska AM, Dobbin K, Ye Y, Qiu TH, Green JE. Effects of pooling mRNA in microarray class comparisons. Bioinformatics 2004;20(18):3318—25.

[39] Tarca AL, Romero R, Draghici S. Analysis of microarray experiments of gene expression profiling. Am J Obstet Gynecol 2006;195(2):373—88.

[40] Jiang Z, Zhou X, Li R, Michal JJ, Zhang S, Dodson MV, et al. Whole transcriptome analysis with sequencing: methods, challenges and potential solutions. Cell Mol Life Sci 2015;72(18):3425—39.

[41] Tang F, Barbacioru C, Wang Y, Nordman E, Lee C, Xu N, et al. mRNA-Seq whole-transcriptome analysis of a single cell. Nat Methods 2009;6(5):377—82.

[42] Zhang W, Yu Y, Hertwig F, Thierry-Mieg J, Zhang W, Thierry-Mieg D, et al. Comparison of RNA-seq and microarray-based models for clinical endpoint prediction. Genome Biol 2015;16:133.

[43] Ostermeier GC, Miller D, Huntriss JD, Diamond MP, Krawetz SA. Reproductive biology: delivering spermatozoan RNA to the oocyte. Nature 2004;429(6988):154.

[44] Nagalakshmi U, Waern K, Snyder M. RNA-Seq: a method for comprehensive transcriptome analysis. Curr Protoc Mol Biol 2010;89. Chapter 4:Unit 4 11 1-3.

[45] Wan Y, Kertesz M, Spitale RC, Segal E, Chang HY. Understanding the transcriptome through RNA structure. Nat Rev Genet 2011;12(9):641—55.

[46] Wolf JB. Principles of transcriptome analysis and gene expression quantification: an RNA-seq tutorial. Mol Ecol Resour 2013;13(4):559—72.

[47] Hrdlickova R, Toloue M, Tian B. RNA-Seq methods for transcriptome analysis. Wiley Interdiscip Rev RNA 2017;8(1).

[48] Conesa A, Madrigal P, Tarazona S, Gomez-Cabrero D, Cervera A, McPherson A, et al. A survey of best practices for RNA-seq data analysis. Genome Biol 2016;17:13.

[49] Mutz KO, Heilkenbrinker A, Lonne M, Walter JG, Stahl F. Transcriptome analysis using next-generation sequencing. Curr Opin Biotechnol 2013;24(1):22—30.

[50] Sheng Q, Vickers K, Zhao S, Wang J, Samuels DC, Koues O, et al. Multi-perspective quality control of Illumina RNA sequencing data analysis. Brief Funct Genomics 2017;16(4):194—204.

[51] Grabherr MG, Haas BJ, Yassour M, Levin JZ, Thompson DA, Amit I, et al. Full-length transcriptome assembly from RNA-Seq data without a reference genome. Nat Biotechnol 2011;29(7):644—52.

[52] Mao S, Sendler E, Goodrich RJ, Hauser R, Krawetz SA. A comparison of sperm RNA-seq methods. Syst Biol Reprod Med 2014;60(5):308—15.

[53] Hamatani T. Human spermatozoal RNAs. Fertil Steril 2012;97(2):275—81.

[54] Lalancette C, Miller D, Li Y, Krawetz SA. Paternal contributions: new functional insights for spermatozoal RNA. J Cell Biochem 2008;104(5):1570—9.

[55] Li C, Zhou X. Gene transcripts in spermatozoa: markers of male infertility. Clin Chim Acta 2012;413(13—14):1035—8.

[56] Krawetz SA, Kruger A, Lalancette C, Tagett R, Anton E, Draghici S, et al. A survey of small RNAs in human sperm. Hum Reprod 2011;26(12):3401—12.

[57] Singh R, Shafeeque C, Sharma S, Singh R, Mohan J, Sastry K, et al. Chicken sperm transcriptome profiling by microarray analysis. Genome 2015;59(3):185—96.

[58] Cai X, Yu S, Mipam T, Yang F, Zhao W, Liu W, et al. Comparative analysis of testis transcriptomes associated with male infertility in cattleyak. Theriogenology 2017;88:28—42.

[59] Karaouzène T, El Atifi M, Issartel J-P, Grepillat M, Coutton C, Martinez D, et al. Comparative testicular transcriptome of wild type and globozoospermic Dpy19l2 knock out mice. Basic Clin Androl 2013;23(1):7.

[60] Kropp J, Carrillo JA, Namous H, Daniels A, Salih SM, Song J, et al. Male fertility status is associated with DNA methylation signatures in sperm and transcriptomic profiles of bovine preimplantation embryos. BMC Genomics 2017;18(1):280.

[61] Legare C, Akintayo A, Blondin P, Calvo E, Sullivan R. Impact of male fertility status on the transcriptome of the bovine epididymis. Mol Hum Reprod 2017;23(6):355–69.

[62] Parthipan S, Selvaraju S, Somashekar L, Arangasamy A, Sivaram M, Ravindra JP. Spermatozoal transcripts expression levels are predictive of semen quality and conception rate in bulls (Bos taurus). Theriogenology 2017;98:41–9.

[63] Selvaraju S, Parthipan S, Somashekar L, Kolte AP, Krishnan Binsila B, Arangasamy A, et al. Occurrence and functional significance of the transcriptome in bovine (Bos taurus) spermatozoa. Sci Rep 2017;7:42392.

[64] Miller D, Tang P-Z, Skinner C, Lilford R. Differential RNA fingerprinting as a tool in the analysis of spermatozoal gene expression. Hum Reprod 1994;9(5):864–9.

[65] Ostermeier GC, Dix DJ, Miller D, Khatri P, Krawetz SA. Spermatozoal RNA profiles of normal fertile men. Lancet 2002;360(9335):772–7.

[66] D'Aurora M, Ferlin A, Garolla A, Franchi S, D'Onofrio L, Trubiani O, et al. Testis transcriptome modulation in Klinefelter patients with hypospermatogenesis. Sci Rep 2017;7:45729.

[67] Neuhaus N, Yoon J, Terwort N, Kliesch S, Seggewiss J, Huge A, et al. Single-cell gene expression analysis reveals diversity among human spermatogonia. Mol Hum Reprod 2017;23(2):79–90.

[68] Noveski P, Popovska-Jankovic K, Kubelka-Sabit K, Filipovski V, Lazarevski S, Plaseski T, et al. MicroRNA expression profiles in testicular biopsies of patients with impaired spermatogenesis. Andrology 2016;4(6):1020–7.

[69] Lin YH, Lin YM, Teng YN, Hsieh TY, Lin YS, Kuo PL. Identification of ten novel genes involved in human spermatogenesis by microarray analysis of testicular tissue. Fertil Steril 2006;86(6):1650–8.

[70] Garrido N, Martinez-Conejero JA, Jauregui J, Horcajadas JA, Simon C, Remohi J, et al. Microarray analysis in sperm from fertile and infertile men without basic sperm analysis abnormalities reveals a significantly different transcriptome. Fertil Steril 2009;91(4 Suppl.):1307–10.

[71] Platts AE, Dix DJ, Chemes HE, Thompson KE, Goodrich R, Rockett JC, et al. Success and failure in human spermatogenesis as revealed by teratozoospermic RNAs. Hum Mol Genet 2007;16(7):763–73.

[72] Jodar M, Kalko S, Castillo J, Ballesca JL, Oliva R. Differential RNAs in the sperm cells of asthenozoospermic patients. Hum Reprod 2012;27(5):1431–8.

[73] Montjean D, De La Grange P, Gentien D, Rapinat A, Belloc S, Cohen-Bacrie P, et al. Sperm transcriptome profiling in oligozoospermia. J Assist Reprod Genet 2012;29(1):3–10.

[74] D'Aurora M, Ferlin A, Di Nicola M, Garolla A, De Toni L, Franchi S, et al. Deregulation of sertoli and leydig cells function in patients with Klinefelter syndrome as evidenced by testis transcriptome analysis. BMC Genomics 2015;16:156.

[75] Garcia-Herrero S, Garrido N, Martinez-Conejero JA, Remohi J, Pellicer A, Meseguer M. Differential transcriptomic profile in spermatozoa achieving pregnancy or not via ICSI. Reprod Biomed Online 2011;22(1):25–36.

[76] Zhao H, Li J, Han B, Li X, Chen J. Improvement of oxidative stress tolerance in Saccharomyces cerevisiae through global transcription machinery engineering. J Ind Microbiol Biotechnol 2014;41(5):869–78.

[77] Kaur P, Kaur G, Bansal MP. Upregulation of AP1 by tertiary butyl hydroperoxide induced oxidative stress and subsequent effect on spermatogenesis in mice testis. Mol Cell Biochem 2008;308(1–2):177–81.

[78] Fatemi N, Sanati MH, Shamsara M, Moayer F, Zavarehei MJ, Pouya A, et al. TBHP-induced oxidative stress alters microRNAs expression in mouse testis. J Assist Reprod Genet 2014;31(10):1287–93.

[79] Syed V, Hecht NB. Rat pachytene spermatocytes down-regulate a polo-like kinase and up-regulate a thiol-specific antioxidant protein, whereas sertoli cells down-regulate a phosphodiesterase and up-regulate an oxidative stress protein after exposure to methoxyethanol and methoxyacetic acid. Endocrinology 1998;139(8):3503–11.

[80] Aitken RJ, Roman SD. Antioxidant systems and oxidative stress in the testes. Oxid Med Cell Longev 2008;1(1):15–24.

[81] Taylor CT. Antioxidants and reactive oxygen species in human fertility. Environ Toxicol Pharmacol 2001;10(4):189–98.

[82] Zini A, Schlegel PN. Identification and characterization of antioxidant enzyme mRNAs in the rat epididymis. Int J Androl 1997;20(2):86–91.

[83] Markey CM, Rudolph DB, Labus JC, Hinton BT. Oxidative stress differentially regulates the expression of gamma-glutamyl transpeptidase mRNAs in the initial segment of the rat epididymis. J Androl 1998;19(1):92–9.

[84] Koziorowska-Gilun M, Gilun P, Fraser L, Koziorowski M, Kordan W, Stefanczyk-Krzymowska S. Antioxidant enzyme activity and mRNA expression in reproductive tract of adult male European Bison (Bison bonasus, Linnaeus 1758). Reprod Domest Anim 2013;48(1):7–14.

[85] Liang M, Wen J, Dong Q, Zhao LG, Shi BK. Testicular hypofunction caused by activating p53 expression induced by reactive oxygen species in varicocele rats. Andrologia 2015;47(10):1175–82.

[86] Monticone M, Tonachini L, Tavella S, Degan P, Biticchi R, Palombi F, et al. Impaired expression of genes coding for reactive oxygen species scavenging enzymes in testes of Mtfr1/Chppr-deficient mice. Reproduction 2007;134(3):483–92.

[87] Agarwal A, Mulgund A, Sharma R, Sabanegh E. Mechanisms of oligozoospermia: an oxidative stress perspective. Syst Biol Reprod Med 2014;60(4):206–16.

[88] Baker BB, Yee JS, Meyer DN, Yang D, Baker TR. Histological and transcriptomic changes in male zebrafish testes due to early life exposure to low level 2,3,7,8-tetrachlorodibenzo-p-dioxin. Zebrafish 2016;13(5):413–23.

[89] Jensen CFS, Ostergren P, Dupree JM, Ohl DA, Sonksen J, Fode M. Varicocele and male infertility. Nat Rev Urol 2017;14.

[90] Paul C, Teng S, Saunders PT. A single, mild, transient scrotal heat stress causes hypoxia and oxidative stress in mouse testes, which induces germ cell death. Biol Reprod 2009;80(5):913–9.

[91] Rockett JC, Mapp FL, Garges JB, Luft JC, Mori C, Dix DJ. Effects of hyperthermia on spermatogenesis, apoptosis, gene expression, and fertility in adult male mice. Biol Reprod 2001;65(1):229–39.

[92] Cong X, Zhang Q, Li H, Jiang Z, Cao R, Gao S, et al. Puerarin ameliorates heat stress-induced oxidative damage and apoptosis in bovine Sertoli cells by suppressing ROS production and upregulating Hsp72 expression. Theriogenology 2017;88:215–27.

[93] Agarwal A, Prabakaran S, Allamaneni SS. Relationship between oxidative stress, varicocele and infertility: a meta-analysis. Reprod Biomed Online 2006;12(5):630–3.

[94] Agarwal A, Hamada A, Esteves SC. Insight into oxidative stress in varicocele-associated male infertility: part 1. Nat Rev Urol 2012;9(12):678–90.

[95] Wang MJ, Ou JX, Chen GW, Wu JP, Shi HJ, O WS, et al. Does prohibitin expression regulate sperm mitochondrial membrane potential, sperm motility, and male fertility? Antioxid Redox Signal 2012;17(3):513–9.

[96] Zhao Y, Li Q, Yao C, Wang Z, Zhou Y, Wang Y, et al. Characterization and quantification of mRNA transcripts in ejaculated spermatozoa of fertile men by serial analysis of gene expression. Hum Reprod 2006;21(6):1583–90.

[97] Lian J, Zhang X, Tian H, Liang N, Wang Y, Liang C, et al. Altered microRNA expression in patients with non-obstructive azoospermia. Reprod Biol Endocrinol 2009;7:13.

[98] Gatta V, Raicu F, Ferlin A, Antonucci I, Scioletti AP, Garolla A, et al. Testis transcriptome analysis in male infertility: new insight on the pathogenesis of oligo-azoospermia in cases with and without AZFc microdeletion. BMC Genomics 2010;11:401.

[99] Garcia-Herrero S, Meseguer M, Martinez-Conejero JA, Remohi J, Pellicer A, Garrido N. The transcriptome of spermatozoa used in homologous intrauterine insemination varies considerably between samples that achieve pregnancy and those that do not. Fertil Steril 2010;94(4):1360–73.

[100] Liu T, Cheng W, Gao Y, Wang H, Liu Z. Microarray analysis of microRNA expression patterns in the semen of infertile men with semen abnormalities. Mol Med Rep 2012;6(3):535–42.

[101] Zhu Z, Li C, Yang S, Tian R, Wang J, Yuan Q, et al. Dynamics of the transcriptome during human spermatogenesis: predicting the potential key genes regulating male gametes generation. Sci Rep 2016;6:19069.

[102] Zhi E, Li P, Chen H, Xu P, Zhu X, Zhu Z, et al. Decreased expression of KIFC1 in human testes with globozoospermic defects. Genes 2016;7(10).

FURTHER READING

[1] Gosalvez J, Tvrda E, Agarwal A. Free radical and superoxide reactivity detection in semen quality assessment: past, present, and future. J Assist Reprod Genet 2017;34(6):697–707.

Chapter 4.3

Oxidative Stress and Sperm Dysfunction: An Insight Into Dynamics of Semen Proteome

Jasmine Nayak, Soumya Ranjan Jena and Luna Samanta
Ravenshaw University, Cuttack, Odisha, India

INTRODUCTION

A steady decline in semen parameter had been observed for more than four decades; nonetheless, the mechanism(s) remain elusive [1]. In males with unexplained infertility, use of routine semen analysis to detect subcellular sperm dysfunctions is futile. Hence, a search for new diagnostic and prognostic sperm function biomarkers and their validation is required. Numerous pathways leading to defective sperm function are linked to reactive oxygen species (ROS), a group of molecules with incompletely reduced oxygen atoms [2,3] that virtually interact with all biomolecules, leading to their altered function.

Nature has bequeathed aerobic organisms with a range of antioxidant defense(s) to thwart the deleterious effects of ROS. However, when their rate of generation exceeds a cell's antioxidant defense, it leads to oxidative stress (OS). Being highly reactive, autocatalytic, and nonspecific, ROS qualify to be good signaling molecules. In all aerobic cells, physiological levels of ROS are essentially upheld [4]. Similarly, optimal sperm function in terms of capacitation, motility, and acrosome reaction is carried out by physiological levels of ROS. In contrast, their overproduction leads to defective sperm function and infertility [5,6]. Whereas both leukocyte and spermatozoa are primary sources of ROS in semen, the spermatozoa are more vulnerable to ROS-induced impairment due to high polyunsaturated fatty acid content and poor antioxidant capacity. More than six decades ago, the first report on detrimental effects of ROS on spermatozoa was published [7]. Subsequent studies established the concept that excessive ROS levels are associated with abnormal semen parameters and sperm function impairment leading to subfertility [2,8−12]. OS originating from diverse etiologies is attributed to be responsible for about two-thirds of the cases of male infertility [13], and seminal OS testing in infertility clinics is gaining acceptance [13,14].

Spermatozoa are essentially silent in terms of transcription and translation, yet the sperm proteome is dynamic and its profile varies from its site of production in the testes through epididymal maturation until the fertilization events. Therefore, studying the sperm proteome in general and with respect to ROS in particular is largely targeted for the discovery of biomarkers to address male factor infertility. This chapter focuses on the proteome profile of spermatozoa under different conditions of male infertility having oxidative predominance as well as oxidatively modified proteins involved in sperm function.

PROTEOMICS: THE TOOLS

The comprehensive analysis including systematic identification and quantification of all the proteins expressed by a cell, tissue, or organism is called proteomics. The last few decades have noticed a tremendous upsurge in the technological advancement of proteomic techniques including tools for separation, identification, and quantification of proteins; and automation of the processes.

Separation of proteins can be based on one or more physical or biochemical parameter such as subcellular location, molecular mass, or the isoelectric point (pI). In certain cases, sample preparation involves the depletion of abundant proteins and enrichment of a specific class of proteins for better analysis. For example, depletion of seminogelins from seminal plasma will enable the analysis of very low abundant proteins more effectively. Similarly, enrichment of phosphoproteins or glycoproteins in spermatozoa lysate will pave the way to the identification of specific proteins that have undergone modifications in a particular pathophysiological state. Proteomic analysis started with two-dimensional gel electrophoresis (2DE) in 1975 [15,16], before the word proteomics was coined [17]. In 2DE, the proteins are first separated by their isoelectric point followed by segregation based on molecular mass. Despite being a very useful method in the past, the major disadvantage of 2DE is poor separation of acidic, basic, hydrophobic, and low abundant proteins and intragel variation. To circumvent this problem, differential in-gel electrophoresis (2D-DIGE) is used. Here, the proteins from each group (e.g., control and experimental) are labeled with different fluorochromes prior to their separation enabling the identification of low abundance proteins and the dynamic range (very low to high abundance of various proteins in a complex mixture) issues due to intragel variation. In both 2DE and 2D-DIGE experiments, the identification of differentially expressed spots (proteins) often involves downstream mass spectrometer (MS)-based protein identification. However, it also has its own limitations; for instance, the problem with separation of hydrophobic proteins and labeling of proteins may be affected when the proteins do not contain accessible lysine (for minimal labeling) or cysteine residues (for saturation labeling).

Subsequently, high throughput identification of proteins involved tandem mass spectrometry preceded by gel-based or gel-free (liquid chromatography) separation of proteins. However, the identification of whole proteins is still limited. Therefore, the proteins are usually cut into peptides for identification and quantification by trypsin as it produces peptides that fall into an optimal mass range. The cleavage is highly specific and current protocols are quite efficient in detecting proteins (generally few cleavage sites are missed) [18]. In MS analysis, the peptides and proteins after separation by chromatography are converted into ions and the proteins or peptides are identified by analyzing their m/z ratio (Fig. 1). The ionization is achieved through the use of soft ionization, usually matrix-assisted laser desorption/ionization (MALDI) and electron spray ionization. Generally, quadrupole (Q) and ion trap mass analyzers filter ions of interest, whereas time of flight and Orbitrap mass analyzers detect mass with high resolution.

Shotgun proteomic platforms couple an ultraperformance liquid chromatographer to a hybrid mass spectrometer (MS/MS) known as LC-MS/MS, having high specificity and sensitivity. This type of chromatography has significantly amplified peptide resolution, decreased coelution, and permitted quantification of a large number of identified peptides. In order to decrease intrasample variability, proteins were labeled with different mass tags such as the isobaric tag for relative and absolute quantitation (iTRAQ), tandem mass tags (TMTs), isotope coded affinity tags, and dimethyl labels for differential marking of samples. However, a paradigm shift in label-free technologies is observed with the development of software packages dedicated to aligning chromatograms from different runs, allowing normalization of data in terms of the amount of protein injected in each run.

Multidimensional protein identification technology (MudPIT) analyzes proteomes without gels. In this approach, protein samples are subject to digestion (either by trypsin or endoproteinase lysC), then the resultant peptide mixtures are resolved by strong cation exchange (SCX) and reversed phase (RP) high performance liquid chromatography, and detected by MS. The MudPIT technique generates an in-depth list of proteins in a given sample, and is sensitive and fast with high reproducibility. However, it lacks the ability to deliver quantitative data [19–21]. From the MS data, protein identification and validation requires a database search using one of several engines available (e.g., Sequest, Mascot, Comet, X!tandem, etc.). Then, based on large protein–protein interaction (PPI) databases such as IntAct [22], BioGRID [23], HPRD [24], and STRING [25], PPI networks are constructed to understand the molecular mechanisms involving the identified proteins. By overlaying identified proteins in any given study to any of the several software suites, such as MetaCore (Thomson Reuters, New York, NY, USA), Ingenuity Pathway Analysis (IPA, QUIAGEN, Redwood City, CA, USA), and the open source platform Cytoscape [26], it is possible to suggest PPI subnetworks in any given study.

A comparative proteomic approach involves complex proteomic fingerprints of healthy and pathophysiological states (and transitions thereof) to distinguish trepidations from the healthy state phenotype before manifestation of the disease state [27]. Thus a reversion to the healthy phenotype may be achieved by therapeutic intervention during the transition-to-disease state. To achieve this goal, a systems biology approach involving comparative proteomics of cells/tissues/body fluids from normal versus diseased states, analysis of protein–protein interactions networks and pathways seems more plausible [27]. Since OS is the common implication in various pathophysiologies such as oligo-, astheno-, and teratozoospermia leading to male infertility, understanding of the dynamic range of protein alterations (which exceeds six orders of magnitude in cells and 10 orders of magnitude in body fluids) in the semen under OS is suggested. This would provide a better insight into the role of ROS in sperm toxicity.

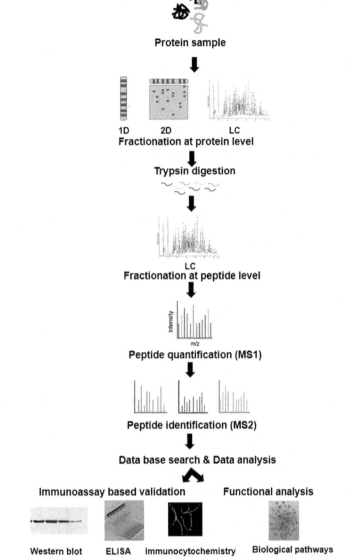

FIGURE 1 Schematic representation of proteomic work flow. *LC*, liquid chromatography.

REACTIVE OXYGEN SPECIES AND SEMEN PROTEOME

Two independent groups have substantially contributed to understanding the alterations in proteome profiling in the sperm and seminal plasma with respect to differences in levels of ROS [28–31], lipid peroxidation [32], and DNA fragmentation [33,34] indices. The initial approaches to study the impact of elevated ROS levels on semen proteome profile was initiated by comparing the proteome of spermatozoa and seminal plasma from men with higher ROS levels than the physiological level (ROS+) with that of men with low or physiological levels of ROS (ROS−). Initially, using 2D-DIGE followed by in-gel digestion of the proteins and LC-MS a total of 31 spots were shown to be differentially expressed with 6 significantly decreased and 25 increased proteins in the ROS− group compared with the ROS+ group. The authors attributed the essential cytoprotective effects against ROS in ROS− spermatozoa to the overabundance of four antioxidant proteins— lactotransferrin isoform-2, lactotransferrin isoform-1, peroxiredoxin-1, and the mitochondrial isoform of Manganese Superoxide Dismutase (Mn-SOD) [28].

In subsequent studies, the samples were subjected to high-throughput LC−MS/MS analysis after in-solution digestion of proteins with trypsin for peptide characterization [29]. The outcome revealed a total of 74 proteins in spermatozoa, out of which 15 proteins with a more than twofold difference were overexpressed (ROS+ group). It is interesting to note that the overexpressed proteins encompassed the histone cluster-1 H2Ba (HIST1H2BA); mitochondrial malate dehydrogenase precursor (MDH2); heat shock proteins (HSP90B1, HSPA5); glutamine synthetase (GLUL); transglutaminase-4 (prostate) (TGM4); glutathione peroxidase-4 isoform A precursor (GPX4); sperm acrosomal membrane protein4 (SPACA4); olfactomedin-4 precursor (OLFM4); and chromosome-20 open reading frame-3 (C20orf3). The majority of these proteins are known to have a role in metabolic regulation and stress management suggesting altered metabolism and adaptive response to counteract the elevated OS. On the other hand, the underexpressed proteins included semenogelin II precursor (SEMG2); peroxiredoxin-6 (PRDX6); clathrin heavy chain-1 (CLTC); eukaryotic translation elongation factor-2 (EEF2); and enolase-1 (ENO1) pointing toward a decline in antioxidant defense. The authors further noticed noteworthy changes in the localization profile of the differentially expressed proteins where the overexpressed proteins were predominantly found in the cellular compartments of intracellular, organelle, macromolecular complex region and mitochondria and the underexpressed proteins were predominate in the cytoplasm, extracellular, plasma membrane, protein complex (e.g., enolase) and the vesicular region (e.g., clathrin heavy chain).

An exclusive abundance of overexpressed proteins in the ROS+ group was found in the endosome, lipid particle, membrane-bound organelles and the microtubules; while the underexpressed proteins were restricted to proteinaceous extracellular matrix only. It may be envisaged that there is cytoplasmic accumulation in the ROS+ group implying maturation failure of the spermatozoa from this group. All these variations were compared simply based on the ROS status without taking into account the fertility status of the donors. Based on these results, a detailed proteomic study was carried out where the proteomic profile of fertile controls having low ROS levels (physiological level; 4−50 relative luminol unit (RLU)/s/10^6 sperm) were compared with those of infertile patients with varied levels of ROS (low: 0−<93 RLU/s/10^6 sperm; medium: >93−500 RLU/s/10^6 sperm; and high: >500 RLU/s/10^6 sperm). The authors reported that among the 305 differentially expressed proteins six proteins with distinct reproductive functions have potential to be developed as biomarkers of OS in spermatozoa. These proteins were identified as calmegin, tripeptidyl peptidase II, dynein intermediate chain-2, axonemal, heat shock 70 kDa protein 4 L, early endosome antigen-1, and plasma serine protease inhibitor [30].

A comparative proteomic profiling of seminal plasma between ROS− (<20 RLU/s/10^6 sperm) and ROS+ (>20 RLU/s/10^6 sperm) samples showed fibronectin I isoform-3 preprotein (FN1), macrophage migration inhibitory factor-1 peptide (MIF) and galectin-3 binding protein (G3BP) to be exclusively expressed in ROS− samples, while cystatin-S precursor (CST4), albumin preprotein (ALB), lactotransferrin (LTF) precursor-1 peptide and prostate-specific antigen isoform-4 (Kalikerin4: KLK4) preprotein were exclusive to the ROS+ group. Of the seven DEPs detected between the groups, prolactin-induced protein (PIP), semenogelin II (SEMG2) precursor, acid phosphatase and prostate short isoform precursor (ACPP) were upregulated in the ROS+ group, while clusterin (CLU) preprotein, zinc alpha-2-glycoprotein 1 (AZGP1), prostate-specific antigen isoform I preprotein (Kalikerin3: KLK3), and semenogelin I (SEMG1) isoform were downregulated [31].

The same authors conducted another in-depth study on a total of 42 infertile men presenting with infertility and 17 proven fertile donors. ROS levels were measured in the seminal ejaculates by a chemiluminescence assay and the infertile men were categorized into three subgroups, low ROS, medium ROS, and high ROS, and compared with fertile men as in the previously described study [30]. Following high throughput LC-MS/MS analysis they reported that proteins involved in biomolecule metabolism, protein folding, and protein degradation are differentially modulated in all three infertile patient groups in comparison to fertile controls. In comparison to the control, the majority of DEP were signal peptides, proteins of the extracellular region, and secreted proteins of the low ROS group; whereas, in medium and high ROS groups, proteins involved in metabolic processes were differentially expressed. In general, proteins involved in metabolism, energy production, protein folding and degradation, as well as stress response proteins were overexpressed and those involved in acute inflammatory responses were underexpressed in all ROS+ infertile groups. Mitochondrial precursor of the trifunctional enzyme subunit alpha (HADHA; a mitochondrial matrix enzyme involved in fatty acid metabolism) was overexpressed across all infertile ROS+ groups; the expression of the protein FAM3D was detected only in the fertile control group. Ingenuity Pathway Analysis revealed that all the 35 focused proteins of a single biological network responsible for protein turnover such as proteases, chaperones, proteins involved in ubiquitination, protein imports into nucleus and mitochondria, and complex macromolecular assembly were overexpressed in the high ROS group. The key protein neprilysin (also known as membrane metallo-endopeptidase; MME) of the network was consistently overexpressed (>2-fold) in all three ROS+ infertile groups. Besides, the identification of mitochondrial electron transport and ATP synthesis proteins and ubiquitination in the seminal plasma; points toward cell damage in ROS+ infertile men. MME and FAM3D along with ROS levels in seminal plasma were suggested to serve as good markers for diagnosis of male infertility.

In another study [32], the authors tried to differentiate the proteome profile of seminal plasma based on semen lipid peroxidation levels in men with normal semen parameters. These authors reported that in men with high lipid peroxidation levels 23 proteins are either absent or underexpressed, while 71 proteins are exclusive or overexpressed. The proteins identified are basically involved in unsaturated fatty acid biosynthesis, oxidant and antioxidant activity, cellular response to heat stress, and immune response. Mucin-5B (MUC5B) was suggested as a potential biomarker of semen OS.

OS and sperm DNA fragmentation are correlated and associated with low pregnancy rates, both in vivo and in vitro. Two important studies tried to identify the seminal protein markers with respect to varied levels of DNA fragmentation. In the first study, 30 DEPs were reported in the high sperm DNA fragmentation group involved in augmentation of innate immune response and decline in lipoprotein remodeling and regulation [33]. In the second study, overexpression of proteins associated with prostaglandin biosynthesis and fatty acid binding were observed in men with high sperm DNA damage. The proteasome subunit alpha type-5 protein (PSMA5) in seminal plasma was suggested as a biomarker of high sperm DNA fragmentation [34]. In all these studies involving spermatozoa and seminal plasma, the main focus was on seminal ROS levels without any categorical distinction between the fertile control group and the infertile group with a particular type or idiopathic infertility. However, a large number of studies were conducted on both spermatozoa and seminal plasma, taking into account a defined specific pathophysiological state such as varicocele, asthenozoospermia (AS), oligozoospermia, teratozoospermia, and so on. In this context, it is appropriate to mention that all these conditions are generally reported to have an augmented level of OS [3,35].

SPERM PROTEOME IN PATHOPHYSIOLOGICAL CONDITION WITH OXIDATIVE PREDOMINANCE

Due to the versatility of proteomic technology, sperm proteomic profiling under different pathophysiological conditions has drawn greater attention in recent years. In the following, reported conditions associated with elevated ROS level in semen are discussed.

Varicocele

Varicocele is one of the major contributors to male factor infertility (20%—40% of infertility cases). Stagnation of testicular microcirculation in varicocele leads to hypoxic-ischemic degenerative changes in testicular cells resulting in compromised semen quality, sperm DNA fragmentation, and infertility, induced by OS [36—38].

The first study comparing men with and without varicocele by 2DE followed by MALDI-TOF revealed that heat shock protein 70 member 5 (HSPA5), mitochondrial ATP synthase subunit delta (ATP5D), superoxide dismutase-1 (SOD1), CLU, Parkinson protein-7 (PARK7), KLK3, PIP, SEMG2, and semenogelin II precursor (SEMG2pre) are underexpressed in the varicocele group, while ACPP was overexpressed [39]. A series of studies was undertaken by Agarwal et al. in order to identify potential sperm biomarkers for varicocele by comparing the spermatozoa proteomic profile of infertile unilateral and bilateral patients with their fertile counterparts [40—43]. When the sperm proteome profile of infertile men with unilateral varicocele was compared with the fertile control, a total of 369 DEPs were reported, of which 38 were unique to the unilateral varicocele group, 14 overexpressed, and 97 underexpressed in the unilateral varicocele group, while 120 proteins were unique to the fertile group [40]. Free radical scavenging was identified as a key biological function that is dismantled in unilateral varicocele as the expression of principal proteins of ROS metabolism such as SOD1, SOD2, PRDX1, TXNRD2, GSRM, DLST, FBP1, FN1, FTH1, LTF, and IQGAP1 were altered [40]. On the other hand, comparison of the infertile bilateral varicocele group with fertile controls demonstrated 58 DEPs where 7 were exclusively observed in sperm from men with bilateral varicocele. Of these, tektin-3 (TEKT3) and T-complex protein-11 homolog (TCP11) were selected and validated as the key sperm biomarkers of infertility in bilateral varicocele [41]. Interestingly, comparison between infertile men with varicocele (unilateral or bilateral) and proven fertile men revealed 99 DEPs, where more than 87% of the DEP involved in major energy metabolism and key sperm functions were underexpressed in the varicocele group. Spermatogenesis, sperm motility, and mitochondrial dysfunction were the key functions affected in the varicocele group. Western blot analysis of five proteins, namely PKAR1A, AK7, CCT6B, HSPA2, and ODF2, involved in stress response and sperm function corroborated the MS results [43].

With an aim to identify varicocele-induced testicular dysfunction, seminal plasma and sperm proteome were compared between adolescents (1) without varicocele, (2) with varicocele and normal semen analysis; and (3) with varicocele and altered semen analysis. Validation of two differentially expressed proteins between these groups confirmed that cysteine-rich secretory protein 3 (CRISP3) is significantly overexpressed in the seminal plasma of adolescents with varicocele and seminal alterations, while the 45 kDa calcium-binding protein (CAB45) is underexpressed in both varicocele groups [44].

An interesting study compared the proteomic profiles of spermatozoa from patients with varicocele and poor sperm quality before and after varicocelectomy. The study reported augmentation of heat shock protein A5 (HSPA5), SOD1, and ATP synthase subunit delta, mitochondrial (ATP5D) after varicocelectomy, signifying their role in sperm quality control [45]. In order to establish the efficacy of varicocelectomy as a treatment option in adolescents with varicocele, seminal plasma of 19 adolescents was compared pre- and postvaricocelectomy, demonstrating that 19 proteins are differentially expressed after the surgery [46].

Asthenozoospermia

Asthenozoospermia (AS) is a common cause of human male infertility characterized by reduced sperm motility; that is, less than 40%. The molecular mechanism behind this impairment is not fully understood in the majority of cases. One of the major causes is the production of ROS, which directly affects sperm motility by production of high concentration of malondialdehyde (MDA) in the semen, which is an end product of lipid peroxidation [47]. Another byproduct of lipid peroxidation, 4-hydroxy nonenal (4HNE), has been demonstrated to form adducts with spermatozoa proteins, particularly cAMP-dependent protein kinase A when exposed in vitro [48].

The most important prerequisite for successful fertilization is sperm motility, which is regulated by cyclic AMP-activated protein kinase-A. It phosphorylates flagella proteins like axonemal dynein and initiates motility [48]. Siva et al. found that sperm proteins responsible for energy and metabolism are expressed at higher levels in asthenozoospermic patients, whereas normozoospermic samples had an elevated level of expression of proteins involved in movement and organization, protein turnover, folding, and stress response [49].

In two independent studies, the whole sperm proteome and sperm tail proteome were compared with normal controls and asthenozoospermic patients. Seventeen proteins [50] and 14 putative protein markers [51] of AS were proposed, respectively. Cytochrome c oxidase subunit 6B (COX6B) and heat shock-related 70 kDa protein-2 (HSPA2) were identified in both studies as putative markers of AS. In order to identify the molecular basis of sperm motility, sperm from normozoospermic men were separated into moderate motile sperm and good motile sperm, and the proteomes from both fractions were compared with that of asthenozoospermic patients. The level of protein tyrosine phosphatase nonreceptor type-14 (PTPN14), a mitochondrial protein, was found to be elevated in the AS patients. Hence it is selected as the most important impaired protein in sperm presenting alterations in motility [52]. Since it is a mitochondrial protein and AS is characterized by OS, it may be considered as a biomarker for progressive motility.

In another study, a total of 741 proteins were identified in seminal plasma of AS patients. Of these proteins, 45 were threefold upregulated and 56 were threefold downregulated in the AS group when compared with healthy donors. Most of these proteins originated from the epididymis and prostate. It was found that downregulation of DJ-1 protein in AS samples was due to high levels of ROS in the seminal plasma of AS patients, affecting semen quality [53]. As DJ-1 is a chaperone, its downregulation in seminal plasma surmises the impaired protein turnover from epididymis and prostate.

By using TMT protein labeling and LC-MS/MS, Amaral et al. performed proteomic profiling considering two complementary approaches to assess the proteins involved in sperm motility. In the first case, comparison between sperm samples differing in motility (asthenozoospermic vs. normozoospermic) was taken into consideration and 80 DEPs were identified. A second comparison between sperm subpopulations of fractionated normozoospermic samples differing in motility (nonmigrated vs. migrated) revealed 93 DEPs. The most interesting finding was that in both comparisons most of the DEPs were similar and included proteins associated with energetic metabolism, protein folding/degradation, vesicle trafficking, the cytoskeleton, and most notably, mitochondrial-related metabolic pathway protein. Therefore, it is obvious to find oxidative predominance in asthenozoospermic cases [54].

Oligozoospermia and Idiopathic Oligoasthenoteratozoospermia

Oligoasthenoteratozoospermia (OAT) is considered one of the common causes of male factor infertility. Various underlying factors have been hypothesized such as chromosomal abnormalities, asymptomatic infection, mitochondrial abnormalities, environmental pollutants, subtle hormonal changes, age, and functional posttesticular organ alteration. Compared to the donors with a proven record of fertility, oligozoospermic patients in the oligoasthenoteratozoospermia and oligoasthenozoospermia groups had significantly elevated ROS levels indicating a positive association between ROS and semen parameters. Thus a common underlying mechanism in these infertile patient groups was suggested [55].

In an attempt to identify proteomic markers of asthenozoospermia, Shen et al. compared the proteome of spermatozoa from normozoospermic individuals with idiopathic asthenozoospermic samples. The differentially expressed proteins GRP78, lactoferrin, SPANXB, PGK2, flagellin, DJ-1, XPA binding protein 2, CAB2, GPX4, and GAPDH in idiopathic asthenozoospermia patients were also involved in ROS metabolism [10].

Proteome profiling of four groups, namely normal sperm count and normal morphology; normal sperm count and abnormal morphology (NA); oligozoospermia and normal morphology (ON); and oligozoospermia and abnormal morphology (OA) revealed 20 DEPs including PIP1 preprotein; zinc alpha-2-glycoprotein-1, and clusterin isoform-1. In the NA group, mucin-6, gastric orosomucoid-1 precursor and acidic epididymal glycoprotein-like isoform-1 precursor were downregulated. On the other hand, in the OA group, prostate specific antigen isoform-1 preprotein and SEMG1 isoform b preprotein were upregulated, while cystatin C precursor was found to be downregulated. Two unique proteins, zinc alpha-2 glycoprotein-1 and tissue inhibitor of metalloproteinase-1 precursor, were upregulated in the ON group while clusterin 1 was downregulated [56].

A study was conducted to compare the protein profile of seminal plasma from infertile men with idiopathic OAT (iOAT) due to OS with that of healthy, fertile men to determine the proteins that are indicative of infertility. A total of 2489 proteins from seminal plasma were identified, out of which 46 proteins may have an influence on infertility due to OS. Twenty-seven of the proteins were common to all iOAT patients and 24 proteins were shown to be 1.5-fold upregulated in iOAT patients compared with the fertile controls. Pathway analysis of these overexpressed proteins in iOAT patients showed the involvement of these proteins in metabolism and inflammation, defense, and stress responses, thus indirectly implying ROS involvement. Understanding the proteins that are indicative of OS and inflammation will help in the selection of new drugs and therapy for the treatment of iOAT infertility [57].

Leukocytospermia

Leukocytes are considered to be an important producer of ROS. Leukocytospermia is a condition defined by the presence of more than 1×10^6 white blood cells/mL of semen [58]. Their abundance is known to produce a detectable amount of ROS, affecting sperm function and lowering the chances of pregnancy. Leukocytospermia affects semen quality with regard to ROS levels by inflicting sperm DNA damage in infertile men. When patients were grouped into no seminal leukocytes ($<10^6$ WBC/mL), men with low-level leukocytospermia ($0.1-1.0 \times 10^6$ WBC/mL), and frank leukocytospermia ($>1.0 \times 10^6$ WBC/mL), in comparison to the no seminal leukocyte group, both low and frank leukocytospermia groups exhibited higher levels of ROS and sperm DNA fragmentation [59]. Further, no significant difference between the two leukocytic groups was observed in terms of ROS level. Albeit no proteomic studies in the strict sense are carried out on leukocytospermic infertile patient semen, but a few studies focused on specific protein to relate the pathway through which it alters fertility status in men particularly in relation to OS. Hagan et al. compared the expression profile of different inflammatory markers in leukocytospermic patients with that of nonleukocytospermic ones. To their surprise they noticed a significantly increased expression of TLR-2/4, COX-2, and Nrf 2 in the sperm head and tail segments of leukocytospermic samples. These findings suggest that TLR-2/4, COX-2, and Nrf 2 can serve as novel biomarkers for inflammation and OS. This can also be a new strategy to diagnose infertile men with idiopathic infertility [60].

Unexplained Infertility

Unexplained male infertility is another end of the problem wherein an infertile patient is presenting with normal semen parameters and normal physical or endocrine attributes. Apart from erectile problems, coital factors, and absence of female factor infertility, immune causes and dysfunctional sperm may contribute to such conditions. Xu et al. reported differentially expressed proteins in sperm of infertile patients whose semen parameters met the World Health Organization guidelines. Using MALDI-TOF/TOF analysis, 24 differentially expressed proteins were identified from the 31 most abundant different protein spots in 2D gels of sperm samples. Following data analysis, the authors categorized these 24 proteins into five functional clusters: (1) sexual reproduction, (2) response to wounding, (3) metabolic process, (4) cell growth and/or maintenance, and (5) uncharacterized. Additionally, 9 of the 24 differentially expressed proteins are involved in a main pathway network including TGF-β1, MYC, β-estradiol, MYCN, and TP53, which are known to be involved in cell–cell communication, proliferation, and differentiation; therefore, they are proposed as potential diagnostic markers of sperm function such as motility, capacitation, acrosomal reaction, and sperm–oocyte communication [61].

Sperm Proteome and Assisted Reproductive Technique Outcome

McReynolds et al. evaluated the sperm proteome of normozoospermic males in relation to in vitro fertilization outcomes in donor oocyte cycles and categorized them into good blastocyst development group and poor blastocyst development group. The analysis reported 49 proteins having statistically significant differential abundance in relation to blastocyst development. Out of these, 29 proteins were underexpressed in the poor blastocyst development group, whereas 20 proteins were overexpressed in comparison to the good blastocyst development group. Stress response proteins, mainly the heat shock proteins (HSPA2, HSPA5, and HSPB1), stress-induced phosphoprotein 1 (STIP1), and CLU, were found to be more abundant in the sperm of the poor blastocyst group [62] Since HSPs are basically involved in stress response alongside their chaperone activity in folding of misfolded proteins and their role in OS management [48,63], their altered expression may be used as a potential biomarker in identification of unexplained male infertility, and thus may play a significant role in causing idiopathic male infertility.

REACTIVE OXYGEN SPECIES—MEDIATED POSTTRANSLATIONAL PROTEIN MODIFICATIONS AND MALE REPRODUCTION

Cellular response to ROS includes both reversible and irreversible redox modification of biomolecules, especially proteins based on the nature and concentration of ROS. A few of the modifications involving ROS such as the activation of protein kinases resulting in phosphorylation of proteins required for capacitation and hyperactivation as well as N-nitrosylation required for capacitation (Fig. 2). Some of the earliest oxidative modifications following an oxidative insult are increased levels of toxic carbonyls, 3-nitrotyrosine (3-NT), and hydroxyl nonenals (HNE). The reaction of oxidants with biomolecules is the molecular basis for sensing alternations in the cellular redox state. Protein oxidation leads to

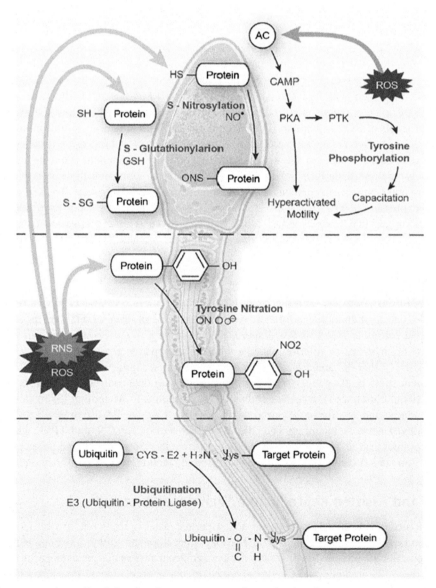

FIGURE 2 Reactive oxygen species mediated alterations in spermatozoa proteins, major site of occurrence on spermatozoa and the affected sperm function. *RNS*, reactive nitrogen species; *ROS*, reactive oxygen species.

aggregation or dimerization of proteins and conformational changes, thereby exposing more hydrophobic residues to an aqueous environment. The accumulation of oxidatively modified protein causes a disruption of cellular function by altering protein expression and gene regulation, protein turnover, modulation of cell signaling, induction of apoptosis and necrosis, and so on, suggesting its role in physiological and pathological conditions.

Phosphorylation

Protein phosphorylation is defined as a covalent addition of the phosphate group to the side chain of tyrosine, serine, and threonine amino acid residues. Phosphorylation is the major posttranslational modification (PTM) that controls epididymal maturation, motility, capacitation, and acrosomal reaction (Fig. 2). During capacitation, influx of calcium into the spermatozoa causes rise in pH, generating a low level of $O_2^{\cdot-}$ and nitric oxide ($NO^{\cdot}$). Both $O_2^{\cdot-}$ and $NO^{\cdot}$ rapidly react to form peroxynitrite ($ONOO^-$), which undergoes homolytic cleavage to form hydroxyl radical ($^{\cdot}OH$) and nitrogen dioxide. This rise in pH and hydroxyl radicals activates adenylyl cyclase, which leads to elevation of intracellular cyclic adenosine monophosphate (cAMP) and protein kinase (PK) A activity [64,65]. ROS are also involved in inhibition of various phosphatases, thus supporting the sperm progression into late stages of capacitation and activation of PK and RAS proteins [66]. The main event in ROS-mediated protein phosphorylation takes place during the late stages of capacitation, which indirectly activates tyrosine kinase activity. During capacitation, synthesis of $O_2^{\cdot-}$ is controlled by extracellular calcium, whereas nitric oxide generation is regulated by both intracellular and extracellular calcium concentration [67]. The activation of these two ROS synthesis has proven to be complex. PKC, protein tyrosine kinase, extracellular-signal-regulated kinase (ERK), phosphatidylinositol 3-kinase (P13K), and PKB (Akt) activation increases $NO^{\cdot}$ levels, while $O_2^{\cdot-}$ production appears to be upstream of $NO^{\cdot}$ production. Reciprocal activation of $NO^{\cdot}$ and $O_2^{\cdot-}$ demonstrates flexibility in the system, thus allowing compensatory action between the two when production of one is impaired [67,68]. In capacitation phosphorylation of tyrosine residues was found predominantly in the region of the fibrous sheath [69] and actin polymerization in the postacrosomal region of the head of the spermatozoa [70]. Actin polymerization is regulated by protein phosphorylation events as inhibitors of PKs prevented it while stimulators of tyrosine phosphorylation in sperm (cAMP, epidermal growth factor, sodium vanadate, H_2O_2, etc.) triggered it [70,71].

ROS-mediated tyrosine phosphorylated protein include AKAP4 (sperm tail protein), AKAP3 (a sperm-specific aldolase related to motility), CABYR (a pyruvate hydrogenase) in the spermatozoa ERK-1 and ERK-2 are also tyrosine phosphorylated during the process of fertilization [72]. In humans, the sperm tail undergoes tyrosine phosphorylation, with the localization being primarily in the principal piece. In OS, molecular chaperones like HSP-90 is phosphorylated at tyrosine residue during capacitation [73,74]. Sperm and egg recognition is a species-specific molecular-driven process. A report suggests that in mice, tyrosine phosphorylation activates sperm-specific surface chaperones during capacitation, which facilitates sperm ZP-recognition [75]. Another study suggests that testis-specific phosphotyrosinated chaperone HSPA2, which regulates the expression of sperm surface receptors, is involved in human sperm-oocyte recognition [76].

The inhibition of AR by superoxide dismutase (SOD) and catalase and stimulation of AR by H_2O_2 (generated by xanthine-xanthine oxidase system) indicate that AR is a ROS-dependent process as capacitation [77].

Thionylation

Protein S-thiolation is a process where protein thiol (SH) groups form mixed disulphides with low-molecular-mass thiols such as glutathione to prevent the irreversible oxidation of cysteine residues on proteins, thereby protecting them under stress conditions such as OS. Glutathione (GSH) is the most abundant and important low-molecular weight thiol within the spermatozoa involved in cell signaling pathways by modulating protein function. OS is reported to induce improper packaging of sperm chromatin. Protamines are unique sperm nuclear proteins that replace histones during spermiogenesis and responsible for sperm chromatin compaction from a solenoid to a toroid structure. Proper inter- [78] and intra-disulphide [79] cross-links between cysteine-rich protamines are responsible for this compaction and stabilization of the sperm nucleus. In the presence of oxidants (ROS), free and accessible thiols on protamines can undergo several modifications. In addition, glutathione peroxidase activity could also be involved in intradisulphide cross-linking of protamines, which requires glutathione [80]. Enzymes that function in energy metabolism are inactivated by S-glutathionylation, thereby impairing energy production during OS.

In a study where sperm were treated with peroxides (tert-butyl hydro-peroxide or tBHP), a dose-dependent increase in S-glutathionylation along with a decrease in progressive and total motility in spermatozoa was noticed [81]. In most cases, elevated levels of ROS have led to the generation of redox-dependent protein modifications, such as tyrosine nitration and S-glutathionylation, causing failure in sperm capacitation. This result implies that excessive OS leads to protein modifications, which could be the reason behind lower motility and fertilization failure. In fact, it is seen in some cases of male infertility and the modification is present all over the sperm cell [81]. Peroxiredoxins (PRDX) are abundant in human semen and are important antioxidant enzymes, which act as ROS scavengers and modulators in ROS-dependent signaling. During elimination of H_2O_2 by PRDXs, the cysteine residues in the active site of the enzyme become oxidized, rendering it inactive and requiring either the thioredoxin/thioredoxin reductase system (for PRDX 1−5) or glutathione/glutathione reductase system mediated by glutathione S-transferase (for PRDX 6) to reactivate the enzyme [82,83]. However, PRDX hyperoxidation (conversion to sulfonated form) is an irreversible process without sulfiredoxin and sestrin1 enzymes. The presence of these later two enzymes has not been reported in semen, thus permanent inactivation of PRDXs in semen under chronic OS cannot be ignored.

In a study it was investigated that PRDX1, PRDX4, PRDX5, and PRDX6 are differentially localized in head, acrosome, mitochondrial sheath, and flagellum of spermatozoa, which could provide protection against ROS [84]. All the reported PRDXs were modified when exposed to H_2O_2. From the results, it is suggested that PRDXs may protect these cells at high levels of H(2)O(2) but could also control H(2)O(2) levels within different cell compartments so that normal sperm activation can occur. Reduced PRDXs and higher levels of PRDX thiol oxidation are correlated negatively with sperm motility and positively with sperm DNA damage and sperm lipid peroxidation in infertile men [85]. It is not known whether PRDX of the seminal plasma is being permanently impacted by OS in a similar fashion due to thiol oxidation of its active site cysteine.

In this conjecture, spermatozoa from normozoospermic healthy individuals were exposed to exogenous hydrogen peroxide, tert-buthyl hydroperoxide, or diethylamine NONOate (DA-NONOate; a nitric oxide: NO• inducer) under capacitating conditions, and then levels of tyrosine phosphorylation and percentage of acrosome reaction (AR) induced by lysophosphatidylcholine (LPC) were determined [81]. Modified sperm proteins from cytosolic, triton-soluble, and triton-insoluble fractions were analyzed by SDSPAGE/immunoblotting and immunocytochemistry with antiglutathione and antinitro tyrosine antibodies. Augmentation in S-glutathionylation levels localized mainly in the cytosolic and triton-soluble fractions of the spermatozoa were observed in response to hydroperoxide exposure. Conversely, an elevation in tyrosine nitrated proteins mainly localized in the triton-insoluble fraction was noticed upon exposure to DA-NONOate. Besides, the exposed spermatozoa showed reduced motility without any observable change in viability. Even under capacitating conditions these oxidant-exposed spermatozoa had tyrosine phosphorylation and AR comparable to that of noncapacitated spermatozoa, implying an impairment of sperm capacitation by OS. The results surmise that OS promotes increase in spermatozoa protein tyrosine nitration and S-glutathionylation, leading to altered motility and the ability to undergo capacitation [81].

S-Nitrosylation

Nitrosylation is considered as an important PTM. NO, despite having an apparently simple diatomic structure, has a wide variety of functions in both physiology and pathology: NO-mediated PTMs such as binding to metal centers; nitrosylation of thiol and amine groups; nitration of tyrosine, tryptophan, amine, carboxylic acid, and phenylalanine groups; and oxidation of thiols (both cysteine and methionine residues) and tyrosine of disrupt cellular signaling processes. However, owing to the greater role of thiol groups in sperm chromatin compaction, nitrosylation of thiols to produce S-nitrosothiol and nitration of tyrosine residues to produce nitrotyrosine has received greater attention [86].

NO increase human sperm motility and capacitation associated with high protein phosphorylation (Fig. 2). NO, besides activating soluble guanylylcyclase, can also modify protein function covalently via S-nitrosylation of cysteine. Besides knowing the sperm it is evidenced they depend on these PTMs to achieve changes in function required for fertilization. In an experiment conducted by Lefievre et al., spermatozoa were incubated with NO donors of different classes. When spermatozoa were incubated with NO donors (S-nitroso-glutathione), 240 S-nitrosylated proteins were identified in spermatozoa via the biotin switch assay combined with MS/MS analysis. On the other hand, spermatozoa treated with glutathione or the untreated samples demonstrated minimal levels of S-nitrosylation. Besides the established targets for S-nitrosylation reported in other cells like tubulin, GST, and HSPs, unique sperm functional proteins such as A-kinase anchoring protein (AKAP) types 3 and 4, voltage-dependent anion-selective channel protein 3, and SEMG 1 and 2 were also reported. These proteins were shown to be localized on the postacrosomal region of the head and throughout the flagellum providing novel insight into the mechanism of action of NO in spermatozoa [87].

The expression pattern of constitutive and inducible nitric oxide synthase (NOS) in spermatozoa isolated from normozoospermic fertile donors and asthenozoospermic infertile patients were characterized by immunohistochemistry. Further, the immunohistochemical expression of citrulline (a marker of NOS activity) and nitrotyrosine (an indicator of peroxynitrite formation) showed cytotoxic effects of NO in spermatozoa. Spermatozoa isolated from normozoospermic fertile donors express augmented NOS constitutively, while in asthenozoospermic samples, expression of inducible NOS and nitrotyrosine was higher. Enhanced NOS activity in sperm from idiopathic asthenozoospermic patients was confirmed from citrulline data. Thus it may be perceived that increased NOS activity and an excess of tyrosine nitration may affect spermatozoa function in idiopathic asthenozoospermia [88].

Carbonylation

Protein carbonylation is defined as the covalent, nonreversible modification of the side chains of cysteine, histidine, and lysine residues by lipid peroxidation end products such as 4-hydroxy, 4-oxoneonenal, and so on, resulting in carbonyl derivatives. During the process of sperm maturation about 85% of the histones are replaced by protamines. Protamines are highly basic protein, rich in amino acid residues like arginine, lysine, and histidine, and containing amino acids that are capable of donating a proton for a hydrogen bond with a DNA phosphate group such as tyrosine, cysteine, serine, glutamine, and threonine [89]. These amino acids (arginine, lysine, and threonine) are more prone to direct metal-catalyzed ROS-mediated oxidative attack resulting in generation of protein carbonyls or Michael adducts between nucleophilic residues and alpha, beta-unsaturated aldehydes [90]. In addition, carbonyl derivatives on lysine, cysteine, and histidine can be formed by secondary reactions with reactive carbonyl compounds on carbohydrates (glycoxidation products), lipids, and advanced glycation/lipoxidation end products (AGE and ALEs) [91]. Furthermore, ROS produced during OS can further damage the peptide backbone, resulting in the generation of protein carbonyls. The process is initiated by hydrogen abstraction from the alpha-carbon in a peptide chain. If two protein radicals are in close proximity, they may cross-link with one another by radical to form peroxide intermediates, leading to rearrangement and subsequent cleavage of the peptide bond to form carbonyl-containing peptides [92]. Spermatozoa of patients having recurrent pregnancy loss without any attributable female factor showed significant elevation in the levels of protein carbonylation and lipid peroxidation together with an increased retention of histones. Therefore, it is opined that histone carrying sites for oxidative modification such as arginine and lysine might be responsible for disturbing the paternal epigenomic control during early stages of embryonic differentiation leading to abortion [93]. The findings were corroborated by a series of recent studies where the lipid peroxidation by-product 4HNE is shown to form adducts with sperm proteins, particularly α-tubulin [94], the molecular chaperone HSPA2 [63], and succinate dehydrogenase (SDHA) [95]. Therefore, the formation of these carbonylated adduct will lead to impairment of functions of these proteins and compromise sperm-oocyte recognition and promote electron leakage from the electron transport chain, thus exacerbating OS experienced by the spermatozoa. Though these preliminary evidences advocate the irreversible protein alteration by carbonylation of sperm proteins, no such MS studies to date identify the carbonylated proteins in spermatozoa under various pathophysiological states.

UBIQUITINATION AND PROTEOLYSIS

One of the most significant protein modifications that occurs in a cell is ubiquitination, which lead to proteolysis. It is a multistep process that links to cellular metabolism and intracellular protein turnover [96]. In the case of spermatozoa and seminal plasma, misfolded and unfolded, oxidized proteins tend to form oligomeric complexes forming protein aggregates, which are then disposed of by the cells. Sutovsky et al. reported that OS augments ubiquitination and has an inverse relationship with sperm parameters [97]. On the other hand, in males with varicocele, unequivocal induction of OS is linked to male infertility [37]. However, Hosseinpour et al. found a lower level of ubiquitination in spermatozoa of varicocele patients despite the presence of OS. The study also found that the levels of ubiquitination have a positive correlation with motility and a negative correlation with morphology [98]. While the results went against Sutovsky et al., it is evident that ubiquitination has a connection to ROS. Perhaps differing levels of ROS result in diverse outcomes in terms of ubiquitination. It will not be out of context to mention here that a study using the GC-2 cell line as a model reported the ubiquitination and degradation of HSPA2 by immunoprecipitation techniques and pharmacological inhibition of proteosomal and lysosomal degradation pathways. Subsequently, the interaction between cochaperone BCL2-associated athanogene 6 that is responsible for stability of HSPA2 by preventing ubiquitination and proteolysis was examined in response to 4HNE exposure via proximity ligation assays. From the results of this study the authors demonstrate a causative link between nonenzymatic PTMs and the relative levels of HSPA2 in the spermatozoa of a specific subclass of infertile males and opined that as a reason for failed sperm-oocyte fusion [99].

There is a well-established relationship between protein oxidation and proteolysis. Studies have shown that there is an increase in protein degradation following oxidative damage [100,101]. When proteins are damaged via oxidation, their native state is altered. The normally folded proteins are disrupted into fragments, cross-linked, or their protein structure changes [102]. The structural changes increase surface hydrophobicity that in turn makes the proteins susceptible to proteolytic attack. In either case, due to OS, proteolytic pathways in sperm are activated in order to prevent possible aggregation of the nonfunctional oxidized proteins [100,101]. It is also assumed that ROS causing modifications alter the proteosomal activity itself, but to what extent is yet to be established [98].

CONCLUDING REMARKS

It is implied from the discussion vide supra that the manifestation of excessive redox-dependent protein modifications is a consequence of ROS overload. Besides, enhanced OS also alters the proteome profile in spermatozoa via diverse mechanisms. The last decade consolidated on identifying proteomic biomarkers and reporting the global oxidative modification of sperm proteome under oxidative predominance. However, the precise molecular mechanism involved in differential expression of sperm proteins under OS and the specific proteins that undergo irreversible oxidative modification in response to ROS overload remains to be elucidated. Moreover, in sperm proteomic studies, only one type of functional modification on proteins in general is considered and proteins with multiple modifications are largely ignored. Moreover, stage-specific changes in a particular type of redox modification in spermatozoa proteins would shed light on the regulatory role ROS play at different maturation stages of spermatozoa. It may be possible that the same protein undergoes varied types of redox regulation in response to different stimuli rendering its pathological manifestation. Therefore, future studies involving redox regulation of the sperm proteome will help integrate the proteome with the sperm metabolome, to address the sperm dysfunction observed in a significant proportion of infertile males.

REFERENCES

[1] Levine H, Jorgensen N, Martino-Andrade A, Mendiola J, Weksler-Derri D, Mindlis I, et al. Temporal trends in sperm count: a systematic review and meta-regression analysis. Hum Reprod Update 2017;23(6):646–59.

[2] Agarwal A, Saleh RA, Bedaiwy MA. Role of reactive oxygen species in the pathophysiology of human reproduction. Fertil Steril 2003;79(4):829–43.

[3] Lavranos G, Balla M, Tzortzopoulou A, Syriou V, Angelopoulou R. Investigating ROS sources in male infertility: a common end for numerous pathways. Reprod Toxicol 2012;34(3):298–307.

[4] Holmstrom KM, Finkel T. Cellular mechanisms and physiological consequences of redox-dependent signalling. Nat Rev Mol Cell Biol 2014;15(6):411–21.

[5] Sharma RK, Agarwal A. Role of reactive oxygen species in male infertility. Urology 1996;48(6):835–50.

[6] Agarwal A, Sharma RK, Nallella KP, Thomas Jr AJ, Alvarez JG, Sikka SC. Reactive oxygen species as an independent marker of male factor infertility. Fertil Steril 2006;86(4):878–85.

[7] Zalata AA, Ahmed AH, Allamaneni SS, Comhaire FH, Agarwal A. Relationship between acrosin activity of human spermatozoa and oxidative stress. Asian J Androl 2004;6(4):313–8.

[8] Aitken RJ, Buckingham D, Harkiss D. Use of a xanthine oxidase free radical generating system to investigate the cytotoxic effects of reactive oxygen species on human spermatozoa. J Reprod Fertil 1993;97(2):441–50.

[9] Aitken RJ. A free radical theory of male infertility. Reprod Fertil Dev 1994;6(1):19–23. discussion-4.

[10] Shen H, Ong C. Detection of oxidative DNA damage in human sperm and its association with sperm function and male infertility. Free Radic Biol Med 2000;28(4):529–36.

[11] Pasqualotto FF, Sharma RK, Nelson DR, Thomas AJ, Agarwal A. Relationship between oxidative stress, semen characteristics, and clinical diagnosis in men undergoing infertility investigation. Fertil Steril 2000;73(3):459–64.

[12] Deepinder F, Cocuzza M, Agarwal A. Should seminal oxidative stress measurement be offered routinely to men presenting for infertility evaluation? Endocr Pract 2008;14(4):484–91.

[13] Tremellen K. Oxidative stress and male infertility—a clinical perspective. Hum Reprod Update 2008;14(3):243–58.

[14] Ko EY, Sabanegh Jr ES, Agarwal A. Male infertility testing: reactive oxygen species and antioxidant capacity. Fertil Steril 2014;102(6):1518–27.

[15] Klose J. Protein mapping by combined isoelectric focusing and electrophoresis of mouse tissues. A novel approach to testing for induced point mutations in mammals. Humangenetik 1975;26(3):231–43.

[16] O'Farrell PH. High resolution two-dimensional electrophoresis of proteins. J Biol Chem 1975;250(10):4007–21.

[17] Wilkins MR, Pasquali C, Appel RD, Ou K, Golaz O, Sanchez JC, et al. From proteins to proteomes: large scale protein identification by two-dimensional electrophoresis and amino acid analysis. Biotechnology 1996;14(1):61–5.

[18] Fannes T, Vandermarliere E, Schietgat L, Degroeve S, Martens L, Ramon J. Predicting tryptic cleavage from proteomics data using decision tree ensembles. J Proteome Res 2013;12(5):2253–9.

[19] Chandramouli K, Qian PY. Proteomics: challenges, techniques and possibilities to overcome biological sample complexity. Hum Genomics Proteomics 2009;2009.

[20] Agarwal A, Bertolla RP, Samanta L. Sperm proteomics: potential impact on male infertility treatment. Expert Rev Proteomics 2016;13(3):285–96.

[21] Agarwal A, Samanta L, Bertolla RP, Durairajanayagam D, Intasqui P. Proteomics in human reproduction: biomarkers for millennials. Springer; 2017.

[22] Orchard S, Ammari M, Aranda B, Breuza L, Briganti L, Broackes-Carter F, et al. The MIntAct project—IntAct as a common curation platform for 11 molecular interaction databases. Nucleic Acids Res 2014;42(Database issue):D358—63.

[23] Stark C, Breitkreutz BJ, Reguly T, Boucher L, Breitkreutz A, Tyers M. BioGRID: a general repository for interaction datasets. Nucleic Acids Res 2006;34(Database issue):D535—9.

[24] Keshava Prasad TS, Goel R, Kandasamy K, Keerthikumar S, Kumar S, Mathivanan S, et al. Human protein reference Database—2009 update. Nucleic Acids Res 2009;37(Database issue):D767—72.

[25] Szklarczyk D, Franceschini A, Wyder S, Forslund K, Heller D, Huerta-Cepas J, et al. STRING v10: protein-protein interaction networks, integrated over the tree of life. Nucleic Acids Res 2015;43(Database issue):D447—52.

[26] Cline MS, Smoot M, Cerami E, Kuchinsky A, Landys N, Workman C, et al. Integration of biological networks and gene expression data using Cytoscape. Nat Protoc 2007;2(10):2366—82.

[27] Turck CW, Falick AM, Kowalak JA, Lane WS, Lilley KS, Phinney BS, et al. The association of biomolecular resource facilities proteomics research group 2006 study: relative protein quantitation. Mol Cell Proteomics 2007;6(8):1291—8.

[28] Hamada A, Sharma R, du Plessis SS, Willard B, Yadav SP, Sabanegh E, et al. Two-dimensional differential in-gel electrophoresis-based proteomics of male gametes in relation to oxidative stress. Fertil Steril 2013;99(5):1216—26. e2.

[29] Sharma R, Agarwal A, Mohanty G, Hamada AJ, Gopalan B, Willard B, et al. Proteomic analysis of human spermatozoa proteins with oxidative stress. Reprod Biol Endocrinol 2013;11:48.

[30] Ayaz A, Agarwal A, Sharma R, Arafa M, Elbardisi H, Cui Z. Impact of precise modulation of reactive oxygen species levels on spermatozoa proteins in infertile men. Clin Proteomics 2015;12(1):4.

[31] Sharma R, Agarwal A, Mohanty G, Du Plessis SS, Gopalan B, Willard B, et al. Proteomic analysis of seminal fluid from men exhibiting oxidative stress. Reprod Biol Endocrinol 2013;11:85.

[32] Intasqui P, Antoniassi MP, Camargo M, Nichi M, Carvalho VM, Cardozo KH, et al. Differences in the seminal plasma proteome are associated with oxidative stress levels in men with normal semen parameters. Fertil Steril 2015;104(2):292—301.

[33] Intasqui P, Camargo M, Del Giudice PT, Spaine DM, Carvalho VM, Cardozo KH, et al. Unraveling the sperm proteome and post-genomic pathways associated with sperm nuclear DNA fragmentation. J Assist Reprod Genet 2013;30(9):1187—202.

[34] Intasqui P, Camargo M, Del Giudice PT, Spaine DM, Carvalho VM, Cardozo KH, et al. Sperm nuclear DNA fragmentation rate is associated with differential protein expression and enriched functions in human seminal plasma. BJU Int 2013;112(6):835—43.

[35] Aitken RJ, Gibb Z, Baker MA, Drevet J, Gharagozloo P. Causes and consequences of oxidative stress in spermatozoa. Reprod Fertil Dev 2016;28(1—2):1—10.

[36] Hamada A, Esteves SC, Agarwal A. Insight into oxidative stress in varicocele-associated male infertility: part 2. Nat Rev Urol 2012; 10(1):26—37.

[37] Agarwal A, Hamada A, Esteves SC. Insight into oxidative stress in varicocele-associated male infertility: part 1. Nat Rev Urol 2012;9(12):678—90.

[38] Cho CL, Esteves SC, Agarwal A. Novel insights into the pathophysiology of varicocele and its association with reactive oxygen species and sperm DNA fragmentation. Asian J Androl 2016;18(2):186—93.

[39] Hosseinifar H, Gourabi H, Salekdeh GH, Alikhani M, Mirshahvaladi S, Sabbaghian M, et al. Study of sperm protein profile in men with and without varicocele using two-dimensional gel electrophoresis. Urology 2013;81(2):293—300.

[40] Agarwal A, Sharma R, Durairajanayagam D, Ayaz A, Cui Z, Willard B, et al. Major protein alterations in spermatozoa from infertile men with unilateral varicocele. Reprod Biol Endocrinol 2015;13:8.

[41] Agarwal A, Sharma R, Durairajanayagam D, Cui Z, Ayaz A, Gupta S, et al. Spermatozoa protein alterations in infertile men with bilateral varicocele. Asian J Androl 2016;18(1):43—53.

[42] Agarwal A, Sharma R, Durairajanayagam D, Cui Z, Ayaz A, Gupta S, et al. Differential proteomic profiling of spermatozoal proteins of infertile men with unilateral or bilateral varicocele. Urology 2015;85(3):580—8.

[43] Agarwal A, Sharma R, Samanta L, Durairajanayagam D, Sabanegh E. Proteomic signatures of infertile men with clinical varicocele and their validation studies reveal mitochondrial dysfunction leading to infertility. Asian J Androl 2016;18(2):282—91.

[44] Zylbersztejn DS, Andreoni C, Del Giudice PT, Spaine DM, Borsari L, Souza GH, et al. Proteomic analysis of seminal plasma in adolescents with and without varicocele. Fertil Steril 2016;99(1):92—8.

[45] Hosseinifar H, Sabbaghian M, Nasrabadi D, Modarresi T, Dizaj AV, Gourabi H, et al. Study of the effect of varicocelectomy on sperm proteins expression in patients with varicocele and poor sperm quality by using two-dimensional gel electrophoresis. J Assist Reprod Genet 2014;31(6):725—9.

[46] Del Giudice PT, da Silva BF, Lo Turco EG, Fraietta R, Spaine DM, Santos LF, et al. Changes in the seminal plasma proteome of adolescents before and after varicocelectomy. Fertil Steril 2013;100(3):667—72.

[47] Walczak-Jedrzejowska R, Wolski JK, Slowikowska-Hilczer J. The role of oxidative stress and antioxidants in male fertility. Cent European J Urol 2013;66(1):60—7.

[48] Bromfield EG, Aitken RJ, Anderson AL, McLaughlin EA, Nixon B. The impact of oxidative stress on chaperone-mediated human sperm-egg interaction. Hum Reprod 2015;30(11):2597—613.

[49] Siva AB, Kameshwari DB, Singh V, Pavani K, Sundaram CS, Rangaraj N, et al. Proteomics-based study on asthenozoospermia: differential expression of proteasome alpha complex. Mol Hum Reprod 2010;16(7):452—62.

[50] Martinez-Heredia J, de Mateo S, Vidal-Taboada JM, Ballesca JL, Oliva R. Identification of proteomic differences in asthenozoospermic sperm samples. Hum Reprod 2008;23(4):783—91.

[51] Hashemitabar M, Sabbagh S, Orazizadeh M, Ghadiri A, Bahmanzadeh M. A proteomic analysis on human sperm tail: comparison between normozoospermia and asthenozoospermia. J Assist Reprod Genet 2015;32(6):853—63.

[52] Chao HC, Chung CL, Pan HA, Liao PC, Kuo PL, Hsu CC. Protein tyrosine phosphatase non-receptor type 14 is a novel sperm-motility biomarker. J Assist Reprod Genet 2011;28(9):851—61.

[53] Wang J, Wang J, Zhang HR, Shi HJ, Ma D, Zhao HX, et al. Proteomic analysis of seminal plasma from asthenozoospermia patients reveals proteins that affect oxidative stress responses and semen quality. Asian J Androl 2009;11(4):484—91.

[54] Amaral A, Paiva C, Attardo Parrinello C, Estanyol JM, Ballesca JL, Ramalho-Santos J, et al. Identification of proteins involved in human sperm motility using high-throughput differential proteomics. J Proteome Res 2014;13(12):5670—84.

[55] Agarwal A, Mulgund A, Sharma R, Sabanegh E. Mechanisms of oligozoospermia: an oxidative stress perspective. Syst Biol Reprod Med 2014;60(4):206—16.

[56] Sharma R, Agarwal A, Mohanty G, Jesudasan R, Gopalan B, Willard B, et al. Functional proteomic analysis of seminal plasma proteins in men with various semen parameters. Reprod Biol Endocrinol 2013;11:38.

[57] Herwig R, Knoll C, Planyavsky M, Pourbiabany A, Greilberger J, Bennett KL. Proteomic analysis of seminal plasma from infertile patients with oligoasthenoteratozoospermia due to oxidative stress and comparison with fertile volunteers. Fertil Steril 2013;100(2):355—66. e2.

[58] World Health O. WHO laboratory manual for the examination and processing of human semen. 2010.

[59] Agarwal A, Mulgund A, Alshahrani S, Assidi M, Abuzenadah AM, Sharma R, et al. Reactive oxygen species and sperm DNA damage in infertile men presenting with low level leukocytospermia. Reprod Biol Endocrinol 2014;12:126.

[60] Hagan S, Khurana N, Chandra S, Abdel-Mageed AB, Mondal D, Hellstrom WJ, et al. Differential expression of novel biomarkers (TLR-2, TLR-4, COX-2, and Nrf-2) of inflammation and oxidative stress in semen of leukocytospermia patients. Andrology 2015;3(5):848—55.

[61] Xu W, Hu H, Wang Z, Chen X, Yang F, Zhu Z, et al. Proteomic characteristics of spermatozoa in normozoospermic patients with infertility. J Proteomics 2012;75(17):5426—36.

[62] McReynolds S, Dzieciatkowska M, Stevens J, Hansen KC, Schoolcraft WB, Katz-Jaffe MG. Toward the identification of a subset of unexplained infertility: a sperm proteomic approach. Fertil Steril 2014;102(3):692—9.

[63] Bromfield E, Aitken RJ, Nixon B. Novel characterization of the HSPA2-stabilizing protein BAG6 in human spermatozoa. Mol Hum Reprod 2015;21(10):755—69.

[64] Yanagimachi R. Fertility of mammalian spermatozoa: its development and relativity. Zygote 1994;2(4):371—2.

[65] de Lamirande E, O'Flaherty C. Sperm activation: role of reactive oxygen species and kinases. Biochim Biophys Acta 2008;1784(1):106—15.

[66] O'Flaherty C, de Lamirande E, Gagnon C. Reactive oxygen species modulate independent protein phosphorylation pathways during human sperm capacitation. Free Radic Biol Med 2006;40(6):1045—55.

[67] de Lamirande E, Lamothe G. Reactive oxygen-induced reactive oxygen formation during human sperm capacitation. Free Radic Biol Med 2009;46(4):502—10.

[68] de Lamirande E, Lamothe G, Villemure M. Control of superoxide and nitric oxide formation during human sperm capacitation. Free Radic Biol Med 2009;46(10):1420—7.

[69] Carrera A, Moos J, Ning XP, Gerton GL, Tesarik J, Kopf GS, et al. Regulation of protein tyrosine phosphorylation in human sperm by a calcium/calmodulin-dependent mechanism: identification of A kinase anchor proteins as major substrates for tyrosine phosphorylation. Dev Biol 1996;180(1):284—96.

[70] Brener E, Rubinstein S, Cohen G, Shternall K, Rivlin J, Breitbart H. Remodeling of the actin cytoskeleton during mammalian sperm capacitation and acrosome reaction. Biol Reprod 2003;68(3):837—45.

[71] Spungin B, Breitbart H. Calcium mobilization and influx during sperm exocytosis. J Cell Sci 1996;109(Pt 7):1947—55.

[72] Visconti PE, Krapf D, de la Vega-Beltran JL, Acevedo JJ, Darszon A. Ion channels, phosphorylation and mammalian sperm capacitation. Asian J Androl 2011;13(3):395—405.

[73] Naz RK, Rajesh PB. Role of tyrosine phosphorylation in sperm capacitation/acrosome reaction. Reprod Biol Endocrinol 2004;2:75.

[74] Ecroyd H, Jones RC, Aitken RJ. Tyrosine phosphorylation of HSP-90 during mammalian sperm capacitation. Biol Reprod 2003;69(6):1801—7.

[75] Asquith KL, Baleato RM, McLaughlin EA, Nixon B, Aitken RJ. Tyrosine phosphorylation activates surface chaperones facilitating sperm-zona recognition. J Cell Sci 2004;117(Pt 16):3645—57.

[76] Redgrove KA, Nixon B, Baker MA, Hetherington L, Baker G, Liu DY, et al. The molecular chaperone HSPA2 plays a key role in regulating the expression of sperm surface receptors that mediate sperm-egg recognition. PLoS One 2012;7(11):e50851.

[77] Zhang H, Zheng RL. Promotion of human sperm capacitation by superoxide anion. Free Radic Res 1996;24(4):261—8.

[78] Saowaros W, Panyim S. The formation of disulfide bonds in human protamines during sperm maturation. Experientia 1979;35(2):191—2.

[79] Balhorn R, Corzett M, Mazrimas JA. Formation of intraprotamine disulfides in vitro. Arch Biochem Biophys 1992;296(2):384—93.

[80] Pfeifer H, Conrad M, Roethlein D, Kyriakopoulos A, Brielmeier M, Bornkamm GW, et al. Identification of a specific sperm nuclei selenoenzyme necessary for protamine thiol cross-linking during sperm maturation. FASEB J 2001;15(7):1236—8.

[81] Morielli T, O'Flaherty C. Oxidative stress impairs function and increases redox protein modifications in human spermatozoa. Reproduction 2015;149(1):113—23.

[82] Manevich Y, Feinstein SI, Fisher AB. Activation of the antioxidant enzyme 1-CYS peroxiredoxin requires glutathionylation mediated by heterodimerization with pi GST. Proc Natl Acad Sci U S A 2004;101(11):3780—5.

[83] Ralat LA, Manevich Y, Fisher AB, Colman RF. Direct evidence for the formation of a complex between 1-cysteine peroxiredoxin and glutathione S-transferase pi with activity changes in both enzymes. Biochemistry 2006;45(2):360—72.

[84] O'Flaherty C, de Souza AR. Hydrogen peroxide modifies human sperm peroxiredoxins in a dose-dependent manner. Biol Reprod 2011;84(2):238–47.

[85] Gong S, San Gabriel MC, Zini A, Chan P, O'Flaherty C. Low amounts and high thiol oxidation of peroxiredoxins in spermatozoa from infertile men. J Androl 2012;33(6):1342–51.

[86] Gow AJ, Farkouh CR, Munson DA, Posencheg MA, Ischiropoulos H. Biological significance of nitric oxide-mediated protein modifications. Am J Physiol Lung Cell Mol Physiol 2004;287(2):L262–8.

[87] Lefievre L, Chen Y, Conner SJ, Scott JL, Publicover SJ, Ford WC, et al. Human spermatozoa contain multiple targets for protein S-nitrosylation: an alternative mechanism of the modulation of sperm function by nitric oxide? Proteomics 2007;7(17):3066–84.

[88] Salvolini E, Buldreghini E, Lucarini G, Vignini A, Di Primio R, Balercia G. Nitric oxide synthase and tyrosine nitration in idiopathic asthenozoospermia: an immunohistochemical study. Fertil Steril 2012;97(3):554–60.

[89] Biegeleisen K. The probable structure of the protamine-DNA complex. J Theor Biol 2006;241(3):533–40.

[90] Levine RL, Stadtman ER. Oxidative modification of proteins during aging. Exp Gerontol 2001;36(9):1495–502.

[91] Nystrom T. Role of oxidative carbonylation in protein quality control and senescence. EMBO J 2005;24(7):1311–7.

[92] Dean RT, Fu S, Stocker R, Davies MJ. Biochemistry and pathology of radical-mediated protein oxidation. Biochem J 1997;324(Pt 1):1–18.

[93] Mohanty G, Swain N, Goswami C, Kar S, Samanta L. Histone retention, protein carbonylation, and lipid peroxidation in spermatozoa: possible role in recurrent pregnancy loss. Syst Biol Reprod Med 2016;62(3):201–12.

[94] Baker MA, Weinberg A, Hetherington L, Villaverde AI, Velkov T, Baell J, et al. Defining the mechanisms by which the reactive oxygen species by-product, 4-hydroxynonenal, affects human sperm cell function. Biol Reprod 2015;92(4):108.

[95] Aitken RJ, Whiting S, De Iuliis GN, McClymont S, Mitchell LA, Baker MA. Electrophilic aldehydes generated by sperm metabolism activate mitochondrial reactive oxygen species generation and apoptosis by targeting succinate dehydrogenase. J Biol Chem 2012;287(39):33048–60.

[96] Chondrogianni N, Petropoulos I, Grimm S, Georgila K, Catalgol B, Friguet B, et al. Protein damage, repair and proteolysis. Mol Aspects Med 2014;35:1–71.

[97] Sutovsky P, Hauser R, Sutovsky M. Increased levels of sperm ubiquitin correlate with semen quality in men from an andrology laboratory clinic population. Hum Reprod 2004;19(3):628–38.

[98] Hosseinpour E, Shahverdi A, Parivar K, Sedighi Gilani MA, Nasr-Esfahani MH, Salman Yazdi R, et al. Sperm ubiquitination and DNA fragmentation in men with occupational exposure and varicocele. Andrologia 2014;46(4):423–9.

[99] Bromfield EG, Aitken RJ, McLaughlin EA, Nixon B. Proteolytic degradation of heat shock protein A2 occurs in response to oxidative stress in male germ cells of the mouse. Mol Hum Reprod 2017;23(2):91–105.

[100] Grune T, Shringarpure R, Sitte N, Davies K. Age-related changes in protein oxidation and proteolysis in mammalian cells. J Gerontol A Biol Sci Med Sci 2001;56(11):B459–67.

[101] Grune T, Merker K, Sandig G, Davies KJ. Selective degradation of oxidatively modified protein substrates by the proteasome. Biochem Biophys Res Commun 2003;305(3):709–18.

[102] Mehlhase J, Grune T. Proteolytic response to oxidative stress in mammalian cells. Biol Chem 2002;383(3–4):559–67.

Chapter 4.4

Metabolomics

Rocío Rivera[1] and Nicolás Garrido[2]

[1]*Instituto Universitario IVI Valencia, València, Spain;* [2]*IVI Foundation, Valencia, Spain*

THE CURRENT SITUATION OF MALE FERTILITY

Currently, infertility affects about 8%−10% of couples at their reproductive age worldwide, and these figures are estimated at around 14% in Europe, similar to other developed countries [1−4]. According to studies from different authors, these percentages vary markedly, depending on different geographic areas as well as time ranges. Among infertile patients, apart from a significant economic burden caused by infertility treatments (if not publicly supported), the main negative health consequences of the infertility are psychological (stress and depression), physical, and social issues [5].

Infertility is typically defined as the inability to achieve a clinical pregnancy after a period of 12 months of regular and unprotected intercourse. This definition has been accepted by the Spanish Society of Fertility, the European Society of Reproduction and Human Embryology [6], and the American Association of Reproductive Medicine. In contrast, the World Health Organization (WHO) stipulates an extended period of 24 months [7]. Usually, patients ask for infertility investigations sooner, and specialists around the globe tend to intervene after 1 year of unfulfilled parenthood.

However, in clinical practice there are factors leading to the reduction of this period when the cause of infertility has specifically been identified such as advanced maternal age, alterations that affect female or male fertility, and so on (Table 1) [8,9]. In addition, waiting for the said formal period of time to pass before treating the couple may negatively impact the reproductive outcomes.

On the other hand, fertility could be defined as the ability to successfully achieve a pregnancy that ends up in a live birth, and its evaluation will be conditioned by the influence of the physiological characteristics of two individuals combined, aggravating the search for risk factors, biomarkers, or treatments that can improve reproductive success rates [9].

Although infertility has historically been almost exclusively related to women and evaluated on them, probably due to cultural reasons, it is roughly estimated that the male factor accounts for approximately 50% of the cases [10] while 30% of all infertility cases are exclusively related to a male infertility factor [3].

In this sense, although the introduction of intracytoplasmic sperm injection in the past led to the thought that one may only need a single sperm to be successful, we now know that the adequacy of the selected sperm will also significantly influence the reproductive success. As a result, the study of the male factor has been gaining increasing interest in the last decades.

ASSISTED REPRODUCTION TECHNIQUES, THEIR OUTCOMES AND LIMITATIONS

During the last few years, worldwide, the number of assisted reproduction treatments has increased annually. It is estimated that since the birth of the first child conceived through assisted reproduction technique (ART), more than 5 million children have been born through these procedures [4]. Therefore, the emergence and great development of ARTs have provided a prodigious advance of the treatments against infertility, increasing the chances of success of infertile couples to conceive [11]. The routine application of advanced technologies to make these treatments more effective is also increasing the knowledge and the available tools to treat infertility.

ART outcomes are still far from perfection or being 100% successful. Results may be highly variable when measured per transfer, per controlled ovarian hyperstimulation (COH), or per patient. They are also highly dependent on the kind of

Oxidants, Antioxidants, and Impact of the Oxidative Status in Male Reproduction. https://doi.org/10.1016/B978-0-12-812501-4.00025-0

TABLE 1 Factors That Advise the Early Study of the Infertile Couple [9]

Female	Male
Age >35 years	Previous genital pathology
Amenorrhea or oligomenorrhea >6 months	Previous urogenital surgery
Pelvic inflammatory disease	Sexually transmitted disease
Pelvic abdominal surgery	Abnormal genial exploration
Tube, uterine, or ovarian pathology	Genetic disease
Endometriosis	
Genetic disease	

ART employed. Usually, the measurement per cumulative rate is a concept recently and increasingly introduced, showing that the live births per transfer may have a wide range between 20% and 40% per COH. When considering the contribution of surplus frozen and thawed embryos from the same cohort transferred in consecutive cycles, the success rate is between 50% and 60%, while the cumulative live-birth rates considering consecutive stimulation cycles can be up to 90%.

This rate of perfection will only be attained when infertility is solved if the laboratory is selecting a single sperm that, after being microinjected into the oocyte, will always result in a healthy embryo that will implant and result in a healthy child. Until this is achieved, a lot of work remains to be done. From the perspective of the gamete and taking into account newborn rates as an indicator of success, even using donated semen and oocytes (the best available gametes) in cycles of artificial insemination or in vitro fertilization, it is clear that not all patients succeed. Frequently, several attempts (inseminations, ovarian stimulations, or embryo transfers, no matter how you measure it) are needed in order to achieve success [12].

Provided that they present the advantage of being almost always in excess compared with oocytes, the spermatozoon is an ideal cell to design strategies that allow us to improve the results of ARTs. However, the decision on which spermatozoon will be used needs to be made by the embryologist in the laboratory. Unlike oocytes, they are not the limiting factor. Hence in many treatments it is necessary to select sperm, and making the best choice may improve outcomes for each patient/performed treatment. Contrarily, with oocytes (where all the cells available will be used) and embryos (since embryo selection tools will improve rates per transfer, but not per patient or ovarian stimulation) the embryologist has to use what is available. In addition, each spermatozoon presents a unique genetic profile and characteristics, giving rise to a wide variety of different sperm phenotypes within the same ejaculates [13], probably some leading to success and others to failure. Those sperm that could potentially succeed will lead to individuals with different phenotypical traits. Thus within an ejaculate millions of different spermatozoa are being able and some unable to fertilize oocytes. Out of this large number of male germ cells, one may only need a few. Hence, choosing them properly will significantly impact the results. In order to select the most capable spermatozoa, we need good diagnostic tools, if possible at a sperm level, permitting first to describe their appropriate molecular characteristics to be successful and second, if possible, to select the best to be employed in ART.

THE RELEVANCE OF MALE FACTOR IN REPRODUCTIVE RESULTS

Since the male factor is responsible for about half of the infertility cases, the study of the male factor, apart from a complete medical history and investigation of sperm characteristics, is an essential part of the analysis of infertile couples. In the early years after the development of intracytoplasmic sperm injection (ICSI), the male factor was pushed to the background [14] since it was thought that it was sufficient to have a single spermatozoon per oocyte obtained after the pick up to be able to perform this technique and to achieve fertilization pregnancy and newborns. However over time the lessons learned after more than 20 years of ICSI are that clinicians and scientists have to acknowledge that a spermatozoon is more than a simple DNA carrier. As a result, insight has grown that if there is failure to achieve 100% success with ARTs, the influence of the sperm and its relevance for the fertilization process has to be investigated; this is reflecting in the number of studies focusing on sperm physiology in the last decade.

Male infertility may be caused or related to various congenital and acquired factors presented at different locations within the male's reproductive tract: congenital or acquired changes or damage at the hypothalamus and pituitary level, leading to endocrine dysfunctions (pregonadal), in the urogenital tract, or failures during spermatogenesis or spermiogenesis to produce competent sperm [15] (gonadal) and postgonadal causes, such as infections, immunological, or environmental factors [16]. It is estimated that about 30% of these cases are pathologies of genetic origin, 50% are nongenetic pathologies and 20% of male infertility has idiopathic origin, with the causes yet unknown. Therefore, the study of male infertility should include, as per the WHO recommendation, a complete medical history, a physical examination and at least two sperm basic analysis or spermiograms [17].

HOW TO ESTIMATE MALE FERTILITY POTENTIAL, ITS LIMITATIONS, AND POTENTIALLY USEFUL TECHNIQUES TO BE APPLIED

To date, the only accepted tool by WHO to assess the male's fertility potential is the basic sperm analysis or spermiogram. However, its value to predict a male's or a semen sample's chances to achieve a successful pregnancy with a baby born are relatively low.

The spermiogram is a relatively simple, fast, informative, and economical technique that can be accompanied by a physical examination and a hormonal and genetic analysis if its result of the patients' anamnesis requires so. However, since it is based on apparent or visual aspects (cell count, motility, and morphology), leaving aside molecular aspects (abnormalities hidden for the human eye, understood as those included in the basic sperm analysis), this diagnostic assessment has a number of limitations [14,18]. Moreover, these molecular aspects can be multiple, as one can extrapolate from all the information available in the literature where one or more molecular features of sperm have been related to fertility status. The technologies to define these sperm characteristics should better comprehend the possibilities of studying several molecular traits in one single experiment or measurement.

Using omics platforms, all classes of biological compounds, epigenetic markers, genes, mRNA, proteins, and metabolites can be analyzed. In other words, the differences are that genomics/transcriptomics enables evaluation of potential information, proteomics permits assessing executed plans, and metabolomics will mostly display the results after these plans' execution [19]. Thus any alteration upstream should be reflected by the metabolomic profile of a cell, tissue, or organ.

Metabolomics is defined as the systematic study of all chemical processes concerning metabolites, providing characteristic chemical fingerprints that specific cellular processes yield, by means of the study of their small-molecule metabolite profiles. Once that is defined, the metabolome represents the group of all metabolites present in a cell, tissue, organ, or organism as the end products or results of cellular processes, including but not exclusive of small-molecule metabolites (such as metabolic intermediates, hormones and other signaling molecules, and secondary metabolites) in a specific moment. In comparison to the analysis of mRNA gene expression or proteomic analyses that provide information about the gene products being expressed within the cell, representing only one single aspect of cellular function, establishing the metabolic profile can give an instantaneous picture of the physiology present. Although the metabolome can be readily defined, it is currently not possible to analyze the entire range of metabolites by a single analytical method and may include several approaches and technologies in order to separate and analyze molecules, depending on the metabolite's characteristics, such as gas chromatography, high-performance liquid chromatography (HPLC), and capillary electrophoresis among the first, and mass spectroscopy, nuclear magnetic resonance (NMR), and others among the second. In the context of metabolomics, a metabolite is usually defined as any molecule less than 1 kDa in size with exceptions, depending on the sample and detection method. The metabolites are all grouped, namely the metabolome, and form a large network of metabolic reactions where outputs from one enzymatic reaction may have inputs into other chemical reactions.

Each omic technology can be put into practice in the assisted reproduction field to define the optimal molecular traits of the cells and tissues involved in reproduction. This biological approach can assist in defining the best spermatozoa and oocyte that can result in fertilization and the best embryo that can implant and result in a live birth, improving assisted reproduction success. The use of genomic, transcriptomic, and proteomic technologies significantly contributed to characterize and better understand human reproductive cells at the molecular level. Metabolomics reflects downstream events of gene expression and is also considered to be more closely related to the actual phenotype rather than either transcriptomics or proteomics as it can be used to directly monitor biochemical activity [20]. However, in contrast to other omic approaches, metabolomics has not been greatly applied in the study and characterization of human sperm cells. Metabolomics has been emerging for several years as a global chemical phenotyping approach offering fascinating descriptive capabilities for addressing life complexity. It facilitates the understanding of the mechanisms of biological and biochemical processes in complex systems and promises new insights into specific research questions [21].

Metabolic profiling or metabolomics is the analysis of various molecular metabolites within cells and fluids using various forms of spectral and analytical approaches, and it attempts to determine metabolites associated with physiologic and pathologic states [22,23]. It offers a significant advantage over the use of the two related fields of study. Smaller variations in gene expression and protein synthesis result in an amplified change in the metabolite profile known as the metabolome [24], and this information can be used to detect subtle cellular events [25]. In fact, metabolomic patterns are the final consequence of biological function and they can directly indicate an aberrant physiological status [26].

EXPLORING MALE FERTILITY BIOMARKERS THROUGH THE OMICS

Research lines in the field of andrology have focused mainly on the search for new tools or tests complementary to the spermiogram, trying to improve its diagnostic capacity along with the development, if possible, of new methods for competent sperm selection that can lead to an increase in success rates in ARTs. In addition, these new methods should be able to define which ejaculate from a single individual, or which sperm within an ejaculate, will present the highest reproductive chances and will improve ART efficiency. Specifically, research has been focused on the search for new infertility biomarkers [27,28] permitting great progress in the knowledge of biochemical and molecular mechanisms that regulate the production of spermatozoa.

The best spermatozoon must have the ability to swim and penetrate the cervical mucus to find and recognize the oocyte, mainly by recognizing the glycoproteins of the zona pellucida and initiating the events that result in an embryo with the ability to implant and grow, resulting in a healthy child [28,29]. In all these processes, several actively participating molecules can be used as biomarkers of sperm function.

To date, several sperm factors seem to be related to male fertility [30,31]. However, none of them has been able to define the exclusive responsibility for this situation, confirming that male infertility can be caused by the combination of different factors. Therefore, it is necessary to carry out studies to determine the key molecular factors in sperm function, standardizing the female factors to determine the relationship between these factors and the ability of sperm to achieve live births.

Several studies have been carried out to identify and understand the molecular mechanisms involved in male infertility. Thus a large number of sperm biomarkers and tests have been described as useful for assessing sperm function [29,32] and among them, those related to DNA integrity, oxidative stress, and expression of RNA profiles are the most studied. Sperm selection techniques used as swim-up or density gradients centrifugation depend on the mobility and morphology of spermatozoa and are not efficient enough to achieve populations of spermatozoa free of DNA damage or oxidation with normal and physiological morphology and competent physiologically. In addition, using ARTs, natural selection of the female reproductive tract is ignored, especially in treatments where ICSI is performed, a technique where reproductive success was thought to be practically independent of sperm functions.

All these facts allow us to conclude that it is necessary to develop new diagnostic tools based on the battery of defined biomarkers. These biomarkers will allow assessment of male fertility potential, to improve diagnostics, to define molecular deficiencies, and, if possible, to use them to separate normal from abnormal spermatozoa capable of fertilizing the oocyte and resulting in embryo and full-term pregnancy [32].

The great breakthrough provoked by the omic sciences, developed mainly on the basis of the findings and knowledge obtained from the Human Genome Project, have revolutionized the classical methods of analysis mainly of multifactorial events, allowing the massive evaluation of hundreds and thousands of genes, proteins, or metabolites in a single experiment. These sciences provide a new dimension of study in any discipline and allow researchers to gain a global vision of biological and molecular processes in a complex and global way [25].

METABOLOMICS IN MALE FERTILITY STUDIES

NMR spectroscopy and coupled technologies such as liquid chromatography-mass spectrometry (LC-MS) and gas chromatography-mass spectrometry (GC-MS) are the main analytical techniques applied in metabolomics analysis of biological fluids [33]. Concretely, 1H-MRS (H magnetic resonance spectroscopy) has provided information about the molecules in live human sperm and may therefore permit the study of the underlying functional biology or metabolomics on them. Given the relatively low concentration of sperm needed to obtain a suitable MRS signal ($\sim 3 \times 10^6$/mL), this could be carried out on sperm from men with oligo-, astheno-, or teratozoospermia. This may lead to the development of new diagnostic tests or ultimately novel treatments for male factor infertility [34].

The aims of metabolomic analysis are to help in the selection of viable spermatozoa to improve ARTs success, to pick out embryos with implantation potential to facilitate single embryo transfer, and to estimate the overall viability of the cohort of embryos [35]. The application of metabolomics to male fertility has been conducted from different perspectives such as the identification of biomarkers of specific traits or conditions in blood, seminal plasma, or semen, particularly focusing on its correlation with fertility in the male; these are scarce, since few articles involve biological samples studied by metabolomic approaches to define the multifactorial aspects of male fertility.

Related to this item, Deepinder et al. [24] reviewed papers concerning seminal plasma metabolomics and its relationship with different fertility-related conditions about 10 years ago and listed the existence of significant differences mainly in oxidative stress biomarkers concentration (−CH, −NH, −OH, and ROH) when comparisons were made between fertile males and idiopathic infertility, and also between those individuals presenting clinical varicocele and vasectomy. Specifically, differences in some metabolites as citrate, lactate, glycerylphosphorylcholine, and glycerylphosphorylethanolamine between donors and infertile males have been found. On the other hand, Deepinder et al. [24] found phosphomonoester and beta-adenosine triphosphate as potential biomarkers to assess testicular failure and ductal obstruction.

In another study analyzing seminal fluid, Gupta et al. [36] used H-NMR spectroscopy in order to determine biomarkers of infertility from 60 healthy, fertile men in comparison with 125 infertile males. Included in this work, for normozoospermic and oligozoospermic patients, lactate, alanine, choline, citrate, glycerophosphocholine, glutamine, tyrosine, histidine, phenylalanine, and uridine were measured. The analysis through linear multivariate discriminant function analysis to determine the molecular signature for each group was performed in a rapid and noninvasive approach.

They identified, among all detected metabolites, alanine, citrate, glycerophosphocholine, tyrosine, and phenylalanine, which can be potentially employed to forecast male infertility with high accuracy of 92.4% in differentiating healthy controls from infertile patients and 92.9% accurately classifying normozoospermic and oligozoospermic samples.

Other approaches included the analysis of serum, looking for minimally invasive sampling to gain insight about the male fertility status with low impact on patients or semen samples. In order to define their metabolic profile linked with sperm function and to find out which potential biomarkers were characterizing bad quality samples, Courant et al. [21] were the first to employ a metabolomic approach with the use of liquid chromatography high resolution mass spectrometry in collected serum samples from men with different semen quality.

They were able to generate the metabolomic fingerprints from Danish young men presenting low, intermediate, or high sperm concentrations, where they found differential metabolites to be involved, and among them, peptides related to the protein complement C3f as putative biomarker. Similarly, Zhang et al. [37] investigated the differential serum metabolic profile in 22 individuals presenting nonobstructive azoospermia in order to identify potential biomarkers to spermatogenic dysfunction compared with 31 healthy controls.

The technology used included high-performance liquid chromatography-tandem mass spectrometry (HPLC-MS/MS), and they found 24 metabolites as potential biomarkers. These metabolites are involved mainly in processes of oxidative stress cell apoptosis in spermatogenesis and energy production also finding some metabolic pathways disrupted in patients with nonobstructive azoospermia, such as those involving D-glutamine and D-glutamate, taurine and hypotaurine, pyruvate, the citrate cycle and alanine, aspartate and glutamate corresponding metabolisms, altered in patients diagnosed with nonobstructive azoospermia.

Another noninvasive sampling approach has been attempted with the evaluation of urinary metabolome to predict male fertility through the amount of sperm production. A differential urinary metabolic profile was determined to identify potential biomarkers indicative of infertility, specifically oligozoospermia [38], in about 300 individuals including 158 fertile and 135 oligozoospermic volunteers. In this study, LC/MC followed by orthogonal projections to latent structures discriminant analysis were applied. Subsequent receiver operating characteristic analysis identified disrupted biological pathways in which specific biomarkers were involved. A number of 10 potential biomarkers such as an increased adenine and methylxanthine, and decreased acylcarnitines, aspartic acid, and leucylproline strongly associated with oligozoospermia were found.

All these studies suggest differential metabolic profiles (in serum, urine, semen), providing novel insights into the pathogenesis underlying male infertility. However, these technologies have also been applied in order to evaluate how sperm condition culture media and how the biological fluids are changed by cell adaptations or response to harm by specific toxins.

As an example of the former, Goodson et al. [39] determined the metabolic substrates used in sperm capacitation culture medium, showing that glucose and fructose may exert their differential effects on capacitation through alterations in redox pathways producing hyperactivation results from the active metabolism of glucose, by using a metabolomic profile characterization in mouse sperm. Other studies, also based on animal experimentation, used blood serum to determine different metabolic patterns from different externally caused reproductive disorders. Huang et al. [26] analyzed arsenic exposure in rats by conducting an integrated proteomics and metabolomics analysis, revealing that this exposure decreased testosterone level and reduced sperm quality. Also, 70 proteins (36 upregulated and 34 downregulated) and 13 metabolites (8 increased and 5 decreased) were found to be altered by arsenic treatment and two of them were specifically related to male reproductive system development and function (spermatogenesis, sperm function, and fertilization). Therefore, these 13 altered metabolites were identified and considered potential biomarkers of fertility that can be affected by arsenic.

As we have seen to date, studies about metabolomic science are more focused on metabolites and the result of oxidative stress [24] or seminal fluid [36], but not on lipids [40]. From the available literature it is clear that these investigations were abandoned due to lack of knowledge of the metabolic pathways and functions at that time. Thanks to omics techniques, the significance of these molecules, which participate in multiple biochemical and structural processes, has been restored. Within the metabolomic field, there has been an important development of the lipidomic profile in recent years. Given the participation of membrane lipids in different events leading to fertilization [41], capacitation, and sperm-oocyte interaction [41,42] as well as their influence on sperm's ability to survive after the freezing/thawing process, we can say that among the molecular factors involved in sperm function, sperm membrane lipids are of particular interest. In fact, changes in the lipid composition of the sperm membrane have been related to decreased sperm quality during cryopreservation [43–45].

In addition, sperm have a very special membrane lipid composition containing very high levels of phospholipids, sterols, glycolipids, and saturated and polyunsaturated fatty acids (PUFAs) that increase its sensitivity to oxidative attack. The proper lipid composition has been positively correlated with sperm quality as fatty acids provide high fluidity to the membrane [46]. Since recent research supports the hypothesis that PUFAs, which are very susceptible to lipid peroxidation, also have antioxidant properties (mainly those of the n-3 series), they are less susceptible to lipid peroxidation [47], which seems contradictory.

Early in the 1980s and 1990s, several studies aimed to find the connection between the lipid composition of the sperm membrane and viability and functionality of spermatozoa. For instance, Nissen et al. [48] reported a significant relationship between DHA content (docosa-hexaenoic-acid) and the count and number of spermatozoa with normal motility. Although lipids are involved in the processes of production and maturation of sperm, motility is the most studied parameter related to lipids to date.

Several studies [49–51] have demonstrated the important role of sperm plasma membrane lipids in seminal quality. Given the susceptibility of PUFAs to oxidative attack, no visible functional alterations in spermatozoa could be directly or indirectly related to oxidative damage, thus reducing the male fertile potential. Therefore, lipid peroxidation could be one of the biochemical factors responsible for the loss of the DHA content in spermatozoa with reduced mobility [48].

As we know, the physiology and molecular characteristics of spermatozoa can vary throughout their maturation in the epididymis and their passage through the entire male reproductive tract until ejaculation [52]. These molecular changes occurring in the epididymis, specifically those occurring in the lipid composition increasing membrane fluidity such as increased phosphatidylcholine content and decreased cholesterol/phospholipid ratio, are related to the induction of sperm motility [53,54]. An increase in cholesterol levels in human spermatozoa with low motility is associated with increased rigidity of the membrane, causing biochemical and functional alterations during the capacitation process [55]. In contrast, PUFAs, which are the most abundant fatty acids in the sperm membrane, improve the mobility of spermatozoa given that they provide fluidity to the sperm membrane. However, at the same time, these lipids make the spermatozoon an easy target for reactive oxygen species (ROS) attack, compromising the cellular integrity and viability of spermatozoa [56].

As we have seen in recent years, oxidative stress as a cause of sperm damage has stimulated interest in being one of the most common causes of male infertility. Many studies focus on mechanisms that trigger the production of ROS [57–59], but it seems that defective spermatozoa themselves are the major source of lipid peroxidation causing the cascade of oxidative damage that affects semen quality [56]. Therefore, the analysis of lipid composition of spermatozoa and the degree of lipid peroxidation could be used as a diagnostic tool to complement the spermiogram.

Few studies have identified the sperm lipid profile limited to describing metabolic compounds with only a few lipids included [20,36,60–64]. For example, Gupta et al. [36] detected 10 metabolites related to male fertility that included glycerophosphocholine, whereas Deepinder et al. [24] identified differences in levels of glycerylphosphorylcholine and glycerylphosphorylethanolamine between donors and infertile patients. Paiva et al. [20] identified some lipids in sperm samples (2-methylglutarate, 2-hydroxy-3-methylvalerate, butyrate, caprate, O-acetylcarnitine, L-acetylcarnitine, and sn-glycero-3-phosphocholine) among thousands of metabolites, and aimed to establish the first comprehensive metabolomic characterization of the human spermatozoa by applying proton NMR (H-NMR) [1] spectroscopy and gas chromatography coupled to mass spectrometry (GC-MS). Using these two complementary strategies, they identified a total of 69 metabolites, of which 42 were identified using NMR, 27 using GC-MS, and 4 using both methods. Afterward, the metabolites were confirmed by two-dimensional homonuclear correlation spectroscopy and heteronuclear single-quantum correlation spectroscopy, indicating that there were overrepresented metabolic pathways including that for carbohydrates as well as for lipids and lipoproteins.

In addition to being able to diagnose a semen sample through lipid analysis and to classify it according to WHO parameters, we herewith provide another approach by creating lipid profiles that are related to reproductive success. These lipid profiles would consist of the description of all the lipids found in spermatozoa of a semen sample from which a pregnancy has been achieved by assisted reproduction. This lipid profile would then have to be compared with the lipid profile in spermatozoa from semen samples that failed to fertilize oocytes.

In our study, we analyzed sperm samples (n = 32) from infertile males undergoing ICSI cycles with normal sperm parameters and total progressive motility >5 mill, 15 of them failing to achieve pregnancy (F) and 17 who succeeded (P). Lipids were separated and analyzed by means of ultraperformance liquid chromatography coupled with mass spectrometry using methanol (MeOH) and methanol/chloroform (MeOH/CHCl$_3$) platforms. A total of 104 different lipids were identified and grouped in 25 different classes. The amount of each class and lipid was compared statistically between groups P and F. Among these 104 lipids, 16 of them were found significantly more abundantly in sperm samples from the F group. Some of the lipids found include ceramides (Cer-03, -05), sphingomyelins (Sphlip-16, -20, -23, -30), 2-monoacylglycerophosphoethanolamines (MAPE13, 14), monoacylglycerophosphoinositol (MAPI03, 04, 06), and 1-monoetherglycerophosphoethanolamine (MEPE09, 12, 14, 15, 19).

Furthermore, when we analyzed the samples according to the chemical class, four subclasses were found to be significantly more abundant in these samples: 1-monoacylglycerophosphoethanolamine, monoetherglycerophosphoethanolamine, 1- monoetherglycerophosphoethanolamine, and lysophosphatidylethanolamine.

This study revealed differences in the lipidomic profile between sperm samples achieving or not achieving pregnancy by means of ICSI. Increasing the knowledge about sperm infertility-related molecular markers is enabling the development of new techniques to assess male fertility status and opens new possibilities to treat patients in vivo and semen samples in vitro in order to overcome these molecular limitations.

CONCLUSIONS

From all the information previously stated, we can conclude that there is an urgent need for sperm quality biomarkers in order to overcome the current limitations of ART results, and given that it has been extensively demonstrated that sperm function is multifactorial, massive analysis techniques seem to be needed in order to characterize sperm molecular profile compatible with fertility.

In this sense, metabolomics seems to be a promising approach, not only to evaluate or forecast the fertility status by sperm analysis, but also in seminal plasma or serum. Currently, there is limited information available with limited usefulness for two reasons. First, metabolomic approaches have been applied to clinical conditions that can be easily determined from other perspectives such as azoospermia or oligozoospermia that can be identified with the classic sperm analysis. Second, there is a lack of robust clinical analyses confirming the predictive ability to forecast live births.

Metabolomics seems the most promising omic science to be applied to investigate male fertility, given that it offers a significant advantage over the use of other omic technologies. Since smaller variations in gene expression and protein synthesis will result in an amplified change in the metabolite profile known as the metabolome, this information can be used to detect subtle cellular events [24].

In conclusion, the use of metabolomic approaches to evaluate male fertility is still experimental and far from being widely incorporated into the clinical arsenal of male fertility evaluation in ART centers. The application of these techniques in assisted reproduction resulted in a better understanding of pathologic processes in male infertility, and potential identification of novel molecular biomarkers related to infertility problems have been described. Eventually, this increases our knowledge to design new diagnostic tests and sperm selection methods to improve the success rates in ARTs.

REFERENCES

[1] Benagiano G, Bastianelli C, Farris M. Infertility: a global perspective. Minerva Ginecol December 2006;58(6):445−57.

[2] Sharlip ID, Jarow JP, Belker AM, Lipshultz LI, Sigman M, Thomas AJ, et al. Best practice policies for male infertility. Fertil Steril May 2002;77(5):873−82.

[3] Thonneau P, Marchand S, Tallec A, Ferial ML, Ducot B, Lansac J, et al. Incidence and main causes of infertility in a resident population (1,850,000) of three French regions (1988−1989). Hum Reprod 1991 Jul;6(6):811−6.

[4] ESHRE. 2014:2016. https:www.eshre.eu/guidelines-and-legañ/ART-fact-sheet.aspx.

[5] Mascarenhas MN, Flaxman SR, Boerma T, Vanderpoel S, Stevens GA. National, regional, and global trends in infertility prevalence since 1990: a systematic analysis of 277 health surveys. PLoS Med 2012;9(12):e1001356.

[6] ESHRE Capri Workshop. Guidelines to the prevalence, diagnosis, treatment and management of infertility. Hum Reprod 1996;11.

[7] Matorras R, Crisol L. Fertilidad e Infertilidad Humanas. In: Matorras R, Coroleu B, Romeu A, Pérez F, editors. Libro Blanco Sociosanitario. "La infertilidad en España: Situación actual y perspectivas". SL, Madrid: Imago Concept & Image Development; 2011. p. 31−42.

[8] Brugo-Olmedo S, Chillik C, Kopelman S. Definición y causas de la infertilidad. RCOG 2003;54:227−48.

[9] Alamá P, Remohí J. Análisis de la Evolución de los Estudios y tratamientos de la infertilidad. In: Matorras R, Coroleu B, Romeu A, Pérez F, editors. Libro Blanco Sociosanitario. "La infertilidad en España: Situación actual y perspectivas". SL: Imago Concept & Image Development; 2011. p. 43−52.

[10] Nallella KP, Sharma RK, Aziz N, Agarwal A. Significance of sperm characteristics in the evaluation of male infertility. Fertil Steril March 2006;85(3):629—34.

[11] Chemes HE, Alvarez Sedo C. Tales of the tail and sperm head aches: changing concepts on the prognostic significance of sperm pathologies affecting the head, neck and tail. Asian J Androl January 2012;14(1):14—23.

[12] Garrido N, Bellver J, Remohi J, Simon C, Pellicer A. Cumulative live-birth rates per total number of embryos needed to reach newborn in consecutive in vitro fertilization (IVF) cycles: a new approach to measuring the likelihood of IVF success. Fertil Steril July 2011;96(1):40—6.

[13] Wang J, Fan HC, Behr B, Quake SR. Genome-wide single-cell analysis of recombination activity and de novo mutation rates in human sperm. Cell July 20, 2012;150(2):402—12.

[14] Lewis SE. Is sperm evaluation useful in predicting human fertility? Reproduction July 2007;134(1):31—40.

[15] Toshimori K, Ito C, Maekawa M, Toyama Y, Suzuki-Toyota F, Saxena DK. Impairment of spermatogenesis leading to infertility. Anat Sci Int September 2004;79(3):101—11.

[16] Khorram O, Patrizio P, Wang C, Swerdloff R. Reproductive technologies for male infertility. J Clin Endocrinol Metab June 2001;86(6):2373—9.

[17] OMS. WHO laboratory manual for the examination and processing of human semen. 5th ed. ilustrada 2010.

[18] Altmae S, Salumets A. A novel genomic diagnostic tool for sperm quality? Reprod Biomed Online May 2011;22(5):405—7.

[19] Silvestri E, Lombardi A, de Lange P, Glinni D, Senese R, Cioffi F, et al. Studies of complex biological systems with applications to molecular medicine: the need to integrate transcriptomic and proteomic approaches. J Biomed Biotechnol 2011;2011:810242.

[20] Paiva C, Amaral A, Rodriguez M, Canyellas N, Correig X, Ballesca JL, et al. Identification of endogenous metabolites in human sperm cells using proton nuclear magnetic resonance ((1) H-NMR) spectroscopy and gas chromatography-mass spectrometry (GC-MS). Andrology May 2015;3(3):496—505.

[21] Courant F, Antignac JP, Monteau F, Le Bizec B. Metabolomics as a potential new approach for investigating human reproductive disorders. J Proteome Res June 7, 2013;12(6):2914—20.

[22] Brison DR, Hollywood K, Arnesen R, Goodacre R. Predicting human embryo viability: the road to non-invasive analysis of the secretome using metabolic footprinting. Reprod Biomed Online September 2007;15(3):296—302.

[23] Singh R, Sinclair KD. Metabolomics: approaches to assessing oocyte and embryo quality. Theriogenology September 1, 2007;68(Suppl. 1):S56—62.

[24] Deepinder F, Chowdary HT, Agarwal A. Role of metabolomic analysis of biomarkers in the management of male infertility. Expert Rev Mol Diagn July 2007;7(4):351—8.

[25] Egea RR, Puchalt NG, Escriva MM, Varghese AC. OMICS: current and future perspectives in reproductive medicine and technology. J Hum Reprod Sci April 2014;7(2):73—92.

[26] Huang Q, Luo L, Alamdar A, Zhang J, Liu L, Tian M, et al. Integrated proteomics and metabolomics analysis of rat testis: mechanism of arsenic-induced male reproductive toxicity. Sci Rep September 2, 2016;6:32518.

[27] Rivera R, Meseguer M, Garrido N. Increasing the success of assisted reproduction by defining sperm fertility markers and selection sperm with the best molecular profile. Expert Rev Obstet Gynecol 2012;7(4).

[28] Garrido N, Remohi J, Martinez-Conejero JA, Garcia-Herrero S, Pellicer A, Meseguer M. Contribution of sperm molecular features to embryo quality and assisted reproduction success. Reprod Biomed Online December 2008;17(6):855—65.

[29] Anton E, Krawetz SA. Spermatozoa as biomarkers for the assessment of human male infertility and genotoxicity. Syst Biol Reprod Med February 2012;58(1):41—50.

[30] Esbert M, Pacheco A, Vidal F, Florensa M, Riqueros M, Ballesteros A, et al. Impact of sperm DNA fragmentation on the outcome of IVF with own or donated oocytes. Reprod Biomed Online December 2011;23(6):704—10.

[31] Meseguer M, Santiso R, Garrido N, Garcia-Herrero S, Remohi J, Fernandez JL. Effect of sperm DNA fragmentation on pregnancy outcome depends on oocyte quality. Fertil Steril January 2011;95(1):124—8.

[32] Said TM, Land JA. Effects of advanced selection methods on sperm quality and ART outcome: a systematic review. Hum Reprod Update 2011;17(6):719—33.

[33] Ebrahimi F, Ibrahim B, Teh CH, Murugaiyah V, Chan KL. NMR-based plasma metabolomic discrimination for male fertility assessment of rats treated with *Eurycoma longifolia* extracts. Syst Biol Reprod Med June 2017;63(3):179—91.

[34] Reynolds S, Calvert SJ, Paley MN, Pacey AA. 1H magnetic resonance spectroscopy of live human sperm. Mol Hum Reprod April 18, 2017;23.

[35] Nagy ZP, Sakkas D, Behr B. Symposium: innovative techniques in human embryo viability assessment. Non-invasive assessment of embryo viability by metabolomic profiling of culture media ('metabolomics'). Reprod Biomed Online October 2008;17(4):502—7.

[36] Gupta A, Mahdi AA, Ahmad MK, Shukla KK, Jaiswer SP, Shankhwar SN. 1H NMR spectroscopic studies on human seminal plasma: a probative discriminant function analysis classification model. J Pharm Biomed Anal January 5, 2011;54(1):106—13.

[37] Zhang Z, Zhang Y, Liu C, Zhao M, Yang Y, Wu H, et al. Serum metabolomic profiling identifies characterization of non-obstructive azoospermic men. Int J Mol Sci January 25, 2017;18(2). https://doi.org/10.3390/ijms18020238.

[38] Zhang J, Huang Z, Chen M, Xia Y, Martin FL, Hang W, et al. Urinary metabolome identifies signatures of oligozoospermic infertile men. Fertil Steril July 2014;102(1):44—53.e12.

[39] Goodson SG, Qiu Y, Sutton KA, Xie G, Jia W, O'Brien DA. Metabolic substrates exhibit differential effects on functional parameters of mouse sperm capacitation. Biol Reprod September 28, 2012;87(3):75.

[40] Nissen HP, Kreysel HW. Analysis of phospholipids in human semen by high-performance liquid chromatography. J Chromatogr August 12, 1983;276(1):29—35.

[41] Flesch FM, Gadella BM. Dynamics of the mammalian sperm plasma membrane in the process of fertilization. Biochim Biophys Acta November 10, 2000;1469(3):197–235.

[42] Kawano N, Yoshida K, Miyado K, Yoshida M. Lipid rafts: keys to sperm maturation, fertilization, and early embryogenesis. J Lipids 2011;2011:264706.

[43] Beirao J, Zilli L, Vilella S, Cabrita E, Schiavone R, Herraez MP. Improving sperm cryopreservation with antifreeze proteins: effect on gilthead seabream (Sparus aurata) plasma membrane lipids. Biol Reprod February 29, 2012;86(2):59.

[44] Kaeoket K, Sang-urai P, Thamniyom A, Chanapiwat P, Techakumphu M. Effect of docosahexaenoic acid on quality of cryopreserved boar semen in different breeds. Reprod Domest Anim June 2010;45(3):458–63.

[45] Maldjian A, Pizzi F, Gliozzi T, Cerolini S, Penny P, Noble R. Changes in sperm quality and lipid composition during cryopreservation of boar semen. Theriogenology January 15, 2005;63(2):411–21.

[46] Niu DM, Wang JJ. Lipids in the sperm plasma membrane and their role in fertilization. Zhonghua Nan Ke Xue July 2009;15(7):651–5.

[47] Garcia BM, Fernandez LG, Ferrusola CO, Salazar-Sandoval C, Rodriguez AM, Martinez HR, et al. Membrane lipids of the stallion spermatozoon in relation to sperm quality and susceptibility to lipid peroxidation. Reprod Domest Anim February 2011;46(1):141–8.

[48] Nissen HP, Kreysel HW. Polyunsaturated fatty acids in relation to sperm motility. Andrologia 1983 ;15(3):264–9.

[49] Lenzi A, Picardo M, Gandini L, Dondero F. Lipids of the sperm plasma membrane: from polyunsaturated fatty acids considered as markers of sperm function to possible scavenger therapy. Hum Reprod Update 1996 ;2(3):246–56.

[50] Force A, Grizard G, Giraud MN, Motta C, Sion B, Boucher D. Membrane fluidity and lipid content of human spermatozoa selected by swim-up method. Int J Androl December 2001;24(6):327–34.

[51] Zhou X, Xia XY, Huang YF. Updated detection of the function of sperm plasma membrane. Zhonghua Nan Ke Xue August 2010;16(8):745–8.

[52] Cooper T. The epididymis, sperm maturation and fertilization. Heidelberg: Springer-Verlag; 1986.

[53] Haidl G, Opper C. Changes in lipids and membrane anisotropy in human spermatozoa during epididymal maturation. Hum Reprod December 1997;12(12]):2720–3.

[54] Rejraji H, Sion B, Prensier G, Carreras M, Motta C, Frenoux JM, et al. Lipid remodeling of murine epididymosomes and spermatozoa during epididymal maturation. Biol Reprod June 2006;74(6):1104–13.

[55] Buffone MG, Verstraeten SV, Calamera JC, Doncel GF. High cholesterol content and decreased membrane fluidity in human spermatozoa are associated with protein tyrosine phosphorylation and functional deficiencies. J Androl 2009 ;30(5):552–8.

[56] Wathes DC, Abayasekara DR, Aitken RJ. Polyunsaturated fatty acids in male and female reproduction. Biol Reprod August 2007;77(2):190–201.

[57] Tartibian B, Maleki BH. Correlation between seminal oxidative stress biomarkers and antioxidants with sperm DNA damage in elite athletes and recreationally active men. Clin J Sport Med March 2012;22(2):132–9.

[58] Santiso R, Tamayo M, Gosalvez J, Meseguer M, Garrido N, Fernandez JL. Simultaneous determination in situ of DNA fragmentation and 8-oxoguanine in human sperm. Fertil Steril January 2010;93(1):314–8.

[59] Thomson LK, Zieschang JA, Clark AM. Oxidative deoxyribonucleic acid damage in sperm has a negative impact on clinical pregnancy rate in intrauterine insemination but not intracytoplasmic sperm injection cycles. Fertil Steril October 2011;96(4):843–7.

[60] Khoshvaght A, Towhidi A, Zare-shahneh A, Noruozi M, Zhandi M, Davachi ND, et al. Dietary n-3 PUFAs improve fresh and post-thaw semen quality in Holstein bulls via alteration of sperm fatty acid composition. Theriogenology March 15, 2016;85(5):807–12.

[61] Schroter F, Jakop U, Teichmann A, Haralampiev I, Tannert A, Wiesner B, et al. Lipid dynamics in boar sperm studied by advanced fluorescence imaging techniques. Eur Biophys J March 2016;45(2):149–63.

[62] van Gestel RA, Brouwers JF, Ultee A, Helms JB, Gadella BM. Ultrastructure and lipid composition of detergent-resistant membranes derived from mammalian sperm and two types of epithelial cells. Cell Tissue Res January 2016;363(1):129–45.

[63] Oresti GM, Penalva DA, Luquez JM, Antollini SS, Aveldano MI. Lipid biochemical and biophysical changes in rat spermatozoa during isolation and functional activation in vitro. Biol Reprod December 2015;93(6):140.

[64] Bernabo N, Greco L, Ordinelli A, Mattioli M, Barboni B. Capacitation-related lipid remodeling of mammalian spermatozoa membrane determines the final fate of male gametes: a computational biology study. OMICS November 2015;19(11):712–21.

Index

Printed in the United States
By Bookmasters